Handbook of Experimental Pharmacology

Volume 261

The *Handbook of Experimental Pharmacology* is one of the most authoritative and influential book series in pharmacology. It provides critical and comprehensive discussions of the most significant areas of pharmacological research, written by leading international authorities. Each volume in the series represents the most informative and contemporary account of its subject available, making it an unrivalled reference source.

HEP is indexed in PubMed and Scopus.

More information about this series at http://www.springer.com/series/164

Wieland Kiess • Matthias Schwab •
Johannes van den Anker
Editors

Pediatric Pharmacotherapy

Springer

Editors
Wieland Kiess
Hospital for Children and Adolescents
Center of Paediatric Research
Department of Women and Child Health
University of Leipzig
Leipzig, Germany

Matthias Schwab
Dr. Margarete Fischer-Bosch-Institute of
Clinical Pharmacology
Robert Bosch Gesellschaft fuer medizinische
Forschung mbH
Stuttgart, Germany

Department of Clinical Pharmacology
University Hospital Tüebingen
Tüebingen, Germany

Johannes van den Anker
Children's Hospital
University of Basel Children's Hospital
Basel, Switzerland

ISSN 0171-2004 ISSN 1865-0325 (electronic)
Handbook of Experimental Pharmacology
ISBN 978-3-030-50493-9 ISBN 978-3-030-50494-6 (eBook)
https://doi.org/10.1007/978-3-030-50494-6

This Springer imprint is published by the registered company Springer Nature Switzerland AG.
The registered company address is: Gewerbestrasse 11, 6330 Cham, Switzerland

Preface

We, as editors, are pleased and proud to present to you "Pediatric Pharmacotherapy" as a new volume of the *Handbook of Experimental Pharmacology*. In 2011, we have published volume 205 of this well-known and highly respected Handbook entitled "Pediatric Clinical Pharmacology." That volume summarized the general aspects of clinical pharmacology and specific methodologies. This new volume is the logical continuation of volume 205 to enrich the understanding of pediatric pharmacotherapy of diseases for not only pediatricians but also representatives of other medical and scientific disciplines as well as general health care providers and learned societies.

Based on the awareness that "*children are not small adults*," it is well accepted that pediatric pharmacotherapy requires data based on prospective clinical trials with the exception of considering various pediatric age groups comprising preterm and term neonates, toddlers, school children, and adolescents. The aim of this volume is to provide 26 state-of-the-art articles arranged into different sections regarding clinically relevant pediatric indications with a strong focus on drug efficacy and safety. We have not systematically and/or completely covered all pharmacotherapy topics for children and adolescents in this volume but have tried to present current therapeutic indications and pharmacological treatments in relation to specific age groups, gender, body composition, and health status. Moreover, rare therapeutic options (e.g. pharmacotherapy in rare skeletal diseases and current and emerging therapies for mucopolysaccharidoses and for mitochondriopathies) should be considered as well. Finally, we have tried to address aspects beyond standard treatment and important information on pharmacodynamics and pharmacokinetics, and pharmacometrics have been included.

We hope that you will share our view that the volume on Pediatric Pharmacotherapy is an essential resource and provides evidence that children are a highly sensitive part of the population who needs specific pharmacological knowledge. The given information shall equip readers to handle complex diseases and treatment strategies.

Leipzig, Germany — Wieland Kiess
Stuttgart-Tübingen, Germany — Matthias Schwab
Basel, Switzerland — John van den Anker

Contents

Antiepileptic Drugs in Pediatrics

Tesfaye Zelleke, Archana Pasupuleti, Dewi Depositario-Cabacar, and Amy Kao

Contents

T. Zelleke · A. Pasupuleti · D. Depositario-Cabacar
Division of Epilepsy and Neurophysiology, Children's National Health System, Washington, DC, USA
e-mail: tzelleke@childrensnational.org; apasupul@childrensnational.org; dcabacar@childrensnational.org

A. Kao (✉)
Division of Epilepsy and Neurophysiology, Children's National Health System, Washington, DC, USA

Center for Behavioral Neurosciences, Children's National Health System, Washington, DC, USA
e-mail: akao@childrensnational.org

W. Kiess et al. (eds.), *Pediatric Pharmacotherapy*,
Handbook of Experimental Pharmacology 261, https://doi.org/10.1007/164_2019_248

Abstract

Epilepsy affects approximately 1% of the population. First-line treatment for epilepsy is the administration of anti-seizure medication, also referred to as antiepileptic drugs (AEDs), although this nomenclature is erroneous as these medications typically do not impact underlying epileptogenic processes; the goal of these medications is to control symptoms. Over 30% of patients are classified as having "medically refractory" epilepsy, i.e., lack of adequate seizure control despite trials of two or three AEDs (Kwan and Brodie, N Engl J Med 342:314–9, 2000). Epilepsy is associated with worse quality of life in children, adolescents, and their families (Cianchetti et al., Seizure 24:93–101, 2015). Patients with epilepsy have a two to three times greater risk of death than the general population, by various causes including sudden unexplained death in epilepsy patients (SUDEP) (Abdel-Mannan et al., Epilepsy Behav 90:99–106, 2019). It is these factors, among others, that have motivated the continued development of AEDs. This chapter will review the history and evolution of AED development, features of specific AEDs with a focus on the newest generation, and examples of AEDs in development.

Keywords

Anticonvulsant · Antiepileptic drug · Antiepileptic medication · Anti-seizure drug · Anti-seizure medication · Drug development · Epilepsy · Pediatric epilepsy · Seizure disorder

1 Evolution of Anti-seizure Medication Development

Epilepsy is a common neurologic disorder affecting about 1% of the population. The first-line treatment for epilepsy is the use of appropriately selected anti-seizure medication.

Potassium bromide was discovered as the first antiepileptic drug (AED) in 1857. The next medication to be available for seizure treatment was phenobarbital in 1912. The discoveries of both bromide and phenobarbital as anti-seizure medications were based on clinical observations. The subsequent availability of animal models opened a new opportunity to test several compounds for anti-seizure activity. The

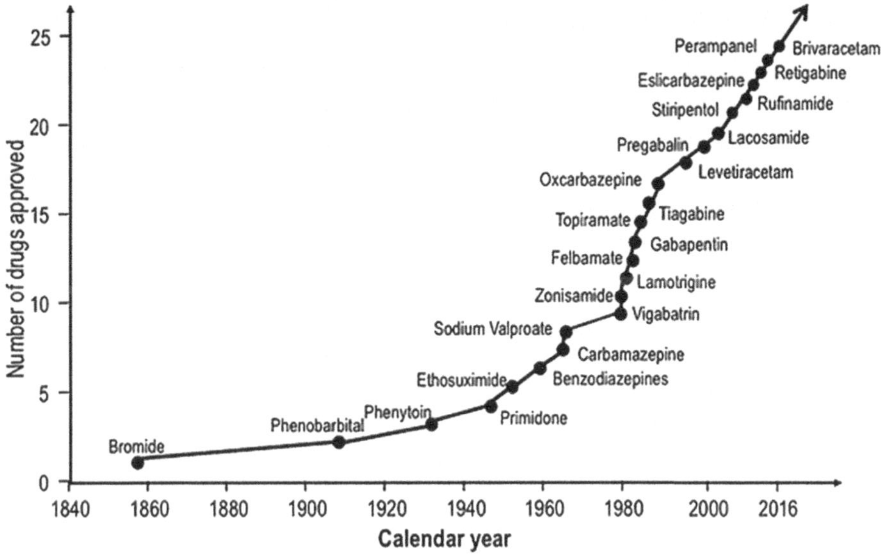

Fig. 1 Year of development of anti-seizure medications (reproduced from Golyala and Kwan 2017)

anti-seizure activity of phenytoin was discovered in 1930 using the electroshock model and electroshock threshold in cats (Rho and White 2018).

The development of algorithms for screening compounds for anti-seizure potentials, spearheaded by the Anticonvulsant Screening Program (ASP), currently known as the Epilepsy Therapy Screening Program (ETSP), of the National Institute of Health/National Institute of Neurologic disorders and Stroke (NIH/NINDS), resulted in development of new anti-seizure medications at a relatively faster pace (Rho and White 2018; Golyala and Kwan 2017). In the past 25 years, over 18 new anti-seizure medications have been introduced (Fig. 1).

At the preclinical stage, medication development is based on targeting seizure mechanisms, creating structural analogues of available anti-seizure medications, and testing of known chemicals for anti-seizure activity (Golyala and Kwan 2017). Various animal models are available to test anti-seizure activity (Rho and White 2018; Golyala and Kwan 2017; Loscher 2017; Bialer and White 2010). Historically, maximal electric shock (MES) and subcutaneous pentylenetetrazol (scPTZ) rodent models have been used. MES may suggest effect in generalized tonic-clonic or partial seizures; scPTZ may suggest effect in nonconvulsive/absence seizures. These models, however, may miss some compounds with anti-seizure activity. Case in point is levetiracetam which failed in both models. Additional animal models were developed to represent broad epilepsy phenotypes, including refractory epilepsy, such as 6 Hz psychomotor seizure model, phenytoin-resistant kindled rat, lamotrigine kindled rat, post-status epilepticus models of temporal lobe epilepsy, and the methylazoxymethanol (MAM) model. Animal models are also available for genetic epilepsies.

Currently the workflow of testing new compounds by the ETSP involves identification and differentiation phases (Kehne et al. 2017). In the initial identification phase, 6 Hz electrical stimulation and MES are used. Additional chronic seizure models are also used and behavioral toxicity is screened. In the differentiation phase, compounds are tested on models of epilepsy – mesial temporal lobe epilepsy model (mice), lamotrigine resistant amygdala kindling model (rat), and post-kainate status epilepticus-induced spontaneous recurrent seizures (rat). Theiler's virus model of acute seizures (viral-encephalitis-induced epilepsy model) can be employed for compounds with unique mechanisms of action or in cases of compelling justifications (Kehne et al. 2017; Loscher 2017).

In the clinical stage of drug development, new compounds are tested as adjunctive therapy first and subsequently as monotherapy (Golyala and Kwan 2017). Since the late 1990s and early 2000s, when several United States governmental acts encouraged and required the research of drugs in the pediatric population, recent expansion of indications to include children have often been based on the extrapolation of efficacy in adult trials in addition to pharmacokinetic data in children (Mulugeta et al. 2016).

New AEDs have similar efficacy as the older AEDs but have improved safety profiles as a group. The challenge remains in developing more effective drugs, drugs which work in intractable epilepsy (Kwan and Brodie 2000), thereby improving quality of life (Cianchetti et al. 2015) and preventing SUDEP (Abdel-Mannan et al. 2019), and drugs which modify the underlying disease, namely, preventing or reversing epileptogenesis (Rho and White 2018).

2 "First-Generation" and "Second-Generation" Antiepileptic Drugs

Although the designations are imprecise and used in a variable fashion, older and newer AEDs are often referred to as "first-" and "second"-generation drugs. The brief summaries below review AEDs in the approximate order of time of development and refer to formal FDA indications as well as consensus-based clinical approaches.

2.1 Phenobarbital

Phenobarbital's mechanism of action is through potentiation of the GABAa receptors by acting as a positive allosteric modulator, gamma-aminobutyric acid (GABA) being the major inhibitory neurotransmitter. It allows the GABAa receptors to remain open longer. At higher concentration, barbiturates such as phenobarbital can directly activate GABAa receptors even in the absence of GABA neurotransmitter.

Phenobarbital is clinically indicated for focal and generalized tonic-clonic seizures. It is often the first-line treatment for neonatal seizures. Phenobarbital has a long half-life, approximately 100 h in newborns and 69 h between 1 and 5 years of age.

Treatment doses: 1–3 mg/kg/day in children and 2–11 mg/kg/day in neonates. This can be administered daily or twice a day (BID).

Drug interactions: Phenobarbital can increase the clearance of other antiepileptic medications including lamotrigine, ethosuximide, felbamate, topiramate, zonisamide, tiagabine, and rufinamide.

Side effects: Sedation, mood change, cognitive effects (slowing), hyperactivity, and aggressiveness in children.

2.2 Phenytoin

Phenytoin has been in use since 1938. Although phenytoin has numerous sites of action, the major anticonvulsant mechanism is thought to be through the sodium channel, by binding to axonal sodium channels and prolonging the channels' inactivated state. This reduces the repetitive firing of neurons during presynaptic stimulation. Phenytoin is clinically indicated for focal and generalized seizures. It is also one of the first-line medications used in status epilepticus.

Treatment doses: For acute management of status epilepticus, dosing is 15–20 mg/kg IV. Maintenance dosing is 5–8 mg/kg/day divided BID or three times a day (TID), with higher dosages required to maintain adequate levels in younger children. Phenytoin is metabolized by the hepatic P450 enzyme system and follows zero-order kinetics; small changes in phenytoin doses can result in disproportionate increases in serum levels.

Drug interactions: Phenytoin is highly protein-bound (approximately 90%). Only the unbound (free) portion is pharmacologically active. The percentage of protein binding depends on albumin concentration, concurrent medication, and renal failure. Substances, such as valproic acid, can compete for binding sites and displace phenytoin, thus increasing phenytoin concentrations and increasing risk for toxicity. Hypoalbuminemia, liver disease, and renal failure can increase levels of unbound phenytoin.

Side effects: Long-term use can lead to gingival hyperplasia, cerebellar atrophy, decreased bone density, and peripheral neuropathy. Acute toxicity includes ataxia, diplopia, and dysarthria.

2.3 Ethosuximide

Ethosuximide treats absence seizures (primary generalized), presumably by blocking T-type calcium channels of thalamic neurons, thus decreasing burst firing of thalamocortical neurons. A multicenter, double-blind, randomized, controlled trial

(Glauser et al. 2010) compared ethosuximide, valproic acid, and lamotrigine in the treatment of childhood absence epilepsy and confirmed historical/clinical consensus that ethosuximide and valproate are more effective than lamotrigine and ethosuximide has fewer adverse attentional effects.

Treatment doses:	Starting dose is approximately 250 mg BID, increasing to maintenance dosing of 20–40 mg/kg/day. Give with food or on a full stomach to avoid gastrointestinal side effects.
Drug interactions:	Valproate has been reported to increase ethosuximide levels.
Side effects:	Most commonly stomach ache or stomach upset. Blood dyscrasias, abnormal liver and renal function tests, and cases of systemic lupus erythematosus and Stevens-Johnson syndrome have been reported.

2.4 Valproate

Valproate is a broad-spectrum antiepileptic discovered in 1967. Its mechanism of action is not fully known, though valproate is thought to work through multiple avenues including potentiation of GABAergic function, inhibition of T-type calcium currents, antagonism of NMDA-receptor neuronal excitation, and inhibition of sodium channels.

Valproate is clinically used to treat multiple seizure types, including generalized seizures (absence, myoclonic, and generalized tonic-clonic), focal seizures, Lennox-Gastaut syndrome (LGS), epileptic encephalopathies, neonatal seizures, and febrile seizures.

Treatment doses:	Starting at 15 mg/kg/day and titrated up to 30 mg/kg/day. Maximum is 60–70 mg/kg/day.
Drug interactions:	Valproate is highly protein-bound and the free fraction increases at higher concentrations. It is a cytochrome P450 inhibitor and as such can interact with multiple medications including other AEDs. Valproate increases serum levels of lamotrigine and phenobarbital. There may be synergy or additive benefit when the combination of valproate and lamotrigine is given (Brodie et al. 1997). Valproate levels are decreased by phenytoin and carbamazepine and increased by felbamate.
Side effects:	Fatigue, weight gain, alopecia, tremor, thrombocytopenia, hepatitis, pancreatitis, and hyperammonemia. Encephalopathy can be caused by polytherapy, metabolic disorders (such as urea cycle, fatty acid disorders, mitochondrial disorders), and liver disease. Young children (under the age of 2 years) are at increased risk of hepatotoxicity.

2.5 Vigabatrin

Vigabatrin is indicated in the United States for infantile spasms in children 1 month to 2 years of age and for adjunctive therapy of refractory complex partial seizures in patients 10 years of age and older. It is particularly beneficial in patients with tuberous sclerosis complex. Vigabatrin is an irreversible GABA transaminase inhibitor, preventing the metabolism of the inhibitory neurotransmitter GABA.

Treatment doses:	For infantile spasms, start at 50 mg/kg/day and titrate to 150 mg/kg/day, divided BID. For complex partial seizures in the pediatric population, start 250 mg BID and titrate to 1,000 mg BID.
Drug interactions:	Vigabatrin may decrease phenytoin levels and increase clonazepam concentrations.
Side effects:	Most commonly fatigue, irritability, insomnia, weight gain, headache, and dizziness. The FDA has required a Risk Evaluation and Mitigation Strategy (REMS) program to ensure that benefits outweigh risks, due to the risk of irreversible bilateral visual field constriction or central retina damage, occurring in >20% of infants treated for infantile spasms, with increased risk with greater duration of exposure (Westall et al. 2014). Diffusion-weighted imaging and T2-hyperintense lesions on brain MRI are seen in approximately 1/3 of pediatric patients, particularly those who are younger and on higher dosing; these resolve with discontinuation of vigabatrin (Pearl et al. 2009) and may resolve even without discontinuation.

2.6 Zonisamide

Zonisamide is indicated as adjunctive therapy for partial seizures in adults. It has been shown to be effective against tonic extension seizures induced by MES, raised the threshold for generalized seizures in the kindled rat, and decreased the length of cortical focal seizures induced by electrical stimulation in cats. It has been shown to block sodium channels and reduce T-type calcium currents.

Treatment doses:	Starting dose of 100 mg (given daily or divided BID), titrated to 400 mg/day. Elimination half-life is approximately 63 h; thus it may take up to 2 weeks to reach steady-state level.
Drug interactions:	Concentrations may be altered by CYP3A4 inducers or inhibitors. Phenytoin, carbamazepine, and valproate increase zonisamide clearance; however, zonisamide does not affect protein binding of phenytoin or carbamazepine.

Side effects: Zonisamide is a sulfonamide, so should not be given to patients with sulfa allergy. Most common side effects are headache, decreased appetite, nausea, dizziness, agitation, insomnia, depression, fatigue, and difficulty with concentration/memory, although perhaps less so than topiramate.

2.7 Lamotrigine

Lamotrigine is a broad-spectrum antiepileptic medication whose primary mechanism of action is through blockade of neuronal sodium channels by stabilization of the inactivated state. It is effective for both focal and generalized seizures and is indicated for adjunctive therapy for partial-onset seizures (POS), primary generalized tonic-clonic seizures, and generalized seizures of LGS in patients 2 years and older, as well as monotherapy in patients aged 16 years and older. However, lamotrigine has been reported to exacerbate myoclonic seizures in some cases.

Drug interactions: Lamotrigine is hepatically metabolized by glucuronyltransferase. Inducers and inhibitors of hepatic metabolism alter lamotrigine levels. Lamotrigine elimination half-life is reduced by carbamazepine, phenobarbital, primidone, and phenytoin. Valproate decreases lamotrigine clearance.

Treatment doses: Monotherapy is 0.3 mg/kg/day for 2 weeks and then 0.6 mg/kg/day for 2 weeks and then increased by 0.6 mg/kg/week every 1–2 weeks until target dose of 4.5–8 mg/kg/day. Maximum dose is 12–15 mg/kg/day. When valproate is added to a regimen with lamotrigine, the starting and maintenance doses of lamotrigine should be reduced by approximately 50%.

Side effects: Dizziness (increased with concomitant use of oxcarbazepine), blurred vision, diplopia, and tremor. Six to ten percent of patients treated with lamotrigine can experience skin rash, leading to a discontinuation of the medication. In order to reduce the risk of skin rash, the recommendation is to start at a low dose and titrate up slowly over 6 weeks.

2.8 Felbamate

Felbamate is indicated for refractory epilepsy, as monotherapy or adjunctive therapy for partial seizures in adults and as adjunctive therapy for children with LGS, after patients have been informed of the risks and given written acknowledgement. Felbamate is effective in MES, scPTZ, and the subcutaneous picrotoxin seizure test.

Treatment doses: Starting dose in children 15 mg/kg/day divided into three or four doses, increasing by 15 mg/kg/day increments to 45 mg/kg/day. Discontinuation, in order to minimize risks, is encouraged if maximum dosing is not effective.

Drug interactions: Felbamate increases phenytoin, valproate, phenobarbital, and the carbamazepine epoxide metabolite. Felbamate is decreased by phenytoin and phenobarbital and increased by carbamazepine.

Side effects: This medication is approached cautiously due to occurrence of aplastic anemia and liver failure. Blood counts, reticulocyte counts, and liver function at baseline and frequently after initiation are recommended. Common side effects however include anorexia, vomiting, insomnia, headache, and somnolence.

2.9 Topiramate

Topiramate is a broad-spectrum AED with likely multiple targets of action, including voltage-gated sodium channels, GABAa receptors, AMPA and kainate subtype of glutamate receptors, and L-type calcium channels. Topiramate is also a type II and IV carbonic anhydrase inhibitor. The pharmacologic actions of topiramate are possibly through effects of channel phosphorylation rather than direct modulation of voltage-gated channels.

Treatment doses: Starting 1–3 mg/kg/day with maximum doses 10–12 mg/kg/day. Slow titration of the medication (advancing 1–2 mg/kg/day every 2 weeks) may decrease the side effects.

Drug interactions: Topiramate is a mild inducer and inhibitor of P450 enzymes. The fraction of metabolized drug may increase when combined with enzyme-inducing drugs.

Side effects: Cognitive effects including memory problems, word finding difficulty, and challenges with verbal fluency. Other potential side effects include renal stones, sedation, paresthesia, decreased appetite and weight loss, and oligohidrosis.

2.10 Oxcarbazepine

Oxcarbazepine is often considered first-line treatment for focal epilepsy as well as focal seizures with secondary generalization. It is chemically similar in structure to carbamazepine, a drug that was first discovered to be effective in patients with epilepsy in the early 1960s. The mechanism of action is on the voltage-gated sodium channels and N-type calcium channels resulting in stabilization of hyperexcited neural membranes.

Treatment doses: Starting dose is 5 mg/kg/day (can be 10 mg/kg/day but this may increase side effects) with a target dose of 15–20 mg/kg/day. It can be titrated up to 50 mg/kg/day, though side effects can often increase beyond treatment with 35 mg/kg/day.

Drug interactions: Oxcarbazepine may increase plasma levels of phenytoin. Oxcarbazepine is metabolized by the CYP3A4 enzyme system and can reduce the effectiveness of hormonal contraceptives. Oxcarbazepine may increase plasma levels of phenytoin. Phenobarbital may decrease oxcarbazepine levels. There is no significant interaction between oxcarbazepine and felbamate, lamotrigine, or valproate.

Side effects: Drowsiness, diplopia, ataxia, rash (rare Stevens-Johnson syndrome), and hyponatremia. The risk of hyponatremia may be seen in 2–3% of children treated with oxcarbazepine. Carbamazepine has been associated with aplastic anemia and agranulocytosis. There is an increased risk of side effects in patients with HLA-B 1502 allele, an allele most prevalent in people with Asian ancestry.

2.11 Levetiracetam

Levetiracetam is approved as adjunctive therapy for myoclonic seizures in patients 12 years and older with juvenile myoclonic epilepsy, for partial seizures in patients 1 month or older, and for primary generalized tonic-clonic seizures in patients older than 5 years with idiopathic generalized epilepsy. The mechanism of action is through binding to the synaptic vesicle protein 2A (SV2A) on secretory vesicle membranes in presynaptic neurons, affecting calcium-dependent neurotransmitter release.

Treatment doses: Starting at 10–20 mg/kg/day, maximum doses 60–80 mg/kg/day. Target dose is generally 30–40 mg/kg/day. Dosing will need to be reduced with renal impairment/failure.

Drug interactions: Limited pharmacokinetic interactions due to minimal plasma protein binding.

Side effects: Somnolence, behavioral problems including aggression, nervousness, and irritability. Pyridoxine may decrease behavioral side effects from levetiracetam.

3 Newest-Generation ("Third-Generation") Medications

3.1 Pregabalin

Pregabalin is a lipophilic analog of GABA, modified to increase diffusion across the blood-brain barrier. It binds to the alpha2-delta subunit of presynaptic voltage-gated calcium channels. It is indicated as adjunctive therapy for partial-onset seizures in patients 4 years of age and older, neuropathic pain associated with diabetic peripheral neuropathy, postherpetic neuralgia, fibromyalgia, and neuropathic pain associated with spinal cord injury. Although evidence is sparse, pregabalin has been used off-label for migraine headaches. Evidence to support off-label use for pain is also lacking; however, there has been a dramatic increase in prescribing of pregabalin, likely driven by the need to decrease opioid use. Increased risk of opioid-related death occurs with concurrent use of opioids and gabapentinoids (Goodman and Brett 2019). Relating to a dramatic increase in deaths associated with misuse of gabapentinoids, in the United Kingdom on April 1, 2019, pregabalin was reclassified as a class C controlled substance (Torjesen 2019).

Treatment doses:	For patients weighing 30 kg or more, initial dose is 2.5 mg/kg/day, increasing to 10 mg/kg/day (maximum 600 mg); for patients 11 kg to less than 30 kg, initial dose is 3.5 mg/kg/day and increased to 14 mg/kg/day. Adjust in patients with reduced renal function.
Drug interactions:	It undergoes negligible metabolism and is not protein-bound, so is unlikely to interact with other medications.
Side effects:	Common side effects included somnolence, increased appetite, and weight.

3.2 Lacosamide

Lacosamide enhances slow inactivation of voltage-gated sodium channels (rather than fast, which other AEDs affect). Oral formulations are indicated for adjunctive or monotherapy for partial-onset seizures in patients 4 years of age and older; intravenous (IV) injection is approved for partial-onset seizures in adults 17 years of age and older. Oral bioavailability is 100%. Because of IV availability, lacosamide is increasingly being used for status epilepticus or acute repetitive seizures.

Treatment doses:	For patients weighing 50 kg or more, initial dosage is 50 mg twice daily, increasing to 150–200 mg twice daily as monotherapy or 100–200 mg twice daily as adjunctive therapy; for patients 30 kg to less than 50 kg, initial dosage is 1 mg/kg twice daily, increasing to maximum 2–4 mg/kg twice daily; and for patients 11 kg to less than 30 kg, initial dosage is

1 mg/kg twice daily, increasing to maximum 3–6 mg/kg twice daily. Dosing should be adjusted in severe renal impairment and mild/moderate hepatic impairment and should be supplemented after hemodialysis. Loading doses by IV have ranged 200–400 mg in adults and 4–10 mg/kg in children (Strzelczyk et al. 2017).

Drug interactions: Strong CYP3A4 and CYP2C9 inhibitors increase lacosamide levels.

Side effects: Dizziness and ataxia are the most frequent. In trials, a small, dose-related increase in PR intervals and asymptomatic first-degree atrioventricular block was seen. A case report of isolated lacosamide overdose describes QRS prolongation (Ng et al. 2019). In patients on medications that affect cardiac conduction (sodium channel, beta, calcium channel, and potassium channel blockers), EKG at baseline and after titration should be obtained. Preclinical data has demonstrated interference of lacosamide with collapsing response mediator protein-2 activity (involved in neuronal differentiation and axonal outgrowth) and decreased brain weight and long-term learning and memory issues in neonatal/juvenile rats (UCB Inc 2018).

3.3 Stiripentol

Stiripentol is used as adjunctive treatment in patients with Dravet syndrome 2 years of age or older. Dravet syndrome (previously called severe myoclonic epilepsy of infancy) is an epileptic encephalopathy most often caused by a mutation in the sodium voltage-gated channel alpha subunit 1 (SCN1A). A randomized, placebo-controlled study showed 67–71% achieved a >50% reduction in convulsive seizures (Chiron et al. 2000). When added to valproate and clobazam, reduction of frequency and severity of seizures was seen; 96% maintained therapy after a median of 8 years (De Liso et al. 2016). Multiple mechanisms of action include (a) enhancement of inhibitory, γ-aminobutyric acid (GABA)ergic neurotransmission (Fisher 2011), (b) inhibition of lactate dehydrogenase which thereby activates ATP-sensitive potassium channels, and (c) blockage of NMDA-sensitive glutamate receptors and voltage-sensitive sodium and calcium channels (Nickels and Wirell 2017).

Treatment doses: 50 mg/kg/day divided BID or TID with a maximum dose of 3 g.

Drug interactions: Stiripentol can increase levels of carbamazepine, phenobarbital, and phenytoin and increases clobazam and norclobazam (clobazam's active metabolite). Phenytoin and phenobarbital decrease levels of stiripentol. Clobazam increases stiripentol levels (Levy et al. 1984; Giraud et al. 2006).

Side effects:	Somnolence, decreased appetite, and agitation, ataxia, weight decreased, hypotonia, nausea, tremor, dysarthria, and insomnia. Serious side effects include neutropenia, thrombocytopenia, and suicidal behavior and ideation (Perez et al. 1999).

3.4 Rufinamide

It is indicated as adjunctive therapy in LGS in patients 1 year or older. Responder rates for total seizures were higher in the rufinamide group (32.7%) versus placebo (10.9%) after a 12-week parallel-group treatment period in a randomized controlled trial (Glauser et al. 2008). Reduction in tonic-atonic seizures was also seen. These results were also seen in Ohtsuka et al. (2014) with a similar decrease in seizure frequency (32.9%). It decreases the recovery of sodium channels from the inactivated state.

Treatment doses:	Starting at 10 mg/kg/day divided BID, increasing to 45 mg/kg/day.
Drug interactions:	Low potential for interactions due to lack of protein binding and metabolism independent of the cytochrome P450 system (Perucca et al. 2008); however, it can decrease levels of carbamazepine and lamotrigine and increase levels of phenobarbital and phenytoin. Valproate can increase rufinamide levels (Critchley et al. 2005).
Side effects:	Decreased appetite, pyrexia, somnolence, nausea, and vomiting. Serious side effects include decreased QTc interval, and hypersensitivity syndrome (Wheless et al. 2009), thus, is contraindicated in patients with Familial Short QT syndrome.

3.5 Eslicarbazepine Acetate

Eslicarbazepine acetate is used for monotherapy and adjunctive treatment of POS in patients 4 years of age or older. Safety and clinical efficacy in adults was seen in five multicenter, randomized, controlled trials, and the data was extrapolated to support pediatric use. A responder rate between 17 and 43% was seen in four phase 3 randomized controlled studies in subjects 16 years or older with refractory partial-onset seizures (Gil-Nagel et al. 2013; Sperling et al. 2015). Its mechanism of action is inhibition of voltage-gated sodium channels; it is related to carbamazepine and oxcarbazepine, but is primarily metabolized to (s)licarbazepine, with greater efficacy and less toxicity compared to the (r) isomer.

Treatment doses:	Once-daily dosing starting at 200 mg daily and then increasing to maximum 1,200 mg/day.
Drug interactions:	Eslicarbazepine can induce the metabolism of drugs that are eliminated by metabolism through CYP3A4 (carbamazepine, phenobarbital, topiramate) or through the UDP-glucuronosyl (lamotrigine). Eslicarbazepine decreases lamotrigine and topiramate levels, increases phenytoin levels, and can decrease plasma levels of oral contraceptives (Bialer and Soares-da-Silva 2012).
Side effects:	Similar profile to oxcarbazepine; dizziness, headache, somnolence, diplopia, nausea/vomiting, rash, hyponatremia (Rolan et al. 2008). Serious side effects include increased PR interval, agitation, anxiety, depression, and increased suicidal ideation (Eddy et al. 2012).

3.6 Perampanel

Perampanel is indicated as monotherapy or adjunctive use in patients 4 years and older for POS with or without secondarily generalized seizures and as adjunctive therapy for primary generalized tonic-clonic seizures in patients 12 years of age and older (Rogawski and Hanada 2013). It acts as a noncompetitive antagonist of the AMPA-type glutamate receptor (Hanada et al. 2011).

Treatment doses:	Starting at 2 mg once at bedtime, increased to 8–12 mg as monotherapy or adjunctive therapy for POS and 8 mg as adjunctive therapy for primary generalized tonic-clonic seizures.
Drug interactions:	Carbamazepine, oxcarbazepine, and phenytoin decrease perampanel levels. Perampanel can increase oxcarbazepine levels. Perampanel enhances metabolism of progesterone. There can be increased fatigue in patients also on levetiracetam, increased irritability in patients also on phenobarbital, and increased likelihood of decreased appetite in patients also on oxcarbazepine (Gidal et al. 2013).
Side effects:	Common side effects include dizziness, somnolence, fatigue, irritability, nausea, headache, and falls (Rugg-Gunn 2014). Serious side effects include depression and increased suicidal ideation.

3.7 Brivaracetam

Brivaracetam is indicated as monotherapy or adjunctive therapy in the treatment of POS in patients aged ≥4 years. Briviact injection is indicated to treat POS in patients aged ≥16 years. Brivaracetam is the (s)-isomer of levetiracetam, with 15–30 times greater affinity for synaptic vesicle protein SV2A (Kaminski et al. 2008).

Treatment doses:	Starting at 50 mg BID and increasing to 100 mg BID (Schoemaker et al. 2017).
Drug interactions:	Decreases carbamazepine levels (von Rosenstiel 2017). There is a negative interaction between brivaracetam and levetiracetam such that the combination may reduce the efficacy (Biton et al. 2014).
Side effects:	Dizziness, somnolence, fatigue, and headaches.

3.8 Cannabidiol/Epidiolex

Epidiolex is a highly purified, plant-derived cannabidiol (CBD) that was approved by the FDA in June 2018 for the treatment of rare severe childhood-onset epilepsies, specifically LGS and Dravet syndrome. Previous studies have shown median reduction of monthly seizures from 48 to 57% in patients with LGS (Thiele et al. 2019) and a greater reduction in frequency of drop seizures with the addition of cannabidiol 10 or 20 mg/kg (Devinsky et al. 2018). CBD was found to reduce the frequency of convulsive seizures in 43% of children with Dravet syndrome by 50% per month, and 5% became seizure-free (Devinsky et al. 2017a, b).

The mode of action is unknown but may be due to multiple mechanisms: (a) antagonism of lipid-activated GPR55 (expressed in excitatory and inhibitory synapses); (b) binding at 5-HT1A receptor; (c) inhibition of adenosine reuptake at voltage-dependent sodium, potassium, and other channels; and (d) antioxidant and anti-inflammatory processes (Sylantyev et al. 2013; Lanuti et al. 2015).

Treatment doses:	Epidiolex comes in a 10 mg/mL suspension in sesame oil. Dosing is 2.5 mg/kg BID. After 1 week, the dose may be increased to 5 mg/kg BID. If further seizure reduction is required, the maximum dose is 10 mg/kg twice daily or 20 mg/kg once per day (Greenwich Biosciences 2018). It has linear pharmacokinetics with a half-life of 56–61 h (Rimmerman et al. 2013).
Drug interactions:	It is metabolized in the liver by cytochrome P450. CBD increases *N*-desmethylclobazam metabolite levels (Devinsky et al. 2017a, b). Studies are ongoing to clarify other medication interactions. A case report described an increase in international normalized ratio (INR) in a patient also on warfarin.

	Elevated liver enzymes were seen more with concomitant valproate intake (Billakota et al. 2019).
Side effects:	Decreased appetite, diarrhea, elevated liver enzymes, fatigue, infections, insomnia, malaise, rash, sedation, and sleep disorder. Serious side effects are aggression, suicidal ideation, new or worsening depression, panic attacks, and liver injury (Devinsky et al. 2018).

3.9 Everolimus

Everolimus is a selective inhibitor of the mammalian target of rapamycin (mTOR) pathway, specifically mTOR complex type II. mTOR is a protein kinase signal transducer that plays a key role in cell growth and proliferation. mTOR dysregulation causes tuberous sclerosis complex (TSC) and has been reported in several models of epileptogenesis (Griffith and Wong 2018). In addition to inhibiting mTOR and downstream effectors of mTOR involved in protein synthesis including hypoxia-inducible factor and vascular endothelial growth factor, mTOR inhibitors prolong opening of calcium and sodium channels, increase potassium channel (Kv1.1) expression, and increase GABA-mediated synaptic activity (Curatolo et al. 2018). Everolimus is approved for certain types of breast cancer, neuroendocrine tumors, advanced renal cell carcinoma, and renal angiomyolipoma in tuberous sclerosis complex, as well as for two neurological conditions. These include:

1. Treatment of patients $\geq$ age 1 year with TSC with subependymal giant cell astrocytoma (SEGA) which cannot be resected. SEGAs often occur near the foramen of Monro and can cause obstructive hydrocephalus. A multicenter, double-blind, placebo-controlled phase 3 trial found that 57% of patients had at least 50% decrease in the sum volumes of all target SEGA lesions, without worsening nontarget or new SEGA lesions, or new/worsening hydrocephalus (Franz et al. 2016).
2. Adjunctive treatment of patients $\geq$2 years with POS and TSC. A phase 3, double-blind, placebo-controlled, three-arm trial (placebo vs low-exposure of 3–7 ng/mL and high exposure of 9–15 ng/mL) demonstrated a dose-related decrease in seizure frequency of $\geq$50% over a 12-week period (French et al. 2016).

The reader is referred to the prescribing information (Novartis 2018), which delineates complex recommendations regarding dosing, drug monitoring, dosing changes/cessation in response to varying severities of adverse reactions, and monitoring of levels related to interactions with P-glycoprotein and CYP3A4 inhibitors/inducers.

Treatment doses:	Dosing for SEGA is 4.5 mg/m^2 once daily, adjusting the dose toward a goal trough level of 5–15 ng/mL. For partial-onset seizures associated with TSC, dosing is 5 mg/m^2 once daily, adjusting the dose with goal trough level 5–15 ng/mL. Adjustments should follow this calculation, with maximum dose increase at any step being 5 mg or less: New dose = current dose × (target concentration divided by current concentration). Half-life is approximately 30 h. Steady state occurs within 2 weeks after once-daily dosing.
Drug interactions:	Everolimus is 75% bound to plasma proteins. It is metabolized via CYP3A4. Regarding anti-seizure medications specifically, concentrations of carbamazepine, clobazam, *N*-desmethylclobazam, and oxcarbazepine increase by approximately 10%. Clonazepam, zonisamide, valproic acid, topiramate, phenobarbital, and phenytoin do not change.
Side effects:	Everolimus has immunosuppressive qualities; thus localized and systemic infections including with opportunistic pathogens have occurred, with an incidence of up to 10% of Grade 3 (severe) and up to 3% of Grade 4 (potentially life-threatening) infections, at higher frequency in children <6 years old. Adverse reactions also include noninfectious pneumonitis, impaired wound healing, myelosuppression, severe hypersensitivity reactions, angioedema, renal failure, metabolic changes (hyperglycemia, hypercholesterolemia, hypertriglyceridemia), and frequently stomatitis (most often within the first 8 weeks; in 44–78% of patients).

More specifically in patients with TSC-associated SEGA, Franz et al. (2016) demonstrated that the most common side effects (≥30% incidence) were stomatitis and respiratory tract infection. The most common Grade 3 or 4 reactions (≥2% incidence) were stomatitis, fever, pneumonia, gastroenteritis, aggression, agitation, and amenorrhea. Most common lab abnormalities were elevated cholesterol and elevated partial thromboplastin time (most common Grade 3–4 abnormality was neutropenia).

In patients with TSC-associated partial-onset seizures, French et al. (2016) demonstrated that the most common side effect was stomatitis (most common Grade 3 or 4 reactions were stomatitis, pneumonia, irregular menses). Drug cessation due to adverse reactions occurred in 5 and 3% of patients in the low trough and high trough groups; the most common being stomatitis (French et al. 2016).

4 Drugs in Development

Many drugs in development aim to modify the underlying disease processes or utilize different mechanisms of action than currently used. The following is not an inclusive list, but exemplifies these approaches.

4.1 Benzodiazepine Formulations

Until May 2019, rectal diazepam was the only FDA-approved non-intravenous therapy for acute repetitive seizures or clusters of seizures. A rectal formulation raises challenges relating to social appropriateness and ease of administration. A new drug application for Nayzilam, a midazolam nasal spray, was accepted by the FDA in 2018 and it received FDA approval in May 2019.

A randomized, double-blind, placebo-controlled, phase 3 study randomized patients admitted to the epilepsy monitoring unit to receive Nayzilam 5 mg or placebo; it found a higher percentage of seizure-free subjects and a longer time to first seizure following treatment with Nayzilam (Van Ess et al. 2017). The open-label extension showed safety with repeated dosing if seizures did not stop within 10 min or if seizures recurred between 10 min and 6 h after first dose; side effects included nasal discomfort, somnolence/fatigue, headache, rhinorrhea/sneezing, and abnormal product taste (Meng et al. 2018). There was also >80% treatment success after one or two doses (Sequeira et al. 2018).

A formulation which delivers alprazolam via inhalation of a thermally generated aerosol is undergoing phase 2b study in adults (A Double-Blind, Placebo-Controlled, Inpatient, Dose-Ranging Efficacy Study of Staccato Alprazolam (STAP-001) in Subjects With Epilepsy With a Predictable Seizure Pattern; clinicaltrials.gov/NCT03478982).

4.2 Bumetanide (NKCC Inhibitor)

Bumetanide is a potent loop diuretic already approved for the treatment of edema associated with congestive heart failure, hepatic and renal disease, including nephrotic syndrome. It also inhibits NKCC1 which is expressed in the brain and is thought to be involved in dysregulated intracellular chloride concentrations in neonatal epilepsy, autism, and traumatic brain injury. Immature neurons have high intracellular chloride, leading GABAa receptor-mediated chloride currents to be depolarizing and excitatory. Bumetanide decreases intracellular chloride, making the action of GABAa receptors more hyperpolarizing.

However, bumetanide poorly penetrates the brain (Loscher 2018). Other challenges include side effects related to its diuretic action and inhibition of the NKCC in the inner ear, leading to hearing loss. A phase 1/2 trial for neonatal seizures was terminated early due to ototoxicity and lack of efficacy (Pressler et al. 2015). Strategies to bypass these issues include the development of lipophilic and uncharged prodrugs, to enter the brain before cleavage to bumetanide.

4.3 Fenfluramine (Amphetamine Derivative)

Fenfluramine was marketed as an appetite suppressant in the treatment of adult obesity, but was removed from the market in 1997 after association with cardiac valve thickening. This association was seen often in combination with phentermine and seemed to be dose-related. Since then, it has been shown to decrease seizure-like behavior in a zebrafish model of Dravet syndrome. Fenfluramine modulates serotonin activity in the brain by disrupting neuronal vesicular storage and inhibiting serotonin reuptake.

A phase 3 trial comparing 0.8 mg/kg/day, 0.2 mg/kg/day, and placebo in pediatric Dravet patients showed a median decrease in monthly convulsive seizure frequency over 14 weeks of 63.9% in the high-dose group versus 17.4% in the placebo group (Lagae et al. 2017). An open-label study using doses of 0.25–1 mg/kg/day (maximum 20 mg/day), with periodic echocardiograms, demonstrated decreased seizure frequency in all nine patients with Dravet, with median reduction 75%; most common adverse reactions were somnolence and anorexia (Schoonjans et al. 2017).

A multicenter trial assessing use of fenfluramine 0.2 and 0.4 mg/kg/day as adjunctive treatment to stiripentol in Dravet was completed in January 2019 (clinicaltrials.gov, NCT02926898). Several studies are ongoing, including an open-label extension trial assessing the long-term safety of 0.2 mg/kg/day (maximum 30 mg/day) in Dravet (clinicaltrials.gov, NCT02823145) and a randomized, double-blind, placebo-controlled trial and open-label extension comparing 0.2 and 0.8 mg/kg/day in Lennox-Gastaut syndrome (clinicaltrials.gov, NCT03355209).

4.4 Ganaxolone (GABAergic)

Progesterone is an endogenous inhibitory neurosteroid. Ganaxolone is a modified (3Beta-methylated) steroid which does not bind steroid receptors but activates synaptic and extrasynaptic GABAA receptors in the brain at sites different from benzodiazepine or barbiturates and potentiates tonic (sustained) and phasic (rapid) inhibition (Younas and Reddy 2018).

Phase 2 studies have demonstrated decrease in seizure frequency in patients with epilepsy associated with protocadherin-19 (PCDH19) (Specchio et al. 2018), CDKL5 mutations, and Lennox-Gastaut syndrome (Devinsky et al. 2017a, b). The presence of low allopregnanolone-sulfate levels in girls with PCDH19 mutations has been correlated with benefit of ganaxolone, suggesting a potential biomarker for response prediction (Sullivan et al. 2018). Ganaxolone and brexanolone (allopregnanolone, an endogenous progesterone metabolite) are being investigated for treatment of super refractory status epilepticus.

4.5 Huperzine

Huperzine (Hup A) is an herbal product derived from the Chinese *Huperzia serrata* club moss which has been used in China for cognitive disorders and is sold in the United States as a supplement for cognitive dysfunction. It acts primarily by acetylcholinesterase inhibition and enhances presynaptic GABAergic tone.

Administration to SCN1A mouse mutants increased their resistance to seizures (Wong et al. 2016). The phase 1 trial with immediate-acting formulation demonstrated nausea and vomiting as peak-related side effects, requiring dosing four to six times a day. An extended release formulation showed less adverse events, with double the dose predicted for significant seizure control being attainable, using a twice/day schedule.

4.6 Ion Channel Modulators

1OP-2198 or XEN1101 is in phase 1 development. It opens the neuronal Kv7.2/7.3 (KCNQ) potassium channel, responsible for slow modulation of the voltage-gated M-current, and has higher potency and selectivity as compared to an earlier Kv7 modulator, ezogabine (Beatch et al. 2018). Production of ezogabine was stopped in 2017 related to side effects (including blue skin and eye discoloration) causing decline in patient initiation.

XEN901 is a selective inhibitor of NaV1.6, sodium channel voltage-gated type 8 alpha subunit, which is highly expressed in excitatory glutamatergic pyramidal neurons. It does not inhibit NaV1.1 (SCN1A; primarily expressed in GABAergic inhibitory interneurons) nor NaV1.5 (expressed in the heart) and thus is unique compared to other sodium channel blockers such as phenytoin or carbamazepine which block all subtypes (and typically exacerbate seizures in patients with SCN1A mutations) (Johnson et al. 2018).

4.7 Metabolic Modulators

Metabolic modulators have been of high interest, contributed to by the resurgence of use and demonstrated benefit of the ketogenic diet.

Decanoic acid is a medium chain fatty acid which is an AMPA (α-amino3-hydroxy-5-methyl-4-isoxazolepropionic acid) receptor antagonist. This is a similar mechanism by which perampanel acts, but at a distinct binding site. These two agents have been shown to be synergistic relating to direct AMPA receptor inhibition, in an ex vivo model of seizure activity, and against seizure-induced activity in human brain slices (Augustin et al. 2018).

2-Deoxyglucose or 2-deoxy-D-glucose (2-DG) differs from glucose by lack of oxygen at the second position and thus inhibits glycolysis because it cannot be converted to fructose-6-phosphate. It potentiates extrasynaptic tonic GABAergic current by activating neurosteroidogenesis and has shown anticonvulsant effects in various seizure models, with the unique property of uptake into brain regions in which there are increased energy demands during seizures or in response to brain injury (Shao and Stafstrom 2017). It has been used as a radiolabeled analog for glucose uptake on positron emission tomography. Phase 3 trials in cancer radiotherapy have occurred.

TAK-935 is a selective inhibitor of cholesterol 24-hydroxylase (CH24H). CH24H converts cholesterol to 24S-hydroxycholesterol, a potentiator of NMDA signaling and inflammation. More than 70% of SCN1A-mutant mice subjected to a hyperthermia-priming seizure and then fed chow with TAK-935, were seizure-free compared to <30% of the control mice, and mortality was prevented (Hawkins et al. 2018). Currently, a multicenter, open-label, pilot study in patients with 15Q duplication syndrome or CDKL5 deficiency disorder is being performed (clinicaltrials.gov/NCT03694275). A randomized, double-blind study in patients with Dravet syndrome or LGS (clinicaltrials.gov/NCT03650452) is recruiting.

Adenosine is an endogenous signaling molecule which inhibits DNA methyltransferase activity and is FDA-approved for the treatment of supraventricular tachycardia. Adenosine kinase is upregulated in animal models of epileptogenesis, with lower levels of adenosine leading to lower seizure threshold and increased DNA methylation. In animal models, increased adenosine prevents progression of epilepsy for up to 3 months. However, due to potential cardiovascular toxicity, delivery directly to the brain is a necessity (Weltha et al. 2018).

References

Abdel-Mannan O, Taylor H, Donner EJ, Sutcliffe AJ (2019) A systematic review of sudden unexpected death in epilepsy (SUDEP) in childhood. Epilepsy Behav 90:99–106

Augustin K, Williams S, Cunninham M et al (2018) Perampanel and decanoic acid show synergistic action against AMPA receptors and seizures. Epilepsia 59:e172–e178

Beatch G, Namdari R, Cadieux J et al (2018) XEN1101, a novel small molecule Kv7.2/7.3 positive allosteric modulator for the treatment of epilepsy, presented at. In: Fourteenth Eilat conference of new antiepileptic drugs and devices (Eilat XIV), Madrid, Spain, May 2018. The Hebrew University of Jerusalem, Jerusalem

Bialer M, Soares-da-Silva P (2012) Pharmacokinetics and drug interactions of eslicarbazepine acetate. Epilepsia 53(6):935–946

Bialer M, White HS (2010) Key factors in the discovery and development of new anti-epileptic drugs. Nat Rev Drug Discov 9(1):68–82

Billakota S, Devinsky O, Marsh E (2019) Cannabinoid therapy in epilepsy. Curr Opin Neurol 32 (2):220–226

Biton V, Berkovic SF, Abou-Khalil B et al (2014) Brivaracetam as adjunctive treatment for uncontrolled partial epilepsy in adults: a phase III, double-blind, randomized, placebo-controlled trial. Epilepsia 55(1):57–66

Brodie MJ, Yeun AWC, The 105 Study Group (1997) Lamotrigine substitution study: evidence for synergism with sodium valproate. Epilepsy Res 26(3):423–432

Chiron C, Marchand MC, Tran A et al (2000) Stiripentol in severe myoclonic epilepsy in infancy: a randomized placebo-controlled syndrome-dedicated trial. STICLO study group. Lancet 356:1638–1642

Cianchetti C, Messina P, Pupillo E et al (2015) The perceived burden of epilepsy: impact on the quality of life of children and adolescents and their families. Seizure 24:93–101

Critchley D, Fuseau E, Perdomo C et al (2005) Pharmacokinetic and pharmacodynamic parameters of adjunctive rufinamide in patients with Lennox-Gastaut syndrome [Abstr]. Epilepsia 46 (Suppl.7):2.351

Curatolo P, Nabbout R, Lagae L et al (2018) Management of epilepsy associated with tuberous sclerosis complex: updated clinical recommendations. Eur J Paed Neurol 22(5):738–748

De Liso P, Chemaly N, Laschet J et al (2016) Patients with Dravet syndrome in the era of stiripentol: a French cohort cross sectional study. Epilepsy Res 125:42–46
Devinsky O, Cross JH, Laux L et al (2017a) Trial of cannabidiol for drug resistant seizures in Dravet syndrome. N Engl J Med 376:2011–2020
Devinsky O, Segal E, Chez M et al (2017b) Open-label trial of ganaxolone in children with Lennox-Gastaut syndrome. American Epilepsy Society annual meeting abstract. https://www.aesnet.org/meetings_events/annual_meeting_abstracts/view/392831
Devinsky O, Patel A, Cross JH, Villanueva V et al (2018) Effect of cannabidiol on drop seizures in the Lennox–Gastaut syndrome. N Engl J Med 378:1888–1897
Eddy CM, Rickards HE, Cavanna AE (2012) Behavioral adverse effects of antiepileptic drugs in epilepsy. J Clin Psychopharmacol 32(3):362–375
Fisher J (2011) The effects of stiripentol on GABAA receptors. Epilepsia 52(Suppl. 2):76–78
Franz DN, Belousova E, Sparagana S et al (2016) Long-term use of everolimus in patients with tuberous sclerosis complex: final results from the EXIST-1 study. PLoS One 11(6):e0158476
French JA, Lawson JA, Yapici Z et al (2016) Adjunctive everolimus therapy for treatment-resistant focal-onset seizures associated with tuberous sclerosis (EXIST-3): a phase 3, randomized, double-blind, placebo-controlled study. Lancet 388:2153–2163
Gidal BE, Ferry J, Majid O et al (2013) Concentration-effect relationships with perampanel in patients with pharmacoresistant partial-onset seizures. Epilepsia 54:1490–1497
Gil-Nagel A, Elger C, Ben-Menachem E et al (2013) Efficacy and safety of eslicarbazepine acetate as add-on treatment in patients with focal-onset seizures: integrated analysis of pooled data from double-blind phase III clinical studies. Epilepsia 54(1):98–107
Giraud C, Treluyer JM, Rey E et al (2006) In vitro and in vivo inhibitory effect of stiripentol on clobazam metabolism. Drug Metab Dispos 34(4):608–611
Glauser T, Kluger G, Sachdeo R et al (2008) Rufinamide for generalized seizures associated with Lennox–Gastaut syndrome. Neurology 70(21):1950–1958
Glauser TA, Cnaan A, Shinnar S et al (2010) Ethosuximide, valproic acid, and lamotrigine in childhood absence epilepsy. N Engl J Med 362(9):790–799
Golyala A, Kwan P (2017) Drug development for refractory epilepsy: the past 25 years and beyond. Seizure 44:147–156
Goodman CW, Brett AS (2019) A clinical overview of off-label use of gabapentinoid drugs. JAMA Intern Med 179(5):695–701
Greenwich Biosciences (2018) Epidiolex prescribing information. https://www.epidiolex.com/sites/default/files/EPIDIOLEX_Full_Prescribing_Information.pdf
Griffith JL, Wong M (2018) The mTOR pathway in treatment of epilepsy: a clinical update. Future Neurol 13(2):49–58
Hanada T, Hashizume Y, Tokuhara N et al (2011) Perampanel: a novel, orally active, noncompetitive AMPA-receptor antagonist that reduces seizure activity in rodent models of epilepsy. Epilepsia 52(7):1331–1340
Hawkins NA, Nishi T, Abrahams BS, During MJ, Kearney JA (2018) TAK-935 reduces seizure frequency and severity and prevents premature lethality in Scn1a+/– Dravet mice. https://www.aesnet.org/meetings_events/annual_meeting_abstracts/view/501989
Johnson JP, Beatch GN, Focken T et al (2018) XEN901, a first-in class subtype selective inhibitor of NAV1.6 voltage gated sodium channels. Presented at fourteenth Eilat conference of new antiepileptic drugs and devices (Eilat XIV), Madrid, Spain, May 2018. The Hebrew University of Jerusalem, Jerusalem
Kaminski RM, Matagne A, Leclerq K et al (2008) SV2A protein is a broad spectrum anticonvulsant target: functional correlation between protein binding and seizure protection in models of both partial and generalized epilepsy. Neuropharmacology 54(4):715–720
Kehne JH, Klein BD, Raeissi S et al (2017) The National Institute of Neurological Disorders and Stroke (NINDS) Epilepsy Therapy Screening Program (ETSP). Neurochem Res 42:1894–1903
Kwan P, Brodie MJ (2000) Early identification of refractory epilepsy. N Engl J Med 342:314–319
Lagae L, Sullivan JE, Cross JH, Devinsky O, Guerrini R et al (2017) ZX008 (fenfluramine) in Dravet syndrome: results of a phase 3, randomized, double-blind, placebo-controlled trial.

American Epilepsy Society annual meeting abstract. https://www.aesnet.org/meetings_events/annual_meeting_abstracts/view/389526
Lanuti M, Talamonti E, Maccarrone M, Chiurchiu V (2015) Activation of GPR55 receptors exacerbate OXDL-induced lipid accumulation and inflammatory responses, while reducing cholesterol efflux from human macrophages. PLoS One 10:e0126839
Levy RH, Loiseau P, Guyot M et al (1984) Stiripentol kinetics in epilepsy: nonlinearity and interactions. Clin Pharmacol Ther 36(5):661–669
Loscher W (2017) Animal models of seizures and epilepsy: past, present, and future role for the discovery of anti-seizure drugs. Neurochem Res 42:1873–1888
Loscher W (2018) Bumetanide and its derivatives. Presented at fourteenth Eilat conference of new antiepileptic drugs and devices (Eilat XIV), Madrid, Spain, May 2018. The Hebrew University of Jerusalem, Jerusalem
Meng T, Sequeira DJ, Van Ess PJ, Pullman WE (2018) Long-term safety experience of Nayzilam™ (USL261; midazolam nasal spray) in subjects with seizure clusters: safety results from the open-label, phase 3 extension of the ARTEMIS-1 study. American Epilepsy Society annual meeting abstract. https://www.aesnet.org/meetings_events/annual_meeting_abstracts/view/501511
Mulugeta Y, Barrett JS, Nelson R et al (2016) Exposure matching for extrapolation of efficacy in pediatric drug development. J Clin Pharmacol 56(11):1326–1334
Ng PC, Schimmel J, Wang GS (2019) Lacosamide overdose: a case of QRS prolongation and seizure. J Emerg Med:1–5. https://doi.org/10.1016/j.jemermed.2019.01.018
Nickels KC, Wirell EC (2017) Stiripentol in the management of epilepsy. CNS Drugs 31 (5):405–416
Novartis (2018) Afinitor prescribing information. https://www.pharma.us.novartis.com/sites/www.pharma.us.novartis.com/files/afinitor.pdf
Ohtsuka Y, Yoshinaga H, Yukiyoshi S et al (2014) Rufinamide as an adjunctive therapy for Lennox-Gastaut syndrome: a randomized double-blind placebo-controlled trial in Japan. Epilepsy Res 108(9):1627–1636
Pearl PL, Vezina LG, Saneto RP et al (2009) Cerebral MRI abnormalities associated with vigabatrin therapy. Epilepsia 50(2):184–189
Perez J, Chiron C, Musial C et al (1999) Stiripentol: efficacy and tolerability in children with epilepsy. Epilepsia 40(11):1618–1626
Perucca E, Cloyd J, Critchley D et al (2008) Rufinamide: clinical pharmacokinetics and concentration-response relationships in patients with epilepsy. Epilepsia 49(7):1123–1141
Pressler RM, Boylan GB, Marlow N et al (2015) Bumetanide for the treatment of seizures in newborn babies with hypoxic ischaemic encephalopathy (NEMO): an open-label, dose finding, and feasibility phase 1/2 trial. Lancet Neurol 14(5):469–477
Rho JM, White HS (2018) Brief history of anti-seizure drug development. Epilepsia 3. (suppl. 2:114–119
Rimmerman N, Ben-Hail D, Porat Z et al (2013) Direct modulation of the outer mitochondrial membrane channel, voltage dependent anion channel 1 (VDAC1) by cannabidiol: a novel mechanism for cannabinoid-induced cell death. Cell Death Dis 4:e949
Rogawski MA, Hanada T (2013) Preclinical pharmacology of perampanel, a selective non-competitive AMPA receptor antagonist. Acta Neurol Scand Suppl 197:19–24
Rolan P, Sargentini-Maier ML, Pigeolet E, Stockis A (2008) The pharmacokinetics, CNS pharmacodynamics and adverse event profile of brivaracetam after multiple increasing oral doses in healthy men. Br J Clin Pharmacol 66(1):71–75
Rugg-Gunn F (2014) Adverse effects and safety profile of perampanel: a review of pooled date. Epilepsia 55(suppl. 1):13–15
Schoemaker R, Wade JR, Stockis A (2017) Brivaracetam population pharmacokinetics in children with epilepsy aged 1 month to 16 years. Eur J Clin Pharmacol 73(6):727–733
Schoonjans A, Paelinck BP, Marchau F et al (2017) Low-dose fenfluramine significantly reduces seizure frequency in Dravet syndrome: a prospective study of a new cohort of patients. Eur J Neurol 24:309–314

Sequeira DJ, Meng T, Pullman WE, Van Ess PJ (2018) Long-term efficacy experience of Nayzilam™ (USL261; midazolam nasal spray) for outpatient treatment of seizure clusters: efficacy results from the open-label, phase 3 extension of the ARTEMIS-1 study. American Epilepsy Society annual meeting abstract. https://www.aesnet.org/meetings_events/annual_meeting_abstracts/view/501543

Shao L, Stafstrom CE (2017) Glycolytic inhibition by 2-deoxy-D-glucose abolishes both neuronal and network bursts in an in vitro seizure model. J Neurophysiol 118:103–113

Specchio N, Masuoka L, Aimetti A, Chez M (2018) Long-term, durable seizure frequency reduction in individuals with CDKL5 deficiency disorder (CDD) treated with ganaxolone. Mutation of the cyclin-dependent kinase-like 5 (CDKL5) gene. American Epilepsy Society annual meeting abstract. https://www.aesnet.org/meetings_events/annual_meeting_abstracts/view/506062

Sperling MR, Abou-Khalil B, Harvey J et al (2015) Eslicarbazepine acetate as adjunctive therapy in patients with uncontrolled partial-onset seizures: results of a phase III, double-blind, randomized, placebo-controlled trial. Epilepsia 56(2):244–253

Strzelczyk A, Zollner JP, Willems LM et al (2017) Lacosamide in status epilepticus: systematic review of current evidence. Epilepsia 58(6):933–950

Sullivan J, Specchio N, Chez M et al (2018) Preliminary evidence of a predictive clinical biomarker in PCDH19-related epilepsy: significant treatment effect of ganaxolone in biomarker-positive patients. American Epilepsy Society annual meeting abstract. https://www.aesnet.org/meetings_events/annual_meeting_abstracts/view/502507

Sylantyev S, Jensen TP, Ross RA, Rusakov DA (2013) Cannabinoid and lysophosphatidylinositol-sensitive receptor GPR55 boosts neurotransmitter release at central synapses. Proc Natl Acad Sci U S A 110:5193–5198

Thiele E, Marsh E, Mzurkiewicz-Beldzinska M et al (2019) Cannabidiol in patients with Lennox-Gastaut syndrome: interim analysis of an open-label extension study. Epilepsia 60:419–428

Torjesen I (2019) Pregabalin and gabapentin: what impact will reclassification have on doctors and patients? BMJ 364:l1107

UCB Inc (2018) Vimpat prescribing information. https://www.vimpat.com/vimpat-prescribing-information.pdf

Van Ess PJ, Braun TL, Sequeira DJ, and Pullman WE (2017) Safety and efficacy of Nayzilam™ (USL261; midazolam nasal spray) for the treatment of intermittent bouts of increased seizure activity in the epilepsy monitoring unit (ARTEMIS-EMU). American Epilepsy Society annual meeting abstract. https://www.aesnet.org/meetings_events/annual_meeting_abstracts/view/349668

von Rosenstiel P (2017) Brivaracetam (UCB 34714). Neurotherapeutics 4(1):84–87

Weltha L, Reemmer J, Boison D (2018) The role of adenosine in epilepsy. Brain Res Bull. https://doi.org/10.1016/j.brainresbull.2018.11.008

Westall CA, Wright T, Cortese F et al (2014) Vigabatrin retinal toxicity in children with infantile spasms an observational cohort study. Neurology 83:2262–2268

Wheless JW, Conry J, Krauss G et al (2009) Safety and tolerability of rufinamide in children with epilepsy: a pooled analysis of 7 clinical studies. J Child Neurol 24(12):1520–1525

Wong JC, Dutton SBB, Collins SD et al (2016) Huperzine a provides robust and sustained protection against induced seizures in Scn1a mutant mice. Front Pharmacol 7:357

Younas I, Reddy DS (2018) A resurging boom in new drugs for epilepsy and brain disorders. Expert Rev Clin Pharmacol 11(1):27–45

Pharmacotherapy of Duchenne Muscular Dystrophy

Eric P. Hoffman

Contents

Abstract

Drug development and pharmacotherapy of rare pediatric diseases have significantly expanded over the last decade, in part due to incentives and financial support provided by governments, regulators, and nonprofit foundations. Duchenne muscular dystrophy (DMD) is among the most common rare pediatric disorders, and clinical trials of therapeutic approaches have seen dramatic expansion. Pharmacotherapeutic standard of care has been limited to off-label prescription of high-dose, daily corticosteroids (prednisone, deflazacort). Deflazacort received FDA approval for DMD in 2016, although the price increases associated with formal FDA approval and the severe side effects associated with corticosteroid use have limited patient/physician uptake and insurance coverage in the USA. In Europe, EMA has given conditional marketing authorization for prescription of Translarna (a stop codon read-through drug prescribed to ~10% of DMD patients), although there is not yet evidence of clinical efficacy. The FDA awarded conditional approval to etiplirsen, an exon-skipping oligonucleotide drug, based on accelerated pathways (increased dystrophin production in patient muscle). Evidence of clinical efficacy remains the focus of post-marketing

E. P. Hoffman (✉)
Department of Pharmaceutical Sciences, School of Pharmacy and Pharmaceutical Sciences, Binghamton University State University of New York, Binghamton, NY, USA
e-mail: ehoffman@binghamton.edu

W. Kiess et al. (eds.), *Pediatric Pharmacotherapy*,
Handbook of Experimental Pharmacology 261, https://doi.org/10.1007/164_2019_256

studies. There are many innovative pharmacotherapies under clinical development for DMD (Phase I, II, and III clinical trials). All are "disease modifying" in the sense that none seek to replace the full-length, normal *DMD* gene or dystrophin protein, but instead either seek to introduce an abnormal "Becker-like" version of the gene or protein or target pathophysiological pathways downstream of the primary defect. It is envisioned that the most significant benefit to DMD patients will be through multidrug approaches simultaneously aiming to introduce partially functional dystrophin in patient muscle while also targeting both chronic inflammation and the fibrofatty replacement of muscle.

Keywords
Becker muscular dystrophy · Corticosteroid · Deflazacort · Disease modifying · Duchenne muscular dystrophy · Dystrophin · Exon skipping · Gene therapy · Prednisone

1 Introduction

Duchenne muscular dystrophy (DMD) is an X-linked recessive disorder that is defined by loss of function mutations in the *DMD* gene leading to loss of the dystrophin protein in the skeletal muscle and heart (Koenig et al. 1987; Hoffman et al. 1987, 1988). Patients with DMD are born apparently healthy but show delayed gross motor milestones, typically leading to clinical ascertainment in early school years (difficulty running or climbing stairs). Diagnostic laboratory tests include grossly elevated serum creatine kinase levels (indicative of muscle damage) and gene mutation testing. The *DMD* gene is the largest identified to date, with 79 exonic regions spanning 2.3 million base pairs of the X chromosome (a typical gene is about 30,000 bp).

Becker muscular dystrophy is a highly variable but generally clinically milder disease compared to DMD and is caused by *DMD* mutations that are compatible with residual dystrophin protein production in patient muscle (partial loss-of-function) in male patients (Hoffman et al. 1989; Arikawa et al. 1991; Kesari et al. 2008; van den Bergen et al. 2014). Becker muscular dystrophy patients show a broad range of clinical severities and progressions of their disease. This variability is only poorly explained by *DMD* gene mutation types or levels of muscle dystrophin. Instead, the rate and extent of fibrofatty replacement of the muscle best explains the severity of symptoms (van den Bergen et al. 2014). The clinical findings in Becker dystrophy have strong implications for DMD therapeutics development, where all dystrophin replacement strategies focus on Becker-like dystrophin and not the introduction of normal full-length dystrophin.

Another clinical diagnostic group of dystrophinopathies is females that are manifesting carriers of the disease (Hoffman et al. 1992; Pegoraro et al. 1995). Due to X-inactivation processes in all female cells, female manifesting carriers of DMD typically show a mosaic pattern of dystrophin expression (dystrophin-positive and dystrophin-negative myofibers), where skewing of X-inactivation toward greater proportions of cells with the mutant DMD gene active leads to loss of most dystrophin from muscle. Most female carriers of DMD are asymptomatic (non-manifesting) and show about 50% each of mutant and normal X chromosomes active in their skeletal muscle and heart. The clinical symptoms of manifesting female carriers are quite variable (similar to Becker dystrophy), from very mild to very severe.

Dystrophin abnormalities in dystrophinopathy patients (DMD, Becker dystrophy, manifesting carriers) are fully manifested biochemically in early fetal life, with both skeletal muscles and heart showing either dystrophin deficiency (DMD) or abnormal quantities or quality of dystrophin (Becker dystrophy, carriers). While the genetic and biochemical defects are "static" and do not change as a function of age, the clinical symptoms are progressive. Thus, dystrophin abnormalities are not sufficient to show severe muscle disease, but instead molecular and cellular events downstream of the primary defect are age-dependent and correlated with clinical symptoms. The histopathological feature best correlated with clinical symptoms is fibrofatty replacement of skeletal muscle (progressive fibrosis) (van den Bergen et al. 2014).

There are thus two general approaches being pursued in the pharmacotherapeutic management of dystrophinopathies: (1) efforts focused on reintroduction of dystrophin in DMD and (2) efforts to slow down the disease progression (e.g., inhibit fibrofatty replacement of muscle). There has been substantial progress on both approaches. However, it is important to note that all dystrophin replacement efforts use highly modified, abnormal dystrophin proteins as the therapeutic agent, not full-length normal dystrophin, and they are likely to slow down disease progression, but unlikely to reverse or cure the disease. For exon skipping, the oligonucleotide drugs exclude an exon flanking a deletion mutation in a DMD patient, resulting in restoration of the mRNA/amino acid translational reading frame and a "Becker-like" dystrophin in DMD patient muscle. With gene therapy, existing viral vectors are able to accommodate only a small fraction of the dystrophin coding sequence and instead focus on micro- or mini-dystrophins. As explained further below, even if there is successful introduction of Becker-like or mini-dystrophins into DMD patient muscle, it is not known the extent to which biochemical rescue will be achieved, how biochemical rescue will translate into improvement of clinical symptoms, and the persistence of this effect.

2 Treatment Goals in DMD: Current Landscape

Studies of muscle biopsies from DMD and healthy age-matched controls in the fetal, newborn/infant (presymptomatic), and childhood (symptomatic) stages have shown that muscle histology and tissue development proceed normally through the fetal period but that the muscle shows a chronic inflammatory state at birth via activation of innate immunity and cell "danger" signals (NFkB pathways) (Chen et al. 2005). The chronic activation of NFkB pathways transitions over years to fibrofatty replacement of muscle (TGFβ pro-fibrotic pathways), and the loss of myofibers in turn correlates with weakness and disability, as noted above.

Potent pharmacological inhibitors of NFkB pathways are the corticosteroid class of drugs. These drugs bind the glucocorticoid receptor (GR; gene name *NR3C1*), where ligand/receptor complexes bind directly to NFkB promoter gene elements and block NFkB gene activation (Hudson et al. 2018). High-dose (0.7–9.0 mg/kg/day) chronic use of corticosteroids (prednisone, deflazacort) has shown efficacy in DMD, improving strength and mobility and delaying loss of ambulation by a few years (Griggs et al. 2016; McDonald et al. 2018). While corticosteroids are clearly effective in DMD, there is considerable variation in practice in terms of prescription and use of corticosteroids due to the high burden of side effects (Griggs et al. 2013; Bello et al. 2015; Cowen et al. 2019). Side effects of concern to patients and their families include stunting of growth, bone fragility, mood changes, weight gain, and increased rate of infections. Loss of bone density and stunting of growth are likely related, as glucocorticoids have profound negative effects on bone growth (Nguyen et al. 2018). Clinical morbidities of loss of bone density include very high rates of bone and vertebral fractures in glucocorticoid-treated DMD boys (Wong et al. 2017; Joseph et al. 2019). Corticosteroid side effects add considerably to healthcare costs (Rice et al. 2018a, b).

As with many indications for corticosteroids, they are prescribed off-label to DMD children, with most physicians choosing to wait until noticeable declines in patient gross motor skills are observed (~4–6 years), in an effort to reduce the burden of side effects at young ages. However, an open-label study of 0.4–2.4-year-old infants with DMD showed that intermittent dosing with corticosteroids (5 mg/kg/day weekends only) led to a slowing of disease progression and some reduction in safety concerns (stunting of growth, Cushingoid features) (Connolly et al. 2019). In 2017, FDA approved deflazacort (Emflaza) for DMD; this was controversial due to the associated cost increases (~$3,000/year prior to approval; ~$60,000/year post-approval) and the greater burden of side effects generally seen with deflazacort compared to prednisone (Bello et al. 2015). The Institute for Clinical and Economic Review (ICER) released a report evaluating the cost-effectiveness of deflazacort (https://icer-review.org/wp-content/uploads/2018/12/ICER_DMD_Draft_Evidence_Report_0522019.pdf).

A second drug for DMD, eteplirsen (exondys-51), was granted accelerated (conditional) approval by the FDA in 2016 based on increased dystrophin protein production in DMD patient muscle (surrogate outcome measure). Eteplirsen is indicated for use in the subset of DMD patients with gene mutations that are amenable to skipping of exon 51 (~12%). The approval was also controversial, as there was disagreement within the FDA and within the medical and scientific communities regarding the rigor and sufficiency of supportive evidence (Railroading at the FDA 2016). Published data from a single clinical trial of 12 DMD patients showed a relatively low level of eteplirsen-induced dystrophin rescue (mean 0.93% of dystrophin levels observed in normal muscle) (Charleston et al. 2018). The relatively small increases in dystrophin protein, coupled with the lack of supportive clinical efficacy data and annual treatment cost (~$800,000), have led to about half

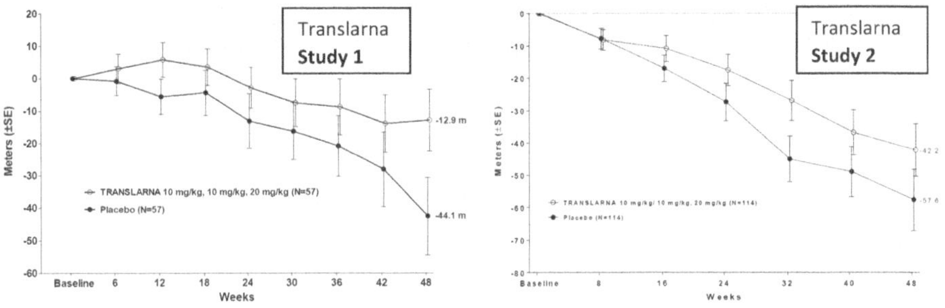

Fig. 1 Comparison of 6-min walk data from Translarna Study 1 and Study 2 (EPAR product information). Two 48-week Translarna (40 mg/kg/day) clinical trials are shown; Study 1 was 5–20 years ambulatory DMD patients, with 57 patients per arm (placebo; 40 mg/kg Translarna); Study 2 was 7–14 years ambulatory DMD patients, with 115 patients per arm. In both studies, Translarna treatment showed a nonsignificant deflection of decline over time of 6-min walk test

of insurance carriers denying coverage for eteplirsen (https://icer-review.org/wp-content/uploads/2018/12/ICER_DMD_Draft_Evidence_Report_0522019.pdf).

In the European Union, the EMA granted conditional approval for Translarna® (ataluren), a small-molecule drug developed to enable read-through of premature stop codons created by nonsense mutations in the mRNA of DMD patients and hence expression of a full-length functional dystrophin protein. PTC Therapeutics Ltd. received conditional marketing authorization for the treatment of ambulatory DMD patients aged 5 years or older who have a nonsense mutation in the dystrophin gene (about 10% of DMD patients). The EPAR product information describes two studies. Study 1 was a 48-week study of 114 patients randomized to Translarna or placebo. Analysis of the primary outcome, 6-min walk test, showed a drug-associated deflection of decline of ~30 m, although this was not statistically significant (Fig. 1). Study 2 was a 48-week study of 228 patients similarly randomized to Translarna or placebo and also used 6-min walk test as the primary outcome. This showed a nonsignificant deflection of decline of ~15 m (Fig. 1). Most Translarna-treated patients were treated with corticosteroids prior to Translarna treatment. EMA considered a confirmatory trial to be a key requirement to support the risk-benefit balance of ataluren. In order to confirm the safety and efficacy of Translarna® in children 5 years or older, a multicenter, randomized, double-blind, 18-month, placebo-controlled study, followed by an 18-month open-label extension, was planned. This study is ongoing. Notably, use of corticosteroids for 12 months is a requirement for enrolment, as is the need to stay on a stable dose of corticosteroids for the duration of the trial, with the anticipated safety concerns of stunting of growth and Cushingoid features.

In summary, the most broadly utilized pharmacotherapy for DMD is daily corticosteroids (daily prednisone or deflazacort), where there is relatively poor adherence to standard of care guidelines due to the burden of side effects of these treatments. Medicines for treatment of mutation-defined subsets of DMD patients have been approved by the FDA (exon 51-amenable mutations; ~12% of DMD patients; exondys 51/eteplirsen) and EMA (stop codon mutations; ~10% of DMD patients; Translarna/ataluren), but neither drug has demonstrated compelling data for clinical efficacy to date.

3 Treatment Goals in DMD: Pharmacotherapies in the Pipeline

The number of drug development programs in DMD has grown exponentially in recent years, with 31 drugs in clinical development at the time of writing (June 2019) (Fig. 2). A summary of the status of these programs is given under categories below.

Exon Skipping The success of Sarepta in obtaining FDA approval for eteplirsen/exondys 51 based on small increases in dystrophin protein content of patient muscle has led to a swell in biotech and pharma interest in pursuing a similar oligonucleotide-based exon-skipping approach, with key variables being variations on oligonucleotide chemistry and different DMD exons targeted. Furthest along is NS Pharma (viltolarsen) that has used the same morpholino chemistry as Sarepta, but

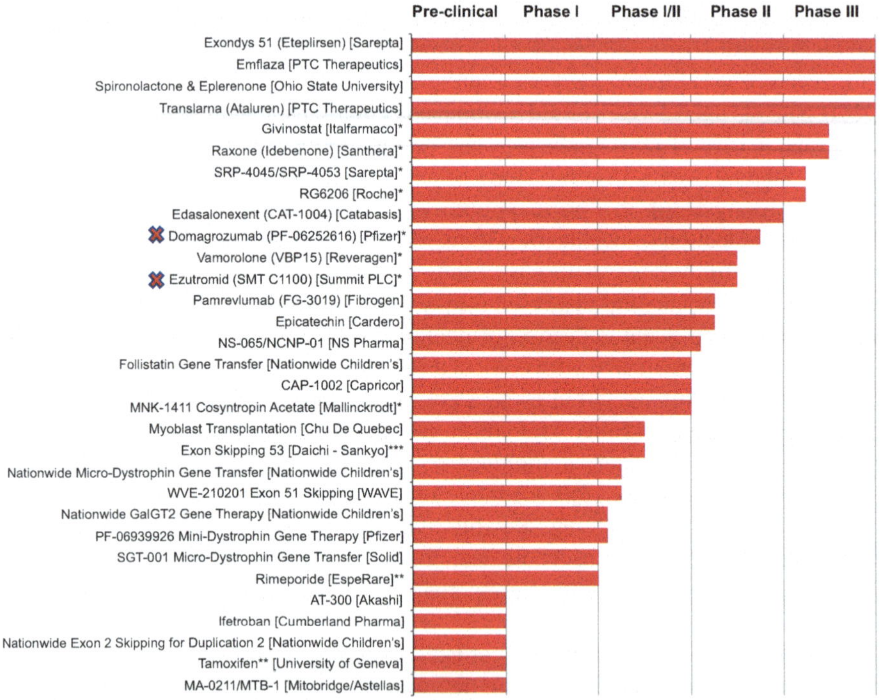

Fig. 2 Clinical-stage drug development programs in DMD as of June 2019. The domagrozumab and SMT C1100 programs have been terminated (marked with X). Taken from https://www.parentprojectmd.org/research/current-research/drug-development-pipeline/

targeted exon 53 instead of eteplirsen's exon 51 (~10% of DMD patients), and used considerably higher doses (80 mg/kg/day; compared to Sarepta's 20 mg/kg/day). Parallel trials in Japan and the USA/Canada have been conducted and shown ~6% mean drug-induced dystrophin levels in patient muscle, levels that are about sixfold those seen with the Sarepta drug. Preliminary studies on viltolarsen have been published (Komaki et al. 2018; Watanabe et al. 2018). Daiichi Sankyo is using a modified 2′-O,4′-C-ethylene-bridged nucleic acid (ENA) chemistry targeting exon 45 (DS-5141) with subcutaneous injections. WAVE is using modified stereopure chemistry targeting exon 51 (WVE-210201). Stereopure oligos have locked chirality that has been optimized for cell delivery and binding to target RNA and may prove more potent and effective. Sarepta is also pursuing additional exons using their morpholino chemistry.

Replacements for Corticosteroids The burden of corticosteroid side effects for DMD patients is severe and the most common reason for discontinuation; alternatives to corticosteroids are under development (Cowen et al. 2019). Furthest along is vamorolone, a dissociative steroidal anti-inflammatory that binds the glucocorticoid and mineralocorticoid receptors, but imparts different activities to the ligand/receptor complexes, leading to retention or improvement of efficacy and lessening of safety concerns (Hoffman et al. 2018, 2019; Conklin et al. 2018). Clinical trials in 48 steroid-naïve DMD boys (4 to <7 years) have shown dose-responsive improvements in gross motor skills and strength. A bifunctional small-molecule drug, edasalonexent, is effective at reducing NFkB pathways and is similarly being developed as an alternative to corticosteroids; Phase 1 data in DMD boys has been published (Finanger et al. 2019). MNK-1411 is a patch delivery of cosyntropin, with the goal of manipulating ACTH/cortisol pathways and thereby replacing corticosteroids.

Viral Vector Delivery A series of proteins are being delivered to DMD muscle using adeno-associated viral vectors (AAV). Most focus on delivering miniature variants of the dystrophin protein (mini- or micro-dystrophins), missing much of the rod domain, with variable retention of other domains. Key variables in dystrophin gene delivery to muscle are (1) serotype of the AAV vector utilized; (2) large-scale AAV viral particle laboratory production methods; (3) the type of dystrophin mini-gene and function of the modified dystrophin (and extent of retained function relative to normal dystrophin); (4) transcriptional promoter driving the mini-gene in the AAV vector; and (5) effectiveness of delivery to muscle and persistence of dystrophin expression. Clinical trials underway include AAV-dystrophin vectors constructed by Nationwide Children's Hospital (Sarepta), Bamboo Therapeutics (Pfizer), and Solid Biosciences. No publications have been released to date on any program.

Nationwide Children's Hospital is also using AAV vectors to deliver follistatin, a modulator of myostatin muscle hypertrophy pathways (see myostatin inhibition below).

There has been considerable attention to applications of CRISPR gene editing technologies to DMD, and preliminary studies in dogs suggest promise (Amoasii et al. 2018). The CRISPR approach edits the DMD patient's gene to restore the reading frame, essentially the same approach as oligonucleotide drug-driven exon skipping. Thus, CRISPR, like exon skipping, aims to change DMD to Becker muscular dystrophy, and this will be carried out using AAV viral vectors. Thus, CRISPR faces many of the same questions and limitations of AAV-mediated dystrophin gene delivery, as noted above. However, one potential advantage of the CRISPR gene editing approach is that it may lead to more permanent changes in the patient's myofiber DNA and thus show a more persistent benefit. That said, any treatment-emergent safety concern observed with CRISPR approaches would not be expected to be reversible as with most other drugs.

Myostatin Inhibition Myostatin is a protein that negatively regulates muscle growth; inhibition of myostatin results in muscle hypertrophy. Modulation of the myostatin pathway has been a strong focus of DMD therapeutics, with the underlying rationale that bigger muscles will provide greater muscle function to DMD patients. There are two key weaknesses to this logic. First, myostatin is already dramatically downregulated in dystrophin-deficient muscle, questioning the value of further downregulation. Second, data from a dog model of dystrophin deficiency (GRMD), where myostatin was decreased by 50% through genetic crossing into the myostatin null bully whippet, showed that reductions in myostatin worsened the phenotype of the dog (Kornegay et al. 2012; Nghiem et al. 2013). Clinical experience with myostatin inhibition in DMD has been unable to show efficacy despite multiple concluded and ongoing clinical trials. Pfizer's domagrozumab program was terminated in 2018 due to a futility analysis, even though the same myostatin antibody improved the *mdx* mouse model of DMD and caused drug-induced muscle hypertrophy in monkeys (St Andre et al. 2017). Ongoing clinical trials in myostatin inhibition include RG6206 antibody (Roche) and follistatin AAV delivery (Nationwide Children's Hospital).

Others Two cell-based clinical trials are underway, one using intravenously delivered mesenchymal stem cells (Capricor's CAP-1002) (Taylor et al. 2019) and myoblast cell trials at Laval University in Quebec. There is considerable evidence of mitochondrial dysfunction in dystrophin-deficient muscle, and clinical studies are underway to determine if bolstering mitochondrial function may show efficacy in DMD (Raxone, Santhera; epicatechin, Cardero; MA-0211, Astellas).

Dystrophin deficiency leads to unstable plasma membranes and ionic imbalance in both skeletal and heart muscles. Modulation of ionic imbalance via eplerenone, a mineralocorticoid receptor antagonist, has shown efficacy in DMD cardiomyopathy (Raman et al. 2015). Vamorolone also shows potent antagonism of the mineralocorticoid receptor similar to eplerenone (distinct from corticosteroids) (Heier et al. 2019). A clinical trial of an inhibitor of the skeletal muscle sodium/proton type 1 exchanger (NHE-1) aims to target similar pathways (rimeporide – Esperare).

Tamoxifen, an estrogen receptor modulator, has shown efficacy in mouse models of DMD (Dorchies et al. 2013), and a double-blind Phase 3 trial has recently begun enrolling patients (NCT03354039).

Two drugs target fibrosis in DMD muscle, with the aim of slowing the transition to fibrofatty replacement associated with muscle weakness. Givinostat is a modulator of histone deacetylases and reduces fibrofatty replacement in DMD muscle (Bettica et al. 2016) (Italfarmaco). Pamrevlumab is a monocslonal antibody targeting connective tissue growth factor (FibroGen).

4 Treatment Goals in Becker Muscular Dystrophy and Female DMD Carriers

Becker muscular dystrophy is defined by a combination of clinical findings (muscular dystrophy in a male that is variable in severity, but milder than DMD), gene mutation findings (*DMD* gene deletion or duplication that is "in-frame" and compatible with dystrophin production), and/or muscle biopsy protein findings (dystrophin that is present in muscle, but of abnormal quantity and/or quality [molecular weight]). Clinically, Becker muscular dystrophy can be just slightly milder than DMD (e.g., loss of ambulation ~20 years of age), through to asymptomatic (elevations of serum creatine kinase in the absence of clinical symptoms – hyperCKemia). Becker muscular dystrophy has an incidence in all world populations similar to DMD, making it one of the more common genetic disorders (incidence of DMD 3.0/100,000 [95% CI 2.33–3.70], BMD 2.2/100,000 [95% CI 1.64–2.88]) (Lefter et al. 2017). About 20% of Becker muscular dystrophy patients report using corticosteroids (Cowen et al. 2019). In general, most Becker dystrophy patients and their physicians feel that the severe side effects outweigh the efficacy of corticosteroids.

There is little in terms of pharmacotherapy development for Becker muscular dystrophy, with no clinical efficacy trials published to date. A clinical trial of givinostat for the treatment of Becker muscular dystrophy is currently recruiting (NCT03238235). Vamorolone may show promise in Becker dystrophy as it is anticipated to reduce dystrophin-targeting microRNAs and thus increase dystrophin levels in muscle (Fiorillo et al. 2015, 2018). Development of experimental therapeutics in Becker muscular dystrophy is poised to expand over the next few years.

The prevalence of female carriers of DMD is about twice the incidence of male DMD boys, or 1 in 2,500 females worldwide. The majority of female carriers are asymptomatic. However, there is increasing recognition of cardiac abnormalities in most female carriers, although these are most commonly imaging findings and are not commonly symptomatic (Adachi et al. 2018). The degree of skeletal muscle and cardiac involvement in female carriers is driven by the skewing of X-inactivation, where a subset of female carriers show the mutation-carrying X active in the majority of cells – e.g., manifesting carriers (Hoffman et al. 1992; Pegoraro et al. 1995). To date, there are no published clinical trials of manifesting carriers and no currently enrolling subjects.

5 Looking Forward

DMD and Becker muscular dystrophy have two somewhat separable components of their disease – the primary defect (dystrophin abnormalities) and the molecular and cellular events driving fibrofatty replacement of muscle and progressive weakness. If gene therapy or CRISPR technologies were able to deliver normal, full-length dystrophin to patient muscle, then it may be possible to provide a curative therapy, particularly if done at an early age (before fibrofatty replacement of muscle occurs). However, none of the existing dystrophin replacement or gene repair strategies to date attempt to introduce a normal dystrophin gene and protein – they instead seek to introduce a Becker dystrophy gene or protein into a DMD child. Given the variable severity of Becker dystrophy, one might expect the efficacy of such approaches to be quite variable in terms of benefit, perhaps on a patient-by-patient basis.

What is most likely to emerge in pharmacotherapy of Duchenne and Becker muscular dystrophies is a multipronged approach, with agents providing rescue of Becker-like dystrophins and additional drugs used in combination addressing both chronic inflammation and the progressive fibrofatty replacement of muscle.

References

Adachi K, Hashiguchi S, Saito M, Kashiwagi S, Miyazaki T, Kawai H, Yamada H, Iwase T, Akaike M, Takao S, Kobayashi M, Ishizaki M, Matsumura T, Mori-Yoshimura M, Kimura E (2018) Detection and management of cardiomyopathy in female dystrophinopathy carriers. J Neurol Sci 386:74–80

Amoasii L, Hildyard JCW, Li H, Sanchez-Ortiz E, Mireault A, Caballero D, Harron R, Stathopoulou TR, Massey C, Shelton JM, Bassel-Duby R, Piercy RJ, Olson EN (2018) Gene editing restores dystrophin expression in a canine model of Duchenne muscular dystrophy. Science 362(6410):86–91

Arikawa E, Hoffman EP, Kaido M, Nonaka I, Sugita H, Arahata K (1991) The frequency of patients having dystrophin abnormalities in a limb-girdle patient population. Neurology 41:1491–1496

Bello L, Gordish-Dressman H, Morgenroth LP, Henricson EK, Duong T, Hoffman EP, Cnaan A, McDonald CM, Investigators CINRG (2015) Prednisone/prednisolone and deflazacort regimens in the CINRG Duchenne natural history study. Neurology 85(12):1048–1055

Bettica P, Petrini S, D'Oria V, D'Amico A, Catteruccia M, Pane M, Sivo S, Magri F, Brajkovic S, Messina S, Vita GL, Gatti B, Moggio M, Puri PL, Rocchetti M, de Nicolao G, Vita G, Comi GP, Bertini E, Mercuri E (2016) Histological effects of givinostat in boys with Duchenne muscular dystrophy. Neuromuscul Disord 26(10):643–649

Charleston JS, Schnell FJ, Dworzak J, Donoghue C, Lewis S, Chen L, Young GD, Milici AJ, Voss J, DeAlwis U, Wentworth B, Rodino-Klapac LR, Sahenk Z, Frank D, Mendell JR (2018) Eteplirsen treatment for Duchenne muscular dystrophy: exon skipping and dystrophin production. Neurology 90(24):e2146–e2154

Chen YW, Nagaraju K, Bakay M, McIntyre O, Rawat R, Shi R, Hoffman EP (2005) Early onset of inflammation and later involvement of TGFbeta in Duchenne muscular dystrophy. Neurology 65(6):826–834

Conklin LS, Damsker JM, Hoffman EP, Jusko WJ, Mavroudis PD, Schwartz BD, Mengle-Gaw LJ, Smith EC, Mah JK, Guglieri M, Nevo Y, Kuntz N, McDonald CM, Tulinius M, Ryan MM, Webster R, Castro D, Finkel RS, Smith AL, Morgenroth LP, Arrieta A, Shimony M, Jaros M, Shale P, McCall JM, Hathout Y, Nagaraju K, van den Anker J, Ward LM, Ahmet A, Cornish

MR, Clemens PR (2018) Phase IIa trial in Duchenne muscular dystrophy shows vamorolone is a first-in-class dissociative steroidal anti-inflammatory drug. Pharmacol Res 136:140–150

Connolly AM, Zaidman CM, Golumbek PT, Cradock MM, Flanigan KM, Kuntz NL, Finkel RS, McDonald CM, Iannaccone ST, Anand P, Siener CA, Florence JM, Lowes LP, Alfano LN, Johnson LB, Nicorici A, Nelson LL, Mendell JR, MDA DMD Clinical Research Network (2019) Twice-weekly glucocorticosteroids in infants and young boys with Duchenne muscular dystrophy. Muscle Nerve 59(6):650–657

Cowen L, Mancini M, Martin A, Lucas A, Donovan JM (2019) Variability and trends in corticosteroid use by male United States participants with Duchenne muscular dystrophy in the Duchenne registry. BMC Neurol 19(1):84

Dorchies OM, Reutenauer-Patte J, Dahmane E, Ismail HM, Petermann O, Patthey-Vuadens O, Comyn SA, Gayi E, Piacenza T, Handa RJ, Décosterd LA, Ruegg UT (2013) The anticancer drug tamoxifen counteracts the pathology in a mouse model of duchenne muscular dystrophy. Am J Pathol 182(2):485–504

Finanger E, Vandenborne K, Finkel RS, Lee Sweeney H, Tennekoon G, Yum S, Mancini M, Bista P, Nichols A, Liu H, Fretzen A, Donovan JM (2019) Phase 1 study of edasalonexent (CAT-1004), an oral NF-κB inhibitor, in pediatric patients with Duchenne muscular dystrophy. J Neuromuscul Dis 6(1):43–54

Fiorillo AA, Heier CR, Novak JS, Tully CB, Brown KJ, Uaesoontrachoon K, Vila MC, Ngheim PP, Bello L, Kornegay JN, Angelini C, Partridge TA, Nagaraju K, Hoffman EP (2015) TNF-α-induced microRNAs control dystrophin expression in Becker muscular dystrophy. Cell Rep 12(10):1678–1690

Fiorillo AA, Tully CB, Damsker JM, Nagaraju K, Hoffman EP, Heier CR (2018) Muscle miRNAome shows suppression of chronic inflammatory miRNAs with both prednisone and vamorolone. Physiol Genomics 50(9):735–745

Griggs RC, Herr BE, Reha A, Elfring G, Atkinson L, Cwik V, McColl E, Tawil R, Pandya S, McDermott MP, Bushby K (2013) Corticosteroids in Duchenne muscular dystrophy: major variations in practice. Muscle Nerve 48(1):27–31

Griggs RC, Miller JP, Greenberg CR, Fehlings DL, Pestronk A, Mendell JR, Moxley RT 3rd, King W, Kissel JT, Cwik V, Vanasse M, Florence JM, Pandya S, Dubow JS, Meyer JM (2016) Efficacy and safety of deflazacort vs prednisone and placebo for Duchenne muscular dystrophy. Neurology 87(20):2123–2131

Heier CR, Yu Q, Fiorillo AA, Tully CB, Tucker A, Mazala DA, Uaesoontrachoon K, Srinivassane S, Damsker JM, Hoffman EP, Nagaraju K, Spurney CF (2019) Vamorolone targets dual nuclear receptors to treat inflammation and dystrophic cardiomyopathy. Life Sci Alliance 2 (1):e201800186

Hoffman EP, Brown RH, Kunkel LM (1987) Dystrophin: the protein product of the Duchenne muscular dystrophy locus. Cell 51:919–928

Hoffman EP, Fischbeck KH, Brown RH, Johnson M, Medori R, Loike JD, Harris JB, Waterston R, Brooke M, Specht L, Kupsky W, Chamberlain J, Caskey CT, Shapiro F, Kunkel LM (1988) Dystrophin characterization in muscle biopsies from Duchenne and Becker muscular dystrophy patients. New Eng J Med 318:1363–1368

Hoffman EP, Kunkel LM, Angelini C, Clarke A, Johnson M, Harris JB (1989) Improved diagnosis of Becker muscular dystrophy by dystrophin testing. Neurology 39:1011–1017

Hoffman EP, Arahata K, Minetti C, Bonilla E, Rowland LP (1992) Dystrophinopathy in isolated cases of myopathy in females. Neurology 42(5):967–975

Hoffman EP, Riddle V, Siegler MA, Dickerson D, Backonja M, Kramer WG, Nagaraju K, Gordish-Dressman H, Damsker JM, McCall JM (2018) Phase 1 trial of vamorolone, a first-in-class steroid, shows improvements in side effects via biomarkers bridged to clinical outcomes. Steroids 134:43–52

Hoffman EP, Schwartz BD, Mengle-Gaw LJ, Smith EC, Castro D, Mah JK, McDonald CM, Kuntz NL, Finkel RS, Guglieri M, Bushby K, Tulinius M, Nevo Y, Ryan MM, Webster R, Smith AL, Morgenroth LP, Arrieta A, Shimony M, Siener C, Jaros M, Shale P, McCall JM,

Nagaraju K, van den Anker J, Conklin LS, Cnaan A, Gordish-Dressman H, Damsker JM, Clemens PR, The Cooperative International Neuromuscular Research Group (2019) Vamorolone trial in Duchenne muscular dystrophy shows dose-related improvement of muscle function. Neurology, in press

Hudson WH, Vera IMS, Nwachukwu JC, Weikum ER, Herbst AG, Yang Q, Bain DL, Nettles KW, Kojetin DJ, Ortlund EA (2018) Cryptic glucocorticoid receptor-binding sites pervade genomic NF-κB response elements. Nat Commun 9(1):1337

Joseph S, Wang C, Bushby K, Guglieri M, Horrocks I, Straub V, Ahmed SF, Wong SC (2019) Fractures and linear growth in a nationwide cohort of boys with Duchenne muscular dystrophy with and without glucocorticoid treatment: results from the UK NorthStar database. JAMA Neurol 76:701. https://doi.org/10.1001/jamaneurol.2019.0242

Kesari A, Pirra LN, Bremadesam L, McIntyre O, Gordon E, Dubrovsky AL, Viswanathan V, Hoffman EP (2008) Integrated DNA, cDNA, and protein studies in Becker muscular dystrophy show high exception to the reading frame rule. Hum Mutat 29(5):728–737

Koenig M, Hoffman EP, Bertelson CJ, Monaco AP, Feener C, Kunkel LM (1987) Complete cloning of the Duchenne muscular dystrophy (DMD) cDNA and preliminary genomic organization of the DMD gene in normal and affected individuals. Cell 50:509–517

Komaki H, Nagata T, Saito T, Masuda S, Takeshita E, Sasaki M, Tachimori H, Nakamura H, Aoki Y, Takeda S (2018) Systemic administration of the antisense oligonucleotide NS-065/NCNP-01 for skipping of exon 53 in patients with Duchenne muscular dystrophy. Sci Transl Med 10(437):eaan0713

Kornegay JN, Childers MK, Bogan DJ, Bogan JR, Nghiem P, Wang J, Fan Z, Howard JF Jr, Schatzberg SJ, Dow JL, Grange RW, Styner MA, Hoffman EP, Wagner KR (2012) The paradox of muscle hypertrophy in muscular dystrophy. Phys Med Rehabil Clin N Am 23(1):149–172

Lefter S, Hardiman O, Ryan AM (2017) A population-based epidemiologic study of adult neuromuscular disease in the Republic of Ireland. Neurology 88(3):304–313

McDonald CM, Henricson EK, Abresch RT, Duong T, Joyce NC, Hu F, Clemens PR, Hoffman EP, Cnaan A, Gordish-Dressman H, Investigators CINRG (2018) Long-term effects of glucocorticoids on function, quality of life, and survival in patients with Duchenne muscular dystrophy: a prospective cohort study. Lancet 391(10119):451–461

Nghiem PP, Hoffman EP, Mittal P, Brown KJ, Schatzberg SJ, Ghimbovschi S, Wang Z, Kornegay JN (2013) Sparing of the dystrophin-deficient cranial sartorius muscle is associated with classical and novel hypertrophy pathways in GRMD dogs. Am J Pathol 183(5):1411–1424

Nguyen KD, Bagheri B, Bagheri H (2018) Drug-induced bone loss: a major safety concern in Europe. Expert Opin Drug Saf 17(10):1005–1014

Pegoraro E, Schimke RN, Garcia C, Stern H, Cadaldini M, Angelini C, Barbosa E, Carroll J, Marks WA, Neville HE, Marks H, Appleton S, Toriello H, Wessel HB, Donnelly J, Bernes SM, Taber JW, Weiss L, Hoffman EP (1995) Genetic and biochemical normalization in female carriers of Duchenne muscular dystrophy: evidence for failure of dystrophin production in dystrophin-competent myonuclei. Neurology 45(4):677–690

Railroading at the FDA (2016) Nat Med 22(11):1193. https://doi.org/10.1038/nm.4234

Raman SV, Hor KN, Mazur W, Halnon NJ, Kissel JT, He X, Tran T, Smart S, McCarthy B, Taylor MD, Jefferies JL, Rafael-Fortney JA, Lowe J, Roble SL, Cripe LH (2015) Eplerenone for early cardiomyopathy in Duchenne muscular dystrophy: a randomised, double-blind, placebo-controlled trial. Lancet Neurol 14(2):153–161

Rice JB, White AG, Johnson M, Wagh A, Qin Y, Bartels-Peculis L, Ciepielewska G, Nelson WW (2018a) Healthcare resource use and cost associated with varying dosages of extended corticosteroid exposure in a US population. J Med Econ 21(9):846–852

Rice JB, White AG, Johnson M, Wagh A, Qin Y, Bartels-Peculis L, Ciepielewska G, Nelson WW (2018b) Quantitative characterization of the relationship between levels of extended corticosteroid use and related adverse events in a US population. Curr Med Res Opin 34(8):1519–1527

St Andre M, Johnson M, Bansal PN, Wellen J, Robertson A, Opsahl A, Burch PM, Bialek P, Morris C, Owens J (2017) A mouse anti-myostatin antibody increases muscle mass and

improves muscle strength and contractility in the mdx mouse model of Duchenne muscular dystrophy and its humanized equivalent, domagrozumab (PF-06252616), increases muscle volume in cynomolgus monkeys. Skelet Muscle 7(1):25
Taylor M, Jefferies J, Byrne B, Lima J, Ambale-Venkatesh B, Ostovaneh MR, Makkar R, Goldstein B, Smith RR, Fudge J, Malliaras K, Fedor B, Rudy J, Pogoda JM, Marbán L, Ascheim DD, Marbán E, Victor RG (2019) Cardiac and skeletal muscle effects in the randomized HOPE-Duchenne trial. Neurology 92(8):e866–e878
van den Bergen JC, Wokke BH, Janson AA, van Duinen SG, Hulsker MA, Ginjaar HB, van Deutekom JC, Aartsma-Rus A, Kan HE, Verschuuren JJ (2014) Dystrophin levels and clinical severity in Becker muscular dystrophy patients. J Neurol Neurosurg Psychiatry 85(7):747–753
Watanabe N, Nagata T, Satou Y, Masuda S, Saito T, Kitagawa H, Komaki H, Takagaki K, Takeda S (2018) NS-065/NCNP-01: an antisense oligonucleotide for potential treatment of exon 53 skipping in Duchenne muscular dystrophy. Mol Ther Nucl Acids 13:442–449
Wong BL, Rybalsky I, Shellenbarger KC, Tian C, McMahon MA, Rutter MM, Sawnani H, Jefferies JL (2017) Long-term outcome of interdisciplinary management of patients with Duchenne muscular dystrophy receiving daily glucocorticoid treatment. J Pediatr 182:296–303

Current and Emerging Therapies for Mucopolysaccharidoses

Florian B. Lagler

Contents

Abstract

Mucopolysaccharidoses (MPSs) are caused by deficiencies of specific lysosomal enzymes that affect the degradation of mucopolysaccharides or glycosaminoglycans (GAGs). Enzyme replacement therapies are available for an increasing number of MPSs since more than 15 years. Together with hematopoietic stem cell transplantation, these enzyme therapies are currently the gold standard of causal treatment in MPS. Both treatments can improve symptoms and prognosis, but they do not cure these severe conditions. The limitations of intravenous enzyme replacement and cell therapy can be

F. B. Lagler (✉)
Institute for Inborn Errors of Metabolism and Department of Paediatrics, Paracelsus Medical University, Salzburg, Austria
e-mail: florian.lagler@pmu.ac.at

W. Kiess et al. (eds.), *Pediatric Pharmacotherapy*,
Handbook of Experimental Pharmacology 261, https://doi.org/10.1007/164_2019_263

summarized as the development of immune reactions against the therapeutic molecules/cells and failure to restore enduring and sufficient drug exposures in all relevant tissues. Thus innovative approaches include small molecules and encapsulated cells that do not induce immune reactions, gene therapy approaches that aim for sustained enzyme expression, and new enzymes that are able to penetrate barriers to drug distribution like the blood-brain barrier. This chapter provides an update on the state of development of these new therapies and highlights current challenges.

Keywords
Cell therapy · Gene therapy · Innovative therapies · Mucopolysaccharidoses · Pharmacology

1 Introduction

Mucopolysaccharidoses (MPSs) are a group of inborn errors of metabolism (IEM) caused by deficiencies of specific lysosomal enzymes that affect the degradation of mucopolysaccharides or glycosaminoglycans (GAGs). The accumulation of GAGs in various organs and tissues of patients affected by MPS leads to a multi-systemic clinical picture with a broad range of clinical signs and symptoms (Neufeld 2001). The clinical descriptions have been published in the first [MPS I-H (Hurler 1920), II (Hunter 1917), and IV (Morquio 1929)] and second [MPS I-S (Scheie et al. 1962), MPS III (Sanfilippo et al. 1963), VI (Maroteaux et al. 1963), VII (Sly et al. 1973)] half of the last century. The identification of the underlying specific enzyme deficiencies founded the basis for the classification of MPS, but moreover it inspired Christian de Duve and Roscoe Brady in the late 1960s (De Duve 1964; Brady 1966) to propose substitution of enzymes as a new therapeutic concept. The mutual cross correction of cultured fibroblasts from patients with MPS I and MPS II in 1968 by the group of Elizabeth Neufeld (Fratantoni et al. 1968) provided the first proof of principle in vitro. Brady succeeded in treating Fabry and Gaucher patients with ceramidetrihexosidase and cerebrosidase isolated from the human placenta, which was a paramount milestone in establishing enzyme replacement therapy (ERT). For technical reasons (low protein abundance, proteolytic degradation, etc.), this protein source could not be used in MPSs (Heartlein and Kimura 2014), but the cloning of the genes coding for the defective enzymes triggered the development of recombinant therapeutic enzymes. So far enzyme products have been marketed for the following mucopolysaccharidoses: MPS I (laronidase; FDA 2003/EMA 2003), MPS II (idursulfase; 2006/2007), MPS IV A (elosulfase alfa; 2014/2014) and MPS VI (galsulfase; 2005/2006), and recently MPS VII (vestronidase alfa, 2017). These therapies, together with hematopoietic stem cell transplantation (HSCT) (only in early detected cases of MPS I), today are the gold standard of causal treatment in MPS. Despite improving symptoms and prognosis, intravenous ERT does not represent a cure for these severe conditions. In this chapter we will discuss the pharmacological principles and limitations of currently available therapies, and we will give an overview on emerging strategies to overcome these limitations.

2 Current Therapies

2.1 Pharmaceutical Characteristics of ERT Medicines

The recombinant lysosomal enzymes for the treatment of MPSs are molecules of approximately 600 amino acid residues and a molecular weight of around 70 kDa. They are similar to the human forms of the enzymes but can be produced in human, animal (e.g., Chinese hamster ovary), or plant cell cultures. All carry a mannose-6-phosphate residue, which binds to target cell surface receptors and facilitates the uptake into the lysosome via 6-mannose-phosphate receptors. The purified enzyme is formulated with sodium chloride, sodium phosphate, and polysorbate 20 to a hydrolysate that has to be diluted in 0.9% saline for infusion. The infusion solution can be used for 24 h.

2.2 Pharmacology of ERT Medicines

Upon intravenous infusion the enzyme is rapidly cleared from the circulation, with plasma half-lives of less than 1 h. In animal distribution studies, the majority of the drug is taken up by the liver. Moreover, there is a substantial uptake into other visceral organs, skin, vasculature, and lymph nodes. Bradytrophic organs like bones are hardly reached as well as the brain and eyes. Although elimination studies are missing, it seems obvious that the main mechanism of plasma clearance is the intracellular uptake via mannose-6-phosphate receptors. The persistence of the enzyme in the lysosomes, which has only been studied in patients and other cells in vitro, is in the range of 0.5–1 week, which is in line with the clinical observation that weekly infusions are more efficient than biweekly. As a consequence, standard treatment is weekly intravenous infusions. Most patients receive the recommended body weight-dependent standard doses, which are in the range of 0.5 mg/kg (Aldurazyme® in MPS II) to 2 mg/kg (Vimizim® in MPS IV A). The infusions are administered over 3–5 h with slowly increasing rates to prevent infusion reactions, which are differently from allergic reactions, and primarily dose dependent. In toxicological and safety studies, local infusion site reactions and generalized immune reactions up to anaphylactoid reactions have been most often observed. In general, the toxicological profile and clinical tolerability is excellent. Most patients develop anti-drug IgG antibodies over time. No clear negative impact on treatment efficacy has been confirmed so far. Acute infusion reactions can present clinically with nausea, diarrhea, rash, urticaria, angioedema, bronchoconstriction, rhinitis, and anaphylaxis. The majority of infusion reactions occur within the first months of treatment, but they can occur at any time. The majority of patients experience some reaction at one point, but most are mild to moderate and manageable with antihistamines and steroids. Like in anaphylactic reactions of other origin, intramuscular adrenaline is the treatment of choice in severe case (grade III and IV) (Lenders et al. 2018; Kim et al. 2017).

2.3 Effects and Limitations of ERT and BMT/HSCT

Enzyme replacement and cell therapy are causal therapies. Ideally, these should restore sufficient enzyme activity to normalize lysosomal function, stop GAG accumulation, and clear stored material without causing relevant inadvertent effects. In reality this is only partly the case. Intravenous ERT and BMT/HSCT can normalize GAG excretion and liver size. However, splenomegaly, cardiac function, walking ability, endurance, airway obstruction and pulmonary function can only be improved to some extent. In general, cardiac valve disease, joint range of motion, skeletal disease, and CNS manifestation seem not to benefit. This can be explained by the following limitations of the two approaches.

2.3.1 Immunoreactivity

For cell therapy immune suppression is a prerequisite. Although this is not the case for enzyme replacement therapy, it is associated with a relevant potential for immune reaction. The spectrum of immune reactions that have been observed upon the administration of recombinant enzymes reaches from silent antibody production to anaphylactic shock. In practically all cases, infusion reactions can be controlled with anti-allergic drugs, yet there is some evidence that in some cases neutralizing antibodies can mitigate therapeutic efficacy (Lenders et al. 2018; Kim et al. 2017).

2.3.2 Low Bioavailability in Certain Tissues

The low vascularization of tissues like bone, cartilage, and cardiac valves and physiological barriers that protect the brain or the eye seem to prevent sufficient concentrations of infused recombinant enzyme at these locations (Lin et al. 2005; Yano et al. 2009). Also cell therapy does not reach all relevant tissues and cells.

2.3.3 Short-Term Exposure

In contrast to the natural continuous enzyme production, the infusion of recombinant enzymes acts as a bolus as it is distributed and eliminated immediately after the infusion has finished (Hendriksz 2016; Ruane et al. 2016; Qi et al. 2014; Xie et al. 2015; Burton et al. 2015). On the one hand, this implies the need for weekly (MPS) or biweekly (other LSDs) infusions, but on the other hand, it has recently been shown that continuous slow release can be more efficacious than boluses (King et al. 2016, 2017).

2.3.4 Late Initiation of Treatment

Besides the inherent limitations of the abovementioned approaches, late initiation of treatment has a major effect on its success. This is because irreversible tissue destructions seem to occur very early in life. Studies in aborted affected fetuses as well as animal studies indicate that GAG accumulation is prevalent even before the 30th week of gestation (Martin and Ceuterick 1983; Wiesmann et al. 1980). If started at birth, however, ERT can normalize GAG storage and reduce pathology even in otherwise hard-to-reach tissues like the cardiac valves, bone, and brain (Dierenfeld et al. 2010). Newborn screening for MPS, as a key measure against late treatment initiation, is currently investigated in a number of pilot programs (Scott et al. 2013; Hopkins et al. 2015; Mechtler et al. 2012), but this is beyond the focus of this review.

3 Emerging Therapies

In the following sections emerging therapies for MPS are introduced. Table 1 summarizes the states of development for each therapy approach and MPS form.

3.1 Intrathecal Enzyme Replacement in MPS I, MPS II, MPS IIIA, and MPS IIIB

A straightforward method to overcome the blood-brain barrier (BBB) is direct injection into the cerebrospinal fluid. It is well established in other indications like treatment of cerebral tumors. The intrathecal space can be accessed by lumbar puncture or subcutaneously implanted drug delivery devices. Several preclinical and clinical studies have been conducted in small and large animals models of MPS I (Munoz-Rojas et al. 2008), II, IIIA, and IIIB patients, respectively. Obviously the ultimate goal is to treat CNS manifestation of these diseases. Clinical trials that evaluate if cognitive decline can be halted or decelerated are currently underway in MPS I, MPS II, MPS IIIA, and MPS IIIB, but conclusive results have not been published so far. Before these pivotal studies could be conducted, several pharmacokinetic and pharmacodynamic characteristics of the drugs had to be clarified. In the following section, this knowledge has been summarized.

3.1.1 What Doses and Intervals Are Needed to Restore Normal Enzyme Activity in Relevant Tissues by Intrathecal Injection?

In different murine and canine (Dickson et al. 2007) MPS models as well as in nonhuman primates, doses have been identified that result in normal enzyme activities in brain parenchyma down to its deep layers, spinal cord, and spinal meninges (Dickson et al. 2007; Kakkis et al. 2004). The injected recombinant enzyme was detectable up to 1–3 months after injection (Munoz-Rojas et al. 2008) and had a brain half-life of 10 days (Kan et al. 2014). These results suggested biweekly or even monthly infusion intervals for use in consecutive clinical trials.

3.1.2 Does the Restored Enzyme Activity Reduce Storage Material and Brain Pathology?

In animal models the concentration of GAGs in brain and meninges, brain vacuolization, and signs of neuroinflammation were reduced with biweekly or monthly infusions. Clinical data from case reports and small studies in adult and pediatric patients with MPS I, II, IIIA, and IIIB indicate that GAGs in CSF are reduced up to 90% (Dickson et al. 2015; Jones et al. 2016; Muenzer et al. 2016).

Table 1 Preclinical and clinical development status of innovative therapies

MPS	Preclinical studies	Clinical trials
Intrathecal enzyme replacement		
MPS I		Case study (Munoz-Rojas et al. 2008) and Phase I study (Dickson et al. 2015)
MPS II		Phase I/II study (Muenzer et al. 2016) and interim results of Phase II/III study (Muenzer et al. 2018)
MPS IIIA		Phase I/II study (Jones et al. 2016)
MPS IIIB		Interim results Phase I/II study (Muschol et al. 2018)
"Trojan horse" approach with fusion proteins		
MPS I	AGT-181 (HIRMAb-IDUA) in nonhuman primates (Boado and Pardridge 2017; Boado et al. 2012)	AGT-181 Phase I (NCT02371226) AGT-181 Phase I/II (NCT03053089) interim results (Giugliani et al. 2018a, b)
MPS II	AGT-182 (HIRMAb-IDS) in nonhuman primates (Boado et al. 2014a)	AGT-182 Phase I (NCT02262338)
MPS IIIA	HIRMAb-SGSH in nonhuman primates (Boado et al. 2014b) cTfRMAb-SGSH in nonhuman primates (Boado et al. 2017)	
MPS IIIB	HIRMAb-LL-NAGLU in nonhuman primates (Boado et al. 2016)	
Nanotechnology		
MPS I	Nanocapsules with Aldurazyme® in MPS I cells (Mühlstein et al. 2013)	
MPS VI	Nanocapsules with Naglazyme® in MPS VI cells (Mayer et al. 2015)	
Gene therapy		
MPS I	Intrathecal AAV-mediated in vivo gene therapy in MPS I dogs (Hinderer et al. 2016; Ellinwood et al. 2011)	SB-318 AAV6/zinc finger nuclease-mediated genome editing NCT02702115
MPS II	Ex vivo gene therapy with lentiviral corrected HSC in MPS II mice (Wakabayashi et al. 2015)	Retroviral in vivo gene therapy (Whitley et al. 1996) SB-913 AAV6/zinc finger nuclease-mediated genome editing NCT03041324
MPS IIIA	Ex vivo gene therapy with lentiviral corrected HSC in MPS IIIA mice (Sergijenko et al. 2013)	Phase I/II intracerebral AAV-mediated in vivo gene therapy (Tardieu et al. 2014; Flanigan et al. 2018)
MPS IIIB	Ex vivo gene therapy with lentiviral corrected HSC in MPS IIIB mice (Holley et al. 2018)	Phase I/II intracerebral AAV-mediated in vivo gene therapy (Tardieu et al. 2017)
MPS VI		Phase I/II systemic AAV-mediated in vivo gene therapy NCT03173521
Microencapsulated cells		
MPS I	Intraperitoneally implanted alpha-L-iduronidase overexpressing cells in MPS I mice (Baldo et al. 2012; Lagranha et al. 2013)	

(continued)

Table 1 (continued)

MPS	Preclinical studies	Clinical trials
MPS II	Intraperitoneally implanted iduronate-2-sulfatase overexpressing myoblasts in MPS II mice (Friso et al. 2005)	
MPS VII	Intraventricularly injected ß-glucuronidase overexpressing fibroblasts in MPS VII mice (Ross et al. 2000)	
Stop codon read-through approach		
MPS I	Chloramphenicol (Quoos Mayer et al. 2013), gentamicin (Kamei et al. 2013; Hein et al. 2004; Keeling et al. 2013), amikacin, lividomycin, paromomycin (Kamei et al. 2013) in MPS I cells	Phase II ataluren EudraCT Number 2015-003105-41
MPS VI	Ataluren, NB30 and NB54 in MPS VI cells (Bartolomeo et al. 2013)	
Pharmacological chaperones		
MPS II	Heparin derivative D2S0 in MPS II cells (Hoshina et al. 2018)	
MPS III	Imino sugars in MPS IIIC mice (Pshezhetsky et al. 2018)	
MPS IV	Imino sugars DLHex-DGJ beta-Gal-inhibitors and isofagomine derivatives in MPS IV cells (Fantur et al. 2010; Suzuki et al. 2014; Thonhofer et al. 2016)	
Genistein (4,5,7-trihydroexyisoflavone)		
MPS III		Case series to randomized controlled studies (Piotrowska et al. 2011; Delgadillo et al. 2011; de Ruijter et al. 2012; Kim et al. 2013)
Pentosan polysulfate (PPS)		
MPS I		Randomized open Phase II study (Hennermann et al. 2016)
Rhodamine B ([9-(2-carboxyphenyl)-6-diethylamino-3-xanthenylidene]-diethylammonium chloride)		
MPS I	Rhodamine in MPS I mice (Derrick-Roberts et al. 2017)	
MPS IIIA	Rhodamine in MPS IIIA mice (Roberts et al. 2006, 2007)	
MPS VI	Rhodamine in MPS VI cells (Roberts et al. 2006)	

MPS mucopolysaccharidosis, *HIRMAb-IDUA* monoclonal antibodies against human insulin receptor fused to iduronidase A, *HIRMAb-IDS* monoclonal antibodies against human insulin receptor fused to iduronate sulfatase A, *cTfRMAb-SGSH* chimeric monoclonal antibodies against the mouse transferrin receptor fused to N-sulfoglucosamine sulfohydrolase, *HIRMAb-LL-NAGLU* monoclonal antibodies against human insulin receptor fused to alpha-N-acetylglucosaminidase, *AAV* adeno-associated virus, *NCT* clinicaltrials.gov-identifier number, *EudraCT* European clinical trials registry identifier number

3.1.3 Do the Drugs Induce Immune Reaction and/or Other Relevant Adverse Reactions?

Currently safety of intrathecal ERT has been studied and reported in a total of 70 [6 MPS I (Munoz-Rojas et al. 2008; Dickson et al. 2015), 49 MPS II (Muenzer et al. 2016, 2018), 12 MPS IIIA (Jones et al. 2016), and 3 MPS IIIB (Muschol et al. 2018)] patients with a maximum follow-up of up to 67 months. No major adverse events have been reported. Serum anti-drug antibodies were a common finding in animal and clinical studies. Antibodies in CSF were only found in patients with substantial serum antibody titres. Thus it was concluded that these presumably crossed the BBB rather than being generated intrathecally. Clinical significance of antibodies has not been reported.

3.1.4 Does Intrathecal ERT Improve the CNS Disease in MPS?

The major motivation for intrathecal ERT is to treat or prevent spinal cord compression and neurocognitive deterioration. Subjective improvement of symptoms associated with spinal cord compression has been observed in a Phase I study of Dickson et al. with intrathecal laronidase in MPS I patients (Dickson et al. 2015). Increased mobility, improved bowel and bladder control, a reduction in crampy leg pain, and reduced sensation of "pins & needles" were reported by patients. Neurological examination showed small gains in the sensory and motor function. Objective study endpoints, however, like CSF GAG reduction, MRI signs for spinal cord compression, somatosensory testing, and a score for activities of daily living, were lacking. The failure to demonstrate efficacy was attributed to the low number of participants ($n = 5$), the lack of sensitive outcome measures for measurement of spinal cord compression, the presence of long-standing (likely irreversible) disease in the subjects, and spinal ligamentous thickening and other contributors to spinal cord compression that would be unlikely to respond to intrathecally delivered enzyme (Dickson et al. 2015).

In the Phase I/II study of Jones et al. with MPS IIIA patients, neurodevelopment (VABS-II, BSID-III, and KABC-II) and gray matter volume were evaluated 22 weeks after intrathecal heparan-N-sulfatase. Of the 12 patients, 4 showed a decline in developmental quotient assessed, 6 were essentially stable, and 2 patients had only a single data point. All except two patients showed reduction in gray matter volume (Jones et al. 2016). The abovementioned studies were primarily designed to proof safety and tolerability; thus it was not entirely unexpected that efficacy could not be statistically proven. In contrast, the randomized controlled Phase II/III trial in children with Hunter syndrome of Muenzer et al. primarily aimed for the proof of efficacy. The effects of monthly intrathecal idursulfase ($n = 32$) on cognitive impairment were assessed with the General Conceptual Ability (GCA) score (part of DAS-II) and the Adaptive Behavior Composite (ABC) score (part of VABS-II) and compared versus no treatment ($n = 16$). The top-line results presented in December 2017 showed no significant improvement of these parameters (Muenzer et al. 2017; Clinicaltrials.gov 2017; Takeda 2017).

So in conclusion it has been shown that intrathecal ERT can be safely used in MPS I, II, IIIA, and IIIB but it remains unclear if the CNS pathology can be reversed or slowed down once developed. This underlines the need for alternative approaches.

3.2 Trojan Horse Approach with Fusion Proteins

Although many therapeutic proteins cannot pass the BBB, it is not a complete barrier for large molecules. Macromolecules like hormones, neurotransmitters, and xenobiotics enter the brain via receptor-mediated active transport systems. This can be utilized by fusing active compounds to antibodies against these receptors. The antibodies act as Trojan horses that transport the therapeutic protein across BBB. Fusion proteins of antibodies against human insulin receptors (HIRMAb) or transferrin receptors (TfRMAb) have been used to develop treatments for MPS I [HIRMAb-IDUA (Boado and Pardridge 2017; Boado et al. 2012)], MPS II [HIRMAb-IDS (Boado et al. 2014a)], MPS IIIA [HIRMAb-SGSH (Boado et al. 2014b), cTfRMAb-SGSH (Boado et al. 2017)] and MPS IIIB [HIRMAb-LL-NAGLU (Boado et al. 2016)]. These studies have indicated that about 1% of intravenously infused enzyme is taken up into the brain, which is considered sufficient to reduce intracellular GAG accumulation. In MPS IIIA mice, GAG accumulation is substantially reduced after treatment with cTfRMAb-SGSH (Boado et al. 2017).

HIRMab in high doses caused hypoglycemia by a weak insulin agonist activity. However, this was not observed when dextrose was added to the infusion (Boado et al. 2012). Moreover, the preclinical studies indicated a good toxicity profile. Currently several clinical trials are ongoing including a Phase I study (NCT02371226) and a Phase I/II (NCT03053089) study with AGT-181 (HIRMAb-IDUA) in 3 and 21 MPS I patients, respectively, extension studies (NCT02597114; NCT03071341), and a Phase I study with AGT-182 (HIRMAb-IDS) in 8 MPS II patients (NCT02262338). Recent reports on preliminary results of a trial with AGT-181 in MPS I patients indicate good effects on GAG levels, on spleen and liver volume, as well as on neurocognitive function (Giugliani et al. 2018a, b).

3.3 Nanotechnology

Another promising strategy to transport enzyme across the BBB is to coat it with polymer-based nanoparticles. The particles conjugate the therapeutic enzyme and build nanocapsules that can pass the BBB by transcytosis and other mechanisms. In vitro studies have been done with arylsulfatase B (Naglazyme® for MPS VI; BioMarin Pharmaceutical) (Mühlstein et al. 2013) and laronidase (Aldurazyme® for MPS I, Genzyme Corporation, Boston, MA, USA) (Mayer et al. 2015).

3.4 Gene Therapy

Gene therapy aims for the correction of genetic sequences in patient cells. In the ex vivo approach, patient cells (e.g., stem cells, fibroblasts, etc.) are gathered, cultured in vitro, corrected genetically, and consecutively reinjected into the patient. In contrast for in vivo gene therapy, the corrected DNA is injected directly into the patient. Most in vivo efforts utilize viral vectors to deliver the corrective genetic material into the target cells. In principle MPSs as well as other lysosomal storage diseases are good candidates for gene therapy approaches. This is because even a relatively small number of corrected cells may be sufficient to produce therapeutic enzyme concentrations in the circulating blood. As in ERT this will result in internalization of enzyme into deficient cells, even if the DNA of these cells was not corrected (Baldo et al. 2014). Like in ERT, another major challenge of systemically administered gene therapy is to reach CNS, bones, and eyes sufficiently (Baldo et al. 2014; Ellinwood et al. 2004). Among many efforts two approaches seem promising for brain targeted gene therapy. First, lentiviral vectors can be used to augment the efficacy of HSCT by inducing overexpression of the therapeutic enzyme. In this sense mouse models of Hunters and Sanfilippo A disease have been successfully treated with autologous HSC transduced with a lentivirus encoding for iduronate-2-sulfatase and N-sulfoglucosamine sulfohydrolase, respectively (Wakabayashi et al. 2015; Sergijenko et al. 2013). Interestingly in contrast to regular HSCT, these modified HSC improved neuropathology significantly. In metachromatic leukodystrophy, another lysosomal storage disease, this strategy has been successfully used in clinical trials (Sessa et al. 2016; Biffi et al. 2013).

Second, adeno-associated viral (AAV) vectors have been directly injected into the brain parenchyma or CSF in many preclinical and some clinical studies. Tardieu et al. (2014, 2017) conducted two Phase I/II studies in 1.5–6 years old children with MPS IIIA and IIIB, respectively. The recombinant AAV vector serotype 2/5 (rAAV2/5) encoding human N-sulfoglycosamine sulfohydrolase (SGSH) or α-N-acetylglucosaminidase (NAGLU) was injected in cerebral and cerebellar white matter with silica glass capillaries. This was well tolerated and induced sustained enzyme production in the brain. After initial specific anti-NAGLU immune response, immunological tolerance was developed. Some cognitive improvement was observed in all patients with the best results in the youngest patient (20 months of age). Another Phase I/II study in MPS IIIA was recently reported by Flanigan et al. using a scAAV9 vector. GAGs in urine and CSF and liver volume were decreased upon gene therapy. Stabilization or improvement of adaptive behavior and cognitive function was observed (Flanigan et al. 2018).

Although larger studies and longer follow-up are needed, these results indicate a window of therapeutic opportunity in early life for this approach. Clinical trials are also underway for MPS II (NCT00004454), IIIB (NCT03300453, NCT03315182), and VI (NCT03173521).

3.5 Cell Microencapsulation

Cell microencapsulation of allogenic cells aims to allow their implantation without the need for immune suppression. By enclosing the cells into a semipermeable membrane, immune reactions can be prevented while exchange of metabolites and nutrients is still possible. Several kinds of microencapsulated cells that have been genetically modified to overexpress the therapeutic enzymes have been studied successfully in MPS types I, II, and VII. In MPS VII mice implantation of microencapsulated β-glucuronidase overexpressing fibroblasts into the lateral ventricles resulted in distribution of the enzyme in most brain areas and the CNS pathology was improved (Ross et al. 2000). Peritoneal application of iduronate-2-sulfatase overexpressing myoblasts reduced GAGs in urine and visceral organs in MPS II mice (Friso et al. 2005). In MPS I mice, encapsulated BHK cells were successfully applied (Baldo et al. 2012), but prednisone was needed to control immune response (Lagranha et al. 2013; Lizzi Lagranha et al. 2017).

3.6 Stop Codon Read-Through

Stop codon read-through (SCRT) therapy aims for genetic correction on the RNA level. Nonsense mutations can induce stop codons that lead to premature termination of the RNA translation and consecutive mRNA degradation by nonsense-mediated mRNA decay (NMD) resulting in truncated dysfunctional peptides. This pathomechanism can be disrupted by inserting amino acids into the sequence, so the stop codon is resolved and full lengths protein can be generated. Several molecules have been shown to apply for SCRT including marketed drugs. Enzyme activity could be increased in MPS fibroblasts and cell lines with chloramphenicol (Quoos Mayer et al. 2013), gentamicin (Kamei et al. 2013; Hein et al. 2004; Keeling et al. 2013), amikacin, lividomycin, and paromomycin (Kamei et al. 2013). Furthermore novel less toxic molecules like PTC124 (ataluren), NB30, and NB54 (paromomycin derivatives) were successfully tried in MPS VI fibroblasts (Bartolomeo et al. 2013) and MPS I cells (Kamei et al. 2013). Ataluren (Translarna®, PTC Therapeutics, South Plainfield, NJ, USA) is market approved for SCRT of nonsense mutations causing Duchenne muscular dystrophy (nmDMD). A Phase II trial with MPS I patients (EudraCT Number 2015-003105-41) is currently being conducted in the United Kingdom. All of these are small molecules that can cross the BBB. However, SCRT is limited to the use in patients with missense mutation.

3.7 Pharmacological Chaperones

Some genetic variants in MPS and many other diseases cause misfolding of the respective enzyme or other protein, respectively. Misfolding leads to an aberrant three-dimensional conformation and consecutively to a reduced function and stability as well as aberrant trafficking of the enzyme. Pharmacological chaperones (PCs) counteract this misfolding pathology by acting as scaffolding for the misfolded proteins. PCs are small molecules that can have advantages over therapeutic proteins in their ability to reach target cells and cell compartments. On the other hand, this approach is limited to patients with amenable mutations that lead to potentially reversible misfolding. In Fabry disease, a pharmacological chaperone (migalastat) has reached market approval. In MPS interesting molecules have been described for MPS II, III, and IV (Takai et al. 2013; Hoshina et al. 2018; Fantur et al. 2010; Suzuki et al. 2014; Thonhofer et al. 2016; Matos et al. 2014), and recently first in vivo experiments in a murine MPS model have been conducted (Pshezhetsky et al. 2018).

3.8 GAG-Reducing Small Molecules

Substrate reduction is an established therapeutic concept in other lysosomal storage diseases like Gaucher disease and Niemann-Pick type C. Partly motivated by the restrictions of ERT to reach the brain, the bones, and the eyes, several small molecules that reduce GAG concentration in urine and tissue have been studied in MPS.

Genistein (4,5,7-trihydroexyisoflavone) is a plant isoflavone, which blocks the epidermal growth factor (EGF)-mediated signal transduction. This pathway regulates the expression of GAG-synthesizing enzymes. Thus the reduction of GAG levels in brains and other organs of genistein-treated MPS III B mice (Malinowska et al. 2010; Piotrowska et al. 2011) was attributed to substrate inhibition. Despite promising preclinical data, clinical studies with 5–10 mg/kg genistein per day, including one placebo-controlled study so far, failed to conclusively confirm effects on neurocognition, whereas safety seems to be good even in high doses (Piotrowska et al. 2011; Delgadillo et al. 2011; de Ruijter et al. 2012; Kim et al. 2013).

Pentosan polysulfate (PPS) is an anti-inflammatory drug approved for the treatment of interstitial cystitis and osteoarthritis (Frohbergh et al. 2014). The rational to use it in MPS is based on its effects on inflammation processes that contribute to bone and joint disease in MPS (Simonaro et al. 2010). PPS improved systemic and joint inflammation, motility, grooming behavior, skull and tracheal malformations (Schuchman et al. 2013), and reduced GAG concentration in urine and tissue of MPS VI rats (Frohbergh et al. 2014). Comparable results were found in MPS I dogs (Simonaro et al. 2016). The underlying mechanism of GAG reduction, however, remains unclear so far. Substrate reduction, increased GAG degradation, direct effects on lysosomal function, and chaperone-like effects may explain this observation (Frohbergh et al. 2014). In a monocentric Phase II study with four MPS I patients, Hennermann et al. found a 24-week treatment with PPS well tolerated. Urinary GAG concentrations and pain were reduced; range of motion was improved (Hennermann et al. 2016).

Rhodamine B ([9-(2-carboxyphenyl)-6-diethylamino-3-xanthenylidene]-diethylammonium chloride) reduced GAG concentration in MPS VI and MPS IIIA skin fibroblasts (Banecka-Majkutewicz et al. 2012; Noh and Lee 2014). Rhodamine

B-treated MPS IIIA mice showed reduced liver size and GAG levels in urine, liver, and brain tissue. Additionally an improvement of the neurological function was proved by water maze experiments (Roberts et al. 2006, 2007). MPS I mice improved in learning and skeletal disease upon Rhodamine B treatment (Derrick-Roberts et al. 2017). Although long-term administration of low-dose Rhodamine B was well tolerated in mice (Derrick-Roberts et al. 2017), safety and efficacy in patients as well as the active mechanism are unknown so far (Giugliani et al. 2012).

Acknowledgment I cordially thank Adriana Montano, PhD, for proofreading.

References

Baldo G, Mayer FQ, Martinelli B, Meyer FS, Burin M, Meurer L, Tavares AMV, Giugliani R, Matte U (2012) Intraperitoneal implant of recombinant encapsulated cells overexpressing alpha-L-iduronidase partially corrects visceral pathology in mucopolysaccharidosis type I mice. Cytotherapy 14:860–867

Baldo G, Giugliani R, Matte U (2014) Gene delivery strategies for the treatment of mucopolysaccharidoses. Expert Opin Drug Deliv 11:449–459

Banecka-Majkutewicz Z, Jakobkiewicz-Banecka J, Gabig-Ciminska M, Wegrzyn A, Wegrzyn G (2012) Putative biological mechanisms of efficiency of substrate reduction therapies for mucopolysaccharidoses. Arch Immunol Ther Exp 60:461–468

Bartolomeo R, Polishchuk EV, Volpi N, Polishchuk RS, Auricchio A (2013) Pharmacological read-through of nonsense ARSB mutations as a potential therapeutic approach for mucopolysaccharidosis VI. J Inherit Metab Dis 36:363–371

Biffi A, Montini E, Lorioli L, Cesani M, Fumagalli F, Plati T, Baldoli C, Martino S, Calabria A, Canale S et al (2013) Lentiviral hematopoietic stem cell gene therapy benefits metachromatic leukodystrophy. Science 341:1233158

Boado RJ, Pardridge WM (2017) Brain and organ uptake in the rhesus monkey in vivo of recombinant iduronidase compared to an insulin receptor antibody-iduronidase fusion protein. Mol Pharm 14:1271–1277

Boado RJ, Hui EK, Lu JZ, Pardridge WM (2012) Glycemic control and chronic dosing of rhesus monkeys with a fusion protein of iduronidase and a monoclonal antibody against the human insulin receptor. Drug Metab Dispos 40:2021–2025

Boado RJ, Ka-Wai Hui E, Zhiqiang Lu J, Pardridge WM (2014a) Insulin receptor antibody-iduronate 2-sulfatase fusion protein: pharmacokinetics, anti-drug antibody, and safety pharmacology in Rhesus monkeys. Biotechnol Bioeng 111:2317–2325

Boado RJ, Lu JZ, Hui EK, Pardridge WM (2014b) Insulin receptor antibody-sulfamidase fusion protein penetrates the primate blood-brain barrier and reduces glycosoaminoglycans in Sanfilippo type A cells. Mol Pharm 11:2928–2934

Boado RJ, Lu JZ, Hui EK, Lin H, Pardridge WM (2016) Insulin receptor antibody-alpha-N-acetylglucosaminidase fusion protein penetrates the primate blood-brain barrier and reduces glycosoaminoglycans in sanfilippo type B fibroblasts. Mol Pharm 13:1385–1392

Boado RJ, Lu JZ, Hui EK, Pardridge WM (2017) Reduction in brain heparan sulfate with systemic administration of an IgG trojan horse-sulfamidase fusion protein in the mucopolysaccharidosis type IIIA mouse. Mol Pharm 15(2):602–608

Brady RO (1966) The sphingolipidoses. N Engl J Med 275:312–318

Burton BK, Berger KI, Lewis GD, Tarnopolsky M, Treadwell M, Mitchell JJ, Muschol N, Jones SA, Sutton VR, Pastores GM et al (2015) Safety and physiological effects of two different doses of elosulfase alfa in patients with morquio a syndrome: a randomized, double-blind, pilot study. Am J Med Genet A 167a:2272–2281

Clinicaltrials.gov (2017) Study of intrathecal idursulfase-IT administered in conjunction with elaprase in pediatric patients with hunter syndrome and early cognitive impairment. https://clinicaltrials.gov/ct2/show/study/NCT02055118

de Ruijter J, Valstar MJ, Narajczyk M, Wegrzyn G, Kulik W, Ijlst L, Wagemans T, van der Wal WM, Wijburg FA (2012) Genistein in Sanfilippo disease: a randomized controlled crossover trial. Ann Neurol 71:110–120

De Duve C (1964) From cytases to lysosomes. Fed Proc:1045–1049

Delgadillo V, O'Callaghan Mdel M, Artuch R, Montero R, Pineda M (2011) Genistein supplementation in patients affected by Sanfilippo disease. J Inherit Metab Dis 34:1039–1044

Derrick-Roberts ALK, Jackson MR, Pyragius CE, Byers S (2017) Substrate deprivation therapy to reduce glycosaminoglycan synthesis improves aspects of neurological and skeletal pathology in MPS I mice. Diseases 5:5

Dickson P, McEntee M, Vogler C, Le S, Levy B, Peinovich M, Hanson S, Passage M, Kakkis E (2007) Intrathecal enzyme replacement therapy: successful treatment of brain disease via the cerebrospinal fluid. Mol Genet Metab 91:61–68

Dickson PI, Kaitila I, Harmatz P, Mlikotic A, Chen AH, Victoroff A, Passage MB, Madden J, Le SQ, Naylor DE (2015) Safety of laronidase delivered into the spinal canal for treatment of cervical stenosis in mucopolysaccharidosis I. Mol Genet Metab 116:69–74

Dierenfeld AD, McEntee MF, Vogler CA, Vite CH, Chen AH, Passage M, Le S, Shah S, Jens JK, Snella EM et al (2010) Replacing the enzyme alpha-L-iduronidase at birth ameliorates symptoms in the brain and periphery of dogs with mucopolysaccharidosis type I. Sci Transl Med 2:60ra89

Ellinwood NM, Vite CH, Haskins ME (2004) Gene therapy for lysosomal storage diseases: the lessons and promise of animal models. J Gene Med 6:481–506

Ellinwood NM, Ausseil J, Desmaris N, Bigou S, Liu S, Jens JK, Snella EM, Mohammed EE, Thomson CB, Raoul S (2011) Safe, efficient, and reproducible gene therapy of the brain in the dog models of Sanfilippo and Hurler syndromes. Mol Ther 19:251–259

Fantur K, Hofer D, Schitter G, Steiner AJ, Pabst BM, Wrodnigg TM, Stutz AE, Paschke E (2010) DLHex-DGJ, a novel derivative of 1-deoxygalactonojirimycin with pharmacological chaperone activity in human G(M1)-gangliosidosis fibroblasts. Mol Genet Metab 100:262–268

Flanigan K, Truxal K, McBride K, McNally K, Kunkler K, Zumberge N, Martin L, Aylward S, Corridore M, Ruiz J et al (2018) A phase 1/2 clinical trial of systemic gene transfer of scAAV9. U1a.HSGSH for MPS IIIA: safety, tolerability, and preliminary evidence of biopotency. Mol Genet Metab 123:S46

Fratantoni JC, Hall CW, Neufeld EF (1968) Hurler and Hunter syndromes: mutual correction of the defect in cultured fibroblasts. Science 162:570–572

Friso A, Tomanin R, Alba S, Gasparotto N, Puicher EP, Fusco M, Hortelano G, Muenzer J, Marin O, Zacchello F (2005) Reduction of GAG storage in MPS II mouse model following implantation of encapsulated recombinant myoblasts. J Gene Med 7:1482–1491

Frohbergh M, Ge Y, Meng F, Karabul N, Solyom A, Lai A, Iatridis J, Schuchman EH, Simonaro CM (2014) Dose responsive effects of subcutaneous pentosan polysulfate injection in mucopolysaccharidosis type VI rats and comparison to oral treatment. PLoS One 9:e100882

Giugliani R et al (2012) Emerging treatment options for the mucopolysaccharidoses. Res Rep Endocr Disord 2:53–64

Giugliani L, Carvalho Doni K, Poswar F, Giugliani R, Boado R (2018a) Somatic effects of AGT-181 in patients with mucopolysaccharidosis I enrolled in a phase I/II clinical trial in Brazil. Mol Genet Metab 123:S53

Giugliani R, Giugliani L, Dalle Corte A, Poswar F, Donis K, Schmidt M, Hunt D, Boado RJ (2018b) Safety and clinical efficacy of AGT-181, a brain penetrating human insulin receptor antibody-iduronidase fusion protein, in a 26-week study with pediatric patients with mucopolysaccharidosis type I. Mol Genet Metab 123:S54

Heartlein MW, Kimura A (2014) Discovery and clinical development of idursulfase (Elaprase®) for the treatment of mucopolysaccharidosis II (Hunter syndrome). In: Pryde DC, Palmer M (eds) Orphan drugs and rare diseases. Royal Society of Chemistry, London, pp 164–182

Hein LK, Bawden M, Muller VJ, Sillence D, Hopwood JJ, Brooks DA (2004) α-L-iduronidase premature stop codons and potential read-through in mucopolysaccharidosis type I patients. J Mol Biol 338:453–462

Hendriksz CJ (2016) Elosulfase alfa (BMN 110) for the treatment of mucopolysaccharidosis IVA (Morquio A Syndrome). Expert Rev Clin Pharmacol 9:1521–1532

Hennermann JB, Gokce S, Solyom A, Mengel E, Schuchman EH, Simonaro CM (2016) Treatment with pentosan polysulphate in patients with MPS I: results from an open label, randomized, monocentric phase II study. J Inherit Metab Dis 39:831–837

Hinderer C, Bell P, Louboutin JP, Katz N, Zhu Y, Lin G, Choa R, Bagel J, O'Donnell P, Fitzgerald CA et al (2016) Neonatal tolerance induction enables accurate evaluation of gene therapy for MPS I in a canine model. Mol Genet Metab 119:124–130

Holley RJ, Ellison SM, Fil D, O'Leary C, McDermott J, Senthivel N, Langford-Smith AWW, Wilkinson FL, D'Souza Z, Parker H et al (2018) Macrophage enzyme and reduced inflammation drive brain correction of mucopolysaccharidosis IIIB by stem cell gene therapy. Brain 141:99–116

Hopkins PV, Campbell C, Klug T, Rogers S, Raburn-Miller J, Kiesling J (2015) Lysosomal storage disorder screening implementation: findings from the first six months of full population pilot testing in Missouri. J Pediatr 166:172–177

Hoshina H, Shimada Y, Higuchi T, Kobayashi H, Ida H, Ohashi T (2018) Chaperone effect of sulfated disaccharide from heparin on mutant iduronate-2-sulfatase in mucopolysaccharidosis type II. Mol Genet Metab 123:118–122

Hunter C (1917) A rare disease in two brothers. Proc R Soc Med 10:104–116

Hurler G (1920) Über einen Typ multipler Abartungen, vorwiegend am Skelettsystem. Z Kinderheilkd 24:220–234

Jones SA, Breen C, Heap F, Rust S, de Ruijter J, Tump E, Marchal JP, Pan L, Qiu Y, Chung JK et al (2016) A phase 1/2 study of intrathecal heparan-N-sulfatase in patients with mucopolysaccharidosis IIIA. Mol Genet Metab 118:198–205

Kakkis E, McEntee M, Vogler C, Le S, Levy B, Belichenko P, Mobley W, Dickson P, Hanson S, Passage M (2004) Intrathecal enzyme replacement therapy reduces lysosomal storage in the brain and meninges of the canine model of MPS I. Mol Genet Metab 83:163–174

Kamei M, Kasperski K, Fuller M, Parkinson-Lawrence EJ, Karageorgos L, Belakhov V, Baasov T, Hopwood JJ, Brooks DA (2013) Aminoglycoside-induced premature stop codon read-through of mucopolysaccharidosis type I patient Q70X and W402X mutations in cultured cells. In: JIMD reports – case and research reports, vol 13. Springer, Berlin, pp 139–147

Kan SH, Aoyagi-Scharber M, Le SQ, Vincelette J, Ohmi K, Bullens S, Wendt DJ, Christianson TM, Tiger PM, Brown JR et al (2014) Delivery of an enzyme-IGFII fusion protein to the mouse brain is therapeutic for mucopolysaccharidosis type IIIB. Proc Natl Acad Sci U S A 111:14870–14875

Keeling KM, Wang D, Dai Y, Murugesan S, Chenna B, Clark J, Belakhov V, Kandasamy J, Velu SE, Baasov T (2013) Attenuation of nonsense-mediated mRNA decay enhances in vivo nonsense suppression. PLoS One 8:e60478

Kim KH, Dodsworth C, Paras A, Burton BK (2013) High dose genistein aglycone therapy is safe in patients with mucopolysaccharidoses involving the central nervous system. Mol Genet Metab 109:382–385

Kim S, Whitley CB, Jarnes Utz JR (2017) Correlation between urinary GAG and anti-idursulfase ERT neutralizing antibodies during treatment with NICIT immune tolerance regimen: a case report. Mol Genet Metab 122:92–99

King B, Hassiotis S, Rozaklis T, Beard H, Trim PJ, Snel MF, Hopwood JJ, Hemsley KM (2016) Low-dose, continuous enzyme replacement therapy ameliorates brain pathology in the neuro-degenerative lysosomal disorder mucopolysaccharidosis type IIIA. J Neurochem 137:409–422

King B, Marshall NR, Hassiotis S, Trim PJ, Tucker J, Hattersley K, Snel MF, Jolly RD, Hopwood JJ, Hemsley KM (2017) Slow, continuous enzyme replacement via spinal CSF in dogs with the paediatric-onset neurodegenerative disease, MPS IIIA. J Inherit Metab Dis 40:443–453

Lagranha VL, de Carvalho TG, Giugliani R, Matte U (2013) Treatment of MPS I mice with microencapsulated cells overexpressing IDUA: effect of the prednisolone administration. J Microencapsul 30:383–389

Lenders M, Schmitz B, Brand SM, Foell D, Brand E (2018) Characterization of drug-neutralizing antibodies in patients with Fabry disease during infusion. J Allergy Clin Immunol 141 (6):2289–2292

Lin HY, Lin SP, Chuang CK, Chen MR, Chen BF, Wraith JE (2005) Mucopolysaccharidosis I under enzyme replacement therapy with laronidase--a mortality case with autopsy report. J Inherit Metab Dis 28:1146–1148

Lizzi Lagranha V, Zambiasi Martinelli B, Baldo G, Avila Testa G, Giacomet de Carvalho T, Giugliani R, Matte U (2017) Subcutaneous implantation of microencapsulated cells overexpressing alpha-L-iduronidase for mucopolysaccharidosis type I treatment. J Mater Sci Mater Med 28:43

Malinowska M, Wilkinson FL, Langford-Smith KJ, Langford-Smith A, Brown JR, Crawford BE, Vanier MT, Grynkiewicz G, Wynn RF, Wraith JE et al (2010) Genistein improves neuropathology and corrects behaviour in a mouse model of neurodegenerative metabolic disease. PLoS One 5:e14192

Maroteaux P, Leveque B, Marie J, Lamy M (1963) A new dysostosis with urinary elimination of chondroitin sulfate B. Presse Med 71:1849–1852

Martin JJ, Ceuterick C (1983) Prenatal pathology in mucopolysaccharidoses: a comparison with postnatal cases. Clin Neuropathol 2:122–127

Matos L, Canals I, Dridi L, Choi Y, Prata MJ, Jordan P, Desviat LR, Perez B, Pshezhetsky AV, Grinberg D et al (2014) Therapeutic strategies based on modified U1 snRNAs and chaperones for Sanfilippo C splicing mutations. Orphanet J Rare Dis 9:180

Mayer FQ, Adorne MD, Bender EA, de Carvalho TG, Dilda AC, Beck RCR, Guterres SS, Giugliani R, Matte U, Pohlmann AR (2015) Laronidase-functionalized multiple-wall lipid-core nanocapsules: promising formulation for a more effective treatment of mucopolysaccharidosis type I. Pharm Res 32:941–954

Mechtler TP, Stary S, Metz TF, De Jesus VR, Greber-Platzer S, Pollak A, Herkner KR, Streubel B, Kasper DC (2012) Neonatal screening for lysosomal storage disorders: feasibility and incidence from a nationwide study in Austria. Lancet 379:335–341

Morquio L (1929) Sur une forme de dystrophie osseuse familialeArchives de medecine des infants. Arch Med Enfants 32:129–135

Muenzer J, Hendriksz CJ, Fan Z, Vijayaraghavan S, Perry V, Santra S, Solanki GA, Mascelli MA, Pan L, Wang N et al (2016) A phase I/II study of intrathecal idursulfase-IT in children with severe mucopolysaccharidosis II. Genet Med 18:73–81

Muenzer J et al (2017) A long-term extension study evaluating intrathecal idursulfase-IT in children with hunter syndrome and cognitive impairment. In: 13th annual WORLD symposium, San Diego

Muenzer J, Burton BK, Harmatz P, Gutiérrez-Solana LG, Ruiz-Garcia M, Jones SA, Guffon N, Inbar-Feigenberg M, Bratkovic D, Wu Y et al (2018) Efficacy and safety of intrathecal idursulfase in pediatric patients with mucopolysaccharidosis type II and early cognitive impairment: design and methods of a controlled, randomized, phase II/III multicenter study. Mol Genet Metab 123:S99–S100

Mühlstein A, Gelperina S, Kreuter J (2013) Development of nanoparticle-bound arylsulfatase B for enzyme replacement therapy of mucopolysaccharidosis VI. Pharmazie 68:549–554

Munoz-Rojas MV, Vieira T, Costa R, Fagondes S, John A, Jardim LB, Vedolin LM, Raymundo M, Dickson PI, Kakkis E et al (2008) Intrathecal enzyme replacement therapy in a patient with mucopolysaccharidosis type I and symptomatic spinal cord compression. Am J Med Genet A 146a:2538–2544

Muschol N, Cleary M, Couce ML, Shaywitz AJ, Cahan H, Grover A, Maricich SM, Melton A, Smith L, de Castro Lopez MJ (2018) ICV-administered BMN 250 (NAGLU-IGF2) is well tolerated and reduces heparan sulfate accumulation in the CNS of subjects with Sanfilippo syndrome type B (MPS IIIB). Mol Genet Metab 123:S102

Neufeld EMJ (2001) The mucopolysaccharidosis. In: Scriver CBA, Sly S et al (eds) The metabolic and molecular basis of inherited disease. McGraw-Hill, New York, pp 3421–3452

Noh H, Lee JI (2014) Current and potential therapeutic strategies for mucopolysaccharidoses. J Clin Pharm Ther 39:215–224

Piotrowska E, Jakobkiewicz-Banecka J, Maryniak A, Tylki-Szymanska A, Puk E, Liberek A, Wegrzyn A, Czartoryska B, Slominska-Wojewodzka M, Wegrzyn G (2011) Two-year follow-up of Sanfilippo Disease patients treated with a genistein-rich isoflavone extract: assessment of effects on cognitive functions and general status of patients. Med Sci Monit 17:Cr196–Cr202

Pshezhetsky AV, Pan X, Héon-Roberts R, Li S-G, Wu HY, Taherzadeh M, De Aragão CDBP, Wood J, Ekins S, Boyd R et al (2018) Chaperone therapy for mucopolysaccharidosis type IIIC. Mol Genet Metab 123:S121–S122

Qi Y, Musson DG, Schweighardt B, Tompkins T, Jesaitis L, Shaywitz AJ, Yang K, O'Neill CA (2014) Pharmacokinetic and pharmacodynamic evaluation of elosulfase alfa, an enzyme replacement therapy in patients with Morquio A syndrome. Clin Pharmacokinet 53:1137–1147

Quoos Mayer F, Alfonso Artigalas O, Lizzi Lagranha V, Baldo G, Vanessa Schwartz I, Matte U, Giugliani R (2013) Chloramphenicol enhances IDUA activity on fibroblasts from mucopolysaccharidosis I patients. Curr Pharm Biotechnol 14:194–198

Roberts AL, Thomas BJ, Wilkinson AS, Fletcher JM, Byers S (2006) Inhibition of glycosaminoglycan synthesis using rhodamine B in a mouse model of mucopolysaccharidosis type IIIA. Pediatr Res 60:309–314

Roberts AL, Rees MH, Klebe S, Fletcher JM, Byers S (2007) Improvement in behaviour after substrate deprivation therapy with rhodamine B in a mouse model of MPS IIIA. Mol Genet Metab 92:115–121

Ross CJ, Bastedo L, Maier SA, Sands MS, Chang PL (2000) Treatment of a lysosomal storage disease, mucopolysaccharidosis VII, with microencapsulated recombinant cells. Hum Gene Ther 11:2117–2127

Ruane T, Haskins M, Cheng A, Wang P, Aguirre G, Knox VW, Qi Y, Tompkins T, O'Neill CA (2016) Pharmacodynamics, pharmacokinetics and biodistribution of recombinant human N-acetylgalactosamine 4-sulfatase after 6 months of therapy in cats using different IV infusion durations. Mol Genet Metab 117:157–163

Sanfilippo S, Podosin R, Langer LJ et al (1963) Mental retardation associated with acid mucpolysacchariduria (heparin sulfate type). J Pediatr 63:837–838

Scheie HG, Hambrick GW Jr, Barness LA (1962) A newly recognized forme fruste of Hurler's disease (gargoylism). Am J Ophthalmol 53:753–769

Schuchman EH, Ge Y, Lai A, Borisov Y, Faillace M, Eliyahu E, He X, Iatridis J, Vlassara H, Striker G (2013) Pentosan polysulfate: a novel therapy for the mucopolysaccharidoses. PLoS One 8:e54459

Scott CR, Elliott S, Buroker N, Thomas LI, Keutzer J, Glass M, Gelb MH, Turecek F (2013) Identification of infants at risk for developing Fabry, Pompe, or mucopolysaccharidosis-I from newborn blood spots by tandem mass spectrometry. J Pediatr 163:498–503

Sergijenko A, Langford-Smith A, Liao AY, Pickford CE, McDermott J, Nowinski G, Langford-Smith KJ, Merry CL, Jones SA, Wraith JE et al (2013) Myeloid/Microglial driven autologous hematopoietic stem cell gene therapy corrects a neuronopathic lysosomal disease. Mol Ther 21:1938–1949

Sessa M, Lorioli L, Fumagalli F, Acquati S, Redaelli D, Baldoli C, Canale S, Lopez ID, Morena F, Calabria A et al (2016) Lentiviral haemopoietic stem-cell gene therapy in early-onset metachromatic leukodystrophy: an ad-hoc analysis of a non-randomised, open-label, phase 1/2 trial. Lancet 388:476–487

Simonaro CM, Ge Y, Eliyahu E, He X, Jepsen KJ, Schuchman EH (2010) Involvement of the Toll-like receptor 4 pathway and use of TNF-α antagonists for treatment of the mucopolysaccharidoses. Proc Natl Acad Sci 107:222–227

Simonaro CM, Tomatsu S, Sikora T, Kubaski F, Frohbergh M, Guevara JM, Wang RY, Vera M, Kang JL, Smith LJ et al (2016) Pentosan polysulfate: oral versus subcutaneous injection in mucopolysaccharidosis type I dogs. PLoS One 11:e0153136

Sly WS, Quinton BA, McAlister WH, Rimoin DL (1973) Beta glucuronidase deficiency: report of clinical, radiologic, and biochemical features of a new mucopolysaccharidosis. J Pediatr 82:249–257

Suzuki H, Ohto U, Higaki K, Mena-Barragan T, Aguilar-Moncayo M, Ortiz Mellet C, Nanba E, Garcia Fernandez JM, Suzuki Y, Shimizu T (2014) Structural basis of pharmacological chaperoning for human beta-galactosidase. J Biol Chem 289:14560–14568

Takai T, Higaki K, Aguilar-Moncayo M, Mena-Barragan T, Hirano Y, Yura K, Yu L, Ninomiya H, Garcia-Moreno MI, Sakakibara Y et al (2013) A bicyclic 1-deoxygalactonojirimycin derivative as a novel pharmacological chaperone for GM1 gangliosidosis. Mol Ther 21:526–532

Takeda (2017) Shire announces top-line results for phase II/III clinical trial in children with hunter syndrome and cognitive impairment. https://www.shire.com/en/newsroom/2017/december/wvdwq3

Tardieu M, Zerah M, Husson B, de Bournonville S, Deiva K, Adamsbaum C, Vincent F, Hocquemiller M, Broissand C, Furlan V et al (2014) Intracerebral administration of adeno-associated viral vector serotype rh.10 carrying human SGSH and SUMF1 cDNAs in children with mucopolysaccharidosis type IIIA disease: results of a phase I/II trial. Hum Gene Ther 25:506–516

Tardieu M, Zerah M, Gougeon ML, Ausseil J, de Bournonville S, Husson B, Zafeiriou D, Parenti G, Bourget P, Poirier B et al (2017) Intracerebral gene therapy in children with mucopolysaccharidosis type IIIB syndrome: an uncontrolled phase 1/2 clinical trial. Lancet Neurol 16:712–720

Thonhofer M, Weber P, Gonzalez Santana A, Tysoe C, Fischer R, Pabst BM, Paschke E, Schalli M, Stutz AE, Tschernutter M et al (2016) Synthesis of C-5a-substituted derivatives of 4-epi-isofagomine: notable beta-galactosidase inhibitors and activity promotors of GM1-gangliosidosis related human lysosomal beta-galactosidase mutant R201C. Carbohydr Res 429:71–80

Wakabayashi T, Shimada Y, Akiyama K, Higuchi T, Fukuda T, Kobayashi H, Eto Y, Ida H, Ohashi T (2015) Hematopoietic stem cell gene therapy corrects neuropathic phenotype in murine model of mucopolysaccharidosis type II. Hum Gene Ther 26:357–366

Whitley CB, McIvor RS, Aronovich EL, Berry SA, Blazar BR, Burger SR, Kersey JH, King RA, Faras AJ, Latchaw RE et al (1996) Retroviral-mediated transfer of the iduronate-2-sulfatase gene into lymphocytes for treatment of mild Hunter syndrome (mucopolysaccharidosis type II). Hum Gene Ther 7:537–549

Wiesmann UN, Spycher MA, Meier C, Liebaers I, Herschkowitz N (1980) Prenatal mucopolysaccharidosis II (Hunter): a pathogenetic study. Pediatr Res 14:749–756

Xie H, Chung JK, Mascelli MA, McCauley TG (2015) Pharmacokinetics and bioavailability of a therapeutic enzyme (idursulfase) in cynomolgus monkeys after intrathecal and intravenous administration. PLoS One 10:e0122453

Yano S, Moseley K, Pavlova Z (2009) Postmortem studies on a patient with mucopolysaccharidosis type I: histopathological findings after one year of enzyme replacement therapy. J Inherit Metab Dis 32(Suppl 1):S53–S57

Current and Emerging Therapies for Mitochondriopathies

Florian B. Lagler

Contents

Abstract

Mitochondrial diseases are a clinically and genetically heterogeneous group of disorders. The underlying dysfunction of the mitochondrial electron transport chain and oxidative phosphorylation is caused by variants of genes encoding mitochondrial proteins. Despite substantial advances in the understanding of the mechanism of these diseases, there are still no satisfactory therapies available. Therapeutic strategies include the use of antioxidants, inducers of mitochondrial biogenesis, enhancers of electron transfer chain function, energy buffers, amino acids restoring NO production, nucleotide bypass therapy, liver transplantation, and gene therapy. Although there are some promising projects underway, to date satisfactory therapies are missing.

F. B. Lagler (✉)
Institute for Inborn Errors of Metabolism and Department of Paediatrics, Paracelsus Medical University, Salzburg, Austria
e-mail: florian.lagler@pmu.ac.at

W. Kiess et al. (eds.), *Pediatric Pharmacotherapy*,
Handbook of Experimental Pharmacology 261, https://doi.org/10.1007/164_2019_264

Keywords
Amino acids · Antioxidants · Electron transfer chain · Energy buffers · Gene therapy · Mitochondrial biogenesis · Mitochondriopathies · Nucleotide bypass · Therapies

1 Introduction

Mitochondrial disorders are the most common cause of inherited neurometabolic diseases (prevalence, 1:4,300) (Chinnery 2014). The underlying dysfunction of the mitochondrial electron transport chain and oxidative phosphorylation is caused by variants of genes encoding mitochondrial proteins (Chinnery 2014). These multi-systemic diseases are clinically, biochemically, and genetically heterogeneous; thus the diagnosis can be challenging. Yet, next-generation sequencing (NGS) improves the rate of early diagnosis and by this opens a new window of opportunity for successful treatment. So far besides symptomatic treatment, mainly approaches to improve oxidative phosphorylation (OXPHOS) and antioxidant capacity like combinations of vitamins and coenzymes have been used. Given the limited efficiency of these current treatments, emerging new therapeutic strategies are of high importance.

2 Current Therapies

Established indications and dosing regimens are summarized in Table 1.

2.1 Improving Electron Transfer Chain (ETC) Function

The mitochondrial ETC function can be improved either by increasing the availability of ETC substrates (dichloroacetate and thiamine) or by enhancing the components of the ETC (CoQ10, idebenone, and riboflavin).

Coenzyme Q10 (ubichinone) transports electrons from complex I to complex II and from there to complex III. Its use is obvious and efficient in primary CoQ10 deficiency, but it was also suggested for other mitochondriopathies. Despite some promising case reports, efficiency on oxidative capacity and lactate levels could not be confirmed in a randomized controlled trial with other mitochondrial disease patients (Glover et al. 2010; El-Hattab et al. 2017).

The CoQ10 analog *idebenone* shares its quinone moiety with CoQ10 but has a much shorter tail with a terminal hydroxyl group and a favorable pharmacokinetic profile. Thus idebenone is more water soluble and shows a rapid absorption from the gut and a large biodistribution. In RCTs with Leber hereditary optic neuropathy (LHON) patients, a positive effect on the visual function, particularly color vision of idebenone, has been observed (El-Hattab et al. 2017; Klopstock et al. 2011, 2013; Rudolph et al. 2013).

Table 1 Current therapies for mitochondrial diseases

Molecules	Doses	Indication
CoQ10	Ubiquinone: 5–30 mg/kg/day (2 doses) Ubiquinol: 2–8 mg/kg/day (2 doses)	Primary CoQ10 deficiency
Idebenone	30–300 mg/dose (3 doses)	LHON
Riboflavin	50–200 mg/day (2–3 doses)	Acyl-CoA dehydrogenase-9 deficiency Multiple acyl-CoA dehydrogenase deficiency
Dichloroacetate	10–25 mg/kg/day (2 doses)	Congenital lactic acidosis
Thiamine	10 mg/kg/day (children) 100–1,000 mg/day (adults)	Leigh disease thiamine transporter deficiency
Arginine	Stroke-like episodes: 500 mg/kg (children)[a] 10 g/m^2 body surface area (adults)[a] Interval: 150–300 mg/kg/day p.o. (3 doses)	MELAS
Lipoic acid	25 mg/kg/day (children) 300–600 mg/day (adults)	MELAS and other mitochondrial disease
Creatine monohydrate	100–300 mg/kg/day divided into three doses (children) 2–10 g/day divided into three doses (adults)	Mitochondrial myopathies

Modified after El-Hattab et al. (2017)

MELAS syndrome mitochondrial encephalomyopathy, lactic acidosis, and stroke-like episodes syndrome, *LHON* Leber hereditary optic neuropathy

[a]Dose is administered within the first 3 h and same dose within 24 h the following 3–5 days

Dichloroacetate increases the catabolism of pyruvate to acetyl-CoA by activation of pyruvate dehydrogenase and therefore improves lactic acidosis in many mitochondrial diseases (Kato et al. 2007). The acetyl-CoA enters the Krebs cycle and by this increases ATP production (oxidative phosphorylation) through the generation of cofactors NADH and FADH2.

Dichloroacetate has been confirmed to reduce lactic acidosis in congenital lactic acidosis (El-Hattab et al. 2017; Parikh et al. 2009).

However, if it also improves the neurological and other clinical outcomes remains controversial to date (Abdelmalak et al. 2013; Barshop et al. 2004; Stacpoole et al. 2006). The safety and tolerability of dichloroacetate are very good in general, but peripheral neuropathy has been observed in individuals with MELAS (mitochondrial encephalomyopathy, lactic acidosis, and stroke-like episodes) syndrome treated with dichloroacetate (El-Hattab et al. 2017; Kaufmann et al. 2006).

Thiamine (vitamin B1) is used in thiamine transporter-2 deficiency, which is caused by mutations in the SLC19A3 gene. Rather high doses of 20 mg/kg/day are needed to treat the neurological symptoms (encephalopathy, Leigh-like syndrome) and lactic acidosis in these patients (Perez-Duenas et al. 2013). As thiamine also enhances pyruvate dehydrogenase activity, it is used in several mitochondrial disorders as monotherapy or in combination, e.g., with CoQ10, carnitine, and vitamins C and E. These combinations can improve lactic acidosis and myopathy in MELAS syndrome and thiamine deficiency (Sato et al. 2000) and symptoms of adult-onset Leigh disease (Mermigkis et al. 2013).

Riboflavin (vitamin B2) promotes the assembly of complexes I and II and catalyzes several enzymatic reactions, e.g., of the ß-oxidation and Krebs cycle. Therefore riboflavin supplementation with the aim to enhance electron transfer has been proposed in a wide range of mitochondriopathies. Evidence from clinical trials that riboflavin supplementation ameliorates symptoms or halts disease progression is only available for complex I (particularly ACAD9 deficiency (Garone et al. 2013; Haack et al. 2010)) and II deficiencies (Bernsen et al. 1993; Bugiani et al. 2006) as well as multiple acyl-CoA dehydrogenase deficiency (Olsen et al. 2007).

2.2 Energy Buffer

Creatine kinase (CK) plays a central role in cellular energy homeostasis. The reversible interconversion of creatine into phosphocreatine generates a pool of rapidly available phosphocreatine for temporal and spatial buffering of ATP levels. This is particularly important in tissues and situation with large and fluctuating energy demands (e.g., muscle and brain). In mitochondrial myopathies the muscle phosphocreatine concentration can be reduced as well as the brain creatine in mitochondrial encephalopathies (Moroni et al. 2002; Tarnopolsky and Parise 1999). Therefore supplementation of creatine monohydrate has been tried as treatment. It improves exercise capacity and strengths in some patients but obviously limited to high-intensity activities (Tarnopolsky et al. 1997), which limit the clinical benefit.

2.3 Antioxidants

Reactive oxidative species (ROS) are generated in small amount during physiological oxidative phosphorylation. Enzymes like glutathione peroxidase and mitochondrial manganese superoxide dismutase scavenge these amounts of ROS under physiological conditions. Under conditions of electron transport chain blockage, ROS production is enhanced, which can cause damage of DNA, proteins, and lipids resulting in cellular dysfunction (Balaban et al. 2005).

Lipoic acid is an organosulfur compound that acts as an essential factor for pyruvate dehydrogenase and has four antioxidant properties: (1) its metal chelating capacity, (2) its ability to scavenge reactive oxygen species (ROS), (3) its ability to regenerate endogenous antioxidants, and (4) its ability to repair oxidative damage. Furthermore it has the capacity to regenerate the endogenous antioxidants vitamin E, vitamin C, and glutathione. Thus it is used in monotherapy and combinations with other oxidants to patients with mitochondrial diseases (Parikh et al. 2009). While the evidence for the efficacy of these vitamins and glutathione alone is limited, the positive effects of lipoic acid on lactic acidosis, urinary oxidative stress markers, and muscle strengths have been shown in a RCT (Rodriguez et al. 2007).

2.4 Restoration of Nitric Oxide Production

Following a number of open-label studies, arginine became the standard treatment for MELAS patients with intravenous infusions during stroke-like episodes and oral arginine during the intervals. This approach led to improved symptoms during episodes and reduced frequency as well as severity of the stroke-like episodes (Koga et al. 2005, 2006, 2007). As MELAS patients have reduced NO concentrations, it is understood that arginine restores adequate NO concentrations and leads to an improved cerebral blood flow. But NO deficiency seems to be an important patho-mechanism not only for stroke-like episodes in MELAS but also for myopathy, lactic acidosis, and diabetes (Koga et al. 2005, 2006, 2007; El-Hattab et al. 2012, 2016; Tengan et al. 2007) and is prevalent in many other mitochondrial diseases like chronic progressive external ophthalmoplegia (CPEO), MERRF (myoclonic epilepsy with ragged red fibers), and MIDD (maternally inherited diabetes and deafness) (Koga et al. 2006; Tengan et al. 2007). Moreover stable isotope studies indicate that citrulline is even more potent as NO precursor than arginine. So far clinical data on the use of citrulline in mitochondriopathy as well as on the use of arginine beyond MELAS are missing.

3 Emerging Therapies

3.1 Stimulation of Mitochondrial Biogenesis

Increasing mitochondrial mass and activity seems a promising approach for improving bioenergetic defects and reduced ATP synthesis in mitochondrial diseases. PGC1 (peroxisome proliferator activated receptor-γ1) plays a major role in mitochondrial biogenesis. PGC1α activates the transcription of OxPhos-related genes and the peroxisomal proliferator activator receptors (PPARs) α, β, and γ, which regulate fatty acid oxidation (Wexler et al. 1997). PBC1α can be modulated pharmacologically (El-Hattab and Scaglia 2013), e.g., by the PPAR agonist bezafibrate, a marketed lipid-lowering drug. Bezafibrate activated mitochondrial biogenesis and increased mitochondrial mass and oxidative phosphorylation in cytochrome c deficient mice (Noe et al. 2013). Improved long-chain fatty acid oxidation, physical activity, and muscle pain were observed in patients with carnitine palmitoyltransferase 2 (CPT2) deficiency. The efficacy and safety of bezafibrate in patients with ETC deficiency are currently being studied in clinical trials.

Resveratrol is a phenol of plant origin. Natural sources of resveratrol include the skin of grapes, blueberries, raspberries, mulberries, and peanuts. Resveratrol activates sirtuins, including SIRT1, which activates PGC1-α. Increased mitochondrial biogenesis upon resveratrol intake has been shown in different mouse models (Komen and Thorburn 2014). *SRT2104* is a novel, first-in-class, highly selective small molecule activator of SIRT1 and was shown to have excellent tolerability and an effect on improved recovery on exercise in elderly individuals (Libri et al. 2012). Both molecules seem promising, but clinical data in mitochondrial diseases are missing.

Aminoimidazole carboxamide ribonucleoside (AICAR) is an intermediate in the generation of inosine monophosphate and an analog of adenosine monophosphate (AMP) that stimulates AMP-dependent protein kinase (AMPK) and by this PGC1-α and mitochondrial biogenesis, as described in mice and in fibroblasts of patients with complex 1 deficiency (Komen and Thorburn 2014; Golubitzky et al. 2011). AICAR is clinically used for the treatment of hyperinsulinemic diabetes, but clinical data on mitochondrial diseases is missing. Moreover performance-enhancing use of AICAR was detected in professional cyclers and other athletes.

Epicatechin is a phenol and catechin prevalent in cacao that increases mitochondrial biogenesis. It is speculated that this effect is mediated via activation of G-protein-coupled estrogen receptor (GPER). In mice epicatechin induces improved exercise performance, fatigue resistance, and enhanced mitochondrial biogenesis (Nogueira et al. 2011). A clinical trial with epicatechin in patients with the mitochondrial disease Friedreich ataxia is currently being conducted (https://clinicaltrials.gov/ct2/show/NCT02660112).

RTA 408 is a synthetic isoprenoid that activates mitochondrial biogenesis via nuclear respiratory factor 2 (Nrf 2) activation (Rai et al. 2015). Based on promising preclinical data (Neymotin et al. 2011), a RCT with RTA 408 in adult patients with mitochondrial myopathy has been started (https://clinicaltrials.gov/ct2/show/NCT02255422).

3.2 Cardiolipin Protection

Elamipretide is a tetrapeptide that binds selectively to cardiolipin, which plays a key role in forming the mitochondrial cristae and other functionally important structures. By its binding to cardiolipin, elamipretide protects cardiolipin from oxidation and the structure and function of the mitochondria (Szeto 2014). A phase 2 trial in 36 patients with primary mitochondrial myopathy showed significantly improved exercise performance in 6-min walking test after 5 days of treatment with elamipretide (Karaa et al. 2018).

4 Gene Therapy

Gene therapy for mitochondrial diseases has been performed in Leber hereditary optic neuropathy (LHON). Adeno-associated virus (AAV) is a feasible vector for the correction of the most common variant in LHON, affecting the mtDNA gene encoding subunit 4 of complex 4 (MT-ND4). In a clinical trial, safety of allotropic gene therapy for LHON was proven. In the treated eyes of 12 patients, the average visual acuity improved (Guy et al. 2017).

References

Abdelmalak M, Lew A, Ramezani R, Shroads AL, Coats BS, Langaee T, Shankar MN, Neiberger RE, Subramony SH, Stacpoole PW (2013) Long-term safety of dichloroacetate in congenital lactic acidosis. Mol Genet Metab 109:139–143

Balaban RS, Nemoto S, Finkel T (2005) Mitochondria, oxidants, and aging. Cell 120:483–495

Barshop BA, Naviaux RK, McGowan KA, Levine F, Nyhan WL, Loupis-Geller A, Haas RH (2004) Chronic treatment of mitochondrial disease patients with dichloroacetate. Mol Genet Metab 83:138–149

Bernsen PL, Gabreels FJ, Ruitenbeek W, Hamburger HL (1993) Treatment of complex I deficiency with riboflavin. J Neurol Sci 118:181–187

Bugiani M, Lamantea E, Invernizzi F, Moroni I, Bizzi A, Zeviani M, Uziel G (2006) Effects of riboflavin in children with complex II deficiency. Brain Dev 28:576–581

Chinnery P (2014) Mitochondrial disorders overview. In: Pagon RA, Adam MP, Ardinger HH, Wallace SE, Amemiya A, Bean LJ (eds) GeneReviews®. University of Washington, Seattle

El-Hattab AW, Scaglia F (2013) Mitochondrial DNA depletion syndromes: review and updates of genetic basis, manifestations, and therapeutic options. Neurotherapeutics 10:186–198

El-Hattab AW, Hsu JW, Emrick LT, Wong LJ, Craigen WJ, Jahoor F, Scaglia F (2012) Restoration of impaired nitric oxide production in MELAS syndrome with citrulline and arginine supplementation. Mol Genet Metab 105:607–614

El-Hattab AW, Emrick LT, Hsu JW, Chanprasert S, Almannai M, Craigen WJ, Jahoor F, Scaglia F (2016) Impaired nitric oxide production in children with MELAS syndrome and the effect of arginine and citrulline supplementation. Mol Genet Metab 117:407–412

El-Hattab AW, Zarante AM, Almannai M, Scaglia F (2017) Therapies for mitochondrial diseases and current clinical trials. Mol Genet Metab 122:1–9

Garone C, Donati MA, Sacchini M, Garcia-Diaz B, Bruno C, Calvo S, Mootha VK, Dimauro S (2013) Mitochondrial encephalomyopathy due to a novel mutation in ACAD9. JAMA Neurol 70:1177–1179

Glover EI, Martin J, Maher A, Thornhill RE, Moran GR, Tarnopolsky MA (2010) A randomized trial of coenzyme Q10 in mitochondrial disorders. Muscle Nerve 42:739–748

Golubitzky A, Dan P, Weissman S, Link G, Wikstrom JD, Saada A (2011) Screening for active small molecules in mitochondrial complex I deficient patient's fibroblasts, reveals AICAR as the most beneficial compound. PLoS One 6:e26883

Guy J, Feuer WJ, Davis JL, Porciatti V, Gonzalez PJ, Koilkonda RD, Yuan H, Hauswirth WW, Lam BL (2017) Gene therapy for leber hereditary optic neuropathy: low- and medium-dose visual results. Ophthalmology 124:1621–1634

Haack TB, Danhauser K, Haberberger B, Hoser J, Strecker V, Boehm D, Uziel G, Lamantea E, Invernizzi F, Poulton J et al (2010) Exome sequencing identifies ACAD9 mutations as a cause of complex I deficiency. Nat Genet 42:1131–1134

Karaa A, Haas R, Goldstein A, Vockley J, Weaver WD, Cohen BH (2018) Randomized dose-escalation trial of elamipretide in adults with primary mitochondrial myopathy. Neurology 90:e1212–e1221

Kato M, Li J, Chuang JL, Chuang DT (2007) Distinct structural mechanisms for inhibition of pyruvate dehydrogenase kinase isoforms by AZD7545, dichloroacetate, and radicicol. Structure 15:992–1004

Kaufmann P, Engelstad K, Wei Y, Jhung S, Sano MC, Shungu DC, Millar WS, Hong X, Gooch CL, Mao X et al (2006) Dichloroacetate causes toxic neuropathy in MELAS: a randomized, controlled clinical trial. Neurology 66:324–330

Klopstock T, Yu-Wai-Man P, Dimitriadis K, Rouleau J, Heck S, Bailie M, Atawan A, Chattopadhyay S, Schubert M, Garip A et al (2011) A randomized placebo-controlled trial of idebenone in Leber's hereditary optic neuropathy. Brain 134:2677–2686

Klopstock T, Metz G, Yu-Wai-Man P, Buchner B, Gallenmuller C, Bailie M, Nwali N, Griffiths PG, von Livonius B, Reznicek L et al (2013) Persistence of the treatment effect of idebenone in Leber's hereditary optic neuropathy. Brain 136:e230

Koga Y, Akita Y, Nishioka J, Yatsuga S, Povalko N, Tanabe Y, Fujimoto S, Matsuishi T (2005) L-arginine improves the symptoms of strokelike episodes in MELAS. Neurology 64:710–712

Koga Y, Akita Y, Junko N, Yatsuga S, Povalko N, Fukiyama R, Ishii M, Matsuishi T (2006) Endothelial dysfunction in MELAS improved by l-arginine supplementation. Neurology 66:1766–1769

Koga Y, Akita Y, Nishioka J, Yatsuga S, Povalko N, Katayama K, Matsuishi T (2007) MELAS and L-arginine therapy. Mitochondrion 7:133–139

Komen JC, Thorburn DR (2014) Turn up the power – pharmacological activation of mitochondrial biogenesis in mouse models. Br J Pharmacol 171:1818–1836

Libri V, Brown AP, Gambarota G, Haddad J, Shields GS, Dawes H, Pinato DJ, Hoffman E, Elliot PJ, Vlasuk GP et al (2012) A pilot randomized, placebo controlled, double blind phase I trial of the novel SIRT1 activator SRT2104 in elderly volunteers. PLoS One 7:e51395

Mermigkis C, Bouloukaki I, Mastorodemos V, Plaitakis A, Alogdianakis V, Siafakas N, Schiza S (2013) Medical treatment with thiamine, coenzyme Q, vitamins E and C, and carnitine improved obstructive sleep apnea in an adult case of Leigh disease. Sleep Breath 17:1129–1135

Moroni I, Bugiani M, Bizzi A, Castelli G, Lamantea E, Uziel G (2002) Cerebral white matter involvement in children with mitochondrial encephalopathies. Neuropediatrics 33:79–85

Neymotin A, Calingasan NY, Wille E, Naseri N, Petri S, Damiano M, Liby KT, Risingsong R, Sporn M, Beal MF et al (2011) Neuroprotective effect of Nrf2/ARE activators, CDDO ethylamide and CDDO trifluoroethylamide, in a mouse model of amyotrophic lateral sclerosis. Free Radic Biol Med 51:88–96

Noe N, Dillon L, Lellek V, Diaz F, Hida A, Moraes CT, Wenz T (2013) RETRACTED: bezafibrate improves mitochondrial function in the CNS of a mouse model of mitochondrial encephalopathy. Mitochondrion 13:417–426

Nogueira L, Ramirez-Sanchez I, Perkins GA, Murphy A, Taub PR, Ceballos G, Villarreal FJ, Hogan MC, Malek MH (2011) (−)-Epicatechin enhances fatigue resistance and oxidative capacity in mouse muscle. J Physiol 589:4615–4631

Olsen RK, Olpin SE, Andresen BS, Miedzybrodzka ZH, Pourfarzam M, Merinero B, Frerman FE, Beresford MW, Dean JC, Cornelius N et al (2007) ETFDH mutations as a major cause of riboflavin-responsive multiple acyl-CoA dehydrogenation deficiency. Brain J Neurol 130:2045–2054

Parikh S, Saneto R, Falk MJ, Anselm I, Cohen BH, Haas R, Medicine Society TM (2009) A modern approach to the treatment of mitochondrial disease. Curr Treat Options Neurol 11:414–430

Perez-Duenas B, Serrano M, Rebollo M, Muchart J, Gargallo E, Dupuits C, Artuch R (2013) Reversible lactic acidosis in a newborn with thiamine transporter-2 deficiency. Pediatrics 131:e1670–e1675

Rai PK, Russell OM, Lightowlers RN, Turnbull DM (2015) Potential compounds for the treatment of mitochondrial disease. Br Med Bull 116:5–18

Rodriguez MC, MacDonald JR, Mahoney DJ, Parise G, Beal MF, Tarnopolsky MA (2007) Beneficial effects of creatine, CoQ10, and lipoic acid in mitochondrial disorders. Muscle Nerve 35:235–242

Rudolph G, Dimitriadis K, Buchner B, Heck S, Al-Tamami J, Seidensticker F, Rummey C, Leinonen M, Meier T, Klopstock T (2013) Effects of idebenone on color vision in patients with leber hereditary optic neuropathy. J Neuroophthalmol 33:30–36

Sato Y, Nakagawa M, Higuchi I, Osame M, Naito E, Oizumi K (2000) Mitochondrial myopathy and familial thiamine deficiency. Muscle Nerve 23:1069–1075

Stacpoole PW, Kerr DS, Barnes C, Bunch ST, Carney PR, Fennell EM, Felitsyn NM, Gilmore RL, Greer M, Henderson GN et al (2006) Controlled clinical trial of dichloroacetate for treatment of congenital lactic acidosis in children. Pediatrics 117:1519–1531

Szeto HH (2014) First-in-class cardiolipin-protective compound as a therapeutic agent to restore mitochondrial bioenergetics. Br J Pharmacol 171:2029–2050

Tarnopolsky MA, Parise G (1999) Direct measurement of high-energy phosphate compounds in patients with neuromuscular disease. Muscle Nerve 22:1228–1233

Tarnopolsky MA, Roy BD, MacDonald JR (1997) A randomized, controlled trial of creatine monohydrate in patients with mitochondrial cytopathies. Muscle Nerve 20:1502–1509

Tengan CH, Kiyomoto BH, Godinho RO, Gamba J, Neves AC, Schmidt B, Oliveira AS, Gabbai AA (2007) The role of nitric oxide in muscle fibers with oxidative phosphorylation defects. Biochem Biophys Res Commun 359:771–777

Wexler ID, Hemalatha SG, McConnell J, Buist NR, Dahl HH, Berry SA, Cederbaum SD, Patel MS, Kerr DS (1997) Outcome of pyruvate dehydrogenase deficiency treated with ketogenic diets. Studies in patients with identical mutations. Neurology 49:1655–1661

GH and IGF-1 Replacement in Children

Roland Pfäffle and Wieland Kiess

Contents

Abstract

In this chapter, we want to give an overview on what we have learned from more than 30 years ago on the use of recombinant human growth hormone (rhGH) and later recombinant human IGF-1 which was introduced for the treatment of short children and what are the safety issues concerned with this treatment. However, rhGH is used not solely in conditions where short stature is the consequence of

R. Pfäffle (✉) · W. Kiess
Department of Pediatric Endocrinology, University Children's Hospital Leipzig, Leipzig, Germany
e-mail: Roland.Pfaeffle@medizin.uni-leipzig.de; rpfaeffle@medizin.uni-leipzig.de

W. Kiess et al. (eds.), *Pediatric Pharmacotherapy*,
Handbook of Experimental Pharmacology 261, https://doi.org/10.1007/164_2019_337

GH deficiency but also in various disorders without a proven GH deficiency. In clinical studies, growth responses to various forms of rhGH therapy were analyzed, adding to our concept about the physiology of growth. Most patients under rhGH treatment show a considerable short-term effect; however, the long-term gain of height in a child obtained by a year-long treatment until final height remains controversial in some of the growth disorders that have been treated with rhGH or IGF-1. Today the first studies on the long-term safety of rhGH treatment have been published and raising some questions whether this treatment is similarly safe for all the patient groups treated with rhGH. Although there is a long-standing safety record for these hormone replacement therapies, in the face of the considerable costs involved, the discussion about the risk to benefit ratio is continuing. Newer developments of rhGH treatment include long-term preparations, which have only to be injected once a week. Although some of these drugs already have proven their non-inferiority to conventional rhGH treatment, we have to await further results to see whether they show improvements in treatment adherence of the patients and prove their long-term safety.

Keywords
Growth hormone · Growth hormone deficiency · Idiopathic short stature · Insulin-like growth factor I · Long-acting growth hormone · Noonan syndrome · Prader-Willi syndrome · Short stature · Small for gestational age · Turner syndrome

Abbreviations

CJD	Creutzfeldt-Jakob disease
EMA	European Medicines Agency
FDA	Food and Drug Administration
GH	Growth hormone, somatropin
GHD	GH deficiency
GHIS	Growth hormone insensitivity syndrome
GHR	Growth hormone receptor
HT	Height
HV	Height velocity
IGFBP-3	Insulin-like growth factor binding protein 3
IGF-I	Insulin-like growth factor 1
IGHD	Isolated growth hormone deficiency
ISS	Idiopathic short stature
NS	Noonan syndrome
PEGylated	(Covalently) bound to polyethylene glycol
PIGFD	Primary insulin-like growth factor 1 deficiency
PTPN11	Protein tyrosine phosphatase, nonreceptor type 11
PWS	Prader-Willi syndrome
rhGH	Recombinant human growth hormone

SDS	Standard deviation (SD) score
SGA	Small for gestational age
SHOX	Short stature homeobox-containing gene
SIR	Standard incidence ratio
SMR	Standard mortality ratio
TS	Turner syndrome

1 Introduction

Growth hormone (somatropin, GH) is a potent metabolic hormone that is important for the metabolism of lipids, carbohydrates, and proteins. In children who have a deficiency of endogenous growth hormone, the use of GH replacement therapy stimulates linear growth and increases growth rate. Human GH (hGH) therapy has been used since the 1950s in children with GHD (Raben 1957), when it was produced by extraction from cadaveric human pituitaries. However, following the occurrence of prion-induced Creutzfeldt-Jakob disease (CJD) in patients treated with contaminated batches of hGH, in 1985, this treatment was halted worldwide. Although the risk was statistically small, there was no means of testing the extract of pooled pituitary glands for the presence of the infecting agent. This decision may also have influenced the upcoming approval of recombinant human GH (rhGH) as a treatment alternative for growth hormone-deficient (GHD) children. Recombinant human insulin has only been approved for some months before, so rhGH is the second biosynthetic molecule, which has been introduced into clinical medicine as a therapeutic agent.

In the late 1970s, recombinant gene technology enabled the expression of the cDNA sequence encoding hGH. Initially, the recombinant protein carried an additional methionine residue at the amino terminus (meth-rhGH). Soon thereafter rhGH was recombinantly expressed in *Escherichia coli* and in eukaryotic cell system was similar to the 22 kd-form of the human growth hormone (Goeddel et al. 1979).

The quantities of rhGH that could be used for the treatment of GHD children increased, and clinicians started studies to optimize treatment strategies with respect to dosing and timing and to study the use of rhGH in short children without GHD. In the years that followed, rhGH treatment was approved for use in various other conditions, including children with chronic renal insufficiency (CRI) in 1993, Turner syndrome (TS) in 1996, Prader-Willi syndrome (PWS) in 2000, short children born small for gestational age (SGA) in 2001, and children with idiopathic short stature (ISS; USA and Canada only) in 2003 (Ranke and Wit 2018) (see Table 1).

In 2005, the European Medicines Agency (EMA) as the first regulatory agency entered a new field when they introduced a legal framework for similar biological medicinal products, also known as biosimilars (Ebbers et al. 2012), which are recombinantly produced macromolecules, which unlike generic drugs cannot be produced and purified following a defined chemical procedure. The "biosimilar" rhGH (Omnitrope®) was the first medicine to be approved via this newly defined

Table 1 Chronology of approvals of rhGH for treatment

Year of approval	Diagnosis	Recommended dose according to approving institution USA (FDA) (μg/kg/day)	Japan (PMDA) mg/kg/week	Europe (EMA) (μg/kg/day)
1985	GHD	23–43	0.175	25–35
1993	Chronic renal failure	50	0.175–0.35	45–50
1996	Turner syndrome	47–67	0.35	45–50
2000	Prader-Willi syndrome	34	0.245	35
2001	Small for gestational age without catch-up growth	67–69	0.23–0.47	35
2003	Idiopathic short stature (ISS)	43–67	Not approved	Not approved
2006	Short stature homeobox-containing gene (SHOX) deficiency	50	Not approved	50
2007	Noonan syndrome	−66	Not approved	Not approved

EMA approval pathway in 2006. The approval of this biosimilar was granted on the basis that it equaled the reference medicine (Genotropin®) in terms of safety, efficacy, and quality. Since this approval, an increasing number of other biosimilar medicines have been approved and used in clinical practice.

2 Pathophysiology of GHD

The GH secretion of a growing child is pulsatile in nature, happening mainly at night, and differs from day to day, as it is affected by numerous factors influencing the regulatory, hypothalamic-pituitary pathways.

Measuring one single GH serum level cannot establish the diagnosis growth hormone deficiency (GHD). Unlike other pituitary hormones, GH is produced in relatively big amounts in the growing child, and already a partial lack of GH secretion might impair longitudinal growth. Although GH secretion evokes many metabolic responses within the organism, these usually have very limited use as reliable surrogate markers for the state of GH deficiency. The best and most often used surrogate markers are serum levels of IGF-I and IGF binding proteins. Although none of them will correlate completely with cumulative GH secretion, and because they are affected by many factors that can influence their production (i.e., general health status, nutrition, liver and kidney function, etc.), these factors are generally used to screen for GHD, as normal levels (e.g., IGF1 > -1.0 SDS) are unlikely in children with GHD.

To make the definitive diagnosis of GHD, however, usually requires two pathological GH stimulation tests. All agents used for provocative testing (insulin, arginine, glucagon, dopamine, etc.) will evoke variable responses of GH secretion (Tillmann et al. 1997; Ghigo et al. 1996).

3 Treatment of GH-Deficient Children with rhGH

The first established indication for the treatment with rhGH is the substitution therapy of GHD. In 1998, the US FDA approved rhGH for the treatment of GHD. GHD should be primarily diagnosed on auxological findings and must biochemically be proven, although this is often difficult and has practical and theoretical limitations.

GH treatment in GHD patients is aimed at normalizing height during childhood and adolescence and to attain an adult height within the normal range. Treatment with rhGH has been proven to be effective in treating short stature in GHD patients, although it has been difficult to show this by the data of controlled studies performed in children with GHD in systematic meta-analyses (Takeda et al. 2010). Controlled trials on GH replacement therapy, however, date back to the very early days of rhGH treatment. With the broader availability of rhGH, treatment has changed entirely to a daily subcutaneous injection to mimic the physiological secretion pattern of human GH. In recent years the average GH dose has also slightly increased. Current consensus guidelines recommend a dose range from 0.025 to 0.05 mg/kg/day, however, where higher doses may be required to attain optimal growth under certain circumstances (Wilson et al. 2003; Growth Hormone Research Society 2001) (Table 2).

Comparing outcomes of studies remains difficult even under standardized GH treatment regimens, as the height gain also relies on various parameters as the severity of GHD, the height and age at start of therapy, and the duration of the

Table 2 Studies in children with GHD treated with rhGH (modified from Ref. (Richmond and Rogol 2010))

Patients *n*	Mean age at start	Mean height SD at start	GH dose mg/kg/day	Mean duration of treatment years	Estimated height gain SD	Reference
13	3.6	−4.1	0.023–0.031	12.2	3.2	(Luca et al. 1996)
18[a]	12.0	−5.6	0.020–0.023	6.2	2.8	(Joss et al. 1983)
25	10.0	−4.5	0.020–0.028	8.6	1.1	(Birnbacher et al. 1998)
88	8.2	−2.9	0.023–0.030	9.9	2.4	(Maghnie et al. 2006)
121	10.8	−3.2	0.043	7.8	2.5	(Blethen 1997)
932	12.0	−2.8	NA	4.9	1.0	(Blethen et al. 1993)
1,034	12.2	−2.8	0.028–0.043	4.6	1.3	(MacGillivray et al. 1998)

[a]These patients were treated with extracted GH

Table 3 Outcome studies in children with SGA treated with rhGH (modified from Ref. (Richmond and Rogol 2010))

Patients *n*	Mean age at start	Mean height SD at start	GH dose mg/kg/day	Mean duration of treatment years	Estimated height gain SD	Reference
28	5.4	−3.6	0.033–0.067	10.0	1.2	(de Zegher and Hokken-Koelega 2005)
54	8.1	−3.0	0.033–0.067	7.8	1.8	(Pareren et al. 2003)
77	10.7	−2.8	0.033	7.0	1.3	(Dahlgren et al. 2005)
91	12.7	−3.2	0.067	2.7	0.6	(Carel et al. 2003)

therapy (Ranke et al. 2010). Therefore, the results of such outcome-studies are listed with some of these important characteristics in Table 3.

4 Treatment of Non-GH-Deficient Children with rhGH

4.1 Children Born Small for Gestational Age (SGA), Without Catch-Up Growth

Most (85–90%) of the children born SGA have a catch-up growth within the first 2 years of their life, although in some children it may take up to 4 years to attain a height within the normal range for their age (Clayton et al. 2007; Lee et al. 2003). For a pediatric endocrinologist, a newborn is small for gestational age (SGA) when the weight and length are below −2 SD for the length of pregnancy.

The FDA in 2001 approved rhGH for the long-term treatment of children with SGA who did not show catch-up growth by the age of 2 years and recommended a dose of up to 0.07 mg/kg/day, whereas the European Medicines Agency (EMA) 1 year later approved the use of rhGH for the treatment of SGA children when they had no catch-up growth up to the age of 4 years and recommended a dose of 0.03 mg/kg/day.

Differences in height gain during treatment of SGA children have also been attributed to factors like parental height, age at the start of therapy, and the duration of therapy. However, the pathophysiological origin of the intrauterine growth retardation, which in many cases remains unsolved, will also affect the response to therapy.

SGA children with IGF-I resistance due to mutations in their IGF-I receptor have high IGF-I serum levels and only show a moderate response to rhGH treatment (Klammt et al. 2011).

The risk to show acute side effects to rhGH treatment seems similar in SGA patients and children with GHD; however, SGA patients have an increased incidence of insulin resistance which temporarily increases under rhGH treatment. They also have a higher risk for the development of metabolic disease in adulthood (Saggese et al. 2013), which should caution the physician not to use higher than the recommended rhGH doses. It therefore seems mandatory to carefully assess the long-term effects of rhGH treatment in these patients (Carel et al. 2012; Sävendahl et al. 2012; Albertsson-Wikland et al. 2016).

4.2 Turner Syndrome

Adult Turner syndrome (TS) patients are in average 20 cm smaller than their female relatives. This growth deficit is attributed to the haploinsufficiency of the SHOX gene, in the pseudoautosomal region of the X chromosome (Rao et al. 1997). Many clinical studies have been performed to estimate the height gain that can be achieved by rhGH treatment in TS patients; however, there exists an uncertainty about the absolute height gain that can be achieved by this treatment. In addition, the timing and dosing of sex steroid replacement therapy at puberty can affect final height in TS patients. A Cochrane Center meta-analysis comprising four studies that compared final height of treated versus untreated patients found a height gain that ranged from 5 to 8 cm (Cave et al. 2003) (Table 4).

Other studies have shown rather consistent results on the height gain using different treatment regimens as outlined in Table 5.

Short-term side effects in TS girls under rhGH treatment seem slightly increased compared to patients with GHD (Bolar et al. 2008); therefore, careful monitoring should be done in this patient group during treatment with rhGH.

4.3 SHOX Deficiency

Short stature in TS patients is mainly attributed to the haploinsufficiency of the SHOX gene on chromosome X. An isolated haploinsufficiency of the SHOX gene, due to a gene deletion or mutation within the gene, is characterized by short stature and may be accompanied other syndromic features like Madelung deformity or disproportionately short extremities. A clinical scoring system was developed to identify those patients, who would most likely profit from a SHOX gene analysis (Rappold et al. 2007). The short stature in TS patients is largely attributed to SHOX gene haploinsufficiency; therefore, it was expected that patients with SHOX deficiency could profit from rhGH therapy. In the prepubertal phase, patients with SHOX deficiency only show a slightly decreased growth rate, but their pubertal growth spurt significantly diminished by a premature growth plate fusion. After the FDA approved rhGH for the treatment of SHOX deficiency in 2006, few reports were published on final height of rhGH-treated SHOX patients; however, the results seem similar to those observed in TS patients (Blum et al. 2013).

Table 4 Outcome studies of girls with TS treated with rhGH (modified from Ref. (Richmond and Rogol 2010))

Patients (number)	Mean age at start (years)	Mean height at start (SD)	GH dose (mg/kg/day)	Mean duration of treatment (years)	Estimated height gain (SD)	Reference
14	10.6	−3.2	0.037–0.111	4.0	1.1	(Carel et al. 1998)
60	9.5	−3.0	0.050	5.9	1.0	(Chernausek et al. 2000)
60	10.9	−2.7	0.047	6.8	0.9	(Pasquino et al. 2005)
68	6.6	−2.8	0.045–0.090	8.6	1.7	(van Pareren et al. 2003)
70	9.3	−3.2	0.054	7.6	1.1	(Rosenfeld et al. 1998)
88	2.0	−1.4	0.050	2.0	1.1	(Davenport et al. 2007)
154	10.3	−3.2	0.050	5.7	1.1	(Stephure and Committee 2005)
188	11.7	−3.7	0.025–0.056	2.4	0.9	(Ranke et al. 2002)
232	9.7	−3.1	0.039–0.051	5.5	1.1	(Quigley et al. 2002)
704	11.9	−3.4	0.043	5.0	1.2	(Soriano-Guillen et al. 2005)

Table 5 Outcome studies of patients with SHOX deficiency treated with rhGH (modified from Ref. (Richmond and Rogol 2010))

Patients (number)	Mean age at start (years)	Mean height at start (SD)	GH dose (mg/kg/day)	Mean duration of treatment (years)	Estimated height gain (SD)	Reference
28	8.3	−3.2	0.037	6.0	1.34	(Blum et al. 2013)
27	7.3	−3.3	0.050	2.0	0.9	(Blum et al. 2007)

4.4 Noonan Syndrome

Noonan syndrome (NS) next to the typical facies and congenital heart defects is characterized by short stature, and the majority of patients have a mutation within the tyrosine-protein phosphatase non-receptor type 11 (PTPN11) gene.

Table 6 Outcome studies of patients with NS treated with rhGH (modified from Ref. (Richmond and Rogol 2010))

Patients *n*	Mean age at start	Mean height SD at start	GH dose mg/kg/ day	Mean duration of treatment years	Estimated height gain SD	Reference
18	8.2	−2.9	0.033–0.066	7.5	1.7	(Osio et al. 2005)
24	7	−3.2	0.025–0.11	7.6	0.6	(Raaijmakers et al. 2008)
29	11	2.7	–0.050	6.4	1.3	(Noordam et al. 2008)

Table 7 Outcome of height in patients with PWS treated with rhGH (modified from Ref. (Richmond and Rogol 2010))

Patients *n*	Mean age at start	Mean height SD at start	GH dose mg/kg/ day	Mean duration of treatment years	Estimated height gain SD	Reference
15	6.8	−1.6	0.037	1	1.2	(Lindgren and Lindberg 2008)
22	6.9	−1.6	0.030–0.060	9.2	1.9	(Lindgren 2006)
35	9.9	−1.1	0.026–0.043	2	0.8	(Myers et al. 2000)
44	4.5	−2.1	0.026–0.043	2	1.6	(Festen et al. 2008)

Children with NS who are treated with rhGH achieved a height of approx. 10 cm exceeding their predicted height (Romano et al. 2009). In the USA rhGH therefore was approved for the treatment of NS children with short stature. So far rhGH has not been approved for treatment of short stature in NS children in Europe.

Because PTPN11 mutations have been found in various malignancies and children with NS have an increased risk for developing malignancies, NS patients treated with rhGH should be carefully monitored for their cardiac function and for a possibly increased incidence of neoplasias (Binder 2009) (Table 6).

4.5 Prader-Willi Syndrome (PWS)

Prader first described patients with PWS in 1956. These patients are characterized by generalized muscular hypotonia and severe feeding problems in early infancy, followed by obesity, growth retardation, hypogonadism, and psychological and behavioral abnormalities. Most of the PWS patients have a deletion or diminished expression of a short segment of chromosome 15 which they inherited from their fathers (Nicholls 1993). It is estimated that this disorder has an incidence of around 1 in 10,000–12,000 newborns (Table 7).

Table 8 Height in patients with ISS treated with rhGH (modified from Ref. (Richmond and Rogol 2010))

Patients *n*	Mean age at start	Mean height SD at start	GH dose mg/kg/day	Mean duration of treatment years	Estimated height gain SD	Reference
68	12.5	−2.7	0.031	4.4	0.5	(Leschek et al. 2004)
50	10.1	−3.2	0.035–0.053	6.5	0.8	(Wit et al. 2005)
80	10.1	−2.7	0.043	5.7	0.7	(Hintz et al. 1999)
29	7.8	−2.1	0.039–0.078	8.0	1.0	(Elder et al. 2008)
126	11.5	−2.7	0.033–0.067	5.9	1.3	(Albertsson-Wikland et al. 2008)

Although only few patients with PWS have GHD, treatment with rhGH has been shown to increase growth and improvement of body composition (see Table 8). Therefore, rhGH treatment of short pediatric PWS patients was approved by the FDA in 2000, and EMA expanded this indication to treat pediatric PWS patients for short stature but also to improve body composition. After the unexplained sudden deaths of several children with PWS under treatment with rhGH, precautions were taken. As all these children suffered from extreme obesity and respiratory abnormalities (Eiholzer 2005), all PWS patients should be thoroughly investigated for the presence of obstructive airway disease prior to rhGH treatment. Obesity is the major problem in patients with PWS with an increased risk of developing type 2 diabetes; therefore, glucose metabolism should be closely monitored in PWS patients treated with rhGH.

4.6 Idiopathic Short Stature (ISS)

In the USA rhGH has also been approved for the treatment of idiopathic short stature (ISS), patients that do not have an otherwise identifiable organic disorder as a cause of their growth impairment, if their height is less than −2.25 SD. These patients most probably constitute a very heterogeneous group of patients. As expected, there is a high variability of responses to treatment among patients with ISS (Table 9).

A Cochrane analysis on the effects of rhGH treatment in ISS found that rhGH treatment increases short-term growth and probably also adult height, although the increase in height does not prevent patients from remaining short in adulthood (Bryant et al. 2007).

Table 9 Incidence of acute side effects

Acute side effect	Estimated incidence
Irritation at injection site	1:10–1:1,000
Exanthema (unspecific)	1:100–1:1,000
Joint or muscle pain	1:100–1:10,000
Headache	1:100–1:1,000
Formation of antibodies against hGH	1:10–1:1,000
Peripheral edema	1:100–1:10,000
Pseudotumor cerebri	1:1,000–1:10,000

5 Dosing of rhGH During Treatment

5.1 Serum IGF-I Serum Levels as Treatment Parameters

Each individual seems to have a different rhGH treatment and shows variable degrees of growth velocity increase during the first years of treatment, accompanied by variable changes in IGF-I serum levels. Usually the rhGH dosage is modified according to body weight or body surface.

IGF-I increases cell proliferation, and clinical studies suggested that elevated serum levels of IGF-I may induce an increased tumor incidence in adults (Samani et al. 2007). So far, however, no clinical study could show that an increased tumor risk is associated with elevated IGF-I level during rhGH treatment in childhood. It is commonly accepted, however, that IGF-I serum levels within the normal range ($\pm$2SD) should not be exceeded during treatment, although it could be demonstrated that children with an IGF-I level in the upper normal range (1.5–2.0 SD) grew better, compared to those that had IGF-I levels in the mid-normal range (Cohen et al. 2007). In summary it seems questionable whether the higher growth rates that can be achieved during initial treatment will result in an improved final height in adulthood.

6 Short- and Long-Term Side Effects of rhGH Treatment

6.1 Short-Term Side Effects of rhGH Treatment

Acute side effects of rhGH treatment occur only rarely, and usually they are benign in nature. It can be summarized that the more severe the GH-deficiency was at the time of diagnosis, the more likely it is that side effects like joint and muscle pain, peripheral edema, or headache will be observed. Usually, a short interruption of treatment or reduction of the applied dose will help to control the symptoms.

The occurrence of antibodies against rhGH is rare, and usually will not interfere with the growth response of the patient. However, patients with GH gene deletions, patients with so called isolated GH deficiency type 1a (IGHD 1a), have the potential to form high titers of GH antibodies that will interfere with the growth response.

6.2 Long-Term Side Effects of rhGH Treatment

The interest in the long-term effects of rhGH treatment has risen in the past decade as rhGH treatment is available now for more than 30 years. In some countries, like in France, a central registry of all patients treated with rhGH was initiated, and initial studies suggested a slightly increased mortality in patients who had received rhGH treatment when compared to an age- and gender-matched population. In about 6,500 patients who received rhGH due to the GHD, SGA, or idiopathic short stature indication, Carel et al. reported a marginal but significant increase in mortality [standard mortality ratio (SMR) of 1.25; 95% confidence interval (CI) 1.0–1.5] (Carel et al. 2012), which was mainly attributable to cardiovascular diseases. Additionally, a dose dependency seemed to be observable, although the number of patients treated with doses in excess of 0.05 mg/kg bodyweight was small. The same group also observed an increased risk for hemorrhagic brain insults (standard incidence ratio, SIR = 1.5 (0.7–2.7)) (Poidvin et al. 2014). These reports raised suspicion, although later meta-analyses from Sweden, Belgium, the Netherlands, and the USA could not confirm these results (Sävendahl et al. 2012; Berglund et al. 2015). These studies have demonstrated how difficult the assessment of long-term treatment risks is in patients who have received rhGH, especially because diagnoses associated with the indications for treatment are very heterogeneous. Also, it could be demonstrated that the morbidity and the mortality risks in patients with short stature due to SGA are inherently different compared to patients with GHD or the general population (Albertsson-Wikland et al. 2016).

7 Long-Acting rhGH Preparations

One of the obstacles associated with rhGH treatment is the necessity of daily injections. This can lead to nonadherence. Nonadherence is suspected to impair the long-term outcome of rhGH treatment in up to 75% of young adults and teenagers (Cutfield et al. 2011).

Numerous innovative pharmaceutical developments have been used to improve rhGH formulations in order to obtain a prolonged effect after administration (Christiansen et al. 2016; Høybye et al. 2015) and thereby to reduce the number of required injections, as the necessity of daily injections seems to be one of the main factors, which interfere with therapy adherence in childhood and adolescence. There are different ways by which these long-acting compounds are modified; six different principles can be differentiated:

1. Depot formulations
2. Fusion proteins of rhGH
3. rhGH molecules bound to albumin
4. rhGH molecules bound to Fab antibodies
5. rhGH molecules covalently bound to polyethylene glycol (PEGylated)
6. Prodrug compounds

Table 10 Different long-acting rhGH formulations under investigation

Technology	Name	Manufacturer	Recommended frequency of injections
Depot	LB03002	LG Life Sciences/ BioPartners	7 days
Depot	CP016	Critical Pharmaceuticals	14 days
Fusion protein	ProFuse GH	Asterion	1 month
Fusion protein	GX-H9	Genexine, Inc.	7–14 days
Fusion protein	LAPSrhGH/ HM10560A	Hanmi Pharmaceutical	7–14 days
Fusion protein	MOD-4023	Pfizer, Inc.	7 days
GH bound to albumin	Somapacitan NNC0195–0092	Novo Nordisk	7 days
GH bound to Fab antibody	AG-B1512	Ahn-Gook Pharmaceutical	14–28 days
PEGylated	BBT-031	Bolder Biotechnology	7 days
PEGylated	Jintrolong	GeneScience Pharmaceuticals	7 days
Prodrug	TransCon ACP-001	Ascendis	7 days

Several long-acting GH formulations have been developed so far, and they have reached different phases within clinical trials (see Table 10). To investigate whether long-acting preparations are effective in treating patients with GHD or idiopathic short stature, clinical trials compare the effect of treatment in respect to growth and to IGF-I serum levels in order to prove non-inferiority to their model-compound rhGH. Although due to the different molecular weights and pharmacokinetics of these formulations, it is difficult to compare these substances directly to their originator compound rhGH, several clinical studies have been performed with a duration of at least 1 year (Chatelain et al. 2017; Zelinska et al. 2017; Luo et al. 2017; Sprogøe et al. 2017; Yuen et al. 2013). Meta-analysis of this data could not find a significant difference between daily rhGH injections and a once weekly high-dose injections of various long-acting rhGH substances in respect to the induced height velocity (HV) and heights (HT SDS) (Yang et al. 2019). The analysis, however, also showed that low-dose long-acting rhGH could not induce a similar HV compared to daily rhGH.

The treatment with long-acting rhGH induced significantly higher IGF-1 serum levels in the first days after injection (Yang et al. 2019), although IGF-I levels stayed within normal limits of ±2SD with one exception (Hwang et al. 2013).

In respect to safety, treatment with high-dose long-acting rhGH was not associated with a higher rate of acute side effects compared to daily injections with rhGH (Yang et al. 2019). In patients receiving long-acting rhGH, the most frequently reported adverse events were injection site pruritus, anemia, hypothyroidism, fever, headache, and vomiting, but these events were classified mostly mild and all resolved spontaneously. Also, no differences were observed in parameters reflecting glucose metabolism serum glucose levels or hemoglobin A1c between patients treated with long-acting rhGH or conventional rhGH therapy.

In conclusion there seems to be no differences between the effects that can be achieved by the treatment between long-acting, mainly weekly injected, rhGH compounds and daily rhGH injections.

However, before long-acting rhGH preparations will be able to significantly improve treatment adherence, multiple inherent obstacles have to be overcome that still exist in the everyday therapy with long-acting rhGH compounds. These include the complexity of preparing the injection, the pain caused by the injections itself, the need for reconstitution of the compound before injection, the type of device that is used for the injections, and others. Future will show whether these obstacles can be overcome.

Although there seems to be no evidence that after an injection of long-acting rhGH, the impact of potentially sustained supraphysiological IGF-1 levels is associated with an increased risk of acute adverse side effects (Christiansen et al. 2016), this does not mean that there are no long-term side effects as have been suggested by other reports (Chan et al. 1998; Hankinson et al. 1998). Therefore, treatment with long-acting rhGH will require close monitoring of the IGF-1 levels during treatment. As long-acting rhGH formulations differ in their pharmacokinetics and the way they influence IGF-1 serum levels, this monitoring needs to consider the pharmacokinetics of each preparation (Christiansen et al. 2016).

8 Treatment with rhIGF-I

A primary deficiency for IGF-I (PIGFD) is a very rare cause for short stature in children and results from primary GH resistance, classically called Laron's syndrome, which is usually caused by mutations in the GH receptor (GHR) or defects within the signaling cascade of the GHR like Stat5b causing the GH insensitivity syndrome (GHIS) (Chernausek et al. 2007). Very rarely GHIS is caused by defects within the signaling IGF-I peptide itself, which are caused by IGF-I gene deletions or mutations.

Even with most modern molecular approaches, the mechanisms causing GHIS in an individual patient cannot be specified.

The following clinical criteria therefore were proposed to define PIGFD:

1. Patients must be very short (height < -3 SD).
2. They should show a normal or even increased GH secretion in classical stimulation tests.
3. They should show a very low IGF-I and IGFBP-3 serum level (<-3 SD), which should not increase during a probatory rhGH treatment.

The last criterion, however, may prove difficult in patients with PIGFD due to IGF-I mutations resulting in a biologically inactive IGF-I as IGF-1 serum levels may be normal when measured in an immunoassay (Netchine et al. 2009).

Both the FDA and EMA approved rhIGF-I (Mecasermin) as an orphan drug for the treatment of PIGFD. Initially rhIGF-I was available in two formulations in the USA, as isolated rhIGF-I (Increlex, mecasermin) and as a protein complex of rhIGF-I bound to IGF-I binding protein-3 (iPlex, mecasermin rinfabate), which after 2007 was no longer available. In theory, the combination of IGF-I and its binding protein IGFBP-3 promised a good option to administer rhIGF-I, because it showed a prolonged bioavailability, whereby the necessity of twice-daily injections of rhIGF-I could be circumvented. Very limited data on the effectiveness of mecasermin rinfabate is available, but this suggests that significantly higher IGF-I doses within the complex would be necessary to induce similar growth rates as obtained in patients treated with rhIGF-I alone.

Studies in patients with GHIS have shown that once- or twice-daily rhIGF-I injections with doses between 40 and 120 μg/kg/day induced a significant increase of growth in children with severe GHIS (Ranke 2015). Long-term treatment with rhIGF-1 can double the growth rate of GHIS patients from an average of 4.0 cm/year before therapy to an average of 9.3 cm/year during the first year, 6.2 cm/year during the second year, and to an average of 4.8 cm/year thereafter. However, the mean height of these patients was very short with −5.6 SDS before treatment and could just be improved to −4.2 SDS after 6 years of rhIGF-I treatment (Chernausek et al. 2007; Backeljauw and Underwood 2001). This increase in height appears small compared to the results that can be obtained in children with GHD by rhGH treatment; however, this has to be seen on the background that patients with severe GHIS can achieve adult heights between −4 and −10 SDS if not treated. At present rhIGF-I treatment only improves adult height in GHIS patients; however, it cannot achieve normal adult height. This may be due in part to the fact that rhIGF-I replacement cannot compensate completely for the missing GH action (Richmond and Rogol 2008), which could be explained by several mechanisms: Firstly, rhIGF-I treatment alone fails to induce IGFBP-3 and ALS production, which results in suboptimal levels of the IGF-I transport complex delivering less IGF-I to target tissues. Secondly, pituitary GH production is suppressed by rhIGF-I administration resulting in decreased levels of GH in the growth plate. Thirdly, this lack of hGH may also impair local IGF-I production within the growth plate.

9 Side Effects of rhIGF-I Treatment

The most frequent adverse event reported in patients treated with rhIGF-I, which can be dangerous, is hypoglycemia due to the insulin-like effect of IGF-1. Although patients with GHIS seem more prone to hypoglycemic episodes, these can be accelerated by rhIGF-I treatment and so severe that hypoglycemic seizures occur. The medication therefore should be divided into two daily injections given shortly before or after a meal or snack to prevent hypoglycemic episodes. Monitoring of preprandial glucose is advised in the initial phase of rhIGF-I treatment and should be continued until the dosage of rhIGF-I is proven to be well-tolerated and effective (Richmond and Rogol 2008). Other side effects of rhIGF-I treatment are the hypertrophy of lymphoid tissue induced by rhIGF-I which can result in hypoacusis and snoring (reported in up to 22% of patients), headache or benign intracranial pressure (approx. 5%), lipohypertrophy at the injection site, and acromegaloid coarsening of the face (which occurs especially around puberty).

10 Conclusion

Since its introduction more than 30 years ago, the indications for rhGH treatment have widened, and it has been shown to increase adult height in several conditions and seems to be a safe therapy during treatment. Carefully designed long-term studies are still needed to assess and weigh the costs (economic, social, and psychological) and benefits (height gain, metabolic changes, and changes in quality of life) of treatment. Also, some of the questions that were raised on the long-term side effects of treatment still need to be addressed in the future. Long-acting substances of rhGH hold the promise to improve treatment adherence of this long-term-treatment; however, this has to be proven and long-term safety issues need to be monitored closely. Treatment with rhIGF-I is a treatment option in patients with PIGFD; however, this diagnosis is very rare, and treatment outcome seems not as those that can be achieved with rhGH in GHD patients.

References

Albertsson-Wikland K, Aronson SA, Gustafsson J, Hagenäs L, Ivarsson SA, Jonsson B et al (2008) Dose-dependent effect of growth hormone on final height in children with short stature without growth hormone deficiency. J Clin Endocrinol Metabol 93:4342–4350

Albertsson-Wikland K, Mårtensson A, Sävendahl L, Niklasson A, Bang P, Dahlgren J et al (2016) Mortality is not increased in recombinant human growth hormone-treated patients when adjusting for birth characteristics. J Clin Endocrinol Metabol 101:2149–2159

Backeljauw PF, Underwood LE (2001) Therapy for 6.5–7.5 years with recombinant insulin-like growth factor I in children with growth hormone insensitivity syndrome: a clinical research center study 1. J Clin Endocrinol Metabol 86:1504–1510

Berglund A, Gravholt C, Olsen M, Christiansen J, Stochholm K (2015) Growth hormone replacement does not increase mortality in patients with childhood-onset growth hormone deficiency. Clin Endocrinol (Oxf) 83:677–683

Binder G (2009) Response to growth hormone in short children with Noonan syndrome: correlation to genotype. Horm Res Paediatr 72:52–56

Birnbacher R, Riedl S, Frisch H (1998) Long-term treatment in children with hypopituitarism: pubertal development and final height. Horm Res Paediatr 49:80–85

Blethen S (1997) Adult height in growth hormone (GH)-deficient children treated with biosynthetic GH. J Clin Endocrinol Metabol 82:418–420

Blethen S, Compton P, Lippe B, Rosenfeld R, August G, Johanson A (1993) Factors predicting the response to growth hormone (GH) therapy in prepubertal children with GH deficiency. J Clin Endocrinol Metabol 76:574–579

Blum WF, Crowe BJ, Quigley CA, Jung H, Cao D, Ross JL et al (2007) Growth hormone is effective in treatment of short stature associated with short stature homeobox-containing gene deficiency: two-year results of a randomized, controlled, multicenter trial. J Clin Endocrinol Metabol 92:219–228

Blum WF, Ross JL, Zimmermann AG, Quigley CA, Child CJ, Kalifa G et al (2013) GH treatment to final height produces similar height gains in patients with SHOX deficiency and Turner syndrome: results of a multicenter trial. J Clin Endocrinol Metabol 98:E1383–E1392

Bolar K, Hoffman AR, Maneatis T, Lippe B (2008) Long-term safety of recombinant human growth hormone in turner syndrome. J Clin Endocrinol Metabol 93:344–351

Bryant J, Baxter L, Cave CB, Milne R (2007) Recombinant growth hormone for idiopathic short stature in children and adolescents. Cochrane Db Syst Rev:CD004440

Carel J-C, Mathivon L, Gendrel C, Ducret J-P, Chaussain J-L (1998) Near normalization of final height with adapted doses of growth hormone in Turner's syndrome. J Clin Endocrinol Metabol 83:1462–1466

Carel J-C, Chatelain P, Rochiccioli P, Chaussain J-L (2003) Improvement in adult height after growth hormone treatment in adolescents with short stature born small for gestational age: results of a randomized controlled study. J Clin Endocrinol Metab 88:1587–1593. https://doi.org/10.1210/jc.2002-021123

Carel J-C, Ecosse E, Landier F et al (2012) Long-term mortality after recombinant growth hormone treatment for isolated growth hormone deficiency or childhood short stature: preliminary report of the French SAGhE study. J Clin Endocrinol Metab 97:416–425. https://doi.org/10.1210/jc.2011-1995

Cave CB, Bryant J, Milne R (2003) Recombinant growth hormone in children and adolescents with Turner syndrome. Cochrane Database Syst Rev 2003(1). Art. No.: CD003887. https://doi.org/10.1002/14651858.CD003887. www.cochranelibrary.com

Chan JM, Stampfer MJ, Giovannucci E, Gann PH, Ma J, Wilkinson P et al (1998) Plasma insulin-like growth factor-I and prostate cancer risk: a prospective study. Science 279:563–566

Chatelain P, Malievsky O, Radziuk K, Senatorova G, Abdou MO, Vlachopapadopolou E et al (2017) A randomized phase 2 study of long-acting TransCon GH vs daily GH in childhood GH deficiency. J Clin Endocrinol Metabol 102:1673–1682

Chernausek SD, Attie KM, Cara JF, Rosenfeld RG, Frane J (2000) Growth hormone therapy of Turner syndrome: the impact of age of estrogen replacement on final height 1. J Clin Endocrinol Metabol 85:2439–2445

Chernausek SD, Backeljauw PF, Frane J, Kuntze J, Underwood LE, Group IG (2007) Long-term treatment with recombinant insulin-like growth factor (IGF)-I in children with severe IGF-I deficiency due to growth hormone insensitivity. J Clin Endocrinol Metabol 92:902–910

Christiansen J, Backeljauw PF, Bidlingmaier M, Biller BM, Boguszewski MC, Casanueva FF et al (2016) Growth Hormone Research Society perspective on the development of long-acting growth hormone preparations. Eur J Endocrinol 174:C1–C8

Clayton P, Cianfarani S, Czernichow P, Johannsson G, Rapaport R, Rogol A (2007) Management of the child born small for gestational age through to adulthood: a consensus statement of the International Societies of Pediatric Endocrinology and the Growth Hormone Research Society. J Clin Endocrinol Metabol 92:804–810

Cohen P, Rogol AD, Howard CP, Bright GM, Kappelgaard A-M, Rosenfeld RG et al (2007) Insulin growth factor-based dosing of growth hormone therapy in children: a randomized, controlled study. J Clin Endocrinol Metabol 92:2480–2486

Cutfield WS, Derraik JG, Gunn AJ, Reid K, Delany T, Robinson E et al (2011) Non-compliance with growth hormone treatment in children is common and impairs linear growth. Plos One 6: e16223

Dahlgren J, Wikland K, Swedish Study Group for Growth Hormone Treatment (2005) Final height in short children born small for gestational age treated with growth hormone. Pediatr Res 57:216–222

Davenport ML, Crowe BJ, Travers SH, Rubin K, Ross JL, Fechner PY et al (2007) Growth hormone treatment of early growth failure in toddlers with Turner syndrome: a randomized, controlled, multicenter trial. J Clin Endocrinol Metabol 92:3406–3416 de Zegher F, Hokken-Koelega A (2005) Growth hormone therapy for children born small for gestational age: height gain is less dose dependent over the long term than over the short term. Pediatrics 115:e458–e462

Ebbers HC, Crow SA, Vulto AG, Schellekens H (2012) Interchangeability, immunogenicity and biosimilars. Nat Biotechnol 30:1186

Eiholzer U (2005) Deaths in children with Prader-Willi syndrome. Horm Res Paediatr 63:33–39

Elder CJ, Barton JS, Brook CGD, Preece MA, Dattani MT, Hindmarsh PC (2008) A randomised study of the effect of two doses of biosynthetic human growth hormone on final height of children with familial short stature. Horm Res Paediatr 70:89–92

Festen DA, van Wijngaarden R, Eekelen M, Otten BJ, Wit JM, Duivenvoorden HJ et al (2008) Randomized controlled GH trial: effects on anthropometry, body composition and body proportions in a large group of children with Prader–Willi syndrome. Clin Endocrinol (Oxf) 69:443–451

Ghigo E, Bellone J, Aimaretti G, Bellone S, Loche S, Cappa M et al (1996) Reliability of provocative tests to assess growth hormone secretory status. Study in 472 normally growing children. J Clin Endocrinol Metabol 81:3323–3327

Goeddel DV, Heyneker HL, Hozumi T, Arentzen R, Itakura K, Yansura DG et al (1979) Direct expression in Escherichia coli of a DNA sequence coding for human growth hormone. Nature 281:281544a0

Growth Hormone Research Society (2001) Consensus guidelines for the diagnosis and treatment of growth hormone (GH) deficiency in childhood and adolescence: summary statement of the GH Research Society. J Pediatr Endocrinol Metabol 14:377–382

Hankinson SE, Willett WC, Colditz GA, Hunter DJ, Michaud DS, Deroo B et al (1998) Circulating concentrations of insulin-like growth factor I and risk of breast cancer. Lancet 351:1393–1396

Hintz RL, Attie KM, Baptista J, Roche A (1999) Effect of growth hormone treatment on adult height of children with idiopathic short stature. N Engl J Med 340:502–507

Høybye C, Cohen P, Hoffman AR, Ross R, Biller B, Christiansen J et al (2015) Status of long-acting-growth hormone preparations – 2015. Growth Horm IGF Res 25:201–206

Hwang J, Lee H, Chung W, Han H-S, Jin D-K, Kim H-S et al (2013) Efficacy and safety of LB03002, a once-weekly sustained-release human GH for 12-month treatment in Korean children with GH deficiency. Eur J Endocrinol 169:179–185

Joss E, Zuppinger K, Schwarz H, Roten H (1983) Final height of patients with pituitary growth failure and changes in growth variables after long term hormonal therapy. Pediatr Res 17: pr1983158

Klammt J, Kiess W, Pfäffle R (2011) IGF1R mutations as cause of SGA. Best Pract Res Clin Endocrinol Metabol 25:191–206

Lee PA, Chernausek SD, Hokken-Koelega AC, Czernichow P, International Small for Gestational Age Advisory Board (2003) International Small for Gestational Age Advisory Board consensus development conference statement: management of short children born small for gestational age, April 24–October 1, 2001. Pediatrics 111:1253–1261

Leschek E, Rose SR, Yanovski JA, Troendle JF, Quigley CA, Chipman JJ et al (2004) Effect of growth hormone treatment on adult height in peripubertal children with idiopathic short stature: a randomized, double-blind, placebo-controlled trial. J Clin Endocrinol Metabol 89:3140–3148

Lindgren AC (2006) Somatropin therapy for children with Prader-Willi syndrome. Treat Endocrinol 5:223–228

Lindgren AC, Lindberg A (2008) Growth hormone treatment completely normalizes adult height and improves body composition in Prader-Willi syndrome: experience from KIGS (Pfizer International Growth Database). Horm Res Paediatr 70:182–187

Luca DF, Maghnie M, Arrigo T, Lombardo F, Messina M, Bernasconi S (1996) Final height outcome of growth hormone-deficient patients treated since less than five years of age. Acta Paediatr 85:1167–1171

Luo X, Hou L, Liang L, Dong G, Shen S, Zhao Z et al (2017) Long-acting PEGylated recombinant human growth hormone (Jintrolong) for children with growth hormone deficiency: phase II and phase III multicenter, randomized studies. Eur J Endocrinol 177:195–205

MacGillivray M, Blethen S, Buchlis J, Clopper R, Sandberg D, Conboy T (1998) Current dosing of growth hormone in children with growth hormone deficiency: how physiologic? Pediatrics 102:527–530

Maghnie M, Ambrosini L, Cappa M, Pozzobon G, Ghizzoni L, Ubertini M et al (2006) Adult height in patients with permanent growth hormone deficiency with and without multiple pituitary hormone deficiencies. J Clin Endocrinol Metabol 91:2900–2905

Myers SE, Carrel AL, Whitman BY, Allen DB (2000) Sustained benefit after 2 years of growth hormone on body composition, fat utilization, physical strength and agility, and growth in Prader-Willi syndrome. J Pediatr 137:42–49

Netchine I, Azzi S, Houang M, Seurin D, Perin L, Ricort J-M et al (2009) Partial primary deficiency of insulin-like growth factor (IGF)-I activity associated with IGF1 mutation demonstrates its critical role in growth and brain development. J Clin Endocrinol Metabol 94:3913–3921

Nicholls RD (1993) Genomic imprinting and uniparental disomy in Angelman and Prader-Willi syndromes: a review. Am J Med Genet 46:16–25

Noordam C, Peer P, Francois I, Schepper DJ, van den Burgt I, Otten B (2008) Long-term GH treatment improves adult height in children with Noonan syndrome with and without mutations in protein tyrosine phosphatase, non-receptor-type 11. Eur J Endocrinol 159:203–208

Osio D, Dahlgren J, Wikland K, Westphal O (2005) Improved final height with long-term growth hormone treatment in Noonan syndrome. Acta Paediatr 94:1232–1237

Pareren Y, Mulder P, Houdijk M, Jansen M, Reeser M, Hokken-Koelega A (2003) Adult height after long-term, continuous growth hormone (GH) treatment in short children born small for gestational age: results of a randomized, double-blind, dose-response GH trial. J Clin Endocrinol Metabol 88:3584–3590

Pasquino A, Pucarelli I, Segni M, Tarani L, Calcaterra V, Larizza D (2005) Adult height in sixty girls with Turner syndrome treated with growth hormone matched with an untreated group. J Endocrinol Invest 28:350–356

Poidvin A, Touzé E, Ecosse E, Landier F, Béjot Y, Giroud M et al (2014) Growth hormone treatment for childhood short stature and risk of stroke in early adulthood. Neurology 83:780–786

Quigley CA, Crowe BJ, Anglin GD, Chipman JJ (2002) Growth hormone and low dose estrogen in turner syndrome: results of a united states multi-center trial to near-final height. J Clin Endocrinol Metabol 87:2033–2041

Raaijmakers R, Noordam C, Karagiannis G, Gregory JW, Hertel NT, Sipilä I et al (2008) Response to growth hormone treatment and final height in Noonan syndrome in a large cohort of patients in the KIGS database. J Pediatr Endocrinol Metabol 21:267–274

Raben M (1957) Preparation of growth hormone from pituitaries of man and monkey. Science 125:883–884

Ranke MB (2015) Treatment with recombinant human insulin-like growth factor-1 in severe primary IGF deficiency and beyond. Horm Res Paediatr 83:358–360

Ranke MB, Wit JM (2018) Growth hormone – past, present and future. Nat Rev Endocrinol 14:285

Ranke PC, Lindberg A, Dorr H, Bettendorf M, Hauffa B et al (2002) Adult height after GH therapy in 188 Ullrich-Turner syndrome patients: results of the German IGLU Follow-up Study 2001. Eur J Endocrinol 147:625–633

Ranke MB, Lindberg A, Board K (2010) Observed and predicted growth responses in prepubertal children with growth disorders: guidance of growth hormone treatment by empirical variables. J Clin Endocrinol Metabol 95:1229–1237

Rao E, Weiss B, Fukami M, Rump A, Niesler B, Mertz A et al (1997) Pseudoautosomal deletions encompassing a novel homeobox gene cause growth failure in idiopathic short stature and Turner syndrome. Nat Genet 16:54–63

Rappold G, Blum WF, Shavrikova EP, Crowe BJ, Roeth R, Quigley CA et al (2007) Genotypes and phenotypes in children with short stature: clinical indicators of SHOX haploinsufficiency. J Med Genet 44:306

Richmond EJ, Rogol AD (2008) Recombinant human insulin-like growth factor-I therapy for children with growth disorders. Adv Ther 25:1276
Richmond E, Rogol AD (2010) Current indications for growth hormone therapy for children and adolescents. Endocr Dev 18:92–108
Romano AA, Dana K, Bakker B, Davis AD, Hunold J, Jacobs J et al (2009) Growth response, near-adult height, and patterns of growth and puberty in patients with Noonan syndrome treated with growth hormone. J Clin Endocrinol Metabol 94:2338–2344
Rosenfeld RG, Attie KM, Frane J, Brasel A, Burstein S, Cara JF et al (1998) Growth hormone therapy of Turner's syndrome: beneficial effect on adult height. J Pediatr 132:319–324
Saggese G, Fanos M, Simi F (2013) SGA children: auxological and metabolic outcomes – the role of GH treatment. J Matern Fetal Neonatal Med 26:64–67
Samani A, Yakar S, LeRoith D, Brodt P (2007) The role of the IGF system in cancer growth and metastasis: overview and recent insights. Endocr Rev 28:20–47
Sävendahl L, Maes M, Albertsson-Wikland K, Borgström B, Carel J-C, Henrard S et al (2012) Long-term mortality and causes of death in isolated GHD, ISS, and SGA patients treated with recombinant growth hormone during childhood in Belgium, The Netherlands, and Sweden: preliminary report of 3 countries participating in the EU SAGhE study. J Clin Endocrinol Metabol 97:E213–E217
Soriano-Guillen L, Coste J, Ecosse E, Léger J, Tauber M, Cabrol S et al (2005) Adult height and pubertal growth in turner syndrome after treatment with recombinant growth hormone. J Clin Endocrinol Metabol 90:5197–5204
Sprogøe K, Mortensen E, Karpf DB, Leff JA (2017) The rationale and design of TransCon growth hormone for the treatment of growth hormone deficiency. Endocr Connect 6:R171–R181
Stephure DK, Committee C (2005) Impact of growth hormone supplementation on adult height in Turner syndrome: results of the canadian randomized controlled trial. J Clin Endocrinol Metabol 90:3360–3366
Takeda A, Cooper K, Bird A, Baxter L, Frampton G, Gospodarevskaya E et al (2010) Recombinant human growth hormone for the treatment of growth disorders in children: a systematic review and economic evaluation. Health Technol Assess (Winch Eng) 14:1–209. iii–iv
Tillmann V, Buckler JM, Kibirige MS, Price DA, Shalet SM, Wales JK et al (1997) Biochemical tests in the diagnosis of childhood growth hormone deficiency 1. J Clin Endocrinol Metabol 82:531–535
van Pareren YK, de Keizer-Schrama SM, Stijnen T, Sas TC, Jansen M, Otten BJ et al (2003) Final height in girls with Turner syndrome after long-term growth hormone treatment in three dosages and low dose estrogens. J Clin Endocrinol Metabol 88:1119–1125
Wilson TA, Rose SR, Cohen P, Rogol AD, Backeljauw P, Brown R et al (2003) Update of guidelines for the use of growth hormone in children: the Lawson Wilkins pediatric endocrinology society drug and therapeutics committee. J Pediatr 143:415–421
Wit JM, Rekers-Mombarg L, Cutler GB, Crowe B, Beck TJ, Roberts K et al (2005) Growth hormone (GH) treatment to final height in children with idiopathic short stature: evidence for a dose effect. J Pediatr 146:45–53
Yang Y, Bai X, Yuan X, Zhang Y, Chen S, Yang H et al (2019) Efficacy and safety of long-acting growth hormone in children with short stature: a systematic review and meta-analysis. Endocrine 65:25–34
Yuen KC, Conway GS, Popovic V, Merriam GR, Bailey T, Hamrahian AH et al (2013) A long-acting human growth hormone with delayed clearance (VRS-317): results of a double-blind, placebo-controlled, single ascending dose study in growth hormone–deficient adults. J Clin Endocrinol Metabol 98:2595–2603
Zelinska N, Iotova V, Skorodok J, Malievsky O, Peterkova V, Samsonova L et al (2017) Long-acting C-terminal peptide–modified hGH (MOD-4023): results of a safety and dose-finding study in GHD children. J Clin Endocrinol Metabol 102:1578–1587

Pharmacotherapy in Rare Skeletal Diseases

Heike Hoyer-Kuhn and Eckhard Schönau

Contents

Abstract

New therapeutic approaches have been established in the field of rare skeletal diseases (e.g., for osteogenesis imperfecta, achondroplasia, hypophosphatemic rickets, hypophosphatasia, and fibrodysplasia ossificans progressiva). After elucidation of the underlying genotypes and pathophysiologic alterations of these diseases, new treatment options have been designed. Most drugs are based on an

H. Hoyer-Kuhn (✉)
Faculty of Medicine, University of Cologne, Cologne, Germany

Department of Paediatrics, University Hospital Cologne, Cologne, Germany
e-mail: heike-katharina.hoyer-kuhn@uk-koeln.de

E. Schönau
Faculty of Medicine, University of Cologne, Cologne, Germany

Department of Paediatrics, University Hospital Cologne, Cologne, Germany

Center for Prevention and Rehabilitation, Unireha, University of Cologne, Cologne, Germany
e-mail: eckhard.schoenau@uk-koeln.de

W. Kiess et al. (eds.), *Pediatric Pharmacotherapy*,
Handbook of Experimental Pharmacology 261, https://doi.org/10.1007/164_2019_305

interaction with the disease-specific cascade of enzymes and proteins involved in the disease. Thereby an approved treatment is available for children with severe forms of hypophosphatasia and hypophosphatemic rickets (asfotase alfa, burosumab). Additionally, there are different phase 3 trials ongoing assessing the efficacy and safety of drugs for osteogenesis imperfecta, achondroplasia, and fibrodysplasia ossificans progressiva (denosumab, vosoritide, palovarotene).

Because all these diseases are rare, the number of investigated patients in the trials is small, and the knowledge about rare side effects and long-term outcome is limited. Therefore it is recommended to treat the patients in specialized centers where the effects of the drugs can be evaluated and data about safety, side effects, and efficacy can be collected.

Based on the fact that most drugs for rare diseases are highly expensive clear indications for start of a treatment, evaluation of the therapy and recommendations how long a treatment has to be administrated are urgently needed.

Keywords
Bisphosphonates · Denosumab · Rare skeletal disease

1 Introduction

A rare disease is defined as a disease which affects less than 1 of 2,500 people. After optimizing diagnostic pathways in rare diseases in general, the possibility to confirm a clinical diagnosis by genetic or biochemical analyses has increased. Due to the elucidation of pathophysiologic pathways of the most frequent rare skeletal diseases, new drugs have been successfully regenerated for rare skeletal diseases (e.g., osteogenesis imperfecta (OI), hypophosphatemic rickets, hypophosphatasia (HPP), achondroplasia, and fibrodysplasia ossificans progressiva (FOP)).

Depending on the pathophysiologic steps of bone metabolism (formation, degradation, adaptation (modeling, remodeling of the bone)), most diseases could be assigned to one of these steps. Disorders as achondroplasia and osteogenesis imperfecta are caused by formation alterations in the growth plates or collagen production and processing – the first step for bone formation (non-mineralized bone matrix also called osteoid). Rickets are caused by an altered mineralization process (reduced amount of calcium and/or phosphate, reduced amount/function of the alkaline phosphatase). Finally remodeling of bones is performed by the interaction of osteoblasts and osteoclasts. Osteocytes work as an interfering factor between osteoblasts and osteoclasts, but the kind of action of the osteocytes is still not fully elucidated. Especially the muscle forces applied to the bones are the most important osteoanabolic stimulus leading to bone formation and remodeling processes which are essential for bone strength (this interaction was described by Harald Frost and analyzed by Eckhard Schoenau in the last 30 years as "functional muscle bone unit," Schoenau and Frost 2002). A schematic overview of these processes, exemplary representation of resulting diseases in case of alterations, and therapeutic options are displayed in Fig. 1 (Hoyer-Kuhn et al. 2017).

Steps during bone formation	Pathophysiology	Disease	Drug used in these diseases
Step 1: Synthesis of Osteoid 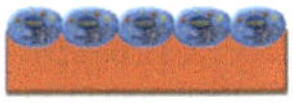	Reduced Stimulation Impaired Synthesis	Osteogenesis Imperfecta	Bisphosphonates Denosumab Antisclerostin
Step 2: Mineralisation 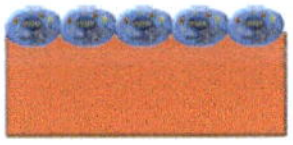	Diseases of Calcium- and Phosphate-metabolism	Hypophosphatemic Rickets Hypophosphatasia	Burosumab Asfotase alfa
Step 3: Remodelling 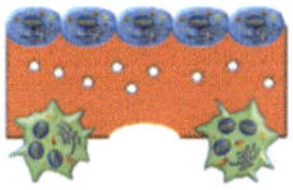	Immobilisation Inflammation Impaired regulation of osteoblasts and osteoclasts	Muscle dystrophy Chronic inflammatory diseases Fibrous dysplasia	Steroids Immunosuppressive drugs Bisphosphonates

Fig. 1 Schematic overview of bone formation and diseases. Schematic overview of the main steps of bone formation. The various diseases manifested through physiological alterations in bone formation, mineralization, and remodeling and the potential drugs that are used in the management of the disease. These drugs don't necessarily target the underlying pathophysiology in the disease but are symptomatic in some diseases

Additionally, alterations of the proteins of bone matrix can cause skeletal diseases. Increased activation of the *ACVR1/ALK2*-Gen (fibrodysplasia ossificans progressiva) cause extraskeletal bone formation (heterotopic ossification) resulting in progressive immobility of the patients accompanied by a reduced life expectancy (Shore et al. 2006).

In fibrous dysplasia (FD), bone growth and modeling/remodeling processes are disturbed leading to additional bone with a woven structure on the long bones/craniofacial bones. In some cases, FD goes along with endocrine disturbances (ovarian cysts in girls, growth hormone excess, hyperthyroidism, precocious puberty, neonatal hypercortisolism) known as McCune-Albright syndrome (Javaid et al. 2019).

2 Drugs

2.1 Supplements

Calcium and vitamine D analoga are used in most bone diseases to assure a normal mineralization process. Usually both drugs are given orally. In case of a high and rapid need of calcium, calcium could also be applicated intravenously as calcium gluconate 10%.

Vitamine D is available as colecalciferol or activated vitamine D calcitriol. Based on the underlying cause of vitamine D deficiency, one or both vitamine D preparations could be supplemented.

In rare bone diseases, a clear pathophysiologic adapted treatment regimen is needed as high doses of supplements also can be contraindicated. In diseases with a reduced availability of minerals like in hypocalcemic or hypophosphatemic rickets, administration of minerals is essential and should be done adapted to the current guidelines (Munns et al. 2016). In other diseases where minerals cannot be incorporated into the bone matrix (HPP or OI), a high dose of minerals are contraindicated due to the risk of nephrocalcinosis (Bishop 2015).

2.2 Antiresorptives

2.2.1 Bisphosphonates

Bisphosphonates are drugs used for decades in adults but also in children with rare bone diseases (Astrom and Soderhall 1998). For children they are still not approved. As off-label use, bisphosphonates have been used in children with osteogenesis imperfecta, fibrous dysplasia, and secondary osteoporosis to reduce number of fractures, decrease chronic pain, and increase bone mineral density and mobility (Glorieux et al. 1995; Astrom and Soderhall 1998; Lala et al. 2000; Plotkin et al. 2003; Chan and Zacharin 2006; Glorieux and Rauch 2006; Land et al. 2006). Bisphosphonates bind to mineralized bone (hydroxyapatites) causing apoptosis of osteoclasts after being resorbed by them. As antiresorptive agents, they only preserve bone but are not osteoanabolic. The reduced bone resorption combined with an intensive physical training inducing bone formation led to an increase in quality of life of the patients during the last decades (Marini et al. 2017).

2.2.2 Denosumab: A RANKL Antibody

Denosumab (a monoclonal RANKL (anti-receptor activator of nuclear factor κB ligand) antibody) was approved in 2009 as treatment option for adults with osteoporosis (Cummings et al. 2009). Denosumab is a fully human monoclonal antibody inhibiting osteoclastic-driven bone resorption by binding to osteoblast-produced RANKL (Fig. 2). It is not approved for children yet. First experiences in childhood are published in the last years for children with OI, FD, and giant-cell tumor (Boyce et al. 2012; Semler et al. 2012b; Shroff et al. 2012; Grasemann et al. 2013; Hoyer-Kuhn et al. 2014a, b, c, 2016b; Wang et al. 2014). Denosumab was only used in an off-label setting in children until today. Results of an international phase 3 trial assessing the safety and efficacy of denosumab in 150 children with OI are awaited in 2020 (NCT02352753).

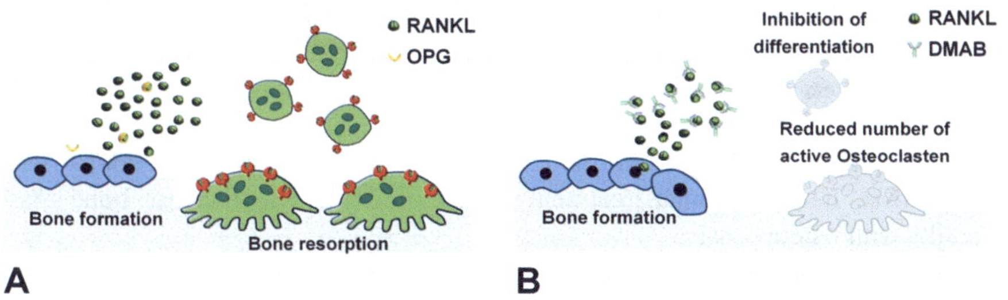

Fig. 2 RANKL/OPG interplay in bone metabolism and denosumab as a blocking agent. RANKL/OPG (receptor activator of NF-κB ligand/osteoprotegerin) interaction in bone formation and bone resorption processes. (**a**) Active RANKL increase differentiation and number of osteoclasts. Therefore bone resorption is increased. (**b**) Denosumab (DMAB) as a monoclonal antibody inactivates RANKL (mimicking the effect of OPG), stops differentiation of pre-osteoclasts, and, thereby, reduces bone resorption

2.3 Monoclonal Antibodies

2.3.1 Denosumab: A RANKL Antibody (See Sect. 2.2.2)

Burosumab: A FGFR23 Antibody

Burosumab is a monoclonal antibody binding to fibroblast growth factor 23 (FGF23) – a highly phosphaturic factor leading to a diminished mineralization of the bones when produced in an increased amount. Burosumab is approved since 2018 in the USA and Europe for treatment of children 1 year and older with confirmed FGF23-associated hypophosphatemic rickets.

Romosozumab: An Anti-sclerostin Antibody

Romosozumab is a monoclonal antibody binding to sclerostin. Thereby it inhibits bone resorption but also increases bone formation. Sclerostin is involved in regulation of bone formation by inhibiting osteoblast differentiation via the WNT pathway (Williams 2014). It was approved for the treatment of adult osteoporosis in the USA recently. In Europe the approval process is still pending. Romosozumab treatment within a phase 3 trial for adults with OI led to an increased cardiovascular risk in adults – therefore it is only approved as "a second-line" approach (Glorieux et al. 2017).

2.4 Anabolic Agents

Osteoanabolic agents are interesting for children as bone growth is altered in most rare skeletal diseases in childhood. Most inherited bone diseases cause a short stature in adulthood. On account of this, it seems compelling to treat children with osteoanabolic agents.

There is no approval for Romosozumab (see Section "Romosozumab: An Anti-sclerostin Antibody") in children. There are no data available in children in the literature yet. Therefore treatment is not recommended outside of clinical trials currently.

Additionally, parathyroid hormone was approved in 2006 for adults with osteoporosis. It is used in a treatment period of 2 years to increase bone mass in adults with osteoporosis.

Based on the fact that an increased risk of developing an osteosarcoma in the growing skeleton was detected in earlier animal experiments, it was not used in children yet.

3 Diseases

3.1 Osteogenesis Imperfecta

Osteogenesis imperfecta (OI; brittle bone disease) is a hereditary bone fragility disorder leading to recurrent fractures. OI is caused in ~90% of the cases by typical autosomal dominant mutations in the genes *COL1A1/2* coding for collagen (Forlino and Marini 2016). Due to the fact that collagen is the base of osteoid formation collagen alterations lead to an increased fracture rate in patients with OI. During the last years, genetic analyses improved. Thereby new genes causing bone fragility syndromes have been detected (Asharani et al. 2012; Semler et al. 2012a; Keupp et al. 2013; Mendoza-Londono et al. 2015; Rauch et al. 2015). Depending on the affected gene, the symptoms might differ, but the increased bone fragility is the characteristic sign in all patients.

OI is a primary osteoporosis caused by a defect of bone formation (Fig. 1). Skeletal signs are recurrent fractures and deformities (mainly of the long bones), vertebral compression fractures, scoliosis, and short stature. Additional symptoms are hypermobility of joints causing atraumatic luxations, hearing impairments (especially during young adulthood), an affection of teeth (dentinogenesis imperfecta), and a discoloration of the sclera (blue-grayish sclera). Because the disease presents with a very wide range of phenotypes, not all symptoms need to be present in the individual patient (Marini et al. 2017).

Therapy requires a multi-modular concept with physical training, surgical procedures, and drug treatment. Physical training (physiotherapy, occupational therapy, rehabilitation) is important for the patients. As described above, the forces applied by the muscles to the bone are the most relevant factors stimulating osteoblasts to produce osteoid (Fricke and Schoenau 2007). A consensus statement of different experts in the field has been published recently (Hoyer-Kuhn et al. 2016a). Additionally, different strategies of muscle training (vibration training, rehabilitation concepts) have shown positive effect on the children (Hoyer-Kuhn et al. 2014b, c).

3.1.1 Bisphosphonates

Drug treatment in children with OI is currently limited to the off-label use of bisphosphonates which is performed in moderate to severely affected children since 20 years.

Pamidronate was the first bisphosphonate used in children with OI. It was proven to increase bone mineral density and to ameliorate chronic bone pain (Glorieux et al. 1998). Depending on the age of the child, it had to be administered 3–6 times per year during a 3-day inpatient stay with a total dose of 9 mg/kg body weight/year. Later neridronate was investigated in randomized trials. It can be given quarterly as an i.v. treatment in a dose of 2 mg/kg body weight/infusion and does not require an overnight stay. Neridronate is frequently used in Europe because it can be administered in an outpatient treatment setting and was investigated in clinical trials in different age groups (Gatti et al. 2005; Antoniazzi et al. 2006; Semler et al. 2011). Neridronate has been shown to have a comparable effect on reshaping of vertebral deformities when given as a single treatment quarterly (Semler et al. 2011). In the USA zoledronic acid is used in different regimes and has shown to be effective even if given only yearly or every 6 months (Panigrahi et al. 2010). Further assessments have proven the reduced costs per patient when treated with zoledronate compared to pamidronate. Oral bisphosphonates like risedronate or alendronate have also been investigated in phase 2/3 trials but are only used in mildly affected patients (Bishop et al. 2013).

3.1.2 Treatment: Denosumab

Elucidation of genetic causes in OI in the last decade offered the possibility to increase knowledge about patients with atypical OI, not caused by mutations in *COL1A1/2*. In 2011 the genetic cause for the previously clinically described OI type VI was discovered (Becker et al. 2011). Patients with this type show a poor response to an antiresorptive treatment with bisphosphonates and on biopsy they present with a high turnover osteoporosis with an increased amount of osteoid (Land et al. 2007). Causative mutations in the gene *SERPINF1* have been described, elucidating a new pathophysiology for OI (Becker et al. 2011). These patients are not affected by a defect of collagen synthesis but show an increased number and activity of osteoclasts. This is mediated via the OPG/RANKL pathway illustrated in Fig. 2. The amount of active RANKL is increased and stimulates maturation and proliferation of osteoclasts.

In these patients a therapy with the monoclonal antibody denosumab was evaluated. Denosumab treatment led to an increase of areal bone mineral density after 12 months in patients with OI type VI and a reduction of chronic pain (Hoyer-Kuhn et al. 2014a). Because this treatment was effective in OI type VI, it was assumed that this antiresorptive treatment might also be superior in children with classical types of OI caused by collagen mutations. Therefore safety and efficacy of denosumab was investigated in a small pilot trial in ten children with classical OI. In these children a positive response even compared to the prior treatment with neridronate was observed without severe side effects during a short treatment period of 12 months (Hoyer-Kuhn et al. 2016b). Currently a phase 3 trial is performed aiming to approve denosumab as the first drug for OI in children (NCT02352753).

It has to be mentioned that there is a significant effect on calcium homoeostasis in patients treated with denosumab. Directly after injection osteoclasts are blocked completely and serum calcium levels can drop significantly. This can last for some weeks requiring oral calcium and vitamine D supplementation. After some months the antibody will be resorbed, and osteoclasts start to differentiate and can cause a rebound hypercalcemia and hypercalciuria. Whether these changes in serum calcium levels will cause side effects like nephrocalcinosis or calcifications of vessels needs to be investigated in the future. During this period of increased bone resorption, some patients suffer from chronic pain located in the joints lasting for 1–2 weeks. This rebound activation of osteoclasts led to a reduction of bone mineral density, and in adults with osteoporosis, an increase of vertebral fractures has been reported after cessation of denosumab. In adults there is a growing discussion how to act to a cessation with denosumab and if a final dose of bisphosphonates might be beneficial to reduce the excessive bone resorption after the end of denosumab treatment (Perosky et al. 2016).

3.1.3 Treatment Anti-sclerostin

Additional to these antiresorptive agents, new substances are under investigation aiming to improve the function of osteoblasts. Sclerostin is involved in adaptation of bone formation by inhibiting osteoblast differentiation via the WNT pathway (Fig. 3). In adults with osteoporosis, anti-sclerostin antibodies are currently investigated as osteoanabolic agent (Glorieux et al. 2017). In OI previous studies in mice showed a positive effect on bone formation when using sclerostin antibodies. BPS804 is a humanized antibody interfering with the WNT pathway by blocking sclerostin. A 21-week phase 2 trial (NCT03216486) in adults with OI showed a good response of serum parameters of bone formation and bone resorption and an increase of lumbar bone mineral density (Glorieux et al. 2017). No data for a longer treatment or on the effect on fracture rate or long-term side effects have been reported yet. Anti-sclerostin and other drugs interfering with the WNT pathway are likely to be investigated in OI during the next years.

3.2 Rickets

Rickets is a condition associated with osteomalacia – a failure of mineralization – and a delay in endochondral ossification at the growth plates of the long bones. Rickets with disturbance of the architecture of the growth plates only occur in children while the growth plates are still open. In adults or after reaching final height with a fusion of the growth plates, rickets are no longer existent, and only features of osteomalacia are found. There are three major factors essential for normal mineralization and organizing of the growth plates: calcium, phosphorus concentrations, and normal levels of alkaline phosphatase. Rickets are divided based on a lack of calcium, phosphorus, or alkaline phosphatase into hypocalcemic rickets, hypophosphatemic rickets, and rickets due to hypophosphatasia.

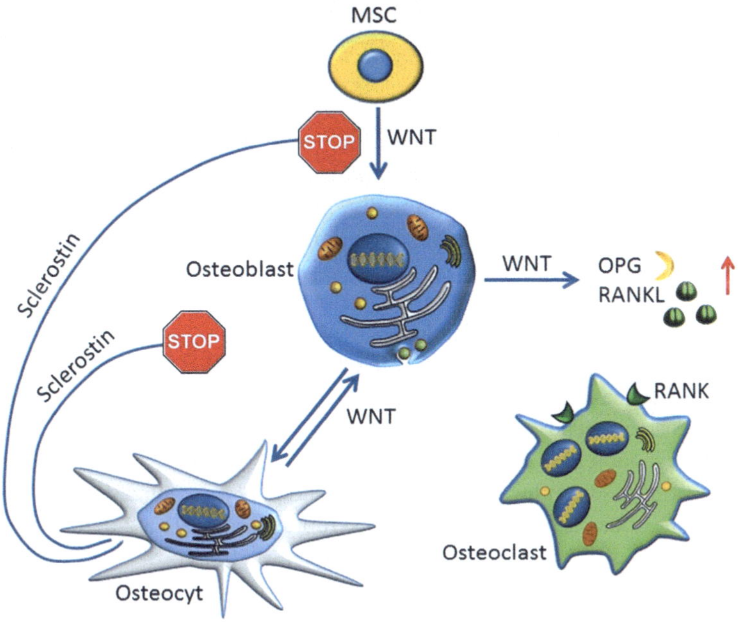

Fig. 3 Schematic presentation of sclerostin effects in bone metabolism. Sclerostin is produced by osteocytes and mesenchymal stem cells (MSC) reducing production of osteoprotegerin (OPG) by inhibiting the WNT signaling pathway. Inactivation of sclerostin by specific antibodies should increase bone mass by increasing bone formation and via the RANKL pathway by reducing activity of osteoclasts

3.2.1 Hypocalcemic Rickets

Hypocalcemic rickets are usually caused by vitamine D deficiency and/or a low calcium intake in the first years of life when growth velocity is high. Hereditary forms are rare and are associated with enzyme defects of the hydroxylation pathway in the kidney and liver for vitamine D activation. Vitamine D deficiency is the most common reason for hypocalcemic rickets in the last years as children are more and more sun protected, spent not enough time outside. In most countries a prophylaxis with vitamine D supplements in the first year of life is recommended.

Children with hypocalcemic rickets present with failure to thrive, bowing of the lower extremities after verticalization, enlarged wrists, rib cage deformities, open anterior fontanelle, and hypocalcemic seizures. On x-ray growth plates of the knees and/or the wrists appear widened and frayed. Additionally, laboratory changes (hypocalcemia, hypovitaminosis D (25-OH vitamine D), and hyperparathyroidism) could be detected.

Treatment Calcium

All children who present with hypocalcemia should receive oral substitution of calcium between 500 and 1,500 mg/day. If necessary calcium could also be given intravenously as calcium gluconate (1–2 mL of a 10% solution per kg body weight) (Munns et al. 2016).

Treatment Vitamine D Analoga

Most regimens for treatment of hypocalcemic rickets include the application of daily doses of 25-OH vitamine D. The amount defers due to national guidelines between 500 IU/day and 2,000 IU/day. Additionally, after healing of rickets, a prophylaxis with 400–600 IU/day (10–15 μg) should be administered during childhood (Munns et al. 2016).

3.2.2 Hypophosphatemic Rickets

In contrast to hypocalcemic rickets, X-linked hypophosphatemic rickets (XLH) is a rare hereditary disease affecting bones and kidneys (incidence 1:20,000). Mutations in the *PHEX* gene lead to a reduced amount of renal phosphate reabsorption mediated by an increased level of fibroblast growth factor 23 (FGF23). Thereby reduced phosphate serum levels could be detected, and mineralization of the growth plates and long bones is altered. Signs and symptoms in XLH are deformities of the legs, a waddling gate, short stature, skeletal pain, and in most cases also affected teeth with dental fistulas (Shimada et al. 2004; Pavone et al. 2015).

Treatment Vitamine D Analoga/Phosphorus

Treatment was based on substitution with oral phosphorus and active vitamine D (phosphate 20–40 mg/kg daily, 1,25(OH)2D 20–30 ng/kg daily in 1–2 dosages, alternatively alfacalcidol 50 ng/kg once per day) at least up to fusion of the growth plates. Phosphorus needs to be administered 5–7 times per day orally (Verge et al. 1991) to store an adequate amount in the body and to reduce the risk of secondary hyperparathyroidism.

Treatment Burosumab

Burosumab as a targeted monoclonal antibody has been approved for children with XLH due to FGFR23 excess. Burosumab is a FGFR23 antibody leading to an increase of renal reabsorption of phosphate and bone mineralization. Thereby it inhibits the phosphaturic function of FGF23 which causes XLH in patients with *PHEX* mutations (Fig. 4). As investigated in pediatric phase 2/3 trials, available burosumab has to be injected every 14 days subcutaneously. Children presented with constant serum phosphate levels and improved bone mineralization when receiving burosumab. Additionally, in a controlled trial, it was shown that burosumab is more effective regarding long bone mineralization than the conservative treatment with phosphate and vitamine D (Whyte et al. 2019). Burosumab was approved by FDA and EMA in 2017/2018.

3.2.3 Hypophosphatasia

Hypophosphatasia (HPP) is a hereditary disorder based on a reduced activity or amount of the alkaline phosphatase (TNSAP; tissue-nonspecific alkaline phosphatase) (Fig. 5). HPP is caused by autosomal recessive or dominant mutations in the

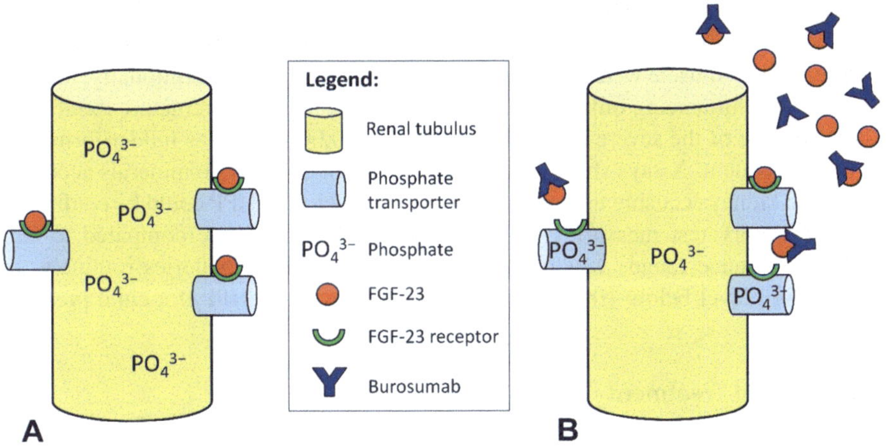

Fig. 4 Pathophysiology and therapeutic approach in hypophosphatemic rickets. (**a**) FGF23 inhibits the renal tubular phosphate transporter resulting in impaired reabsorption of phosphate from the renal tubule. (**b**) Burosumab (an antibody that binds FGF23) prevents FGF23-mediated inhibition of the phosphate transporter, thereby allowing the reabsorption of phosphate

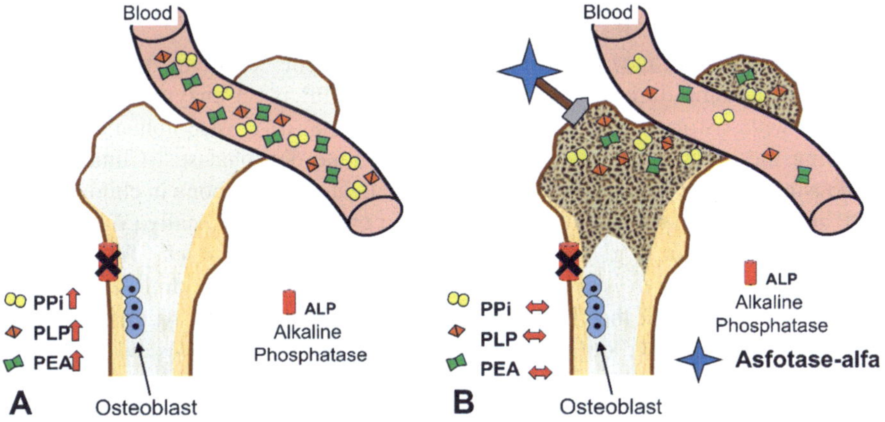

Fig. 5 Pathophysiology and therapeutic approach in hypophosphatasia. (**a**) Hypophosphatasia is characterized by a deficiency in alkaline phosphatase, leading to phosphate metabolites [pyrophosphate (PPi), pyridoxal phosphate (PLP), phosphoethanolamine (PEA)] accumulating in blood vessels, and impaired bone mineralization. (**b**) In the presence of asfotase alfa, a recombinant enzyme mimicking the effect of alkaline phosphatase, phosphate metabolites are incorporated into the osteoid, therefore allowing bone mineralization. While the genetic defect that inhibits alkaline phosphatase is still present, serum phosphate levels decrease, allowing for improved mineralization of bone

ALPL gene characterized by a very wide spectrum of severity (Hofmann et al. 2014). The spectrum reaches from perinatal lethal forms to types which only present during adulthood with muscle weakness and early onset osteoarthritis. Additionally, there is one subtype influencing only the teeth of the patients causing premature tooth loss. The incidence of the severe cases is estimated 1:100,000, whereas milder forms are far more frequent. X-rays show typical rickets-like pattern, while minerals accumulate in the kidneys causing nephrocalcinosis. A suspicion of HPP could be confirmed by a laboratory test measuring a reduced alkaline phosphatase compared to age adapted reference ranges which are not provided by all laboratories routinely. A double-digit level below 100 U/mL is highly suspicious of HPP if a child presents with rickets.

Conventional Treatment

Targeted treatment options have not been available in HPP up to now. To avoid side effects of a standard rickets treatment approach with supplements as vitamine D and calcium in HPP, a specific diagnosis should be achieved as early as possible. Supplementation of minerals (calcium, phosphate, and vitamine D) should be kept at a necessary minimum to avoid deficiencies and due to the risk of nephrocalcinosis. Bisphosphonates are also contraindicated in HPP (Whyte 2016).

Treatment: Asfotase Alfa

A recently approved new therapeutic option for patients suffering from musculoskeletal symptoms during childhood caused by HPP is an enzyme replacement therapy with asfotase alfa (Fig. 5). Asfotase alfa is a recombinant enzyme imitating the function of "tissue-nonspecific alkaline phosphatase." Clinical trials demonstrated that asfotase alfa improved mineralization of the bone in children with HPP and increased survival in severely affected children dramatically (Whyte et al. 2012). Asfotase alfa is given subcutaneously 2–3 times per week. Treatment of severe affected children is recommended. In milder affected children, a treatment should be considered if the child presents with skeletal problems. At this particular time, it has to be pointed out that there are no long-term experiences available yet.

3.3 Achondroplasia

Achondroplasia is the most common skeletal dysplasia. It is characterized by a disproportioned short stature (long trunk, short limbs) with a final height of less than 130 cm (Pauli 2019). The estimated incidence is 1:10,000 to 1:30,000 affected newborns.

The disease is caused by activating mutations in the *FGFR3* gene coding for the FGFR3 receptor in chondrocytes. Gain of function of the FGFR3 receptor leads to an increased inhibition of proliferation and differentiation of the chondrocytes in the growth plates of the long bones (Fig. 6). Thereby growth of the long bones is disturbed leading to the phenotype of disproportioned short stature. In 90% of affected patients, one typical autosomal dominant mutation could be detected by

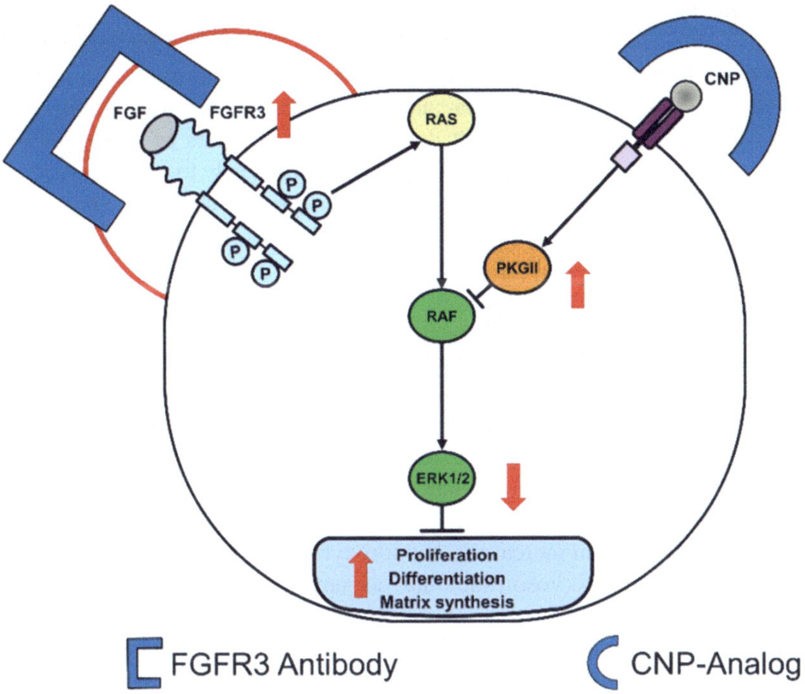

Fig. 6 Therapeutic approaches in achondroplasia. The differentiation of chondrocytes in the growth plates is regulated by an inhibiting pathway in the chondrocytes. As first step FGF (fibroblast growth factor) activates the receptor (fibroblast growth factor receptor 3 = FGFR 3). Using the "Ras-ERK pathway," the proliferation of chondrocytes is reduced. This signaling is mediated by Ras (Rat sarcoma protein) and RAF (rapidly accelerated fibrosarcoma) finally influencing ERK1/2 (extracellular signal-regulated kinases). New therapeutic approaches target this inhibiting pathway. FGFR3 antibodies block the whole cascade, while CNP analoga (C-type natriuretic peptide) interact via a cascade including PKGII (cGMP-dependent protein kinase-2) directly with ERK1/2. Both agents will lead to a reduced inhibition and will therefore increase the proliferation of chondrocytes

Sanger sequencing. Additionally, patients present with a macrocephaly, hypoplasia of the midface, hypermobility of the joints, muscular hypotonia, and recurrent middle ear infections (Ceroni et al. 2018). The most severe symptom during the first years is a reduced diameter of the foramen magnum at the cervical-spinal junction. This can lead to a compression of the spinal cord with the need of neurosurgical intervention.

Currently therapeutic interventions are only symptomatic with focus on prevention of complications. Patients are followed neurologically and regarding their growth during childhood. Disease-specific growth charts can be used to follow height of children (Del Pino et al. 2019). Beside the neurosurgical intervention in case of spinal cord compressions, orthopedic monitoring is necessary to detect deformities leading to disability.

3.3.1 Treatment: Growth Hormone

A treatment with growth hormone has been investigated with ambiguous results. In Japan growth hormone is approved for treatment of achondroplasia, but it is not approved by EMA or FDA. A meta-analysis of 558 children treated with growth hormone showed a catch-up growth during the first 2 years of treatment with a decrease of growth velocity afterward. In the end this leads to an improvement of height of 1 SD during the first 2 years, but no results of final height are presented. Especially no convincing data about the influence on disproportion or foramen magnum stenosis are available (Miccoli et al. 2016).

3.3.2 Treatment: Vosoritide

Drugs addressing the disturbed signaling in the chondrocytes of patients with achondroplasia are currently under investigation in clinical trials. The opposite signaling of FGFR3-mediated intracellular signaling in the chondrocytes is mediated by C-type natriuretic peptide (CNP) (Fig. 6). CNP is inhibiting the intracellular cascade of the FGFR3 receptor-mediated "Ras-ERK pathway." The hypothesis is that CNP analoga could inhibit the FGFR3-mediated inhibition of chondrocyte proliferation leading to an increase in chondrocyte proliferation and differentiation. Therefore CNP analoga (vosoritide) are currently investigated in clinical trials (NCT03197766). First data of a phase 2 trial with an extension period over 42 months showed an increase of growth velocity in children 5–14 years (Savarirayan et al. 2019). Vosoritide needs to be administered subcutaneously. No results about final height and the effect on the foramen magnum are available yet. Additionally, it is not known, how this treatment will affect limb and trunk proportions.

3.4 Fibrodysplasia Ossificans Progressiva

Fibrodysplasia ossificans progressiva (FOP) is a very rare skeletal disease caused by mutations in *ACVR1*, coding for "activin receptor-like kinase-2" (ALK2) affecting the "bone morphogenetic protein (BMP) type I" receptor (Fig. 7) (Shore et al. 2006).

The increased activation of the receptor causes a phosphorylation of SMAD proteins stimulating intranuclear transcription factors. These transcription factors initiate the production of cartilage tissue which later mineralizes and will be transformed into solid bone. Actually, there are only 1,000 affected people diagnosed worldwide. In these patients intramuscular injections, traumata, and muscular injuries can cause a rapid formation of bone tissue everywhere in the body called flare-up. During childhood most patients develop heterotopic ossification in the upper extremities, shoulders, and neck with resulting immobility of the joints. Finally many of them die due to respiratory insufficiency and cardiac decompensation due to the increased rigidity of the thorax. Life expectancy of the patients is limited to a mean of 30–45 years. Diagnosis is difficult, but already directly after birth malformations of the big toe are visible in nearly all patients.

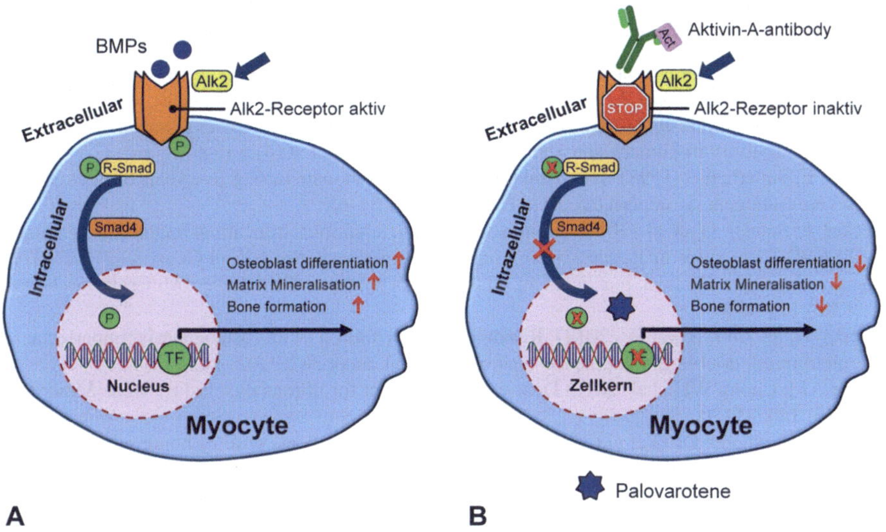

Fig. 7 Pathophysiology of fibrodysplasia ossificans progressive and therapeutic approach. (**a**) Molecular pathway in fibrodysplasia ossificans progressiva showing the intracellular cascade involved in extraskeletal ossification. (**b**) Palovarotene is a retinoic acid receptor gamma agonist that inactivates downstream the intracellular signaling of the Alk2 (activin receptor-like kinase-2) receptor which normally interacts with bone morphogenetic protein (BMP). This leads to reduced intracellular signaling by different smad molecules. The hypothesis is that palovarotene thereby diminishes osteoblast differentiation and heterotopic ossification

Therapeutic options are still limited and focus on prevention of traumata, e.g., avoiding intramuscular injections. In case of a flare-up, treatment with high-dose corticosteroids has shown to reduce the occurrence of new ossifications (level of evidence expert opinion, case series).

3.4.1 Treatment: Palovarotene

Palovarotene belongs to retinoic acid receptor gamma agonists (RAR gamma), inhibiting the increased activation of the ALK2 receptor and consequently intracellular signaling (Fig. 7b). This should suppress the formation of new bone tissue in extraskeletal regions. The first results of previous trials showed a reduction of new heterotopic ossifications and a reduction of chronic pain in 40 patients older 6 years of age. Currently a phase 3 study with palovarotene is performed in children and adults with FOP (NCT03312634). Dosage and treatment duration are still under investigation. There are different approaches to reduce the gain of function of the ALK2 receptor from which palovarotene is the substance most advanced in the clinical development program. An activin A antibody is currently tested in a phase 2 trial (NCT03188666).

References

Antoniazzi F, Zamboni G et al (2006) Early bisphosphonate treatment in infants with severe osteogenesis imperfecta. J Pediatr 149(2):174–179

Asharani PV, Keupp K et al (2012) Attenuated BMP1 function compromises osteogenesis, leading to bone fragility in humans and zebrafish. Am J Hum Genet 90(4):661–674

Astrom E, Soderhall S (1998) Beneficial effect of bisphosphonate during five years of treatment of severe osteogenesis imperfecta. Acta Paediatr 87(1):64–68

Becker J, Semler O et al (2011) Exome sequencing identifies truncating mutations in human SERPINF1 in autosomal-recessive osteogenesis imperfecta. Am J Hum Genet 88(3):362–371

Bishop N (2015) Clinical management of hypophosphatasia. Clin Cases Miner Bone Metab 12(2):170–173

Bishop N, Adami S et al (2013) Risedronate in children with osteogenesis imperfecta: a randomised, double-blind, placebo-controlled trial. Lancet 382(9902):1424–1432

Boyce AM, Chong WH et al (2012) Denosumab treatment for fibrous dysplasia. J Bone Miner Res 27(7):1462–1470

Ceroni JRM, Soares DCQ et al (2018) Natural history of 39 patients with Achondroplasia. Clinics (Sao Paulo) 73:e324

Chan B, Zacharin M (2006) Maternal and infant outcome after pamidronate treatment of polyostotic fibrous dysplasia and osteogenesis imperfecta before conception: a report of four cases. J Clin Endocrinol Metab 91(6):2017–2020

Cummings SR, San Martin J et al (2009) Denosumab for prevention of fractures in postmenopausal women with osteoporosis. N Engl J Med 361(8):756–765

Del Pino M, Fano V et al (2019) Height growth velocity during infancy and childhood in achondroplasia. Am J Med Genet A 179(6):1001–1009

Forlino A, Marini JC (2016) Osteogenesis imperfecta. Lancet 387(10028):1657–1671

Fricke O, Schoenau E (2007) The 'Functional Muscle-Bone Unit': probing the relevance of mechanical signals for bone development in children and adolescents. Growth Hormon IGF Res 17(1):1–9

Gatti D, Antoniazzi F et al (2005) Intravenous neridronate in children with osteogenesis imperfecta: a randomized controlled study. J Bone Miner Res 20(5):758–763

Glorieux FH, Rauch F (2006) Medical therapy of children with fibrous dysplasia. J Bone Miner Res 21(Suppl 2):P110–P113

Glorieux FH, Travers R et al (1995) Pamidronate treatment in children with fibrous dysplasia and osteogenesis imperfecta. Bone 17(6):611–611

Glorieux FH, Bishop NJ et al (1998) Cyclic administration of pamidronate in children with severe osteogenesis imperfecta. N Engl J Med 339(14):947–952

Glorieux FH, Devogelaer JP et al (2017) BPS804 anti-sclerostin antibody in adults with moderate osteogenesis imperfecta: results of a randomized phase 2a trial. J Bone Miner Res 32 (7):1496–1504

Grasemann C, Schundeln MM et al (2013) Effects of RANK-ligand antibody (denosumab) treatment on bone turnover markers in a girl with juvenile Paget's disease. J Clin Endocrinol Metab 98(8):3121–3126

Hofmann C, Girschick H et al (2014) Unexpected high intrafamilial phenotypic variability observed in hypophosphatasia. Eur J Hum Genet 22(10):1160–1164

Hoyer-Kuhn H, Netzer C et al (2014a) Two years' experience with denosumab for children with osteogenesis imperfecta type VI. Orphanet J Rare Dis 9(1):145

Hoyer-Kuhn H, Semler O et al (2014b) Effect of denosumab on the growing skeleton in osteogenesis imperfecta. J Clin Endocrinol Metab 99(11):3954–3955

Hoyer-Kuhn H, Semler O et al (2014c) A specialized rehabilitation approach improves mobility in children with osteogenesis imperfecta. J Musculoskelet Neuronal Interact 14(4):445–453

Hoyer-Kuhn H, Bartz-Seel J et al (2016a) Diagnostik und therapie der osteogenesis imperfecta. Monatsschr Kinderheilkd 165(4):333–346

Hoyer-Kuhn H, Franklin J et al (2016b) Safety and efficacy of denosumab in children with osteogenesis imperfect--a first prospective trial. J Musculoskelet Neuronal Interact 16(1):24–32
Hoyer-Kuhn H, Rehberg M et al (2017) Angeborene skeletterkrankungen. Monatsschr Kinderheilkd 165(8):663–671
Javaid MK, Boyce A et al (2019) Best practice management guidelines for fibrous dysplasia/ McCune-Albright syndrome: a consensus statement from the FD/MAS international consortium. Orphanet J Rare Dis 14(1):139
Keupp K, Beleggia F et al (2013) Mutations in WNT1 cause different forms of bone fragility. Am J Hum Genet 92(4):565–574
Lala R, Matarazzo P et al (2000) Pamidronate treatment of bone fibrous dysplasia in nine children with McCune-Albright syndrome. Acta Paediatr 89(2):188–193
Land C, Rauch F et al (2006) Effect of intravenous pamidronate therapy on functional abilities and level of ambulation in children with osteogenesis imperfecta. J Pediatr 148(4):456–460
Land C, Rauch F et al (2007) Osteogenesis imperfecta type VI in childhood and adolescence: effects of cyclical intravenous pamidronate treatment. Bone 40(3):638–644
Marini JC, Forlino A et al (2017) Osteogenesis imperfecta. Nat Rev Dis Primers 3:17052
Mendoza-Londono R, Fahiminiya S et al (2015) Recessive osteogenesis imperfecta caused by missense mutations in SPARC. Am J Hum Genet 96(6):979–985
Miccoli M, Bertelloni S et al (2016) Height outcome of recombinant human growth hormone treatment in achondroplasia children: a meta-analysis. Horm Res Paediatr 86(1):27–34
Munns CF, Shaw N et al (2016) Global consensus recommendations on prevention and management of nutritional rickets. J Clin Endocrinol Metab 101(2):394–415
Panigrahi I, Das RR et al (2010) Response to zolendronic acid in children with type III osteogenesis imperfecta. J Bone Miner Metab 28(4):451–455
Pauli RM (2019) Achondroplasia: a comprehensive clinical review. Orphanet J Rare Dis 14(1):1
Pavone V, Testa G et al (2015) Hypophosphatemic rickets: etiology, clinical features and treatment. Eur J Orthop Surg Traumatol 25(2):221–226
Perosky JE, Khoury BM et al (2016) Single dose of bisphosphonate preserves gains in bone mass following cessation of sclerostin antibody in Brtl/+ osteogenesis imperfecta model. Bone 93:79–85
Plotkin H, Rauch F et al (2003) Effect of pamidronate treatment in children with polyostotic fibrous dysplasia of bone. J Clin Endocrinol Metab 88(10):4569–4575
Rauch F, Fahiminiya S et al (2015) Cole-Carpenter syndrome is caused by a heterozygous missense mutation in P4HB. Am J Hum Genet 96(3):425–431
Savarirayan R, Irving M et al (2019) C-type natriuretic peptide analogue therapy in children with achondroplasia. N Engl J Med 381(1):25–35
Schoenau E, Frost HM (2002) The "muscle-bone unit" in children and adolescents. Calcif Tissue Int 70(5):405–407
Semler O, Beccard R et al (2011) Reshaping of vertebrae during treatment with neridronate or pamidronate in children with osteogenesis imperfecta. Horm Res Paediatr 76(5):321–327
Semler O, Garbes L et al (2012a) A mutation in the 5′-UTR of IFITM5 creates an in-frame start codon and causes autosomal-dominant osteogenesis imperfecta type V with hyperplastic callus. Am J Hum Genet 91(2):349–357
Semler O, Netzer C et al (2012b) First use of the RANKL antibody denosumab in osteogenesis imperfecta type VI. J Musculoskelet Neuronal Interact 12(3):183–188
Shimada T, Kakitani M et al (2004) Targeted ablation of Fgf23 demonstrates an essential physiological role of FGF23 in phosphate and vitamin D metabolism. J Clin Invest 113(4):561–568
Shore EM, Xu M et al (2006) A recurrent mutation in the BMP type I receptor ACVR1 causes inherited and sporadic fibrodysplasia ossificans progressiva. Nat Genet 38(5):525–527
Shroff R, Beringer O et al (2012) Denosumab for post-transplantation hypercalcemia in osteopetrosis. N Engl J Med 367(18):1766–1767
Verge CF, Lam A et al (1991) Effects of therapy in X-linked hypophosphatemic rickets. N Engl J Med 325(26):1843–1848

Wang HD, Boyce AM et al (2014) Effects of denosumab treatment and discontinuation on human growth plates. J Clin Endocrinol Metab 99(3):891–897

Whyte MP (2016) Hypophosphatasia – aetiology, nosology, pathogenesis, diagnosis and treatment. Nat Rev Endocrinol 12(4):233–246

Whyte MP, Greenberg CR et al (2012) Enzyme-replacement therapy in life-threatening hypophosphatasia. N Engl J Med 366(10):904–913

Whyte MP, Carpenter TO et al (2019) Efficacy and safety of burosumab in children aged 1-4 years with X-linked hypophosphataemia: a multicentre, open-label, phase 2 trial. Lancet Diabetes Endocrinol 7(3):189–199

Williams BO (2014) Insights into the mechanisms of sclerostin action in regulating bone mass accrual. J Bone Miner Res 29(1):24–28

Pharmacotherapy of Children and Adolescents with Type 1 Diabetes Mellitus

Thomas M. Kapellen

Contents

Abstract

Insulin treatment in children and adolescents with autoimmune type 1 diabetes has changed tremendously in the last 20 years with the knowledge of DCCT trial regarding near-normal glucose levels on the micro- and macrovascular outcome. Intensified insulin therapy is now standard of care. Carb counting however was introduced systematically only recently in several countries. In industrialized countries most patients in this age group are treated with continuous subcutaneous insulin injections. Nowadays this is combined with continuous subcutaneous glucose measurement commencing sensor-augmented pump therapy. Predictive low glucose suspend reduces the frequency of hypoglycemic events. Still not available for children is a commercially available closed loop system. However, treatment goals are still frequently not reached especially in the group of adolescents. Therefore several additive drugs are tested to improve treatment results. There are new insulins with faster and longer action profile in the pipeline to better mimic physiologic insulin profiles. Smart insulins may be able to mimic reaction on blood sugar levels. The broad facet of treatment modalities helps

T. M. Kapellen (✉)
Hospital for Children and Adolescents, University of Leipzig, Leipzig, Germany
e-mail: thomas.kapellen@medizin.uni-leipzig.de

W. Kiess et al. (eds.), *Pediatric Pharmacotherapy*,
Handbook of Experimental Pharmacology 261, https://doi.org/10.1007/164_2019_245

pediatric diabetes teams to individualize therapy and so improve patients' health-related quality of life.

Keywords
Adolescents · Children · CSII · Insulin treatment · Long-acting insulin · Rapid-acting insulin · Sensor-augmented pump therapy

1 Introduction

Type 1 diabetes mellitus (T1D) is one of the most common metabolic disorders in childhood and adolescence, with increasing incidence. In Germany a 3.4% yearly increments of newly diagnosed children below the age of 14 years can be found with highest increase in very young children (Bendas et al. 2015). Overall approximately 96,000 children below 15 years develop T1D all over the word yearly (Meyer-Davis et al. 2018). From the estimated 500,000 children and adolescents with T1D worldwide, about 26% come from Europe and another 22% from North America and the Caribbean States. In Asia the prevalence is much lower (Meyer-Davis et al. 2018).

Due to chronic autoimmune destruction of insulin-producing pancreatic beta cells, affected type 1 diabetes patients suffer from partial or in most cases absolute insulin deficiency. Banting and Best first purified pancreatic extract and injected it in a 14-year-old boy with T1D almost 100 years ago (in 1921). Eli Lilly in the USA and 1 year later Novo Nordisk in Europe began to produce this "normal insulin" from animal pancreas (Quianzon and Cheikh 2012). Because multiple daily injections were needed about every 4–6 h to control blood glucose levels, the development of a longer-acting insulin was required to improve the practicability of insulin treatment and quality of life. In the 1930s protamine was added by Hagedorn, and in the same years, zinc was added by Scott and Fisher. Isophane neutral protamine Hagedorn (NPH) lasted up to 24 h and could be mixed with normal insulin. Zinc NPH mixtures had an even longer action. In 1982 the first recombinant human insulin preparations became available on the market.

With longer survival of patients with T1D, chronic microvascular and macrovascular complications became more evident. The DCCT trial showed a linear relation of blood glucose control and these diabetic complications. Intensive insulin treatment with multiple daily injections (MDI) or continuous subcutaneous insulin injection (CSII) could dramatically reduce diabetic retinopathy and nephropathy compared to a conventional diabetes treatment with less frequent injections (The Diabetes Control and Complications Trial Research Group 1993). So intensified insulin treatment with the goal of near-normal glucose values is the standard treatment for T1D in any age today. However in many patients hypoglycemia is the limiting factor for getting close to normal blood glucose values 24 h a day. Therefore several modifications in insulin pharmacokinetics were accomplished with changes in the amino acid chains or due to adding of fatty acids. These so-called analog insulins showed either shorter or longer action and could reduce the rate of hypoglycemic events in intensively treated T1D patients (Quianzon and Cheikh 2012).

2 Insulin Therapy in Children and Adolescents with Type 1 Diabetes Mellitus

After diagnosis of type 1 diabetes mellitus, insulin treatment should be immediately started to avoid development of ketosis or ketoacidosis. For intensified insulin treatment, several short-acting and long-acting insulins with different action profiles are available on the market (Table 1).

Multiple daily insulin injection treatment (MDI) with either insulin pens or syringes is still the most common treatment regimen worldwide (Danne et al. 2018). Continuous subcutaneous insulin injection (CSII) or insulin pump treatment is rapidly increasing especially in young children (Sherr et al. 2016).

Both treatment regimens combine a so-called mealtime bolus with a basal insulin or a continuous delivered basal rate. The mealtime bolus is usually calculated by carbohydrate counting. In Germany carbohydrates are counted by units, and one unit stands for 10–12 g carbohydrates, whereas in most other countries, carbohydrates are counted by grams. In Table 2 usual mealtime factors for different age groups are shown.

Table 1 Available insulin preparations with their suggested action profiles regarding start of action, peak, and duration when injected s.c.

Insulin type	Onset of action (h)	Peak of action (h)	Duration of action (h)
Mealtime insulin (rapid/short acting)			
Ultrarapid-acting analog (faster aspart)	0.05–0.2	1–3	3–5
Rapid analog insulin (aspart, lispro, glulisine)	0.15–0.35	1–3	3–5
Regular insulin (short acting)	0.5–1	2–4	4–8
Basal insulin (intermediate/long acting)			
NPH insulin	2–4	4–12	12–24
Glargine	2–4	8–12	22–24
Detemir	1–2	4–7	20–24
Glargine U300	2–6	Minimal peak	30–36
Degludec	0.5–1.5	Minimal peak	>42

Table 2 Mealtime bolus factors for 10 g carbohydrates (CU) at different times a day (personal experience and can vary individually and depends on pubertal stage)

Daytime (years)	0–5	5–12	10–18
Morning (IE/CU)	0.8	0.8–1.5	1.0–2.5
Snack (IE/CU)	0.6	0.6–1.2	1.0–2.0
Lunch (IE/CU)	0.6	0.6 ± 1.2	1.0–2.0
Tea snack (IE/CU)	0.5	0.8–1.2	1.0–2.5
Dinner (IE/CU)	0.6	0.8–1.5	1.0–2.5
Midnight snack (IE/CU)	0.5	0.5–1.2	1.0–2.0

Table 3 Correction bolus factors for 1 unit of rapid-acting insulin lower the blood glucose level by *x* mmol/L at different times a day (personal experience can vary individually and depends on pubertal stage and metabolic control)

Daytime (years)	0–5	5–10	10–15
Daytime (mmol/L)	8–15	3–8	1–4
Nighttime (mmol/L)	16–20	6–15	2–6

The short- or rapid-acting insulins are also used for correction of higher blood sugar levels. Therefore patients usually calculate with a correction factor. This correction factor depends on the age and the time of correction. Insulin sensitivity is higher in lower age and in the night hours compared to the day. Usually we recommend half of the correction dose for the night. Table 3 shows usual correction factors depending on age and time of the day.

In general insulin requirement is age dependent. At onset a child usually needs 0.7–1.0 Units per kg bodyweight. Toddlers have a lower requirement of about 0.5–0.7 U/kgbw. In remission phase the insulin demand can decrease below 0.5 U/kgbw. In adolescence the requirement often will go above 1.0 up to 2.0 U/kgbw.

3 Rational for Different Insulins

Short-acting regular insulin is still the cheapest insulin on the market and so the widest available over the globe (Danne et al. 2018). It can be used in MDI and is also approved for the use in insulin pumps. It should be injected 20–30 min before meal because of its later onset of action compared to rapid-acting analogs. That is the major disadvantage especially when used in toddlers and younger children with unknown carbohydrate intake. When regular insulin is used, a larger meal and a snack after 2–3 h are regularly covered by the duration of the insulin action. If the snack is missed, hypoglycemia can occur.

Short-acting regular insulin can be combined with any basal insulin. In low-income countries, it is frequently combined with NPH twice or three times daily (Fig. 1a).

Because of the nonphysiological onset of action and the duration of action of regular insulin, *rapid-acting analog insulins* were developed. Three different rapid-acting insulins are on the market (aspart, glulisine, lispro). No clinical significant differences regarding hypoglycemia, metabolic control results, and action profile have been observed in either adult or pediatric population (Home 2012; Philotheou et al. 2011). However the advantages of rapid-acting analog insulin compared to regular insulin are still under debate. A Cochrane review showed a slightly weighted difference in HbA1c of 0.1% in favor of rapid-acting analogs in MDI and 0.2% in favor of rapid-acting analogs when used in CSII in adult patients with type 1 diabetes. This review could not find significant differences in the frequency of severe hypoglycemia (Fullerton et al. 2016). There is no Cochrane analysis for children

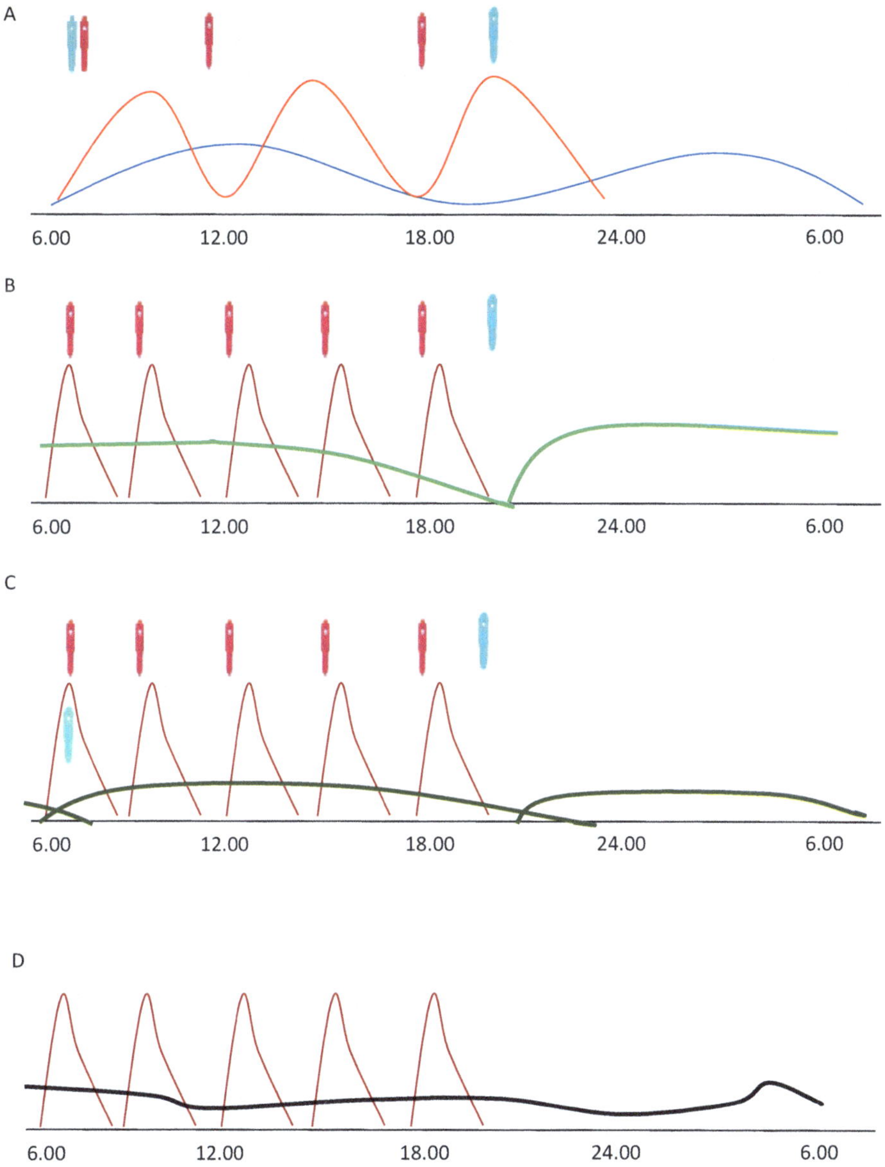

Fig. 1 Different insulin regimens with different short- and long-acting insulins. (**a**) Regular insulin (red lines) for mealtime bolus and a snack and NPH insulin (blue lines) twice or three times daily (not shown). (**b**) Rapid-acting analog and glargine: Rapid-acting analog (red lines) for mealtime bolus and glargine (green line). (**c**) Rapid-acting analog and detemir: Rapid-acting analog (red lines) for mealtime bolus and detemir (dark green line). (**d**) CSII: red lines = mealtime bolus. Black line = basal rate (variable programmable every hour to get individualized basal profile)

available. However data about the use of rapid-acting analogs for postprandial injection are available (Danne et al. 2003). Although preprandial injection of rapid analog insulin is recommended to avoid high postprandial glucose excursions in toddlers with unknown food intake, postprandial injection may be safer to avoid hypoglycemia. In practice for every single meal or snack, rapid-acting analog should be injected immediately before the meal. If hyperglycemia is present, the analog should be injected at least 15–20 min before the meal to correct the higher blood glucose. In most insulin pumps, rapid-acting analog insulin is used.

Ultrarapid-acting analog insulins try to imitate the physiological action profile of prandial insulin action with a faster and steeper increase of action than rapid analogs when administered subcutaneously. In regular insulin and rapid analogs, the limiting factor for resorption and start of action is the dissociation from a hexamer into dimers and monomers. The ultrafast insulin aspart realizes this faster dissociation by adding niacin amide and L-Arginine. It has been approved in the USA and Europe for adults with type 1 diabetes in 2017. Approval for children is awaited. In adults subcutaneous injection of ultrafast aspart resulted in a twice as fast detection of insulin compared to aspart. The insulin concentration within the first 30 min after injection was doubled. These effects were even more pronounced in CSII (Heise et al. 2017). In children and adolescents, the same pharmacokinetic characteristics were seen (Fath et al. 2017). Clinical trial data in adults however are still sparse especially regarding the effect on metabolic control and hypoglycemia. With BioChaperone Lispro another ultrafast acting insulin is in the pipeline that was however also only tested in adults with type 1 diabetes (Anderson et al. 2018). It could also show reduced postprandial blood glucose excursions in the first 2 h after a meal in this adult study population.

4 Basal Insulins

As mentioned above the oldest basal insulin is *NPH*. The unclear solution of regular insulin and protamine has to be mixed before use to get a reproducible action profile. NPH that has not been mixed thoroughly has a high variability in action that varies up to twofold (Lucidi et al. 2015). Therefore appropriate resuspension takes up to 1 min and 30 s, a time that is quite long and not realistic for most patients. Within-subject variability is also higher than with long-acting analogs. With its peak of action, the use is limited because of higher risk of nocturnal hypoglycemia especially in adolescents with the need for pronounced insulin action in the early morning (dawn phenomenon).

The first basal analog that was approved is *insulin glargine*. Changes in the molecular structure shift the isoelectric point from a pH of 5.4 to 6.7 making the molecule less soluble at physiological pH. In the neutral pH of subcutaneous space, higher-order aggregates form. These result in a slow and almost peakless dissolution and absorption. Action lasts for about 24 h with a slight waning effect after about 20 h of action. A recent meta-analysis that compared long-acting insulin analogs with NPH in type 1 diabetes showed a reduction of nocturnal hypoglycemia

(RR 0.66, 95% CI 0.57; 0.76) and a slight better HbA1c without a significant reduction of severe hypoglycemia (Laranjeira et al. 2018). However data in children are quite different with one Finnish retrospective study that could not find a difference between glargine and NPH concerning either HbA1c or hypoglycemia (Päivärinta et al. 2008). Danne et al. compared NPH and glargine in preschool children in a randomized trial with continuous subcutaneous glucose monitoring and detected more asymptomatic but less symptomatic hypoglycemia in the glargine group (Danne et al. 2013). The higher strength formulation insulin *glargine U 300* has a flatter and longer action profile than the original U 100 glargine. In adults in most studies no significant difference in hypoglycemia and nocturnal hypoglycemia was found. However in a study with continuous subcutaneous glucose monitoring, a reduced rate of nocturnal hypoglycemia and an overall smoother glucose course with less steep postprandial excursions could be found in adults (Bergenstal et al. 2017). For children trials for approval are ongoing.

Insulin detemir is an insulin analog in which a fatty acid (myristic acid) is bound to a lysine amino acid at position B29. It is quickly absorbed and then bound to albumin in the blood through its fatty acid at position B29. It then slowly dissociates from this complex resulting in a long-acting profile (see Table 1). It is usually injected once or (more often) twice daily in pediatric patients. Thalange et al. found a significant reduction of overall and nocturnal hypoglycemia compared to NPH in a long-duration (52 weeks) randomized clinical trial in children without effect on HbA1c (Thalange et al. 2013). A slight less weight gain (like in many adult studies) was observed compared to NPH. The mechanism of detemir on weight is not understood yet. Some authors and many clinicians can observe a slightly higher dosage of detemir compared with NPH and especially when changing from glargine (up to 25%) (Abali et al. 2015).

In the novel *insulin degludec*, the addition of hexadecanedioic acid to lysine at B29 allows the formation of multi-hexamers in s.c. tissue. A slow and stable release of monomers lasts for up to 40 h. Therefore the ultra-long action profile should allow a less stringent timing of basal insulin administration from day to day that could fit more into the daily life of an adolescent or young adult. In a randomized controlled trial comparing degludec with detemir in 350 children and adolescents or 26 weeks showed no significant differences in Hba1c and rates of hypoglycemia. However a significantly lower fasting plasma glucose could be found (Thelange et al. 2015).

There are a number of premixed insulins available on the market primarily composed to make insulin therapy easier for older patients with type 2 diabetes. Recently a premixed detemir/aspart was tested in a clinical trial. The option of less frequent injections is paid by less flexible meals. Premixed insulins are not supported by the philosophy of modern basal bolus principles to achieve best glycemic control and more flexible life. However in adolescents with worse metabolic control such strategies might improve the situation.

Insulin treatment should whenever possible be adapted to the daily life of patients and family and not vice versa. Therefore all thinkable combinations of insulin are allowed to reach best metabolic control and high quality of life.

Patients should be systematically taught about action profiles of different insulins and about timing of insulin injections. Insulin absorption is influenced by several factors including the injection site, age, fat mass, dose of insulin (slower absorption in larger doses), body temperature, and insulin concentration. Devices for warming the injection site are available. Adequate storage of insulin is important. Freezing, direct sunlight exposition, or warming should be avoided. Unused insulin should be stored in a refrigerator. When used, insulin cartridges should be discarded after 4 weeks at room temperature and after 3 months when stored in the refrigerator. Usual injection sites for insulin are the abdomen, front and lateral thigh, buttock, and lateral aspects of the arm (not in small children). Cleaning or disinfection of the injection sites is not necessary. However rotation of the sites is very important to avoid lipohypertrophy/lipohypotrophy.

Nowadays usually *pen injector devices* are used for MDI in pediatric population. For pediatric patients with low insulin requirement, dosage in half units should be available and is provided by most manufacturers currently. A few pen devices have a memory function that can sometimes be linked to an app. Still syringes are available also in ½ unit marks. In syringes insulin can be self-mixed. In this case of self-mixing, the compatibility of the different mixed agents should be proven (e.g., regular insulin with NPH). The recommended needle length for children and adolescents is now between 4 and 6 mm (Danne et al. 2018). If there is enough s.c. fat, lifting of the skin fold is not necessary. For patients with fear of injections or needles, alternatively *subcutaneous indwelling catheters* (e.g., i-port) can be used if an insulin pump is no alternative for these patients. These catheters can improve metabolic control in children with injection problems (Burdik et al. 2009). These catheters can like pump catheters stay for 2–3 days in place and have than to be replaced. If basal and short-acting insulin will be injected in the same catheter, a minimal interval of 60 min between the two insulin types can avoid negative effects on insulin absorption. In some cases automatic injection devices could help with injection fear. *Jet injectors* that bring insulin into the subcutaneous tissue with high pressure can cause a variable injection depth and therefore may influence pharmacokinetics. In a recent study in healthy young adults, jet injection showed comparable pharmacokinetic profiles and glucose-lowering effects compared to pen injection (Engwerda et al. 2017).

5 Insulin Pump Therapy

Continuous subcutaneous insulin infusion (CSII) or insulin pump therapy is increasingly used in pediatric population. In Germany now more than 50% of children and adolescents and more than 90% of children below 5 years use CSII (Holl and Prinz 2019). Insulin pump therapy with a continuous basal insulin supply and mealtime or correction boluses whenever needed is currently the most physiological way to imitate insulin maintenance. Beneath these features many so-called smart pumps offer a bolus calculator to more accurate dose insulin amounts needed for carbohydrates and correction of higher blood sugars. The possibility to increase or decrease basal rates in special situations like active sports, acute illnesses, or physiologically higher insulin demand with menstrual circle adds another feature to improve metabolic control. In a large nationwide German prospective population-based cohort, CSII proved to be the favorable insulin therapy for children, adolescents, and young adults. In the matched analysis of this cohort, almost 10,000 patients with CSII were compared to a propensity score matched group of almost 10,000 MDI users. Pump use was associated with a significant reduction of severe hypoglycemia (9.55 vs. 13.97 per 100 patient years) and a significant reduction of diabetic ketoacidosis (3.64 vs 4.26 per 100 patient years). Glycated hemoglobin was also significantly lower with CSII (8.04% vs 8.22%) (Karges et al. 2017). On the other hand, health-related quality of life could be shown to be improved in children and families of children with type 1 diabetes after switching from MDI to CSII (Mueller-Godeffroy et al. 2018). In this study children 8–11 years and caregivers in all age groups reported substantially improved patient-reported outcomes and burden from diabetes treatment.

Dosing of pumps is quite similar to that of MDI despite a slightly lower need of insulin (about 15% less with CSII). Basal rates are much lower in CSII than when a basal insulin is used and can either be hourly programmed age and weight dependent with dosage sliding scales or in block dosing (this is very country specific) (Kapellen et al. 2015; Bachran et al. 2012).

Patients and caregivers must be aware of the consequences of catheter problems regarding ketoacidosis management and should be supplied with either a ketone meter or urine ketone strips and a management plan. Diabetes teams that care for children and adolescents with CSII should provide a 24 h helpline to support families in these situations (Kapellen et al. 1998).

6 Sensor-Augmented Pump Therapy

The combination of CSII with continuous subcutaneous glucose measurement (CGM) offers with different algorithms a more sophisticated and semiautomated pump therapy. The so-called sensor-augmented pump therapy (SAP) is clearly related to the time a sensor is worn or not worn. Especially in adolescents the potential beneficial effect was countersteered by low sensor use (Bergenstal et al. 2010). Pumps that shut down basal insulin supply in hypoglycemia improved the frequency of hypoglycemic events and could reduce severe hypoglycemia. Predictive low glucose suspend algorithms more sophisticatedly stop basal insulin supply before a hypoglycemia will even occur (Beato-Vibora et al. 2018). As a consequence of these achievements, a so-called *hybrid closed loop* system was developed. This system can not only react on low but also on high blood sugar levels and with its algorithm adopt basal rate in both ways increasing and decreasing it to improve the glucose time in range. The first approved system was brought on the market in September 2016 in the USA (Medtronic 670G) first for adults and then for children above the age of 6 years (Forlenza et al. 2019). Marketing in Europe started in autumn 2018; however not in every country the system is available. Other systems are on the way. With the Cambridge algorithm, Tauschmann et al. could show an improvement of metabolic control in a wide age range in patients with type 1 diabetes and worse metabolic control (Tauschmann et al. 2018). So we can expect a quantity of new combinations of insulin pumps combined with sensor and different algorithms that could make life with diabetes easier for families and patients.

7 Non-insulin Adjunctive Therapy

Many adolescents develop insulin resistance due to several mechanisms. On one hand children and adolescents have a higher risk to develop overweight and obesity (Kapellen et al. 2013). On the other side, a physiological insulin resistance occurs in adolescence due to pubertal hormonal changes. There is a long and ongoing discussion about adding *metformin* to the insulin treatment. A meta-analysis in children and adolescents with type 1 diabetes does not support evidence for an improvement in glycemic control with addition of metformin. However there can be seen a slight reduction in total daily insulin dose and BMI (Khalifah et al. 2017). A randomized controlled trial in overweight and obese adolescents could show similar results with some patients that benefit more from weight loss (Libman et al. 2015). On the other hand, about 36% of patients reported about gastrointestinal adverse events. Recently a randomized controlled trial in adults with type 1 diabetes with addition of metformin and a study duration of at least 3 years show beneficial effect on cardiovascular risk factors but again not on glycemic control (Petrie et al. 2017). The authors found a reduction in intima media thickness, BMI, and LDL cholesterol and an increase in eGFR.

Glucagon-like peptide-1 (GLP1) is an intestinal hormone that is secreted with meal stimulus (incretine). GLP1 stimulates insulin secretion in a glucose-like manner. Furthermore it inhibits glucagon secretion, slows gastric emptying, and induces satiety. There is seen an improvement of beta cell survival and proliferation with GLP1 stimulation. Additionally peripheral insulin sensitivity is improved together with reduced hepatic glucose production (Unger 2013; Tosur et al. 2018).

GLP1 is rapidly degraded after secretion by dipeptidyl peptidase-4 (DPP4), whereas *GLP1 agonists* are not degraded and so can activate GLP1 receptors longer than physiologically. On the other hand, *DPP4 inhibitors* would enhance the endogenous GLP1 activity. Both kinds of incretin enhancers are widely used in patients with type 2 diabetes. Several meta-analyses did not show significant effects on metabolic control if both substance classes are used additionally to insulin in patients with type 1 diabetes (Tosur et al. 2018). GLP1 agonists were associated with weight loss and decreased daily insulin requirement. However there were seen significant gastrointestinal side effects. There is no published data on children or adolescents, but studies are ongoing. DPP4 inhibitors seem to have even more limited benefits for patients with type 1 diabetes.

Sodium-glucose cotransporters are mainly located in the intestinal mucosa (SLGT1) and the renal proximal tubule (SGLT2). Sodium-glucose cotransporter 2 (SGLT2) inhibitors primarily increase the glucose excretion by blocking reabsorption in the proximal tubule. This leads to lower plasma glucose and a modest reduction in HbA1c, weight, and blood pressure (Tosur et al. 2018; Riddle and Cefalu 2018). Dosing is typically once daily oral without dose titration. With increased glucosuria typical side effects occur like urinary or genital irritation or urinary tract infections. In large clinical trials of patients with type 2 diabetes and increased cardiovascular risk, the use of SGLT2 inhibitors has shown favorable effects on heart failure, cardiovascular death, and progression of albuminuria (Zinman et al. 2015; Neal et al. 2017). So enthusiastic wider clinical use is found in patients with type 2 diabetes without knowing the underlying mechanisms leading to the cardiovascular benefits. Several larger studies in adults with type 1 diabetes analyzed the benefits and possible side effects of adding SGLT2 inhibitors to insulin treatment (Riddle and Cefalu 2018). The results of all studies with different substances were quite similar. A median HbA1c reduction of 0.25–0.52% could be achieved. Weight was reduced by 2.2–4.5 kg compared to placebo. Diabetic ketoacidosis as a known side effect however was found in a dose-dependent manner in 1.5–6.0% compared to 0–1.9% in the placebo group. Better glycemic control was achieved without increased risk for hypoglycemia. However the DKA risk is quite challenging especially if one might assume that the risk would be even higher in a clinical and non-trial setting with less frequent patient visits. The problem might even be more striking because the DKA in SGLT2 inhibitor treatment is not a typical T1DM DKA. Blood glucose levels are only moderately increased without other typical DKA symptoms. So for patients with type 1 diabetes, new strategies for detecting and managing this normoglycemic DKA have to be established. Trials in children and adolescents are on the way to start. With the knowledge of side effects, very well-elaborated teaching strategies are needed, and in the future those patients that benefit most with an acceptable rate of possible side effects have to be identified for a personalized medicine.

In conclusion treatment of children and adolescents with type 1 diabetes has to be an individualized pharmacotherapy discussing all treatment possibilities including technological support with patients and families. Quite frequently this treatment will change over the time when children are growing and can better express their own wishes. Beneath good metabolic control, quality of life has always to be considered as children and adolescents will have their disease lifelong.

References

Abali S, Turan S, Atay Z, Güran T, Haliloglu B, Bereket A (2015) Higher insulin detemir doses are required for the similar glycemic control: comparison of insulin detemir and glargine in children with type 1 diabetes mellitus. Pediatr Diabetes 16:361–366

Anderson G, Meiffren G, Lamers D, DeVries JH, Ranson A, Seroussi C, Alluis B, Gaudier M, Soula O, Heise T (2018) Ultra-rapid BioChaperone Lispro improves postprandial blood glucose excursions vs lispro in a 14-day crossover treatment study in people with type 1 diabetes. Diabetes Obes Metab 20:2627–2632

Bachran R, Beyer P, Klinkert C, Heidtmann B, Rosenbauer J, Holl RW (2012) Basal rates and circadian profiles in continuous subcutaneous insulin infusion (CSII) differ for preschool children, prepubertal children, adolescents and young adults. Pediatr Diabetes 13:1–5

Beato-Vibora PI, Quiros-Lopez C, Lazaro-Martin L, Martin-Frias M, Barrio-Castellanos R, Gil-Poch E, Arroyo-Diez FJ, Gimenez-Alvarez M (2018) Impact of sensor-augmented pump therapy with predictive low glucose suspend function on glycemic control and patient satisfaction in adults and children with type 1 diabetes. Diabetes Technol Ther 20:738–743

Bendas A, Rothe U, Kiess W, Kapellen TM, Stange T, Manuwald U et al (2015) Trends in incidence rates during 1999-2008 and prevalence in 2008 of childhood type 1 diabetes mellitus in Germany-model based national estimates. PLoS One 16:10

Bergenstal RM, Tamborlane W, Ahmann A, Buse JB, Dailey G, Davis SN, Joyce C, Peoples T, Perkins BA, Welsh JB, Willi SM, Wood MA, STAR 3 Study Group (2010) Effectiveness of sensor-augmented insulin-pump therapy in type 1 diabetes. N Engl J Med 363:311–320

Bergenstal RM, Bailey TS, Rodbard D, Ziemen M, Guo H, Muehlen-Bartmer I, Ahmann AJ (2017) Comparison of insulin glargine 300 units/mL and 100 units/m Lind adults with type 1 diabetes: continuous glucose monitoring profiles and variability using morning and evening injections. Diabetes Care 40:554–560

Burdik P, Cooper S, Horner B, Cobry E, McFann K, Chase HP (2009) Use of a subcutaneous injection port to improve glycemic control in children with type 1 diabetes. Pediatr Diabetes 10:116–119

Danne T, Aman J, Schober E, Deiss D, Jacobsen JL, Friberg HH, Jensen LH, ANA 1200 Study Group (2003) A comparison of postprandial and preprandial administration of insulin aspart in children and adolescents with type 1 diabetes mellitus. Diabetes Care 26:2359–2364

Danne T, Philotheou A, Goldman D, Guo X, Cali A, Johnston P (2013) A randomized trial comparing the rate of hypoglycemia – assessed using continuous glucose monitoring – in 125 preschool children with type 1 diabetes treated with insulin glargine or NPH insulin (the PRESCHOOL study). Pediatr Diabetes 14:593–601

Danne T, Phillip M, Buckingham BA, Jarosz-Chobot P, Saboo B, Urakami T, Battelino T, Hanas R, Codner E (2018) ISPAD clinical practice guidelines 2018: insulin treatment in children and adolescents with diabetes. Pediatr Diabetes 19(Suppl 27):115–135

The Diabetes Control and Complications Trial Research Group (1993) The effect of intensive treatment of diabetes on the development and progression of long-term complications in insulin dependent diabetes mellitus. N Engl J Med 329:977–986

Engwerda EE, Tack CJ, de Galan BE (2017) Pharmacokinetic and pharmacodynamic variability of insulin when administered by jet injection. J Diabetes Sci Technol 11:947–952

Fath M, Danne T, Biester T, Erichsen L, Kordonouri O, Haahr H (2017) Faster-acting insulin aspart provides faster onset and greater early exposure vs insulin aspart in children and adolescents with type 1 diabetes mellitus. Pediatr Diabetes 18:903–910

Forlenza GP, Pinhas-Hamile O, Liljenquist DR, Shulman DI, Bailey TS, Bode BW, Wood MA, Buckingham BA, Kaiserman KB, Shin J, Huang S, Lee SW, Kaufman FR (2019) Safety evaluation of the MiniMed 670G system in children 7-13 years of age with type 1 diabetes. Diabetes Technol Ther 21:11–19

Fullerton B, Siebenhofer A, Jeitler K, Horvath K, Semlitsch T, Berghold A, Plank J, Pieber TR, Gerlach FM (2016) Short acting insulin analogues versus regular human insulin for adults with type 1 diabetes. Cochrane Database Syst Rev:CD012161

Heise T, Pieber TR, Danne T, Erichsen L, Haahr H (2017) Pharmacodynamic characteristics of fast-acting insulin aspart in adults with type 1 diabetes. Clin Pharmacokinet 56:551–559

Holl RW, Prinz N (2019) Versorgung von Kindern und Jugendlichen mit Diabetes – aktuelle Situation und Veränderungen der letzten 23 Jahre. In: Deutscher Gesundheitsbericht Diabetes 2019. Herausgeber Deutsche Diabetesgesellschaft. Kirchheim Verlag, Mainz. ISSN 1614-824X

Home PD (2012) The pharmacokinetics and pharmacodynamics of rapid-acting insulin analogues and their clinical consequences. Diabetes Obes Metab 14:780–788

Kapellen TM, Dost A, Leludas C, Kiess W (1998) Patient acceptance and use of an emergency telephone hotline service in pediatric diabetes care. Diabetes Care 21:1365

Kapellen TM, Gausche R, Dost A, Wiegand S, Flechtner-Mors M, Keller E, Kiess W, Holl RW, for the DPV-Science-Initiative of the German Competence Network Diabetes and the German Competence Network Obesity (Consortium LARGE) (2013) Children and adolescents with type 1 diabetes in Germany are more overweight than healthy controls: results comparing DPV database and CrescNet database. J Pediatr Endocrinol Metab 7:1–6

Kapellen TM, Heidtmann B, Lilienthal E, Rami-Merhar B, Engler-Schmidt C, Holl RW (2015) Continuous subcutaneous insulin infusion in neonates and infants below 1 year: analysis of initial bolus and basal rate based on the experiences from the German working group for pediatric pump treatment. Diabetes Technol Ther 17:872–879

Karges B, Schwandt A, Heidtmann B, Kordonouri O, Binder E, Schierloh U, Boettcher C, Kapellen T, Rosenbauer J, Holl RW (2017) Association of insulin pump therapy versus insulin injection therapy with severe hypoglycemia, ketoacidosis, and glycemic control among children, adolescents, and young adults with type 1 diabetes. JAMA 318:1358–1366

Khalifah RA, Alnhdi A, Alghar H, Alanazi M, Florez ID (2017) The effect of adding metformin to insulin therapy for type 1 diabetes mellitus children: a systematic review and metaanalysis. Pediatr Diabetes 18:664–673

Laranjeira FO, de Anrade KR, Figueiredo AC, Silva EN, Pereira MG (2018) Long acting insulin analogues for type 1 diabetes: an overview of systematic reviews and meta-analysis of randomized controlled trials. PLoS One 13:e0194801

Libman IM, Miller KM, DiMeglio LA, Bethin KE, Katz ML, Shah A, Simmons JH, Haller MJ, Raman S, Tamborlane WV, Coffey JK, Saenz AM, Beck RW, Nadeau KJ, for the T1D Exchange Clinic Network Metformin RCT Study Group (2015) Effect of metformin added to insulin on glycemic control among overweight/obese adolescents with type 1 diabetes. JAMA 314(21):2241–2250

Lucidi P, Porcellati F, MarinelliAndreoli A, Carriero I, Cioli P, Bolli GB, Fanelli CG (2015) Pharmacokinetics and pharmacodynamics of NPH in Type 1 diabetes: the importance of appropriate resuspension before subcutaneous injection. Diabetes Care 38:2204–2210

Meyer-Davis EJ, Kahkoska AR, Jefferies C, Dabelea D, Balde N, Gong CX, Aschner P, Craig ME (2018) ISPAD clinical practice guidelines 2018: definition, epidemiology and classification of diabetes in children and adolescents. Pediatr Diabetes 19(Suppl 27):7–19

Mueller-Godeffroy E, Vonthein R, Ludwig-Seibold C, Heidtmann B, Boettcher C, Kramer M, Hessler N, Hilgard D, Lilienthal E, Ziegler A, Wagner VM, on behalf of the German working group for Pediatric Pump Therapy (agip) (2018) Psychosocial benefits of insulin pump therapy in children with type 1 diabetes and their families: the pumpkin multicenter randomized controlled trial. Pediatr Diabetes 19:1471–1480

Neal B, Perkovic V, Mahaffey KW, CANVAS Program Collaborative Group et al (2017) Canagliflozin and cardiovascular and renal events in type 2 diabetes. N Engl J Med 377:644–657

Päivärinta M, Tapainen P, Veijola R (2008) Basal insulin switch from NPH to glargine in children and adolescents with type 1 diabetes. Pediatr Diabetes 9:83–90

Petrie JR, Chaturvedi N, Ford I, Brouwers MC, Greenlaw N, Tillin T, Hramiak I, Hughes AD, Jenkins AJ, Klein EK, Klein R, Ooi TC, Rossing P, Stehouwer CD, Sattar N, Colhoun HM, on behalf of REMOVAL Study Group (2017) Cardiovascular and metabolic effects of metformin in patients with type 1 diabetes (REMOVAL): a double-blind, randomised, placebo-controlled trial. Lancet Diabetes Endocrinol 5:597–609

Philotheou A, Arslanian S, Blatniczky L, Peterkova V, Souhami E, Danne T (2011) Comparable efficacy and safety of insulin glulisine and insulin lispro when given as part of basal bolus regimen in a 26-week trial in pediatric patients with type 1 diabetes. Diabetes Technol Ther 13:327–334

Quianzon CC, Cheikh I (2012) History of insulin. J Community Hosp Intern Med Perspect 2(2). https://doi.org/10.3402/jchimp.v2i2.18701

Riddle MC, Cefalu WT (2018) SGLT inhibitors for type 1 diabetes: an obvious choice or too good to be true? Diabetes Care 41:2444–2447

Sherr JL, Hermann JM, Campbell F, Foster NC, Hofer SE, Allgrove J, Maahs DM, Kapellen TM, Holman N, Tamborlane WV, Holl RW, Beck RW, Warner JT (2016) Use of insulin pump therapy in children and adolescents with type 1 diabetes and its impact on metabolic control: comparison of results from three large transatlantic paediatric registries. Diabetologia 59:87–91

Tauschmann M, Thabit H, Bally L, Allen JM, Hartnell S, Wilinska ME, Ruan Y, Sibayan J, Kollman C, Cheng P, Beck RW, Acerini CL, Evans ML, Dunger DB, Elleri D, Campbell F, Bergenstal RM, Criego A, Shan VN, Leelaranthna L, Hovorka R, APCam11 Consortium (2018) Closed loop delivery in suboptimal controlled type 1 diabetes: a multicentre, 12 week randomized trial. Lancet 392:1321–1329

Thalange N, Bereket A, Larsen J, Hiort LC, Peterkova V (2013) Insulin analogues in children with type 1 diabetes: a 52-week randomized clinical trial. Diabet Med 30:216–225

Thelange N, Deeb L, Iotova V, Kawamura T, Klingensmith G, Philotheou A, Silverstein J, Tumini S, Ocampo Francisco A-M, Kinduryte O, Danne T (2015) Insulin degludec in combination with bolus insulin aspart is safe and effective in children and adolescents with type 1 diabetes. Pediatr Diabetes. 16:164–176

Tosur M, Redondo MJ, Lyons SK (2018) Adjuvant pharmacotherapies to insulin for the treatment of type 1 diabetes. Curr Diab Rep 18:79

Unger J (2013) Rational use of GLP1 receptor agonists in patients with type 1 diabetes. Curr Diab Rep 13:663–668

Zinman B, Wanner C, Lachin JM et al (2015) Empagliflozin, cardiovascular outcomes, and mortality in type 2 diabetes. N Engl J Med 373:2117–2128

Pharmacotherapy of Children and Adolescents with Type 2 Diabetes Mellitus

Thomas M. Kapellen

Contents

Abstract

Increasing obesity and overweight has led to increased prevalence of type 2 diabetes mellitus (T2D) in adolescents and young adults all over the world. Overweight naturally reduces insulin sensitivity. The following permanent insulin resistance can be found even in younger obese children. Beta-cell insufficiency following high insulin production over years leads to impaired glucose tolerance and later type 2 diabetes mellitus. In children and adolescents, the diagnosis of T2D is often made by screening very obese patients with oral glucose tolerance test. Usually in these patients, few or no diabetes symptoms are found. As frequently found in pediatric pharmacotherapy, only a few of the modern substances used in adults are available for pediatric patients with type 2 diabetes

T. M. Kapellen (✉)
Hospital for Children and Adolescents, University of Leipzig, Leipzig, Germany
e-mail: thomas.kapellen@medizin.uni-leipzig.de

W. Kiess et al. (eds.), *Pediatric Pharmacotherapy*,
Handbook of Experimental Pharmacology 261, https://doi.org/10.1007/164_2019_266

mellitus. The essential change in lifestyle for weight reduction is difficult in this age group with often rather disappointing results.

Keywords
Adolescents · Pharmacotherapy · Type 2 diabetes · Youth

1 Introduction

Type 2 diabetes mellitus (T2D) is increasing in many countries all over the world (Reinehr et al. 2010; Zeitler et al. 2018; Dabelea et al. 2014; Chan et al. 1993; Wei et al. 2002). Very informative data are available from the USA. In 2001 the prevalence of adolescents below the age of 20 years was 0.34/1,000 (95% CI, 0.31–0.37); in 2009 about 0.46/1,000 (95% CI, 0.43–0.49) adolescents with T2D were diagnosed. A higher prevalence could be found in ethnic minorities. In American Indian youth, the highest prevalence could be found (1.20 pro 1,000) followed by black youth (1.06 pro 1,000) and Hispanics (0.79 pro 1,000) compared to a prevalence of 0.17/1,000 in white youth. These data show an increment of 30.5% in prevalence in 8 years (Dabelea et al. 2014). For Hispanics and black youth, prevalence of type 2 diabetes is equal to prevalence of type 1 diabetes in the USA.

In Asiatic countries incidence of T2D in youth is even higher than type 1 diabetes incidence (Chan et al. 1993; Wei et al. 2002, 2003; Sugihara et al. 2005; Ramachandran et al. 2003). Obesity is a risk factor for the development of T2D; however in Japan 30% of the pediatric T2D population has normal weight (Sugihara et al. 2005); in Taiwan normal weight T2D youth is even higher (about 50%) (Ramachandran et al. 2003). In a national screening program in Taiwan in children and adolescents between 6 and 18 years, the incidence of type 2 diabetes was 6.5/100,000 compared to an incidence of type 1 diabetes of 1.5/100,000 (Wei et al. 2003).

There is data showing an earlier onset of diabetes-induced microvascular and macrovascular complications in youth with type 2 diabetes mellitus (Zeitler et al. 2018; Rodriguez et al. 2006; Copeland et al. 2011). Therefore a strict metabolic control has to be reached in young type 2 patients.

2 Principles of Treatment of Youth-Onset Type 2 Diabetes Mellitus

Type 2 diabetes mellitus disproportionally affects those with fewer socioeconomic resources and in Asia especially affluent population. This complicates diabetes education and compliance of patients and families.

Like in type 1 diabetes, management goals are near-normal glucose without hypoglycemia. Education to self-management is mandatory. First goal should be weight loss. Often families do not know the link between weight and glucose metabolism (Copeland et al. 2013).

Frequently a weight loss of 5–10% will lead to normal glucose levels without pharmacotherapy. Therefore lifestyle intervention is the first step in therapy of T2D

(Zeitler et al. 2018). Behavioral changes are mandatory usually for the whole family. Small steps and increments are helpful for the compliance. Group-oriented education and treatment is more beneficial in obese patients. Reward systems can help to achieve permanent changes. Dietary modifications should focus on elimination of soft drinks. Fruit and vegetable intake should be increased at the same time. Convenience foods are frequently high caloric and should also be avoided. Portions should be reduced and eating out of home (take away) should be limited. Dietary education should include interpretation of food tables.

Exercise is the third column in diabetes and weight management. Regular exercise improves glucose control and reduces insulin resistance and cardiovascular risk factors (alone without weight loss) (American Diabetes Association 2018). Reduction of sedentary habits like TV time and computer-related activities can be achieved by a daily exercise program. Often group activities of obese children and adolescents can help to activate this group of patients and avoid shame.

3 Pharmacotherapy

Pharmacotherapy is still limited due to limited approval of antidiabetic drugs in this age group.

In the actual ISPAD guideline, the initial treatment of type 2 diabetes mellitus should include metformin and/or insulin depending on the presentation of the patient at onset (Zeitler et al. 2018). The formal recommendations are shown in Table 1. The goal of initial treatment should be to attain an Hba1c below 7.0% regarding the newest ISPAD guideline (Zeitler et al. 2018). This can frequently be reached by

Table 1 Initial treatment at onset depending on clinical presentation (adapted to ISPAD recommendations and personal experience)

Metabolic status and symptoms	Recommended therapy
No clinical symptoms, patient was found to be diabetic by lab parameters like oral glucose tolerance test, or elevated HbA1c (6.5–7.0%)	Education and lifestyle intervention for 3 months without pharmacotherapy Depending on compliance add metformin
Metabolic stable patient HbA1c < 8.5% No symptoms	Metformin begin with 500–1,000 mg for 7–14 days Titrate on tolerability and GI symptoms by 500–1,000 mg every 1–2 weeks up to a maximal dose of 1,000 mg BID or 850 mg TID or 2,000 mg extended release metformin (where available) once daily
Patients with ketosis/ketonuria/ketoacidosis **or** HbA1c >8.5%	At least initial insulin Several regimens possible (see chapter T1D) Often once-daily intermediate or basal insulin (0.25–0.5 U/kg starting dose) is effective At the same time, metformin can be started unless acidosis is present

metformin alone or in combination with basal insulin. A treat to target strategy more likely ensures good long-term metabolic control than a treat to failure strategy. Therefore therapy should be intensified when the target Hba1c is not reached or tends to increase. An overview of the potential drugs is given in Table 2.

4 Insulin Therapy in Children and Adolescents with Type 2 Diabetes Mellitus

As discussed in the chapter of type 1 diabetes, several insulin regimens are possible. In patients with ketoacidosis or high HbA1c, we usually start with an intensified insulin treatment after initial DKA scheme with intravenous insulin. The so-called multiple daily insulin injection (MDI) treatment with either insulin pens or syringes is still the most common treatment regimen worldwide. This treatment regimen combines a so-called mealtime bolus with a basal insulin. The mealtime bolus is usually calculated by carbohydrate counting. The short or rapid acting insulins are also used for correction of higher blood sugar levels. Therefore patients usually calculate with a correction factor. This correction factor depends on the age and the time of correction (see chapter type 1 diabetes).

Usually T2D patients are very insulin resistant at the initiation of insulin therapy. This resistance has to be overcome by quite high doses (sometimes more than 1.5 U/kg). By adding metformin (after acidosis is resolved) insulin can often be reduced gradually.

In general most patients can be treated with basal insulin alone after some days (Table 1). In 90% of youth with type 2 diabetes, insulin can be weaned off with increasing metformin (Kelsey et al. 2016).

5 Metformin

Metformin is a biguanide that acts through AMP kinase in the liver, muscle, and fat and improves glycemia through reduction of hepatic glucose production by decreasing gluconeogenesis and by stimulating peripheral glucose uptake (Lentferink et al. 2018). Fatty oxidation is increased in skeletal muscles. Several studies have shown weight loss potential both in adults and children (Lentferink et al. 2018). Insulin sensitivity is improved, and metformin could be preventive in the development of T2D in adults (Lentferink et al. 2018). Treatment with metformin has little to no risk for hypoglycemia. However intestinal side effects are seen frequently but can be limited by slowly dose titration with initial treatment in the evening. Abdominal pain, diarrhea, and nausea are often only transient at initiation of metformin. Patients should be carefully informed about the possible side effects to improve compliance. A known risk of lactacidosis in this age group is even lower than in adults. The risk is increased in renal impairment, cardiac or respiratory insufficiency, and longer fasting periods. Therefore treatment should be paused during gastrointestinal illnesses and perioperative (Zeitler et al. 2018). Metformin is frequently used in PCOS. It has

Table 2 Drugs for treatment of type 2 diabetes in youth (Maloney et al. 2019)

Substance	Approval	Results in clinical trials	Hypoglycemia	Effects on weight
Metformin	Yes for children from 10 years	HbA1c reduction improves fasting glucose	Not likely	BMI reduction in most studies at least for the first 6 months
Insulin	No age limit	Hba1c reduction improves fasting glucose	Highest risk	Weight gain likely
Thiazolidinediones	Not approved <18 years	HbA1c reduction of 0.5–1.3% in adults lowest failure rates in combination with metformin in adolescents	Low risk	Weight gain likely up to 3–4 kg
Sulfonylurea	Not approved <18 years in all countries approved for neonatal diabetes	HbA1c reduction of 1.5–2% in adults Glimepiride pediatric trial: Not superior to metformin	High risk	Weight gain likely
Alpha-glucosidase inhibitors	Not approved <18 years No studies in youth	HbA1c reduction on long term 0.5–1.0% Frequent side effect: flatulence	Not likely	Weight neutral
Incretin mimetics (GLP-1 receptor agonists)	Not approved <18 years several studies make near approval likely	HbA1c reduction of 0.5–1.9% lowers fasting plasma glucose Same pharmacodynamics in youth like in adults In combination with metformin in adolescents, HbA1c difference was 1.06% at the cost of more gastrointestinal side effects	Low risk	Liraglutide −2.5 kg
DPP-IV inhibitors	Not approved <18 years	HbA1c reduction of 0.58–0.72% in adults Studies in youth underway	Very low risk	Slight weight gain in trials (0.5–1.0 kg)
Sodium-glucose cotransporter 2 (SGLT2) inhibitors	Not approved <18 years	HbA1c reduction of 1.0–1.2% in adults Studies in youth underway	Low risk	Weight loss up to 3 kg in trials

the potential to normalize ovulatory abnormalities and hence increases the pregnancy risk.

Jones et al. published the first randomized controlled study on metformin in adolescents with T2D from the USA and Russia. With metformin 1,000 mg BID, a significant improvement of fasting plasma glucose and HbA1c (7.5% vs 8.6%) could be reached compared to placebo. Side effects were mainly gastrointestinal (Jones et al. 2002). In the TODAY study in 699 participants, metformin in combination with rosiglitazone had a significant better effect on HbA1c and insulin sensitivity than metformin alone in a randomized controlled trial over 6 months (TODAY Study group 2013). In type 2 diabetic youth with an Hba1c higher than 6.3% at diagnosis, an early metformin failure is more likely.

6 Sulfonylurea

Sulfonylurea and meglitinides bind to receptors on the K+/ATP channel. This binding leads to close the K+ channel. The closure enables insulin secretion (Bowman et al. 2018). In adults sulfonylurea are still used in first line if the patient has no cardiovascular disease or chronic kidney disease and a cheap drug should be considered. Pricing however is very different between countries (Davies et al. 2018). Sulfonylureas have a long binding to the receptors, whereas metiglinides have intermediate equilibration and binding times. This leads to less frequent hypoglycemia in modern sulfonylurea or Metiglinides what is preferable. Metiglinides can be dosed before a meal and titrated on the demand regarding the amount of carbohydrate uptake.

Only data of one trial with glimepiride was conducted in youth with type 2 diabetes mellitus. Glimepiride reduced HbA1c in the same way like metformin (−0.54% vs −0.71%). In the glimepiride group, a weight gain was seen, whereas in the metformin group, a weight loss could be found. Safety profile even regarding hypoglycemia was not different between the two treatment groups (Gottschalk et al. 2007).

There is different approval status in different countries. Sulfonylurea are well proven and approved for the treatment of neonatal diabetes with mutations at the K+/ATP Channel (Bowman et al. 2018).

7 Thiazolidinediones

Thiazolidinediones (TZD) act by activating PPARs (peroxisome proliferator-activated receptors). This is followed by an upregulation of a number of specific genes and decreasing transcription of others. The main effect is an increase in the storage of fatty acids in adipocytes. The decreased amount of fatty acids in the circulation leads to an upregulation of the oxidation of carbohydrates more specifically glucose. Insulin sensitivity is increased especially in the muscle, adipose tissue, and liver. In adults a reduction of HbA1c of 0.5–1.3% can be reached. Side effects of

TZD however are weight gain, anemia, and fluid retention. A slightly higher risk of bladder cancer was seen in one meta-analysis. Results of some studies showed an increased risk of cardiovascular disease, whereas others showed protection (Mannucci et al. 2008). These studies led to a period of market restriction especially in the USA. These restrictions are removed now. In the actual adult guideline for pharmacological treatment of type 2 diabetes, sulfonylurea like TZD are recommended as first-line treatment if the patient has no cardiovascular disease or chronic kidney disease, and a cheap drug should be considered (Davies et al. 2018).

In the TODAY study, rosiglitazone in combination with metformin showed significantly fewer patients with treatment failure (38.6%) in the observation period of 5 years compared to metformin plus lifestyle intervention (46.6%) and metformin alone (51.7%). The addition of rosiglitazone thus decreased the risk of treatment failure by 23% (TODAY Study group 2013). In a closer look into the result showed that the combination of rosiglitazone with metformin in preventing treatment failure was more effective in girls than in boys. Racial differences were also seen with metformin monotherapy being least effective in non-Hispanic blacks (Gandica and Zeitler 2016). There is still no market authorization below the age of 18 years.

8 α-Glucosidase Inhibitors

Alpha-glucosidase inhibitors (acarbose, miglitol) sometimes referred to as starch blockers reduce the absorption of carbohydrates in the small intestine. Major side effects are flatulence and diarrhea. This substance group is no further recommended in adult guidelines (Davies et al. 2018). There is no data of clinical trials in adolescents.

9 Glucagon-Like Peptide-1 Receptor Agonists (GLP-1 RA, Incretin Mimetics)

Glucagon-like peptide-1 (GLP1) is an intestinal hormone that is secreted with meal stimulus (incretine). GLP1 stimulates insulin secretion in a glucose-like manner. Furthermore it inhibits glucagon secretion, slows gastric emptying, and induces satiety. There is seen an improvement of beta-cell survival and proliferation with GLP1 stimulation. Additionally peripheral insulin sensitivity is improved together with reduced hepatic glucose production (Unger 2013; Tosur et al. 2018).

GLP 1 is rapidly degraded after secretion by dipeptidyl peptidase-4 (DPP4), whereas GLP 1 agonists are not degraded and so can activate GLP1 receptors longer than physiologically. Incretin mimetics are widely used in adult type 2 patients. They are recommended as first-line treatment when weight loss and minimizing the risk of hypoglycemia are the treatment goals. From cardiovascular outcome studies, GLP-1 RA have a high benefit regarding the primary endpoints cardiovascular death, nonfatal myocard infarction, and nonfatal stroke [LEADER trial, (Marso et al. 2018)]. GLP-1 RA have to be injected subcutaneously. Different preparations have to be injected from BID (exenatide) to once daily (liraglutide, lixisenatide) up to once a week (semaglutide, dulaglutide, exenatide extended release). Several side effects are known. Most common are nausea, vomiting, and diarrhea; all tend to diminish over time. There is a minimal risk for hypoglycemia. Associations with the risk for gallbladder events are known (Davies et al. 2018).

In children and adolescents, pharmacokinetics and pharmacodynamics for liraglutide are similar to adults (Klein et al. 2014). Tamborlane et al. tested the efficacy of liraglutide added to metformin with or without basal insulin to improve metabolic control. One hundred thirty-five patients (10–17 years old) were randomized to either liraglutide up to 1.8 mg/day (66) or placebo. At 26 weeks HbA1c decreased by 0.64% in the liraglutide treatment and increased by 0.42% in the placebo group. Fasting plasma glucose decreased similarly with liraglutide compared to an increase in the controls. Overall the gastrointestinal side effects were seen more frequently in the liraglutide treatment group. A significant BMI reduction could not be shown (Tamborlane et al. 2019). In a short-term trial in obese adolescents, liraglutide was efficacious to reduce BMI compared to placebo (Mastrandrea et al. 2019). Liraglutide is likely to be approved for use in children and adolescents soon.

10 Dipeptidyl Peptidase-4 Inhibitors (DPP4 Inhibitors)

GLP 1 is rapidly degraded after secretion by dipeptidyl peptidase-4 (DPP4). Inhibitors of DPP4 can consecutively increase the availability of endogenous GLP 1 activity. DPP 4 inhibitors are oral administered. Their potential to lower glucose is moderate with reduction of 0.5% in HbA1c (Zeitler et al. 2018; Davies et al. 2018). Weight effect is neutral and the risk of hypoglycemia is low. In combination with sulfonylurea however, the risk for hypoglycemia is increased by 50% compared to sulfonylurea therapy alone. So for adults these substances (as monotherapy) are recommended if compelling need to minimize hypoglycemia.

In children and adolescents, no study results have been published, but trials are on the way.

11 Sodium-Glucose Cotransporter 2 Inhibitors (SGLT2 Inhibitors)

Sodium-glucose cotransporters are mainly located in the intestinal mucosa (SLGT1) and the renal proximal tubule (SGLT2). Sodium-glucose cotransporter 2 (SGLT2) inhibitors primarily increase the glucose excretion by blocking reabsorption in the proximal tubule. This leads to lower plasma glucose and a modest reduction in HbA1c, weight, and blood pressure (Tosur et al. 2018; Riddle and Cefalu 2018). Dosing is typically once-daily oral without dose titration. With increased glucosuria typical side effects occur like urinary or genital irritation or urinary tract infections. In large clinical trials of patients with type 2 diabetes and increased cardiovascular risk, the use of SGLT2 inhibitors has shown favorable effects on heart failure, cardiovascular death, and progression of albuminuria (Zinman et al. 2015; Neal et al. 2017). Enthusiastic wider clinical use is found in patients with type 2 diabetes without knowing the underlying mechanisms leading to the cardiovascular benefits. Blood pressure can be reduced like weight without increasing risk of hypoglycemia. In type 1 diabetes, increased rates of DKA are found. This could not be confirmed in large adult type 2 diabetes trials. Typical side effects due to the excretion of glucose over the urinary tract are mycotic genital infections. Fracture risk and the risk of lower limb amputation were higher with canagliflozin (Davies et al. 2018). In adults SGLT2 inhibitors are recommended for first-line treatment in patients with cardiovascular or kidney disease and if weight loss is a primary objective. Recently there was shown similar pharmacokinetics and exposure-response on dapagliflozin of adolescents compared to adults with type 1 diabetes (Busse et al. 2019). Again there are no studies in type 2 diabetes in youth published yet, but several are underway.

12 Conclusions

Type 2 diabetes in youth does more rapidly deteriorate compared to adults. A greater proportion of adolescents with T2D come from ethnical minorities or low-income families. Metformin in combination with lifestyle intervention is the first-line treatment with all limitations due to motivational problems for changes of lifestyle in this population. A treatment failure is more frequently and earlier seen in this age compared to adults. So far only insulin and in some countries sulfonylureas are approved for this age group. Most likely GLP1-RA will be approved soon. Other therapeutic options are tested in trials. Recruitment however is very difficult because of several problems including low prevalence, low cooperation in this population to participate in trials, and high dropout rates. So competent authorities in Europe and the USA should think about alternative solutions like extrapolation from adult data combined with pharmacokinetic and pharmacodynamic data of adolescents or non-controlled efficacy and safety studies.

References

American Diabetes Association (2018) 4. Lifestyle management: standards of medical care in diabetes-2018. Diabetes Care 41(suppl 1):S38–S50

Bowman P, Sulen A, Barbetti F et al (2018) Effectiveness and safety of long-term treatment with sulfonylureas in patients with neonatal diabetes due to KCNJ11 mutations: an international cohort study. Lancet Diabetes Endocrinol 6:637–646

Busse D, Tang W, Scheerer M, Danne T, Biester T, Sokolov V, Boulton D, Parkinson J (2019) Comparison of pharmacokinetics and exposure-response relationship of dapagliflozin between adolescents/young adults and adult patients with type 1 diabetes mellitus. Br J Pharamcol 85 (8):1820–1828

Chan JC, Cheung CK, Swaminathan R, Nicholls MG, Cockram CS (1993) Obesity, albuminuria and hypertension among Hong Kong Chinese with non-insulin-dependent diabetes mellitus (NIDDM). Postgrad Med J 69:204–210

Copeland KC, Zeitler P, Geffner M, Guandalini C, Higgins J, Hirst K et al (2011) Characteristics of adolescents and youth with recent-onset type 2 diabetes: the TODAY cohort at baseline. J Clin Endocrinol Metab 96:159–167

Copeland KC, Silverstein J, Moore KR, Prazar GE, Raymer T, Shiffman RN, Springer SC, Thaker VV, Anderson M, Spann SJ, Finn SK (2013) American academy of pediatrics, management of newly diagnosed type 2 diabetes mellitus (T2DM) in children and adolescents. Pediatrics 131:364–382

Dabelea D, Mayer-Davis EJ, Saydah S, Imperatore G, Linder B, Divers J, Bell R, Badaru A, Talton JW, Crume T, Liese AD, Merchant AT, Lawrence JM, Reynolds K, Dolan L, Liu LL, Hamman RF, SEARCH for Diabetes in Youth Study (2014) Prevalence of type 1 and type 2 diabetes among children and adolescents from 2001 to 2009. JAMA 311:1778–1778

Davies MJ, D'Alessio DA, Fradkin J et al (2018) Management of hyperglycaemia in type 2 diabetes, 2018. A consensus report by the American Diabetes Association (ADA) and the European Association for the Study of diabetes (EASD). Diabetologia 61:2461–2498

Gandica R, Zeitler P (2016) Update on youth onset type 2 diabetes: lessons learned from treatment options for type 2 diabetes in adolescents and youth clinical trial. Adv Pediatr Infect Dis 63:195–209

Gottschalk M, Danne T, Vlajnic A, Cara JF (2007) Glimepiride versus metformin as monotherapy in pediatric patients with type 2 diabetes. A randomized, single-blind comparative study. Diabetes Care 30:790–794

Jones K, Arslanian S, McVie R, Tomlinson M, Park J-S (2002) Metformin improves glycaemiccontrol in children with type 2 diabetes. Diabetes Care 25:89–94

Kelsey MM, Geffner ME, Guandalini C et al (2016) Presentation and effectiveness of early treatment of type 2 diabetes in youth: lessons from the TODAY study. Pediatr Diabetes 17 (3):212–221

Klein DJ, Battelino T, Chatterjee DJ et al (2014) Liraglutide's safety, tolerability, pharmacokinetics and pharmacodynamics in pediatric type 2 diabetes: a randomized double blind, placebo controlled trial. Diebetes Technol Ther 16:679–687

Lentferink YE, Knibbe CA, van der Vorst MM (2018) Efficacy of metformin treatment with respect to weight Reduction in children and adults with obesity: a systematic review. Drugs 78:1887–1901

Maloney A, Rosenstock J, Fonseca V (2019) A model-based meta-analysis of 24 antihyperglycemic drugs for type 2 diabetes: comparison of treatment effects at therapeutic doses. Clin Pharmacol Ther 105:1213–1223

Mannucci E, Monami M, Lamanna C, Gensini GF, Marchionni N (2008) Pioglitazone and cardiovascular risk. A comprehensive meta-analysis of randomized clinical trials. Diabetes Obes Metab 10:1221–1238

Marso SP, Daniels GH, Brown-Frandsen K et al (2018) Liraglutide and cardiovascular outcomes in type 2 diabetes. N Engl J Med 375:311–322

Mastrandrea LD, Witte L, Carlsson Petri KC, Hale PM, Hedman HK, Riesenberg RA (2019) Liraglutide in a paediatric (7-11y) population with obesity: a randomized, double-blind, placebo-controlled short term trial to assess safety, tolerability, pharmacokinetiks, and pharmacodynamics. Pediatr Obes 14:e12495

Neal B, Perkovic V, Mahaffey KW et al CANVAS Program Collaborative Group (2017) Canagliflozin and cardiovascular and renal events in type 2 diabetes. N Engl J Med 377:644–657

Ramachandran A, Snehalatha C, Satyavani K, Sivasankari S, Vijay V (2003) Type 2 diabetes in Asian-Indian urban children. Diabetes Care 26:1022–1025

Reinehr T, Kiess W, Kapellen T, Wiegand S, Holl RW (2010) Children with diabetes mellitus type 2 in Europe: an underserved population. Arch Dis Child 95:954

Riddle MC, Cefalu WT (2018) SGLT inhibitors for type 1Diabetes: an obvious choice or too good to be true? Diabetes Care 41:2444–2447

Rodriguez BL, Fujimoto WY, Mayer-Davis EJ, Imperatore G, Williams DE, Bell RA et al (2006) Prevalence of cardiovascular disease risk factors in U.S. children and adolescents with diabetes: the SEARCH for diabetes in youth study. Diabetes Care 29:1891–1896

Sugihara S, Sasaki N, Kohno H, Amemiya S, Tanaka T, Matsura N, The Committee for Medical Treatment of Childhood-Onset Type 2 Diabetes Mellitus, The Japanese Society for Pediatric Endocrinology (2005) Survey of current medical treatments for childhood onset type 2 diabetes mellitus in Japan. Clin Pediatr Endocrinol 14:65–75

Tamborlane WV, Barrientos-Perez M, Fainberg U et al (2019) Liraglutide in children and adolescents with type 2 diabetes. N Engl J Med. https://doi.org/10.1056/NEJMoa1903822

TODAY Study Group (2013) Effects of metformin, metformin plus rosiglitazone, and metformin plus lifestyle on insulin sensitivity and β-cell function in TODAY. Diabetes Care 36:1749–1757

Tosur M, Redondo MJ, Lyons SK (2018) Adjuvant pharmacotherapies to insulin for the treatment of type 1 diabetes. Curr Diab Rep 18:79

Unger J (2013) Rational use of GLP1 receptor agonists in patients with type 1 diabetes. Curr Diab Rep 13:663–668

Wei JN, Sung FC, Li CY, Chang CH, Lin RS, Lin CC, Chiang CC, Chuang LM (2002) Low birth weight and high birth weight infants are both at an increased risk to have type 2 diabetes among schoolchildren in Taiwan. Diabetes Care 26:343–348

Wei JN, Sung FC, Lin CC, Lin RS, Chiang CC, Chuang LM (2003) National surveillance for type 2 diabetes mellitus in Taiwanese children. JAMA 290:1345–1350

Zeitler P, Arslanian S, Fu J, Pinhas-Hamiel O, Reinehr T, Tandon N, Urakami T, Wong J, Maahs DM (2018) ISPAD guideline type 2 diabetes (T2D) in youth. Pediatr Diabetes 19(Suppl 27):28–46. https://doi.org/10.1111/pedi.12719

Zinman B, Wanner C, Lachin JM et al (2015) Empagliflozin, cardiovascular outcomes, and mortality in type 2 diabetes. N Engl J Med 373:2117–2128

Biologicals in the Treatment of Pediatric Atopic Diseases

Maike vom Hove, Martina P. Neininger, Thilo Bertsche, and Freerk Prenzel

Contents

The authors "Maike vom Hove" and "Martina P. Neininger" shared first authorship.

The authors "Thilo Bertsche" and "Freerk Prenzel" shared senior authorship.

M. vom Hove · F. Prenzel (✉)
Hospital for Children and Adolescents, Leipzig University Medical Center, Leipzig, Germany
e-mail: freerk.prenzel@uniklinik-leipzig.de

M. P. Neininger · T. Bertsche
Drug Safety Center, Institute of Pharmacy, Leipzig University, Leipzig, Germany

W. Kiess et al. (eds.), *Pediatric Pharmacotherapy*,
Handbook of Experimental Pharmacology 261, https://doi.org/10.1007/164_2019_307

Abstract

The management of atopic diseases such as severe asthma, severe atopic dermatitis, and severe food allergy in childhood is challenging. In particular, there are safety concerns regarding the use of high-dose corticosteroids. The recent development of biologicals and their approval for the treatment of children offer a new, very promising, and more personalized therapy option. Omalizumab, mepolizumab, and dupilumab are currently approved as add-on treatments of severe asthma in children and have been shown to be effective in improvement of asthma control and reduction of exacerbations. Dupilumab is the only biological approved for the treatment of atopic dermatitis in adolescents so far. It has been demonstrated to significantly improve symptoms of atopic dermatitis.

However, safety data for biologicals used in atopic diseases in children and adolescents are still very limited. Biologicals are generally considered to be safe in adults. These data are often extrapolated to children. Additionally, data for long-term use are lacking. Thus, the safety profiles of those biologicals cannot yet be conclusively assessed.

Keywords

Adverse drug reactions · Allergic rhinitis · Anti-IgE · Anti-IL-4R · Anti-IL-5 · Asthma · Atopic dermatitis · Benralizumab · Biologicals · Children · Drug safety · Dupilumab · Food allergies · Mepolizumab · Omalizumab · Reslizumab

1 Asthma

In case of severe asthma with uncontrolled symptoms and recurrent exacerbations under treatment with high-dose inhaled corticosteroids and another controller medication biologicals offer a more personalized add-on treatment. So far, biologicals approved for the treatment of asthma in children are omalizumab $\geq$6 years, mepolizumab $\geq$6 years, and dupilumab $\geq$12 years.

1.1 Anti-immunoglobulin E (IgE)

Omalizumab is an anti-IgE humanized monoclonal antibody. It was the first biological approved for the treatment of severe persistent allergic asthma in adults and adolescents $\geq$12 by the US Food and Drug Administration (FDA) in 2003 and by the European Medicines Agency (EMA) in 2005. In 2009 (EMA) and 2016 (FDA), it was also approved for children $\geq$6 years of age.

Mechanism of action: Omalizumab binds to the Fc-part of circulating IgE, preventing it from interacting with FcεRI receptors on basophils and mast cells, downregulating their FcεRI expression, and inhibiting the effector cells form mediator release (Holgate et al. 2005).

Pharmacokinetics: After subcutaneous injection, time to peak serum level is 6–8 days. The average absolute bioavailability is 62%. In asthmatic patients, half-life serum elimination is about 17–23 days. Omalizumab is eliminated via degradation in the liver reticuloendothelial system and the endothelial cells (Lowe et al. 2009; Xolair – U. S. Food and Drug Administration 2013).

Use: Add-on treatment for patients $\geq$6 years with severe persistent allergic asthma, who suffer from frequent respiratory symptoms and severe exacerbations even though being treated with high doses of inhaled steroids and inhaled long-acting β_2-agonists. Further therapy conditions are (1) allergy to a perennial allergen (confirmed by positive skin prick test or specific serum IgE); (2) for patients $\geq$12 years, a reduced lung function with FEV1 $\leq$ 80% predicted; and (3) serum IgE and body weight have to be within the dosing range (GINA 2019; Xolair – European Medicines Agency 2009).

Application: The dose and frequency of application are determined by body weight and baseline serum IgE. Dependent on these measurements 75 – maximum 600 – mg omalizumab can be given every 2–4 weeks. It is administered via subcutaneous injection.

The full protective effect can be expected 4–6 weeks after initiating the treatment with omalizumab (Teach et al. 2015). At least 4 months is suggested as initial trial (GINA 2019).

An extension of the dosing interval by about 1/3, after having reached a stable condition during a 4-month treatment period, has been shown to result in the maintenance of asthma control in the majority of adult patients (Bölke et al. 2019).

During the treatment with omalizumab and for up to 12 months after the interruption of treatment, the serum IgE levels remain elevated. Therefore, a renewed testing of serum IgE for dose determination during this time period is not possible (Xolair – European Medicines Agency 2009).

Efficacy: Clinical trials of asthmatic children and adolescents treated with omalizumab as add-on therapy demonstrated a significantly reduced number of exacerbations (Berger et al. 2003; Busse et al. 2011; Milgrom et al. 2001; Teach et al. 2015) and reduced rate of hospitalization (Deschildre et al. 2013; Lanier et al. 2009; Pitrez et al. 2017). Furthermore, a reduction of respiratory symptoms and improvement in asthma control have been shown (Busse et al. 2011; Deschildre et al. 2013).

Regarding the health-related quality of life, a significant benefit of omalizumab compared to placebo was reported in pediatric patients with moderate-to-severe allergic asthma (Lemanske et al. 2002).

Under treatment with omalizumab, the likelihood of dosage reduction of inhaled corticosteroids is increased (Busse et al. 2011; Deschildre et al. 2013; Milgrom et al. 2001; Normansell et al. 2014).

The PROSE study demonstrated a reduced susceptibility to infections with rhinovirus in asthmatic children treated with omalizumab, resulting in a decrease of viral respiratory infections and viral asthma exacerbations (Esquivel et al. 2017; Teach et al. 2015).

Observational studies in children treated with omalizumab over a 2-year period showed an ongoing benefit with a continually decreasing exacerbation rate, still reduced dose of inhaled corticosteroids (as in the 1 year of treatment), and a normalized lung function (Deschildre et al. 2013, 2015; Odajima et al. 2017). This continued benefit has been confirmed by an observational study over a 6-year treatment period (Folqué et al. 2019). Thus, the prolonged use of omalizumab does not result in an efficacy loss.

1.2 Anti-interleukin-5 (IL-5) and Anti-IL-5 Receptor (IL-5R)

IL-5 plays a major role in the differentiation, maturation, and activation of eosinophils (Clutterbuck et al. 1989).

Mepolizumab is an anti-interleukin-5 (IL-5) humanized monoclonal antibody.

It was approved by the FDA to treat severe eosinophilic asthma in patients ≥12 years in 2015 and by the EMA to treat children ≥6 years in 2018.

Mechanism of action: Mepolizumab binds free IL-5, inhibiting it from activating the IL-5 receptor on eosinophils and basophils. Thus, mepolizumab hinders the signaling of IL-5 and limits the survival, proliferation, and activation of eosinophils (Kouro and Takatsu 2009).

Pharmacokinetics: Following subcutaneous injection, time to peak serum level is 4–8 days. The absolute bioavailability is about 76%. The mean half-life is 16–22 days. After accounting for bodyweight and bioavailability, pharmacokinetics in children was approximately consistent with adults and adolescents (Nucala – European Medicines Agency 2015).

Use: Add-on treatment for patients ≥6 years with severe eosinophilic asthma (Nucala – European Medicines Agency 2015).

Recommended eligibility criteria: Treatment with high-dose inhaled corticosteroids and an additional controller medication; two or more severe exacerbations in the last year and/or dependency on systemic corticosteroids. Optimal benefit is expected in patients with baseline blood eosinophils ≥150 μg or ≥300 cells/μl in the past 12 months (Nucala – European Medicines Agency 2015; Ortega et al. 2016).

Patients with uncontrolled asthma and ≥150/μl eosinophils are the most likely to benefit from a therapy with mepolizumab (Busse 2019).

Application: Mepolizumab is administered subcutaneously. Adolescents 12–17 years receive 100 mg, and children 6–11 years receive 40 mg every 4 weeks (Nucala – European Medicines Agency 2015).

Efficacy: The approval of mepolizumab in children (6–12 years) was based on the effectiveness data gained in the pharmacokinetics/pharmacodynamics study in 36 children with severe eosinophilic asthma (6–12 years) and on the data of adolescents in the mepolizumab severe asthma pivotal program. A similar efficacy regarding the exacerbation rate and improvement in asthma control has been shown for children and adolescents/adults (Gupta et al. 2018). Further efficacy data for children are still lacking.

The MENSA trial showed that mepolizumab can significantly reduce the risk for asthma exacerbations and improve asthma control in adolescents (>12 years) and adults with severe eosinophilic asthma (Ortega et al. 2016). Furthermore, an improvement in the health-related quality of life (Chupp et al. 2017) and a reduced hospitalization rate due to severe exacerbations were reported (Yancey et al. 2017).

In the long-term use (84 weeks), an ongoing and stable effect regarding the reduced exacerbation rate was shown (Lugogo et al. 2016).

Information regarding the optimal duration of treatment is scarce. For patients treated with mepolizumab during 1 year, worsening of asthma control and a de novo increase of the eosinophil count already 3 months after discontinuation were observed (Haldar et al. 2014; Ortega et al. 2019). For adults with severe eosinophilic asthma, effectiveness during a treatment period up to 4.5 years has been shown (Khatri et al. 2019).

Reslizumab is an anti-IL-5 humanized monoclonal antibody.

It was approved by the FDA and EMA as add-on therapy in adults with severe eosinophilic asthma in 2016. It is not approved for children and adolescents.

Mechanism of action: Reslizumab attaches and neutralizes IL-5, hindering it from stimulating the proliferation and survival of eosinophils and inhibiting signaling (Cinqaero – European Medicines Agency 2016).

Pharmacokinetics: The peak serum concentration is expected at the end of the infusion. Reslizumab has a half-life of about 24 days. Reslizumab is degraded by widely distributed enzymes (Cinqaero – European Medicines Agency 2016).

Use: Add-on treatment in severe eosinophilic asthma, uncontrolled on high-dose inhaled corticosteroids, and an additional controller medication in adults (Cinqaero – European Medicines Agency 2016). Further recommended eligibility criteria:

Three or more severe exacerbations in the last year and blood eosinophils ≥400 μg (Cooper et al. 2018).

Application: The drug is administered as intravenous infusion (3 mg/kg body weight) every 4 weeks (Cinqaero – European Medicines Agency 2016).

Efficacy: In studies including adolescents ≥12 years and adults with uncontrolled asthma and an eosinophil count of ≥400 μg, a reduction of the exacerbation rate, improvement in lung function, and quality of life were reported (Bjermer et al. 2016; Castro et al. 2015; Corren et al. 2016).

Improvements in lung function and asthma control were sustained during a study period of 24 months, indicating long-term efficacy of reslizumab in adult patients with moderate-to-severe eosinophilic asthma (Murphy et al. 2017). No data are available for children aged up to 11 years.

In a subgroup analysis of 39 adolescents from 12 to 17 years, a paradoxal increase in asthma exacerbations was observed (Cinqaero – U.S. Food and drug administration 2016).

Benralizumab is an anti-IL-5 receptor humanized monoclonal antibody.

Benralizumab was approved by the FDA for patients ≥12 years with severe asthma in 2017 and by the EMA for adult patients in 2018.

Mechanism of action: It binds to the α-subunit of the IL-5 receptor (IL-5R). IL-5R is expressed on eosinophil and basophil progenitor and mature cells. Benralizumab inhibits IL-5 receptor signaling and induces cytotoxicity of eosinophils and basophils (Ghazi et al. 2012).

Pharmacokinetics: The absolute bioavailability is about 59%. Benralizumab has a half-life of approximately 15 days and is degraded by proteolytic enzymes widely distributed in the body (Fasenra – European Medicines Agency 2018).

Use: Add-on maintenance treatment of adult patients with severe eosinophilic asthma, uncontrolled on high-dose inhaled corticosteroids and long-acting β_2-agonists (Fasenra – European Medicines Agency 2018).

Application: 30 mg of benralizumab is administered via subcutaneous injection every 4 weeks for the first three doses, afterward every 8 weeks.

Efficacy: In adolescents ≥12 and adults with severe, uncontrolled asthma, and an eosinophil count of ≥300 μg, benralizumab improved pulmonary function and reduced the rate of exacerbations and asthmatic symptoms (Bleecker et al. 2016; FitzGerald et al. 2016).

Long-term efficacy over a time period of 1 year has been demonstrated (Busse et al. 2019).

Data for children aged up to 11 years are not available. In a subgroup analysis of 108 adolescents aged 12–17 years, no effect on the asthma exacerbation rate was noted (Fasenra – European Medicines Agency 2018).

1.3 Anti-interleukin-4 Receptor (IL-4R)

Dupilumab is a humanized monoclonal antibody targeting interleukin-4 receptor (IL-4R). The treatment of asthma in adolescents ≥12 years with dupilumab was approved by the FDA in 2018 and by the EMA in 2019.

Mechanism of action: Dupilumab binds to the α-subunit of interleukin-4 receptor, inhibiting IL-4 and IL-13 signaling. IL-4 and IL-13 recruit eosinophils, activate Th2 cells, animate IgE production, and inhibit the differentiation of keratinocytes. Thus, they play a major role in type 2 inflammation as in asthma and atopic dermatitis (Vakharia and Silverberg 2019).

Pharmacokinetics: After subcutaneous injection, time to peak serum level is 7 days. The absolute bioavailability is 64%. The metabolic pathway of dupilumab has not been characterized. Since dupilumab is a human monoclonal IgG4 antibody, it is expected to be degraded into small peptides and amino acids via catabolic pathways (Shirley 2017).

Use: Add-on treatment for patients ≥12 years with severe asthma and type 2 inflammation characterized by elevated eosinophils and/or elevated levels in the fraction of exhaled nitric oxide (FE_{NO}), which is uncontrolled under high-dose inhaled steroids plus another controller medication (Duxipent – European Medicines Agency 2017).

Application: Dupilumab is administered via subcutaneous injection. Patients with severe eosinophilic/type 2 asthma receive an initial dose of 400 mg, followed by 200 mg every 2 weeks. Patients with severe asthma and dependence on oral corticosteroids or with an additional moderate-to-severe atopic dermatitis receive an initial dose of 600 mg, followed by 300 mg every 2 weeks (Duxipent – European Medicines Agency 2017).

Efficacy: In the QUEST trial, adolescents $\geq$12 years and adults with uncontrolled asthma (107 of 1,902 patients were adolescents aged 12–17 years) were analyzed. The patients who received dupilumab showed an improved lung function, better asthma control, and lower rates of exacerbations compared to placebo-treated patients. In the subgroup analysis, patients with higher baseline levels of eosinophils ($\geq$150 cells/μl and $FE_{NO} \geq 25$ ppb) profited the most. For patients with eosinophils <150 cells/μl and FE_{NO} <25 ppb, no significant improvement of lung function or exacerbations was noted (Castro et al. 2018).

Thus, it can be concluded that the presence of type T2 inflammation (indicated by high eosinophils and FE_{NO}) makes it more likely for dupilumab to be effective (Busse 2019).

In the VENTURE trial, adolescents $\geq$12 years and adults with oral glucocorticoid-dependent severe asthma were treated with dupilumab. Severe exacerbations as well as the dose of oral glucocorticoids were significantly reduced under treatment. Furthermore, an improvement of the lung function was shown (Rabe et al. 2018).

Reduced rate of exacerbations and improved lung function were also reported in uncontrolled moderate-to-severe asthma in adults (Wenzel et al. 2013, 2016).

2 Atopic Dermatitis

Atopic dermatitis is the most common chronic inflammatory skin disease in children, affecting up to 20% of children and adolescents worldwide. Approximately 33% are diagnosed with moderate-to-severe disease (Silverberg and Simpson 2013).

2.1 Anti-interleukin-4 receptor

Dupilumab was approved by the FDA and EMA in 2019 for the treatment of moderate-to-severe atopic dermatitis in patients aged $\geq$12 who are candidates for systemic therapy (Duxipent – European Medicines Agency 2017).

Dosage and application in atopic dermatitis in adolescents: For adolescents with a body weight of <60 kg, an initial dose of 400 mg is applied subcutaneously (two 200 mg injections), followed by 200 mg every 2 weeks.

For adolescents with a body weight of $\geq$60 kg, an initial dose of 600 mg is applied subcutaneously (two 300 mg injections), followed by 300 mg every 2 weeks.

It is recommended to combine dupilumab with daily emollients and when needed to add topical anti-inflammatory agents (Wollenberg et al. 2018).

Efficacy: For adults with moderate-to-severe atopic dermatitis treated with dupilumab in two phase 3 trials, a significant improvement in the investigators global assessment (IGA), eczema area and severity index (EASI) score, pruritus, and quality of life was reported (Simpson et al. 2016). Furthermore, long-term efficacy on improved signs and symptoms of atopic dermatitis during a time period of 76 weeks has been reported (Deleuran et al. 2019).

In a phase 3 trial with 251 adolescents (12–17 years) with moderate-to-severe atopic dermatitis, a significant improvement in measures of overall disease severity, skin clearing, reduction in itch, and improved quality of life compared to placebo was seen (Simpson et al. 2019).

Efficacy data in children <12 years are scarce. In a small case series of children (7–15 years) with severe atopic dermatitis treated with dupilumab during an average time of 8.5 months, a significant improvement has been reported (Treister and Lio 2019).

First results from a phase 3 trial in children 6–11 years of age with severe atopic dermatitis showed a significant improvement in overall disease severity, skin clearing, reduced itching, and improved health-related quality of life (Sanofi Press Release 2019).

2.2 Further Biologicals in the Treatment of Atopic Dermatitis

So far, no other biological agent is approved for the therapy of atopic dermatitis in children and adolescents.

For the treatment with omalizumab, no consistent evidence of efficacy was found so far. Hence, the therapy is not recommended (Wang et al. 2016; Wollenberg et al. 2018).

The use of mepolizumab showed only modest improvement in clinical symptoms in atopic dermatitis so far. Therefore, its application is recommended only in well-selected patients, who do not respond to standard therapy (Oldhoff et al. 2005; Wollenberg et al. 2018).

Lebrikizumab and tralokinumab are humanized monoclonal antibody against IL-13. Nemolizumab is a monoclonal antibody targeting IL-31 receptor. A significant clinical improvement in adults with moderate-to-severe atopic dermatitis was shown in the first trials investigating these substances (Eichenfield 2017; Ruzicka and Mihara 2017; Wollenberg et al. 2019).

3 Food Allergies

So far, there is no FDA- or EMA-approved therapy for the prevention of severe reactions due to food allergies. In 2018, the FDA granted breakthrough therapy designation for omalizumab for the prevention of severe allergic reaction due to accidental ingestion of food in patients with food allergies (Vickery 2019). An upcoming clinical trial will investigate omalizumab monotherapy as an adjunct to multifood oral immunotherapy (Sampson et al. 2019).

In several randomized placebo-controlled trials, the efficacy of omalizumab in combination with oral immunotherapy in children has been examined.

A significant improvement in efficacy and safety of multifood oral immunotherapy under omalizumab therapy in children 4–15 years with multifood allergies was described in a phase 2 clinical trial (Andorf et al. 2018). In children (6–14 years) with severe cow's milk allergy, the treatment with a combination of oral immunotherapy and omalizumab leads to desensitization of all treated children compared to none in the untreated group (Takahashi et al. 2017).

Contrarily, in a randomized double-blind placebo-controlled study of omalizumab combined with oral immunotherapy for the treatment of cow's milk allergy in patients aged 7–32 years, a significant improvement in safety but not in efficacy was noted. Furthermore, after 8 weeks of avoidance, an increased reactivity to cow's milk was noted again (Wood et al. 2016). In a retrospective observational study of children with severe food allergies, treated with omalizumab for severe asthma, a significant increase in the food allergen threshold was noted. Furthermore, anaphylactic reactions due to accidental food ingestion were significantly lower (Fiocchi et al. 2019).

4 Allergic Rhinitis

Allergic rhinitis is a symptomatic reaction of the nose induced by an IgE-mediated inflammation of the nasal mucosa due to allergen exposure in a sensitized patient (Bousquet et al. 2001). For the treatment of allergic rhinitis in adults or children, no biological is approved so far.

Efficacy of omalizumab compared to placebo in uncontrolled allergic rhinitis in adult patients has been shown in several studies. It significantly improved health-related quality of life and nasal symptoms and decreased rescue medication use (Tsabouri et al. 2014).

Nevertheless, compared to other pharmacotherapies, the benefits are small; hence it is not recommended as monotherapy in allergic rhinitis. But in patients with polyallergic rhinitis and increased risk of anaphylactic reactions, it can be used in combination with allergen immunotherapy (Wise et al. 2018).

In a study with adult patients treated for uncontrolled asthma and comorbid perennial allergic rhinitis with 300 mg dupilumab every 2 weeks, a significant improvement of nasal symptoms as runny nose, sneezing, nasal blockage, and postnasal discharge was reported. No significant effect was seen in patients treated with 200 mg every 2 weeks (Weinstein et al. 2018).

5 Drug Safety

5.1 General Aspects of Adverse Drug Reactions

Biologicals used in atopic diseases seem to have a comparatively good benefit-risk ratio – at least in adults. Most adverse drug reactions are at placebo level in this patient group (Chipps et al. 2017; Farne et al. 2017; Xiong et al. 2019). Since trials

Table 1 Adverse events of omalizumab according to (Busse et al. 2011)

Adverse event	Placebo (number of patients [%] from $n = 211$)	Omalizumab 100 mg (number of patients [%] from $n = 208$)
All adverse events	47% (100)	39% (82)
Eyes, ears, nose, and throat	3% (6)	1% (2)
Gastrointestinal	1% (2)	5% (10)
Hematological	12% (6)	0% (1)
Anaphylactic	3% (6)	0% (1)
Infection	19% (22)	8% (17)
Injection site	3% (6)	4% (8)
Musculoskeletal	1% (3)	1% (3)
Nervous system	3% (7)	1% (3)
Psychiatric	1% (2)	0% (0)
Respiratory	22% (47)	16% (34)
Skin	9% (19)	8% (16)
Others	9% (19)	13% (27)

for pediatric use are scarce, data are sometimes extrapolated from adult use without sufficient clinically relevant data.

A review judged *omalizumab* to be a safe therapy for the treatment of severe asthma in children (Ahmed and Turner 2019). This statement was based on at least ten randomized controlled trials in children. The most commonly reported adverse reactions were headaches and injection site reactions, including injection site pain, swelling, erythema, and pruritus during clinical trials in adult and adolescent patients $\geq$12 years. In clinical trials in children 6 to $<$12 years of age, the most commonly reported adverse reactions were headache, pyrexia, and upper abdominal pain. Most of the reactions were mild or moderate in severity (Xolair – European Medicines Agency 2009). An overview of adverse drug events in children found in the ICATA study is presented in Table 1.

For the approval of *mepolizumab* in children and adolescents, 36 pediatric patients (aged 6–11 years) and 25 adolescents (aged 12–17 years) received mepolizumab (Nucala – European Medicines Agency 2015). Although not finally assessable yet, the safety profile is expected to be comparable between adolescents and adults (Deeks 2016). The most frequently reported adverse reactions were headache, injection site reactions, back pain, and fatigue (Deeks 2016).

The safety profile of *reslizumab* and *benralizumab* has not yet been established in children and adolescents aged up to 17 years due to paucity of data. The most commonly reported adverse events were worsening asthma, headache, nasopharyngitis, upper respiratory tract infections, and sinusitis (Bjermer et al. 2016; Bleecker et al. 2016). The most frequently observed adverse drug reactions in *dupilumab* treatment were upper respiratory tract infection (14%), injection site erythema (13%), and headache (10%) (Wenzel et al. 2016). Serious adverse events (SAE) were reported in up to 8% of patients. The most frequent SAE was pneumonia

(Castro et al. 2018). Injection site reactions occurred in up to 26% of patients. Those reactions were strongly dose-related (Wenzel et al. 2016). Patients suffering from severe atopic dermatitis treated with dupilumab are at an increased risk for conjunctivitis (Akinlade et al. 2019). The International Eczema Council developed a consensus on the management of dupilumab-associated conjunctivitis including lubricating eye drops, ointments or oral antihistamines, and referral to ophthalmologists in severe cases requiring corticosteroid, ciclosporin, or tacrolimus eye drops (Thyssen et al. 2019).

5.2 Hypersensitivity

Hypersensitivity reactions such as bronchospasm, rash, urticaria, angioedema, and hypotension have been observed in the treatment of children and adolescents with biologicals. Due to the limited data available, the risk profile of the biologicals cannot be fully characterized. In omalizumab, a delayed onset of symptoms and a protracted progression have been observed (Limb et al. 2007). Allergic reactions may also occur after a long period of treatment. In a meta-analysis of 1,380 children (aged 6–11 years), anaphylaxis was not more frequent in omalizumab compared to placebo (Rodrigo and Neffen 2015), and a recent review reported an overall incidence rate of 0.2% (Chipps et al. 2017). In mepolizumab and benralizumab, delayed reactions after hours and days have been observed, whereas in benralizumab the onset of symptoms usually occurs within 20 min after infusion. Serious life-threatening anaphylactic reactions were only very rarely or never documented (Bleecker et al. 2016; FitzGerald et al. 2016; Lugogo et al. 2016; Pavord et al. 2012).

In case of a severe hypersensitivity reaction, the respective biological should be discontinued (Cinqaero – European Medicines Agency 2016; Deeks 2016; Duxipent – European Medicines Agency 2017; Fasenra – European Medicines Agency 2018; Nucala – European Medicines Agency 2015; Xolair – European Medicines Agency 2009).

5.3 Serum Sickness

Especially in omalizumab, serum sickness has been reported as a delayed type III allergic reaction. This typically occurs 1–5 days after administration of the first or one of the subsequent injections but also after a longer period of treatment. Typical symptoms of serum sickness are arthritis/arthralgia, rash (urticaria or other forms), fever, and lymphadenopathy. Prevention and treatment of this disease involve H1-antihistamines and glucocorticosteroids (Xolair – European Medicines Agency 2009).

5.4 Eosinophil Count Increase

Eosinophilia occurred in 4% of patients treated with dupilumab (Castro et al. 2018). Thereof, 8% showed clinical symptoms. Transient increase of eosinophil counts has been observed in 14% of patients (Rabe et al. 2018). Higher eosinophil counts before the initiation of dupilumab treatment seem to be associated with a higher risk for transient increase of eosinophil counts during treatment (Wenzel et al. 2016). Rarely, Churg-Strauss syndrome (allergic eosinophilic granulomatous vasculitis) or systemic hypereosinophilic syndrome has been reported in the treatment with omalizumab. Usually, those disorders occur when a systemic glucocorticosteroid therapy is reduced.

5.5 Immunogenicity

Antibodies to every therapeutic antibody were found. However, the clinical relevance cannot finally be assessed. For mepolizumab, in up to 8% of the patients, antibodies against the active ingredient have been documented including also data from children of 6 to 11 years of age (Pavord et al. 2012). The majority of those patients showed only a transient presence of antibodies. Patients treated with benralizumab and reslizumab developed antidrug antibodies in 15% and 13%, respectively. Antidrug antibodies to dupilumab were reported in 5% of patients (Rabe et al. 2018). For all biologicals, no association with serious adverse events or reduced efficacy was found (Bel et al. 2014; Bleecker et al. 2016; FitzGerald et al. 2016; Murphy et al. 2017; Rabe et al. 2018).

5.6 Immunoglobulin E Increase

The total amount of immunoglobulin E is increased during omalizumab therapy. The increase can last for 1 year after discontinuation. Therefore, dosage calculations have to be based on the initial immunoglobulin E amount, if the discontinuation period was shorter than 1 year (Xolair – European Medicines Agency 2009).

5.7 Helminth Infections

Since eosinophils are involved in the immune response to some helminth infections, caution is advised in patients with a high risk of parasitic infections. It is recommended to sufficiently treat a helminth infection before initiating a therapy with biologicals. If helminthiasis occurs during antibody therapy and does not sufficiently respond to antihelminth therapy, discontinuation of antibody treatment is recommended (Deeks 2016). A placebo-controlled study showed a slight increase in the infection rate during treatment with omalizumab in patients with a chronically high risk of helminth infection. In a broad spectrum of clinical studies, helminth infection was not uncommon with ≤ 1 out of 1,000 patients. Therefore, caution is advised in patients at high risk of helminth infection, particularly when travelling to endemic areas. For benralizumab, patients with helminth infections were excluded from clinical trials. For reslizumab, no helminth infections were documented (Murphy et al. 2017).

5.8 Infections and Vaccinations

In patients treated with mepolizumab, herpes zoster virus infections have been detected (Deeks 2016). This led to the recommendation to vaccinate against varicella before the initiation of mepolizumab treatment. Dupilumab, however, seems to be associated with a lower risk for clinically relevant herpes viral infections (Eichenfield et al. 2019). The summary of product characteristics recommends not to vaccinate with live or live-attenuated vaccines simultaneously with dupilumab as there are no safety data available (Duxipent – European Medicines Agency 2017).

5.9 Adolescents of Childbearing Age

At least in animal experiments, biologicals such as omalizumab and mepolizumab penetrate the placental barrier. Their risk potential for the fetus is unknown. Biologicals should therefore not be used during pregnancy unless there is an urgent need to do so.

5.10 Drug-Drug Interactions

Clinically relevant drug-drug interactions, including those with the anti-asthmatic therapy, are currently not reported for omalizumab and mepolizumab. The efficacy of drugs for the treatment of parasitic infections may be indirectly reduced (see Sect. 9.7).

5.11 Limitations for Benefit-Risk Considerations

Due to the rather small number of patients and short duration of studies, evidence on the safety of biologicals in the treatment of atopic diseases is still very limited, particularly for pediatric use (Henriksen et al. 2018; Menzella et al. 2016). Data from adolescents and adults are often extrapolated to children aged 6–11 years (Chipps et al. 2017). In particular, data for long-term use are lacking. Considering their higher life span compared to adults, these safety data are urgently needed in the management of pediatric atopic diseases. For omalizumab and mepolizumab, evidence suggests that there is no difference in the safety profile between short-term and long-term treatment (Chipps et al. 2017; Khatri et al. 2019). However, especially to determine the risk of long-term adverse events such as malignancy in children, studies with a longer duration and including a relevant number of pediatric patients are needed (Chipps et al. 2017).

References

Ahmed H, Turner S (2019) Severe asthma in children – a review of definitions, epidemiology, and treatment options in 2019. Pediatr Pulmonol 54:778–787. https://doi.org/10.1002/ppul.24317

Akinlade B, Guttman-Yassky E, de Bruin-Weller M, Simpson EL, Blauvelt A, Cork MJ, Prens E, Asbell P, Akpek E, Corren J, Bachert C, Hirano I, Weyne J, Korotzer A, Chen Z, Hultsch T, Zhu X, Davis JD, Mannent L, Hamilton JD, Teper A, Staudinger H, Rizova E, Pirozzi G, Graham NMH, Shumel B, Ardeleanu M, Wollenberg A (2019) Conjunctivitis in dupilumab clinical trials. Br J Dermatol. https://doi.org/10.1111/bjd.17869

Andorf S, Purington N, Block WM, Long AJ, Tupa D, Brittain E, Rudman Spergel A, Desai M, Galli SJ, Nadeau KC, Chinthrajah RS (2018) Anti-IgE treatment with oral immunotherapy in multifood allergic participants: a double-blind, randomised, controlled trial. Lancet Gastroenterol Hepatol 3:85–94. https://doi.org/10.1016/S2468-1253(17)30392-8

Bel EH, Wenzel SE, Thompson PJ, Prazma CM, Keene ON, Yancey SW, Ortega HG, Pavord ID (2014) Oral glucocorticoid-sparing effect of mepolizumab in eosinophilic asthma. N Engl J Med 371:1189–1197. https://doi.org/10.1056/NEJMoa1403291

Berger W, Gupta N, McAlary M, Fowler-Taylor A (2003) Evaluation of long-term safety of the anti-IgE antibody, omalizumab, in children with allergic asthma. Ann Allergy Asthma Immunol 91:182–188. https://doi.org/10.1016/S1081-1206(10)62175-8

Bjermer L, Lemiere C, Maspero J, Weiss S, Zangrilli J, Germinaro M (2016) Reslizumab for inadequately controlled asthma with elevated blood eosinophil levels: a randomized phase 3 study. Chest 150:789–798. https://doi.org/10.1016/j.chest.2016.03.032

Bleecker ER, FitzGerald JM, Chanez P, Papi A, Weinstein SF, Barker P, Sproule S, Gilmartin G, Aurivillius M, Werkström V, Goldman M (2016) Efficacy and safety of benralizumab for patients with severe asthma uncontrolled with high-dosage inhaled corticosteroids and long-acting β2-agonists (SIROCCO): a randomised, multicentre, placebo-controlled phase 3 trial. Lancet 388:2115–2127. https://doi.org/10.1016/S0140-6736(16)31324-1

Bölke G, Church MK, Bergmann K-C (2019) Comparison of extended intervals and dose reduction of omalizumab for asthma control. Allergo J Int 28:1–4. https://doi.org/10.1007/s40629-018-0087-6

Bousquet J, van Cauwenberge P, Khaltaev N (2001) Allergic rhinitis and its impact on asthma. J Allergy Clin Immunol 108:S147–S334. https://doi.org/10.1067/mai.2001.118891

Busse WW (2019) Biological treatments for severe asthma: a major advance in asthma care. Allergol Int 68:158–166. https://doi.org/10.1016/j.alit.2019.01.004

Busse WW, Morgan WJ, Gergen PJ, Mitchell HE, Gern JE, Liu AH, Gruchalla RS, Kattan M, Teach SJ, Pongracic JA, Chmiel JF, Steinbach SF, Calatroni A, Togias A, Thompson KM, Szefler SJ, Sorkness CA (2011) Randomized trial of omalizumab (anti-IgE) for asthma in inner-city children. N Engl J Med 364:1005–1015. https://doi.org/10.1056/NEJMoa1009705

Busse WW, Bleecker ER, FitzGerald JM, Ferguson GT, Barker P, Sproule S, Olsson RF, Martin UJ, Goldman M, Yañez A, Fernández M, Tolcachier A, Belloni J, Taborda J, de Salvo M, Maspero J, Victorio C, Navarta MC, Grilli M, Rodríguez P, Otaola M, Cambursano V, Malamud P, Stok A, Arce G, Roza O, Scherbovsky F, Elias P, Saez MS, Peters M, Phillips M, Upham J, Gibson P, Thien F, Douglass J, Thomas P, Bardin P, Sajkov D, Hew M, Langton D, Pez A, Fritscher C, Hetzel J, Mattos W, Stelmach R, Antila M, Fernandes AL, Metev H, Ivanov Y, Bogdanova A, Markova AD, Peneva M, Veselinova R, Petkova T, Petrova V, Shopova E, Ivanova Y, Yotsova R, Kirkova G, Petrova G, Dachev S, Sotirova K, Stoyanova M, Yakov O, Ilieva-Fartunova V, Lemiere C, Laviolette M, Yang W, Pek B, Killorn WP, Poirier C, Chouinard G, Melenka L, Leigh R, Nair P, Dorscheid D, Martin J, Pavie J, Rosenblut A, Cartagena C, Quilodran C, Muñoz S, Malkusova I, Veverka J, Holub S, Mares J, Kozel R, Kopecka D, Zindr V, Cerva P, Chanez P, Bourdin A, Devouassoux G, Taille C, de Blay F, Goupil F, Leroyer C, Gourcerol D, Didi T, Didier A, Garcia G, Bonniaud P, Vasram RR, Lommatzsch M, Harnest U, Linnhoff A, Keller C, Hoheisel G, Förster K, Schultz T, Schenkenberger I, Kirschner J, Schmoller T, Zielen S, Kornmann M, Beck E, Volgmann L,

Dichmann R, Overlack A, Winkler J, Mikloweit P, Ballenberger S, Rolke M, Korn S, Pabel H, Hoffmann M, Feimer J, Rabe K, Deckelmann R, Welte T, Ohbayashi H, Hozawa S, Shimoda T, Yoshida M, Nagakura T, Kamei T, Sano Y, Kagami S, Takahashi H, Haida M, Kimura G, Nakamura H, To Y, Shinkai M, Shimokawaji T, Kudo M, Shijyubo N, Tochigi T, Kato M, Tanaka A, Gon Y, Sasaki N, Ohdaira T, Omori C, Takahashi T, Takeuchi S, Nakajima K, Makita H, Kaneko M, Furuta K, Taniguchi M, Inobe Y, Miki H, Nakamura Y, Miyazawa N, Yano S, Iijima M, Yamato T, Diaz J, Matsuno A, Felix E, Guerreros A, Daly A, Rodriguez Chariarse F, Salazar D, Castro S, Chavez W, Estrella R, Aquino T, Atienza T, Samoro R, Isidro MGD, Kuna P, Antczak A, Bednarek M, Mądra-Rogacka D, Hofman T, Jutel M, Pisarczyk-Bogacka E, Kot A, Mróz R, Czupryńska-Borkowska M, Żurowska-Gębala M, Dyczek A, Jasieniak-Pinis G, Wojnowski P, Trębas-Pietraś E, Dobryniewska M, Stobiecki M, Tarnowska-Matusiak M, Magner A, Kolczyński A, Kachel T, Bartuzi Z, Majorek-Olechowska B, Śliwiński P, Balicka V, Hajoł E, Stachera J, Rachel M, Michnar M, Tałałaj J, Springer E, Napora P, Grzelewski T, Bijata-Bronisz R, Świderska A, Mincewicz G, Sankowski Z, Fijołek T, Kwaśniewski A, Jerzyńska J, Cygler J, Olesiejuk R, von Steiner I, Machowiak W, Filipek K, Piskorz P, Uhryn E, Nittner-Marszalska M, Rybicka-Liszewska E, Bodzenta-Łukaszyk A, Chełmińska M, Krupa-Borek I, Skucha W, Płoszczuk A, Mihaescu T, Petrui ID, Savu A, Apti G, Toma C, Trailescu A, Sokurenko S, Trofimov V, Leshchenko I, Shaporova N, Ilyashevich I, Stitsenko I, Vizel A, Ilkovich Y, Tikhanov D, Goncharova S, Ezhov A, Ignatova G, Izmozherova N, Berdnikova N, Goryachkina L, Popova V, Bolieva L, Rebrov A, Nosov V, Magnitskaya O, Nedogoda S, Abrosimov V, Molotkov A, Reshedko G, Smirnov M, Osipenko M, Pavlysh E, Myasoedova S, Lenskaya L, Chistyakov V, Vishneva E, Uon L, Zateyschikova A, Laleko S, Pak T, Bruning A, Naidoo V, Reddy J, van Zyl Smit R, Park H-S, Cho YJ, Cho S-H, Lee SH, Lee BJ, Kim JS, Cho YS, Park C-S, Kim M-K, Koh Y-I, Kim J-H, Lee SY, Lee SP, Park JW, Yoo KH, Yoon H, Lee J, Hur G-Y, Lee SK, Kim H, Ramos Barbón D, Laffond Yges E, Martínez Moragón E, Arias Guillen M, Saura Vinuesa A, Sánchez-Toril López F, Velasco Garrido JL, García-Cosio Piqueras B, Pérez de Llano L, Valero Santiago AL, Rubio MC, Bjermer L, Lundbäck B, Gemicioglu B, Bavbek S, Ediger D, Erdinc M, Hanta I, Nayci S, Arinc S, Iashyna L, Mostovoy Y, Ostrovskyy M, Kuryk L, Lemko I, Ospanova T, Moskalenko L, Korzh O, Blazhko V, Krakhmalova O, Romaniuk L, Dytyatkovs'ka Y, Yakovenko O, Gavrysyuk V, Burhan H, Saralaya D, Scott S, Morice A, Jackson-Voyzey E, Win T, Nasser S, Harrison R, Chaudhuri R, Nordstrom M, De P, Masoli M, Mansur A, Gunstone A, Niven R, Harrison T, Babu S, Bhuchar S, Kureishy S, Zwetchkenbaum J, Kaplan L, Bleecker E, Reyes S, Fakih F, Heuer M, Klein R, Marcus M, Hussain I, Tanus T, Raissy H, Alpizar S, Rodriguez H, Gleich G, Bridges T, Pouzar J, Steven G, Matz J, Krstevska S, Ziworitin D, Kaplan A, Sublett J, DeAngelo J, Darter A, Agaiby J, Hagan J, Davis E, Siri D, Mcevoy C, Dharma C, Karimjee N, Kelsen S, Frade M, Silverthorn A, Kline J, Averill F, Ruiz J, Robinette E, Shaikh Z, Aguilar C, Nish W, Alvarez G, Ismail Y, Parikh P, Leong M, Murphy D, Garcia F, Goldsobel A, Blanco A, Campbell E, Perez G, Chupp G, Bates T, Perez V, Wenzel S, Shenoy K, Katial R, Bernstein D, Parikh N, Sims W, Ferguson G, Pham D, George A, Beasley R, Perez G, Garver R, Garcia-Portela M, Wong S, Soong W, Guillot R, Hudes G, Arif A, Binker J, Villareal M, Ziegner U, Ojile J, Goswami S, Piniella C, Segal I, Zafra H, Lee M, Tarpay M, Panuto J, Merchant R, Springsteen P, Scialla T, Shapero P, Allen K, Moss M, Cruz H, Rumbyrt J, Boyd A, Nathan R, Bernstein J, Jacobs J, Ginchansky E, Johnston J, Baxter B, Johnson T II, Apaliski S, Corder C, Fuentes D, Diaz J, Ngo C, Le L (2019) Long-term safety and efficacy of benralizumab in patients with severe, uncontrolled asthma: 1-year results from the BORA phase 3 extension trial. Lancet Respir Med 7:46–59. https://doi.org/10.1016/S2213-2600(18)30406-5

Castro M, Zangrilli J, Wechsler ME, Bateman ED, Brusselle GG, Bardin P, Murphy K, Maspero JF, O'Brien C, Korn S (2015) Reslizumab for inadequately controlled asthma with elevated blood eosinophil counts: results from two multicentre, parallel, double-blind, randomised, placebo-controlled, phase 3 trials. Lancet Respir Med 3:355–366. https://doi.org/10.1016/S2213-2600(15)00042-9

Castro M, Corren J, Pavord ID, Maspero J, Wenzel S, Rabe KF, Busse WW, Ford L, Sher L, FitzGerald JM, Katelaris C, Tohda Y, Zhang B, Staudinger H, Pirozzi G, Amin N, Ruddy M, Akinlade B, Khan A, Chao J, Martincova R, Graham NMH, Hamilton JD, Swanson BN, Stahl N, Yancopoulos GD, Teper A (2018) Dupilumab efficacy and safety in moderate-to-severe uncontrolled asthma. N Engl J Med 378:2486–2496. https://doi.org/10.1056/NEJMoa1804092

Chipps BE, Lanier B, Milgrom H, Deschildre A, Hedlin G, Szefler SJ, Kattan M, Kianifard F, Ortiz B, Haselkorn T, Iqbal A, Rosén K, Trzaskoma B, Busse WW (2017) Omalizumab in children with uncontrolled allergic asthma: review of clinical trial and real-world experience. J Allergy Clin Immunol 139:1431–1444. https://doi.org/10.1016/j.jaci.2017.03.002

Chupp GL, Bradford ES, Albers FC, Bratton DJ, Wang-Jairaj J, Nelsen LM, Trevor JL, Magnan A, ten Brinke A (2017) Efficacy of mepolizumab add-on therapy on health-related quality of life and markers of asthma control in severe eosinophilic asthma (MUSCA): a randomised, double-blind, placebo-controlled, parallel-group, multicentre, phase 3b trial. Lancet Respir Med 5:390–400. https://doi.org/10.1016/S2213-2600(17)30125-X

Cinqaero – European Medicines Agency (2016) EPAR – product information. https://www.ema.europa.eu/en/medicines/human/EPAR/cinqaero. Accessed Aug 2019

Cinqaero – U.S. Food and Drug Administration (2016) Summary review on reslizumab. Reference ID 3895552. https://www.accessdata.fda.gov/drugsatfda_docs/nda/2016/761033Orig1s000SumR.pdf. Accessed Aug 2019

Clutterbuck EJ, Hirst EM, Sanderson CJ (1989) Human interleukin-5 (IL-5) regulates the production of eosinophils in human bone marrow cultures: comparison and interaction with IL-1, IL-3, IL-6, and GMCSF. Blood 73:1504–1512

Cooper K, Frampton G, Harris P, Rose M, Chorozoglou M, Pickett K (2018) Reslizumab for treating asthma with elevated blood eosinophils inadequately controlled by inhaled corticosteroids: an evidence review group perspective of a NICE single technology appraisal. Pharmacoeconomics 36:545–553. https://doi.org/10.1007/s40273-017-0608-z

Corren J, Weinstein S, Janka L, Zangrilli J, Garin M (2016) Phase 3 study of reslizumab in patients with poorly controlled asthma: effects across a broad range of eosinophil counts. Chest 150:799–810. https://doi.org/10.1016/j.chest.2016.03.018

Deeks ED (2016) Mepolizumab: a review in eosinophilic asthma. BioDrugs 30:361–370. https://doi.org/10.1007/s40259-016-0182-5

Deleuran M, Thaçi D, Beck LA, de Bruin-Weller M, Blauvelt A, Forman S, Bissonnette R, Reich K, Soong W, Hussain I, Foley P, Hide M, Bouaziz J-D, Gelfand JM, Sher L, Schuttelaar MLA, Wang C, Chen Z, Akinlade B, Gadkari A, Eckert L, Davis JD, Rajadhyaksha M, Staudinger H, Graham NMH, Pirozzi G, Ardeleanu M (2019) Dupilumab shows long-term safety and efficacy in moderate-to-severe atopic dermatitis patients enrolled in a phase 3 open-label extension study. J Am Acad Dermatol. https://doi.org/10.1016/j.jaad.2019.07.074

Deschildre A, Marguet C, Salleron J, Pin I, Rittié J-L, Derelle J, Taam RA, Fayon M, Brouard J, Dubus JC, Siret D, Weiss L, Pouessel G, Beghin L, Just J (2013) Add-on omalizumab in children with severe allergic asthma: a 1-year real life survey. Eur Respir J 42:1224–1233. https://doi.org/10.1183/09031936.00149812

Deschildre A, Marguet C, Langlois C, Pin I, Rittié J-L, Derelle J, Abou Taam R, Fayon M, Brouard J, Dubus JC, Siret D, Weiss L, Pouessel G, Beghin L, Just J (2015) Real-life long-term omalizumab therapy in children with severe allergic asthma. Eur Respir J 46:856–859. https://doi.org/10.1183/09031936.00008115

Duxipent – European Medicines Agency (2017) EPAR – product information. https://www.ema.europa.eu/en/documents/product-information/dupixent-epar-product-information_en.pdf. Accessed Aug 2019

Eichenfield L (2017) Lebrikizumab improves patient-reported outcomes (PROs) in a phase 2 study in patients with atopic dermatitis. J Am Acad Dermatol 76:AB423. https://doi.org/10.1016/j.jaad.2017.06.133

Eichenfield LF, Bieber T, Beck LA, Simpson EL, Thaçi D, de Bruin-Weller M, Deleuran M, Silverberg JI, Ferrandiz C, Fölster-Holst R, Chen Z, Graham NMH, Pirozzi G, Akinlade B, Yancopoulos GD, Ardeleanu M (2019) Infections in dupilumab clinical trials in atopic dermatitis: a comprehensive pooled analysis. Am J Clin Dermatol 20:443–456. https://doi.org/10.1007/s40257-019-00445-7

Esquivel A, Busse WW, Calatroni A, Togias AG, Grindle KG, Bochkov YA, Gruchalla RS, Kattan M, Kercsmar CM, Khurana Hershey G, Kim H, Lebeau P, Liu AH, Szefler SJ, Teach SJ, West JB, Wildfire J, Pongracic JA, Gern JE (2017) Effects of omalizumab on rhinovirus infections, illnesses, and exacerbations of asthma. Am J Respir Crit Care Med 196:985–992. https://doi.org/10.1164/rccm.201701-0120OC

Farne HA, Wilson A, Powell C, Bax L, Milan SJ (2017) Anti-IL5 therapies for asthma. Cochrane Database Syst Rev 9:CD010834. https://doi.org/10.1002/14651858.CD010834.pub3

Fasenra – European Medicines Agency (2018) EPAR – product information. https://www.ema.europa.eu/en/documents/product-information/fasenra-epar-product-information_en.pdf. Accessed Aug 2019

Fiocchi A, Artesani MC, Riccardi C, Mennini M, Pecora V, Fierro V, Calandrelli V, Dahdah L, Valluzzi RL (2019) Impact of omalizumab on food allergy in patients treated for asthma: a real-life study. J Allergy Clin Immunol Pract 7:1901–1909.e5. https://doi.org/10.1016/j.jaip.2019.01.023

FitzGerald JM, Bleecker ER, Nair P, Korn S, Ohta K, Lommatzsch M, Ferguson GT, Busse WW, Barker P, Sproule S, Gilmartin G, Werkström V, Aurivillius M, Goldman M (2016) Benralizumab, an anti-interleukin-5 receptor α monoclonal antibody, as add-on treatment for patients with severe, uncontrolled, eosinophilic asthma (CALIMA): a randomised, double-blind, placebo-controlled phase 3 trial. Lancet 388:2128–2141. https://doi.org/10.1016/S0140-6736(16)31322-8

Folqué MM, Lozano J, Riggioni C, Piquer M, Álvaro M, Machinena A, Giner MT, Domínguez O, Jiménez-Feijoo RM, Dias da Costa M, Plaza AM (2019) 'Real-life' experience in asthmatic children treated with omalizumab up to six-years follow-up. Allergol Immunopathol (Madr) 47:336–341. https://doi.org/10.1016/j.aller.2018.09.009

Ghazi A, Trikha A, Calhoun WJ (2012) Benralizumab – a humanized mAb to IL-5Rα with enhanced antibody-dependent cell-mediated cytotoxicity – a novel approach for the treatment of asthma. Expert Opin Biol Ther 12:113–118. https://doi.org/10.1517/14712598.2012.642359

GINA (2019) Adolscents and adults with difficult-to-treat and severe asthma. https://ginasthma.org/severeasthma/

Gupta A, Steinfeld J, Price R, Azmi J, Bradford E, Yancey S (2018) Mepolizumab for severe eosinophilic asthma: a comparison of efficacy in children, adolescents, and adults. Eur Respir J 52:PA5447. https://doi.org/10.1183/13993003.congress-2018.PA5447

Haldar P, Brightling CE, Singapuri A, Hargadon B, Gupta S, Monteiro W, Bradding P, Green RH, Wardlaw AJ, Ortega H, Pavord ID (2014) Outcomes after cessation of mepolizumab therapy in severe eosinophilic asthma: a 12-month follow-up analysis. J Allergy Clin Immunol 133:921–923. https://doi.org/10.1016/j.jaci.2013.11.026

Henriksen DP, Bodtger U, Sidenius K, Maltbaek N, Pedersen L, Madsen H, Andersson EA, Norgaard O, Madsen LK, Chawes BL (2018) Efficacy, adverse events, and inter-drug comparison of mepolizumab and reslizumab anti-IL-5 treatments of severe asthma – a systematic review and meta-analysis. Eur Clin Respir J 5:1536097. https://doi.org/10.1080/20018525.2018.1536097

Holgate S, Casale T, Wenzel S, Bousquet J, Deniz Y, Reisner C (2005) The anti-inflammatory effects of omalizumab confirm the central role of IgE in allergic inflammation. J Allergy Clin Immunol 115:459–465. https://doi.org/10.1016/j.jaci.2004.11.053

Khatri S, Moore W, Gibson PG, Leigh R, Bourdin A, Maspero J, Barros M, Buhl R, Howarth P, Albers FC, Bradford ES, Gilson M, Price RG, Yancey SW, Ortega H (2019) Assessment of the long-term safety of mepolizumab and durability of clinical response in patients with severe eosinophilic asthma. J Allergy Clin Immunol 143:1742–1751.e7. https://doi.org/10.1016/j.jaci.2018.09.033

Kouro T, Takatsu K (2009) IL-5- and eosinophil-mediated inflammation: from discovery to therapy. Int Immunol 21:1303–1309. https://doi.org/10.1093/intimm/dxp102

Lanier B, Bridges T, Kulus M, Taylor AF, Berhane I, Vidaurre CF (2009) Omalizumab for the treatment of exacerbations in children with inadequately controlled allergic (IgE-mediated) asthma. J Allergy Clin Immunol 124:1210–1216. https://doi.org/10.1016/j.jaci.2009.09.021

Lemanske RF, Nayak A, McAlary M, Everhard F, Fowler-Taylor A, Gupta N (2002) Omalizumab improves asthma-related quality of life in children with allergic asthma. Pediatrics 110:e55. https://doi.org/10.1542/peds.110.5.e55

Limb SL, Starke PR, Lee CE, Chowdhury BA (2007) Delayed onset and protracted progression of anaphylaxis after omalizumab administration in patients with asthma. J Allergy Clin Immunol 120:1378–1381. https://doi.org/10.1016/j.jaci.2007.09.022

Lowe PJ, Tannenbaum S, Gautier A, Jimenez P (2009) Relationship between omalizumab pharmacokinetics, IgE pharmacodynamics and symptoms in patients with severe persistent allergic (IgE-mediated) asthma. Br J Clin Pharmacol 68:61–76. https://doi.org/10.1111/j.1365-2125.2009.03401.x

Lugogo N, Domingo C, Chanez P, Leigh R, Gilson MJ, Price RG, Yancey SW, Ortega HG (2016) Long-term efficacy and safety of mepolizumab in patients with severe eosinophilic asthma: a multi-center, open-label, phase IIIb study. Clin Ther 38:2058–2070.e1. https://doi.org/10.1016/j.clinthera.2016.07.010

Menzella F, Lusuardi M, Galeone C, Taddei S, Facciolongo N, Zucchi L (2016) Mepolizumab for severe refractory eosinophilic asthma: evidence to date and clinical potential. Ther Adv Chronic Dis 7:260–277. https://doi.org/10.1177/2040622316659863

Milgrom H, Berger W, Nayak A, Gupta N, Pollard S, McAlary M, Taylor AF, Rohane P (2001) Treatment of childhood asthma with anti-immunoglobulin E antibody (omalizumab). Pediatrics 108:E36. https://doi.org/10.1542/peds.108.2.e36

Murphy K, Jacobs J, Bjermer L, Fahrenholz JM, Shalit Y, Garin M, Zangrilli J, Castro M (2017) Long-term safety and efficacy of reslizumab in patients with eosinophilic asthma. J Allergy Clin Immunol Pract 5:1572–1581.e3. https://doi.org/10.1016/j.jaip.2017.08.024

Normansell R, Walker S, Milan SJ, Walters EH, Nair P (2014) Omalizumab for asthma in adults and children. Cochrane Database Syst Rev:CD003559. https://doi.org/10.1002/14651858.CD003559.pub4

Nucala – European Medicines Agency (2015) EPAR – product information. https://www.ema.europa.eu/en/documents/product-information/nucala-epar-product-information_en.pdf. Accessed Aug 2019

Odajima H, Ebisawa M, Nagakura T, Fujisawa T, Akasawa A, Ito K, Doi S, Yamaguchi K, Katsunuma T, Kurihara K, Teramoto T, Sugai K, Nambu M, Hoshioka A, Yoshihara S, Sato N, Seko N, Nishima S (2017) Long-term safety, efficacy, pharmacokinetics and pharmacodynamics of omalizumab in children with severe uncontrolled asthma. Allergol Int 66:106–115. https://doi.org/10.1016/j.alit.2016.06.004

Oldhoff JM, Darsow U, Werfel T, Katzer K, Wulf A, Laifaoui J, Hijnen DJ, Plötz S, Knol EF, Kapp A, Bruijnzeel-Koomen CAFM, Ring J, de Bruin-Weller MS (2005) Anti-IL-5 recombinant humanized monoclonal antibody (mepolizumab) for the treatment of atopic dermatitis. Allergy 60:693–696. https://doi.org/10.1111/j.1398-9995.2005.00791.x

Ortega HG, Yancey SW, Mayer B, Gunsoy NB, Keene ON, Bleecker ER, Brightling CE, Pavord ID (2016) Severe eosinophilic asthma treated with mepolizumab stratified by baseline eosinophil thresholds: a secondary analysis of the DREAM and MENSA studies. Lancet Respir Med 4:549–556. https://doi.org/10.1016/S2213-2600(16)30031-5

Ortega H, Lemiere C, Llanos J-P, Forshag M, Price R, Albers F, Yancey S, Castro M (2019) Outcomes following mepolizumab treatment discontinuation: real-world experience from an open-label trial. Allergy Asthma Clin Immunol 15:37. https://doi.org/10.1186/s13223-019-0348-z

Pavord ID, Korn S, Howarth P, Bleecker ER, Buhl R, Keene ON, Ortega H, Chanez P (2012) Mepolizumab for severe eosinophilic asthma (DREAM): a multicentre, double-blind, placebo-controlled trial. Lancet 380:651–659. https://doi.org/10.1016/S0140-6736(12)60988-X

Pitrez PM, de Souza RG, Roncada C, Heinzmann-Filho JP, Santos G, Pinto LA, Jones MH, Stein RT (2017) Impact of omalizumab in children from a middle-income country with severe therapy-resistant asthma: a real-life study. Pediatr Pulmonol 52:1408–1413. https://doi.org/10.1002/ppul.23845

Rabe KF, Nair P, Brusselle G, Maspero JF, Castro M, Sher L, Zhu H, Hamilton JD, Swanson BN, Khan A, Chao J, Staudinger H, Pirozzi G, Antoni C, Amin N, Ruddy M, Akinlade B, Graham NMH, Stahl N, Yancopoulos GD, Teper A (2018) Efficacy and safety of dupilumab in glucocorticoid-dependent severe asthma. N Engl J Med 378:2475–2485. https://doi.org/10.1056/NEJMoa1804093

Rodrigo GJ, Neffen H (2015) Systematic review on the use of omalizumab for the treatment of asthmatic children and adolescents. Pediatr Allergy Immunol 26:551–556. https://doi.org/10.1111/pai.12405

Ruzicka T, Mihara R (2017) Anti-interleukin-31 receptor a antibody for atopic dermatitis. N Engl J Med 376:2093. https://doi.org/10.1056/NEJMc1704013

Sampson HA, Berin MC, Plaut M, Sicherer SH, Jones S, Burks AW, Lindblad R, Leung DYM, Wood RA (2019) The Consortium for Food Allergy Research (CoFAR): the first generation. J Allergy Clin Immunol 143:486–493. https://doi.org/10.1016/j.jaci.2018.12.989

Sanofi Press Release (2019) Dupixent® (dupilumab) showed positive topline results in phase 3 trial of children aged 6 to 11 years with severe atopic dermatitis. https://www.sanofi.com/-/media/Project/One-Sanofi-Web/Websites/Global/Sanofi-COM/Home/media-room/press-releases/2019/2019-08-06-07-05-00-1897265-en.pdf. Accessed Aug 2019

Shirley M (2017) Dupilumab: first global approval. Drugs 77:1115–1121. https://doi.org/10.1007/s40265-017-0768-3

Silverberg JI, Simpson EL (2013) Association between severe eczema in children and multiple comorbid conditions and increased healthcare utilization. Pediatr Allergy Immunol 24:476–486. https://doi.org/10.1111/pai.12095

Simpson EL, Bieber T, Guttman-Yassky E, Beck LA, Blauvelt A, Cork MJ, Silverberg JI, Deleuran M, Kataoka Y, Lacour J-P, Kingo K, Worm M, Poulin Y, Wollenberg A, Soo Y, Graham NMH, Pirozzi G, Akinlade B, Staudinger H, Mastey V, Eckert L, Gadkari A, Stahl N, Yancopoulos GD, Ardeleanu M (2016) Two phase 3 trials of dupilumab versus placebo in atopic dermatitis. N Engl J Med 375:2335–2348. https://doi.org/10.1056/NEJMoa1610020

Simpson EL, Paller AS, Siegfried EC, Boguniewicz M, Sher L, Gooderham MJ et al (2019) Efficacy and safety of dupilumab in adolescents with uncontrolled moderate to severe atopic dermatitis: a phase 3 randomized clinical trial. JAMA Dermat. https://doi.org/10.1001/jamadermatol.2019.3336

Takahashi M, Soejima K, Taniuchi S, Hatano Y, Yamanouchi S, Ishikawa H, Irahara M, Sasaki Y, Kido H, Kaneko K (2017) Oral immunotherapy combined with omalizumab for high-risk cow's milk allergy: a randomized controlled trial. Sci Rep 7:17453. https://doi.org/10.1038/s41598-017-16730-6

Teach SJ, Gill MA, Togias A, Sorkness CA, Arbes SJ, Calatroni A, Wildfire JJ, Gergen PJ, Cohen RT, Pongracic JA, Kercsmar CM, Khurana Hershey GK, Gruchalla RS, Liu AH, Zoratti EM, Kattan M, Grindle KA, Gern JE, Busse WW, Szefler SJ (2015) Preseasonal treatment with either omalizumab or an inhaled corticosteroid boost to prevent fall asthma exacerbations. J Allergy Clin Immunol 136:1476–1485. https://doi.org/10.1016/j.jaci.2015.09.008

Thyssen JP, de Bruin-Weller MS, Paller AS, Leshem YA, Vestergaard C, Deleuran M, Drucker AM, Foelster-Holst R, Traidl-Hoffmann C, Eyerich K, Taieb A, Su JC, Bieber T, Cork MJ, Eichenfield LF, Guttman-Yassky E, Wollenberg A (2019) Conjunctivitis in atopic dermatitis patients with and without dupilumab therapy – international eczema council survey and opinion. J Eur Acad Dermatol Venereol 33:1224–1231. https://doi.org/10.1111/jdv.15608

Treister AD, Lio PA (2019) Long-term off-label dupilumab in pediatric atopic dermatitis: a case series. Pediatr Dermatol 36:85–88. https://doi.org/10.1111/pde.13697

Tsabouri S, Tseretopoulou X, Priftis K, Ntzani EE (2014) Omalizumab for the treatment of inadequately controlled allergic rhinitis: a systematic review and meta-analysis of randomized clinical trials. J Allergy Clin Immunol Pract 2:332–340.e1. https://doi.org/10.1016/j.jaip.2014.02.001

Vakharia PP, Silverberg JI (2019) New and emerging therapies for paediatric atopic dermatitis. Lancet Child Adolesc Health 3:343–353. https://doi.org/10.1016/S2352-4642(19)30030-6

Vickery BP (2019) Can omalizumab monotherapy benefit real-world food allergy patients? Lessons from an observational study. J Allergy Clin Immunol Pract 7:1910–1911. https://doi.org/10.1016/j.jaip.2019.05.007

Wang H-H, Li Y-C, Huang Y-C (2016) Efficacy of omalizumab in patients with atopic dermatitis: a systematic review and meta-analysis. J Allergy Clin Immunol 138:1719–1722.e1. https://doi.org/10.1016/j.jaci.2016.05.038

Weinstein SF, Katial R, Jayawardena S, Pirozzi G, Staudinger H, Eckert L, Joish VN, Amin N, Maroni J, Rowe P, Graham NMH, Teper A (2018) Efficacy and safety of dupilumab in perennial allergic rhinitis and comorbid asthma. J Allergy Clin Immunol 142:171–177.e1. https://doi.org/10.1016/j.jaci.2017.11.051

Wenzel S, Ford L, Pearlman D, Spector S, Sher L, Skobieranda F, Wang L, Kirkesseli S, Rocklin R, Bock B, Hamilton J, Ming JE, Radin A, Stahl N, Yancopoulos GD, Graham N, Pirozzi G (2013) Dupilumab in persistent asthma with elevated eosinophil levels. N Engl J Med 368:2455–2466. https://doi.org/10.1056/NEJMoa1304048

Wenzel S, Castro M, Corren J, Maspero J, Wang L, Zhang B, Pirozzi G, Sutherland ER, Evans RR, Joish VN, Eckert L, Graham NMH, Stahl N, Yancopoulos GD, Louis-Tisserand M, Teper A (2016) Dupilumab efficacy and safety in adults with uncontrolled persistent asthma despite use of medium-to-high-dose inhaled corticosteroids plus a long-acting β2 agonist: a randomised double-blind placebo-controlled pivotal phase 2b dose-ranging trial. Lancet 388:31–44. https://doi.org/10.1016/S0140-6736(16)30307-5

Wise SK, Lin SY, Toskala E, Orlandi RR, Akdis CA, Alt JA, Azar A, Baroody FM, Bachert C, Canonica GW, Chacko T, Cingi C, Ciprandi G, Corey J, Cox LS, Creticos PS, Custovic A, Damask C, DeConde A, DelGaudio JM, Ebert CS, Eloy JA, Flanagan CE, Fokkens WJ, Franzese C, Gosepath J, Halderman A, Hamilton RG, Hoffman HJ, Hohlfeld JM, Houser SM, Hwang PH, Incorvaia C, Jarvis D, Khalid AN, Kilpeläinen M, Kingdom TT, Krouse H, Larenas-Linnemann D, Laury AM, Lee SE, Levy JM, Luong AU, Marple BF, McCoul ED, McMains KC, Melén E, Mims JW, Moscato G, Mullol J, Nelson HS, Patadia M, Pawankar R, Pfaar O, Platt MP, Reisacher W, Rondón C, Rudmik L, Ryan M, Sastre J, Schlosser RJ, Settipane RA, Sharma HP, Sheikh A, Smith TL, Tantilipikorn P, Tversky JR, Veling MC, Wang DY, Westman M, Wickman M, Zacharek M (2018) International consensus statement on allergy and rhinology: allergic rhinitis. Int Forum Allergy Rhinol 8:108–352. https://doi.org/10.1002/alr.22073

Wollenberg A, Barbarot S, Bieber T, Christen-Zaech S, Deleuran M, Fink-Wagner A, Gieler U, Girolomoni G, Lau S, Muraro A, Czarnecka-Operacz M, Schäfer T, Schmid-Grendelmeier P, Simon D, Szalai Z, Szepietowski JC, Taïeb A, Torrelo A, Werfel T, Ring J (2018) Consensus-based European guidelines for treatment of atopic eczema (atopic dermatitis) in adults and children: part II. J Eur Acad Dermatol Venereol 32:850–878. https://doi.org/10.1111/jdv.14888

Wollenberg A, Howell MD, Guttman-Yassky E, Silverberg JI, Kell C, Ranade K, Moate R, van der Merwe R (2019) Treatment of atopic dermatitis with tralokinumab, an anti-IL-13 mAb. J Allergy Clin Immunol 143:135–141. https://doi.org/10.1016/j.jaci.2018.05.029

Wood RA, Kim JS, Lindblad R, Nadeau K, Henning AK, Dawson P, Plaut M, Sampson HA (2016) A randomized, double-blind, placebo-controlled study of omalizumab combined with oral immunotherapy for the treatment of cow's milk allergy. J Allergy Clin Immunol 137:1103–1110.e11. https://doi.org/10.1016/j.jaci.2015.10.005

Xiong X-F, Zhu M, Wu H-X, Fan L-L, Cheng D-Y (2019) Efficacy and safety of dupilumab for the treatment of uncontrolled asthma: a meta-analysis of randomized clinical trials. Respir Res 20:108. https://doi.org/10.1186/s12931-019-1065-3

Xolair – European Medicines Agency (2009) EPAR – product information. https://www.ema.europa.eu/en/medicines/human/EPAR/xolair#overview-section. Accessed Aug 2019

Xolair – U. S. Food and Drug Administration (2013) Clinical pharmacology review. https://www.fda.gov/media/88330/download

Yancey SW, Ortega HG, Keene ON, Mayer B, Gunsoy NB, Brightling CE, Bleecker ER, Haldar P, Pavord ID (2017) Meta-analysis of asthma-related hospitalization in mepolizumab studies of severe eosinophilic asthma. J Allergy Clin Immunol 139:1167–1175.e2. https://doi.org/10.1016/j.jaci.2016.08.008

Dermatology Part 2: Ichthyoses and Psoriasis

Michael Sticherling

Contents

M. Sticherling (✉)
Psoriasis-Center, Deutsche Zentrum für Immuntherapie, Erlangen, Germany
e-mail: Michael.Sticherling@uk-erlangen.de

W. Kiess et al. (eds.), *Pediatric Pharmacotherapy*,
Handbook of Experimental Pharmacology 261, https://doi.org/10.1007/164_2019_345

Abstract
Acute and chronic inflammatory skin diseases are frequent in childhood and may be hereditary or acquired. In this context, ichthyosis is rather a symptom than a defined disease as scaling is accompanying a number of disorders and is mostly consequence of a disrupted skin barrier. Ichthyosis is the basic pathogenic trait of atopic dermatitis but on the other side describes a group of rare hereditary diseases. These may only affect the skin or comprise several internal symptoms as well. Psoriasis is another scaling inflammatory skin disease with classical sharply demarcated erythematosquamous plaques and with a distinct immunogenetic background. It comprises several clinical subsets, some of which are characteristic for children and demanding in both diagnostics and therapy. Comorbid diseases point towards a systemic inflammatory response and require ample, often systemic treatment. Both ichthyosis and psoriasis may be topically treated including emollients with and without humectants as well as active agents like corticosteroids, vitamin D derivatives, and calcineurin inhibitors. In moderate to severe diseases, systemic treatment should be applied using methotrexate, ciclosporin, fumarates, or biologics. Their use should be critically discussed yet if necessary and indicated be applied to avoid chronic physical and psychological damage to the affected children.

Keywords
Ichthyosis · Psoriasis · Systemic therapy · Topical therapy · UV-therapy

1 Introduction

Chronic inflammatory skin diseases pose major therapeutic challenges, especially when present in children and adolescents. Apart from aspects like reduction of quality of life and a major influence on physical and emotional development of the affected children, only few therapeutic agents are evaluated and even fewer licensed for use in this delicate age period. Many skin diseases may be treated by external or topical agents only, yet more severe and chronic disease is often better treated systemically. With the advent of novel, well-tolerated, and effective systemic agents, the use of topical therapy has diminished. However, in many cases it is still needed to increase clinical effectivity and to treat residual or undulating limited skin manifestations.

2 Ichthyoses

Ichthyoses represent a group of very heterogeneous skin diseases with a distinct genetic background which are characterized by increased and mostly disseminated scaling (Yoneda 2016; Takeichi and Akiyama 2016). Quite a few are already present at birth (congenital) and perpetuate through childhood or even adulthood. Clinical manifestations vary from mild to severe or even life-threatening. Apart from skin involvement, internal manifestations and malformations may be associated.

Four groups of ichthyoses are differentiated: (1) isolated, that is, skin-restricted, noncongenital ichthyoses, (2) associated congenital ichthyoses, (3) isolated congenital ichthyoses, and (4) associated non-congenital ichthyoses. Among these, autosomal dominant *ichthyosis vulgaris* is the most common disease with a prevalence of 1:250. It is related to a mutation at 1q21 which codes for the structural protein filaggrin. Grayish scaling is found on the trunk and extensor surfaces of extremities sparing the folds of arms and legs. The handlines are often prominent. Around half of the cases are associated with atopic diseases (atopic dermatitis and other forms of eczema, rhinoconjunctivitis, and asthma bronchiale). *X-chromosomal recessive ichthyosis* has an incidence of 1:2,000 among boys with an underlying genetic deficit of steroid sulfatase. A fine scaling can be seen immediately after birth. After vanishing until the age of 3–4 months, dark brown rhomboid scales remain to be seen on extremities and trunk, often suggesting lack of hygiene to the patient's surrounding. Palms and soles are always spared, but folds may be involved. Among *associated noncongenital ichthyoses*, Refsum syndrome and multiple sulfatase deficiency show only mild scaling, but associated internal organ, ophthalmological and neurological symptoms have to be excluded.

In contrast, *isolated congenital ichthyoses*, comprising lamellar and epidermolytic ichthyoses, are present at birth already, with distinct scaling, some accompanied by erythroderma which may fade in early childhood. The genetic background is not known for all disease subsets. *Epidermolytic ichthyoses* are very rare with a prevalence of less than 1:100,000 and comprise bullous ichthyosiform erythroderma Brocq and ichthyosis bullosa Siemens, both associated with specific keratin-mutations (Peter Rout et al. 2019). Clinically *Brocq-type ichthyosis* shows both erythroderma and massive bullous manifestations, which regress in early childhood and evolve into spinular keratoses. In contrast, *Siemens type ichthyosis* lacks erythroderma, but shows formation of bullae after even minor trauma as well as circumscribed keratoses, mainly on the limbs sparing the trunk except the umbilical area.

Associated congenital ichthyoses comprise among others Sjögren-Larsson and Tay as well as Netherton syndrome, again associated with ichthyosiform erythroderma at birth. Other clinical associations include mental retardation (Sjögren-Larsson), increased rate of skin cancer (Tay and other trichothiodystrophy syndromes) and atopic diseases as well as immune defects (Netherton syndrome) which have to be included into therapeutic decisions.

Apart from intensive and regular topical rehydrating and keratolytic treatment for all ichthyoses, systemic retinoids are efficient and should individually be discussed for congenital ichthyoses (Mazereeuw-Hautier et al. 2019a, b; Cortés et al. 2019). Systemic corticosteroids and immunomodulatory agents should not be used, however, if indicated topical or systemic antibiotic treatment in addition to ample skin dressings for erosions and bullous manifestations.

3 Psoriasis

Psoriasis is one of the most common human inflammatory skin diseases afflicting 1.5–2% of the Caucasian population (Lowes et al. 2007). Epidemiologically, two peaks of incidence have been described, one in the third decade of life with a distinct hereditary, familial background, and a more severe course and a second peak in the fourth to fifth decade with a variable clinical course (Swanbeck et al. 1995). However, 20 percent of all psoriasis patients have the first manifestation of their diseases before the twentieth birthday with obvious consequences on their physical, emotional, and socioeconomic development (Augustin et al. 2010). At the same time, therapeutic approaches in childhood and adolescence are limited, and only few agents are licensed for this age.

The disease spectrum may grossly be divided into plaque and pustular psoriasis. Around 80% of all cases in adulthood present as *plaque psoriasis or psoriasis vulgaris* apparently with a similar percentage in childhood based on comparably limited epidemiological data available for this age (Benoit and Hamm 2007; Augustin et al. 2010; Chiam et al. 2011; Svendsen et al. 2016). Psoriasis plaques are sharply demarcated, distinctly red, and covered by medium-sized to coarse scales. Predilections sites are the extensor surfaces of extremities, the scalp and external meatus of the ear, as well as behind the auricle, at the umbilicus and at the rima ani. This is quite in contrast to atopic dermatitis which is diffusely demarcated, of pale red color, and covered by fine scaling. The synonymous term flexural dermatitis for AD is misleading as this location is mainly found in school age, whereas young children and adolescents show extensor surfaces predominantly involved. Similarly, napkin psoriasis is sharply demarcated and more common than napkin AD. Facial and palmar manifestations are rare in adult psoriasis, but characteristic for childhood. *Nail involvement* with nail pitting, salmon patches, and onycholysis is found in about 30% of juvenile patients and may indicate psoriasis arthritis where severe nail involvement is common (80%) but may also be present as minimal and only manifestation in familial, otherwise noninvolved cases (Pourchot et al. 2017).

A specific subtype in childhood is *guttate psoriasis* with oval, slightly elevated plaques of around 10 millimeter diameter, of yellow-reddish color, and covered by only mild scaling (Svendsen et al. 2016). They appear as an exanthema mainly on the trunk 1–2 weeks after viral or bacterial infections, characteristically after streptococcal tonsillitis and will vanish within the course of several weeks or few months (Thorleifsdottir et al. 2016, 2017; Rachakonda et al. 2015). The effects of tonsillectomy are discussed controversially, but surgical indication should be liberal. Oral antibiotic treatment may be advisable in acute cases, and for a limited period, effects of long-term antibiotic treatment are, however, much debated (Dogan et al. 2008; Owen et al. 2001; Horton et al. 2016).

In addition, vaccinations have been suspected to initiate or exacerbate skin manifestations (Gunes et al. 2015; Kokolakis et al. 2010). All recommended childhood vaccinations can and should be administered as long as there is no active skin disease (Groot et al. 2015; Heijstek et al. 2011). Ongoing and well-tolerated topical and systemic therapy do not pose a contraindication. However, any live vaccines should be administered before starting systemic immunomodulatory treatment or only after interrupting therapy for an interval depending on the agent used.

Guttate psoriasis may present as a single bout of disease, recidivate after further infections, may persist or even evolve into classical plaque psoriasis either in childhood or later life especially when the family history for psoriasis is positive. Many cases of childhood psoriasis may not be diagnosed at all, but treated as atopic dermatitis and mycosis, the classical and much more frequent differential diagnoses.

Twenty percent of psoriasis patients show *pustular psoriasis* with the most common subtype of *pustulosis palmoplantaris (PPP)* on palms and soles which is sharply demarcated at the edges of hand and feet where palmar borders dorsal skin. The simultaneous presentation of pain, erythema, and sterile pustules turning yellowish-brown when drying and coarse, partly circular scaling is characteristic. Classical plaque psoriasis may be present at other body sites in rare cases. Despite the circumscribed area involved, ample use of hands and feet in everyday life is severely hampered and demands efficient treatment. *Generalized pustular psoriasis* (GPP) is rare (2% of all adult cases), yet a severe disease with fever and a distinct reduction of general condition (Liao et al. 2002; de Oliveira et al. 2010). Differential diagnosis should include other pustular exanthemas due to infections or drug reactions. *Acrodermatitis continua suppurativa Hallopeau* with acral and periungual pustules and redness is often associated with acral bone erosions and arthritis.

Psoriasis arthritis (PsA) of childhood is included in the group of juvenile idiopathic arthritis (JIA) and covers classical peripheral as well as axial arthritis. In contrast to adult psoriasis where PsA presents after around 10 years of skin involvement in 75% of cases, the majority of childhood cases present before and even without any distinct skin manifestations. PsA is found in 30% of adult cases; comparable data for childhood psoriasis are hardly available. Details of this disease subset are covered in other chapters of this book but need to be addressed here as concomitant PsA distinctly influences therapeutic decisions on psoriatic skin disease (Cellucci et al. 2016; Ringold et al. 2013).

Similarly, *comorbid diseases* as found and extensively studied in adult psoriasis are relevant in childhood and have obvious impact on disease severity and therapeutic choices. Metabolic (diabetes mellitus, dyslipidemia, increased body weight) and cardiovascular diseases (esp. arterial hypertension) are more prevalent in childhood compared to healthy, age-related controls (Skinner et al. 2015; Tollefson et al. 2018; Kara et al. 2019; Osier et al. 2017). In adult disease, a two- to fivefold increase of comorbidities could be shown in different ethnic populations. If both psoriasis and comorbidities are mutually influencing each other or are results of shared, yet independent or parallel pathogenic pathways is still a matter of debate.

Disease severity is well defined in adult psoriasis, and several instruments for physician- and patient-based quantification are available, some validated or consented. A widely accepted approach to quantify disease severity and to monitor effective treatment is the psoriasis area and severity index (PASI) which summarizes redness, infiltration, scaling, and distribution on the skin surface in a numerical scale between zero (no skin manifestations) and 72 (maximal disease severity) (Fredriksson and Pettersson 1978; Langley and Ellis 2004; van Geel et al. 2017; Finlay 2005). Alternatively the percentage of affected body surface area (BSA) can be used. For life quality aspects, the dermatological life quality index (DLQI) is well-established and – though not psoriasis-specific – most widely used (Finlay and Khan

1994; Lewis-Jones and Finlay 1995; Beattie and Lewis-Jones 2006). PASI and BSA have not been validated for children: however, an adaptation of DLQI for ages 4–16 years is available (CDLQI) (Lewis-Jones and Finlay 1995).

Moreover, patient perception of disease severity, its impact on every day aspects as well as patient expectations towards therapy and its appreciation are currently discussed intensively for adults. A number of patient related outcomes (PRO) have become available recently for practical use. For adult treatment decisions, a PASI and/or BSA and DLQI above ten have been consented to discriminate between mild and moderate/severe disease defining the need for systemic treatment. In addition, distinct manifestations at visible (scalp, face, nails) or delicate sites (intertriginous, anogenital) are a criterion for disease severity as is the number and severity of comorbid diseases. In most cases, PsA will demand systemic treatment.

Treatment goals regarding efficacy in induction therapy have been consented for adults with a reduction of initial PASI after 12–16 weeks by at least 75% (PASI75) or a PASI 50–75 and DLQI ≤ 5 (Mrowietz et al. 2011). These may be adapted to children by using the CDLQI.

Psoriasis treatment options can be separated into three groups, (1) topical treatment, (2) treatment with ultraviolet (UV) light, and (3) systemic treatment (Peter Rout et al. 2019) (Table 1). Many of them may be combined to increase efficacy; some should not be combined which in many cases demands broad dermatological expertise (Bruner et al. 2003; van de Kerkhof 2015; van Geel et al. 2015). Therefore it is the decision of both patient/parents and physician based on individual parameters which treatment and when to initiate and how long to use. German and European guidelines for adult psoriasis and recently for juvenile psoriasis are available which critically cover the different treatment options (Nast et al. 2015, 2018; Eisert et al. 2019a, b). Decisions depend on the severity of the disease as described above, response to previous treatments, duration of disease-free state off treatment, expectations towards time to response and extent of response (disease-free state, minimal disease, or distinct improvement). Long-term response and tolerability have to be taken into account when treating a chronic inflammatory skin disease. In children and adolescents, such considerations have to be done even more critically than compared to adult patients (Sticherling et al. 2011; Ståhle et al. 2010; de Jager et al. 2010).

Table 1 The three main therapeutic approaches to psoriasis

Topical	UV	Systemic
Salicylic acid	Narrow band UV-B (311 nm)	Fumarates
Urea	Broad spectrum UV-B	Methotrexate
Corticosteroids	Photochemo-therapy (PUVA)	Ciclosporin
Vitamin D3 analogues	Balneophototherapy Bath-PUVA	Retinoids
Vitamin A analogues (Tazaroten)	Balneophototherapy Salt solution baths + UV-B	Apremilast
Dithranol		Biologics
Tar		

Currently there is no cure for psoriasis, yet available options allow at least distinct improvement of psoriasis manifestations and long-term suppression of exacerbation. This will differentially be discussed with the individual agents and approaches below; however when doing so, off-label status and local or national health imbursement regulations have to be taken into account.

4 Topical Therapy

Topical treatment, also referred to as local or external, plays an important role even with very effective and well-tolerated systemic treatments currently available and even more so in childhood psoriasis (Brune et al. 2003; Albrecht et al. 2011; Fluhr et al. 2000; Mason et al. 2013; van de Kerkhof 2015; Stein Gold 2016). It may be used as monotherapy in limited disease, in combination with systemic treatment or UV light to improve or accelerate clinical responses or when other modalities are contraindicated. Topical products usually contain (1) emollients as basic formulation, (2) humectants, (3) keratoplastic/keratolytic agents, and (4) active agents. In the following, the various therapeutic agents are differentially discussed for use in ichthyoses and psoriasis.

4.1 Emollients

Apart from active ingredients, the appropriate emollient is of prime importance for the efficacy of topical therapy as the penetration of agents through stratum corneum and epidermis is not only facilitated but enhanced by appropriate base composition. As an example, the same steroid compound may clinically be differently resorbed and thus differently potent depending on the formulation of emollient. Most commonly used emollients are white soft paraffin (petrolatum) apart from liquid paraffin, lanolin, castor oil, cetyl and stearyl alcohols, silicone oils, cocoa and shea butter, isopropyl myristate and palmitate, as well as polyethylene glycols. Special care is advised for juvenile patients by avoiding fragrances, artificial colors, and chemical conservation.

Numerous vehicles are available from creams to lotions, ointments, gels, foams, sprays, and shampoos. Young patients and their parents should be educated in the correct application of topical agents with respect to the frequency and duration of daily application and the maximal body surface area to be treated. A “fingertip unit” is easy to communicate and defines the optimal 500 mg of topical that should be applied to one hand size area of skin which in turn is equivalent to about 1% of adolescent or adult body surface area.

Based on the activity of skin inflammation (water in oil for subacute and chronic, oil in water base for acute disease), the affected body site (face versus extremities, skin folds versus free integument), and skin type (dry, oily, mixed skin) as well as season of the year (oil in water base in summer, water in oil in winter), galenic formulations have to be individually adapted.

4.2 Humectants

The skin barrier function is impaired in both psoriasis and ichthyosis resulting in increased transepidermal water loss and epidermal hyperproliferation and dyskeratosis. Therefore skin moisturization is of prime importance in addition to active anti-inflammatory agents. Humectants are often added to increase or maintain moisture in skin, most popular among them glycerol, sorbitol, polyethylene glycols, and urea (Gelmetti 2009; Lindh and Bradley 2015). Urea is a low molecular weight organic compound which is used in concentrations from 2 to 10% for rehydration of skin as well as for increasing the penetration of active agents like corticosteroids (Celleno 2018; Pan et al. 2013; Friedman et al. 2016; Fluhr et al. 2000). Mild skin irritation, especially at sensitive sites like face and folds, is the major unwanted effects and is especially relevant in children. Therefore concentrations below 2% should be used or glycerol as an alternative humectant.

4.3 Keratolytic/Keratoplastic Agents

Epidermal hyperproliferation and dyskeratosis are characteristic for psoriasis and ichthyoses. Therefore, initially excessive scaling material should be removed to enable penetration of active agents. The most common agent is salicylic acid which shows keratinolytic activity at concentrations above 5%, whereas lower concentrations are antiseptic (Madan and Lewitt 2014). Salicylic acid should, however, not be used in children younger than 12 years because of possible relevant resorption and intoxication. Similarly, modern topical combinations, with corticosteroids to increase their penetration into the skin, are only evaluated in adults and should be used cautiously in childhood. Alternative keratolytic agents are propylene glycol and dimethicon. The keratolytic activity of urea is only found well above a concentration of 5% which restrict its use in children (Eisert et al. 2019a, b).

4.4 Active Topical Agents

Most of the currently available topical agents are very effective and their clinical use is well-established; however, their evidence levels regarding efficacy and tolerability in childhood are limited (Table 2). Long-term topical treatment of larger skin areas will challenge the compliance of young patients, especially in adolescence as it takes time to apply in addition to tolerate greasiness and stickiness, skin irritation, as well as odor and the risk of contact sensitization. Continuous and widespread use of topical agents like corticosteroids and vitamin D derivatives may result in relevant systemic resorption which can be overcome by de-escalation and proactive treatment protocols as outlined below or by combination with other topical agents, with UV light or systemic treatment.

Table 2 Topical and systemic therapy for ichthyoses and psoriasis

	Plaque psoriasis	Guttate psoriasis	Pustular psoriasis	Ichthyosis vulgaris	X-chrom. recessive ichthyosis	Epidermolytic ichthyosis	Associated congenital ichthyosis
Topical							
Emollients	++	++	+	++	++	++	++
Topical GCS	++	++	+	–	–	–	–
Topical Calcineurin-inhibitors	+	+	–	–	–	–	–
Topical vitamin D	++	+	–	–	–	–	–
Topical vitamin A	(+)	–	(+)	–	–	–	–
Dithranol	+	++	–	–	–	–	–
Tars	(+)	–	–	(+)	(+)	–	–
Systemic							
Systemic GCS	(+)	–	+	–	–	–	–
Fumarate	–	–	–	–	–	–	–
Methotrexate (MTX)	+	(+)	++	–	–	–	–
Ciclosporin	+	(+)	+		–	–	–
Acitretin	+	(+)	+	(+)	–	+	+
Biologics					–	–	–
Adalimumab	++	–	(+)	–	–	–	–
Etanercept	+	–	(+)	–	–	–	–
Biosimilars	(+)	–		–	–	–	–

–not recommended (+) may be used, no evidence + recommendation ++ high recommendation

5 Topical Corticosteroids

Corticosteroids (CS) are until today the most effective and reliable anti-inflammatory agents available in medicine. Their clinical effects are mediated by intracellular corticoid receptors resulting in altered levels of inflammatory cytokines, adhesion molecules, and lipid mediators. The potency of topical corticosteroids has been classified into three to seven classes, numbered by decreasing potency in the USA, by increasing potency in Europe (Table 3).

With regard to their long-term local and systemic side effects, they should, however, very cautiously be used in chronic, recidivating inflammatory diseases like psoriasis and atopic dermatitis and for no longer than 4–8 weeks (Eisert et al. 2019a, b; Sticherling et al. 2011; Ståhle et al. 2010; de Jager et al. 2010). Especially childhood skin is prone to local side effects even after short-term use and with regard to the special relation of body surface to body volume of children which will result in relevant systemic resorption (Kragballe et al. 1991; Ruiz-Maldonado et al. 1982; van de Kerkhof 2015). Topical steroids should be used for induction therapy only and be slowly tapered by decreasing the application frequency upon improvement ("de-escalation"). Continued use over weeks or months twice a week at the sites which were originally involved ("proactive treatment") may spare steroid dose as well as reduce the number and severity of flares.

Topical corticosteroids have been pharmacologically improved over the years by increasing their lipophilicity through esterification, thus limiting their activity to the skin organ by inactivation within the epidermis. This holds true especially for mometasone and methylprednisolone aceponate or the development of novel formulations like sprays or foams. Hydrocortisone may be used in early childhood and delicate locations like the face and groin; otherwise class two agents are to be preferred. Prednisone is not topically effective. Corticosteroids are available in diverse vehicles which allows their appropriate use at any body site including sensitive areas like the face and folds as well as in a sensitive patient group like children.

Table 3 Topical corticosteroids listed by potency in Europe and the USA

Europe	USA		Corticosteroid compound (examples)
I	VII	Mildest	Hydrocortisone
	VI	Mild	Prednicarbate
II	V	Medium	Methylprednisolone aceponate Betamethasone valerate Triamcinolone acetonide
III	IV	Potent	Betamethasone dipropionate
	III	Very potent	Mometasone furoate
	II	Super potent	Halobetasol propionate
IV	I	Super high	Clobetasol proprionate

6 Vitamin D Analogues

Synthetic topical vitamin D-analogues are able to modulate keratinocyte proliferation and differentiation as well as inflammatory processes by intracellular receptor-driven mechanisms directly regulating pertinent genes. Calcipotriene (USA), called calcipotriol in Europe and Canada, is probably one of the best studied topical agents by GCP-criteria (Guenther et al. 2002; Kragballe et al. 2006; Park et al. 1999; van de Kerkhof et al. 2002). Available data for children are, however, limited (Eisert et al. 2019a, b). Clinical application may often have to be discontinued especially in children due to frequent skin irritation. Otherwise contact sensitization is rare and cancerogenic properties absent. Three different agents (calcipotriol, tacalcitol, calcitriol) are available as solution, cream, and ointment (Guenther et al. 2002; Weindl et al. 2006). Because of systemic resorption with hypercalcemia and hypercalciuria, vitamin D analogues should only be used on less than 30% of the body surface for maximally 8 weeks. Their efficacy can be increased by combination with UV light; however, simultaneous use of lactic and salicylic acid should be avoided as vitamin D analogues destabilize in their presence.

7 Topical Vitamin A Analogues

The acetylene retinoid tazarotene is a third-generation topical retinoid licensed for psoriasis in adults aged above 18 years in the USA and acne vulgaris in patients above the age of 12 (Weinstein et al. 2003; Weindl et al. 2006). However, tazarotene is currently not available in many countries. The agent binds to the retinoic acid receptors ß and gamma with a resulting decrease of epidermal proliferation and de-differentiation. Skin irritation is often limiting its clinical use. No more than 10–20% of body surfaces should be treated at a time. Altogether systemic retinoids like acitretin are more effective in chronic and hyperproliferative (scaling) skin manifestations and should be considered in chronic and widespread disease. Their effects in ichthyoses are not evaluated.

8 Topical Calcineurin-Inhibitors

Calcineurin inhibitors downregulate intracellular calcineurin resulting in a decreased production of interferon gamma, IL-2, and IL-4 by T-lymphocytes. Two topical macrolide calcineurin inhibitors, pimecrolimus and tacrolimus, are licensed for atopic dermatitis only (Steele et al. 2005); however, good clinical effects were seen for plaque psoriasis as well as in inverse locations of psoriasis in a number of case compilations and controlled studies (Brune et al. 2007; Castellsague et al. 2018; Eichenfield et al. 2002; Malecic and Young 2016). Initial burning sensations and pruritus may subside under continuous treatment. Long-term date does not support a black box warning on the risk of lymphoma following prolonged use of topical calcineurin inhibitors (Paghdal and Schwartz 2009). Topical calcineurin inhibitors may represent an alternative to corticosteroids at sensitive sites and in sensitive populations like children.

9 Dithranol

Dithranol (anthralin, cignolin) is a synthetic derivative of a natural mixture of plant ingredients, which has been used in medicine for centuries (Eisert et al. 2019b; Körber et al. 2019; Saraswat et al. 2007). Neither is it resorbed, mutagenic, and cancerogenic nor does it cause contact sensitization. Short *contact therapy* at increasing concentrations of 0.1–3% is applied over weeks starting with a few minutes to be subsequently rinsed off (Eisert et al. 2019a). In contrast *long-contact therapy* is started at lower concentrations of 0.01% and left on for 8–12 h. Mild skin irritation is intended but may limit its use with children where on the other side guttate psoriasis responds exceptionally well. Major additional disadvantages are reversible dark discoloration of the skin, hair, and nails and washable discoloration of clothing as well as sanitary fittings. As for conservation reasons, 1% salicylic acid is regularly added to the ointment; combination with vitamin D analogues should therefore be avoided. Dithranol is mainly used in a hospital setting for induction therapy of mild to moderate psoriasis (Eisert et al. 2019a). However, dithranol appears to have the longest disease-free interval among all other psoriasis treatments.

10 Tars

The various tar preparations (coal, wood tar) show (Sekhon et al. 2018) anti-inflammatory, antipruritic, and antiproliferative as well as antibacterial and antifungal activity (Paghdal and Schwartz 2009). Coal tar is available as crude tar or liquor carbonis detergens (LCD) and mostly sold over the counter. The *World Health Organization's List of Essential Medicines* rates tars among the most effective and safe medicines. A reduction of DNA synthesis as well as mitotic activity may normalize epidermal keratinization with positive clinical results on psoriasis and other epidermal hyperkeratotic diseases. In the USA crude coal tar (2–4% in petrolatum) is combined with artificial ultraviolet radiation (either broad or narrowband UVB) for the treatment of psoriasis as described by the American dermatologist William H. Goeckerman (1884–1954) and is regarded as safe and efficacious (Zhu et al. 2016; Kortuem et al. 2010). (Mild) irritation at the sites of application, folliculitis, and photosensitivity in addition to smell and discoloration of the skin and clothing limit its use especially in children. Conflicting data are available on carcinogenesis which is not relevant in short-term use (Eisert et al. 2019a; Paghdal and Schwartz 2009). In children, tars should be used with special care and only in cases when topical alternatives are neither available nor applicable (Eisert et al. 2019a).

11 Novel Topical Agents and Skin Delivery Systems

Progress in the development of topical agents has been limited over the last decade (Eisert et al. 2019a; Körber et al. 2019). New galenic formulations or penetration promotors may improve local treatment in the future. Novel agents currently in phase 2 and 3 studies include Janus and tyrosine kinase (JAK and TYK inhibitors) as well as phosphodiesterase 4 (PDE4) inhibitors (Svendsen et al. 2016) with good therapeutic responses together with good to fair tolerability. Oral counterparts have already been licensed for rheumatoid and psoriasis arthritis.

12 Treatment with Ultraviolet Light

Ultraviolet light (UV) belongs to the broad spectrum of light emitted by the sun with wave lengths from 180 to 400 nm (Table 4). It comprises UVC (180–280 nm), UVB (280–320 nm), and UVA (320–400 nm) (Table 5). Belonging to electromagnetic radiation, the wavelength correlates to the depth of invasion into material or tissues. UVC is therefore efficiently filtered by the upper atmosphere and ozone layer, whereas UVB and A reach the Earth's surface and unprotected human skin. UVB is penetrating to the epidermal-dermal layer and UVA down to the middle dermis. Similarly, UVA light may penetrate glass panes and will be present until dawn, whereas UVB light will maximally reach the Earth's surface at midday. Around 11 o'clock in the morning and 3 o'clock in the afternoon, maximal UV irradiation is seen, and both adults and especially children should avoid direct sun exposure at that time. UV protection can be achieved by just staying out of the sun in the shade, by protective clothes, and by using chemical or physical UV protection, the latter recommended for children.

Biologically, UV light was shown to exert distinct immunological reactions on all resident and migratory cells of the skin (keratinocytes, endothelial cells, fibroblasts, Langerhans cells, T-cells) mostly resulting in a localized and temporary downregulation of immune mechanisms. Therefore the human skin exploits UV light to counteract constantly ongoing allergic and autoimmune processes. At least four different skin types are differentiated according to the color of the skin, hair, and eyes, erythema time and the degree of tanning after UV exposure. The most frequent skin types II and III in North Europe show an erythema time of unprotected skin of around 30 min. The skin is, however, able to counteract UV exposure to some extent

Table 4 Wave lengths of total sun light

Sun light	Wavelength (nm)
Ultraviolet light	180–400
Visible light	400–800
Infrared light	800–3,000

Table 5 Distribution of wave lengths within the ultraviolet spectrum

Ultraviolet light	Wavelength (nm)
UV-C	180–280
UV-B	280–320
UV-A	320–400
UV-A2	320–340
UV-A1	340–400

through production of melanin by melanocytes, by thickening of the epidermis and especially stratum corneum as well as active repair of UV-induced cell and DNA damage. With overdrive of these protective or reparative mechanisms, acute and chronic UV effects have to be anticipated. Sunburn is probably the most frequent human skin disease and may comprise a clinical range of mild erythema to blister formation. Repetitive sunburns in childhood are related to the incidence of malignant melanoma. Chronic and repetitive UV exposure will result in earlier and more pronounced skin aging as well as a higher rate of skin cancer, predominantly basal cell carcinoma, and squamous cell carcinoma. Though these tumors are very rare in children, they can be expected under massive immunosuppression or defective UV repair as in xeroderma pigmentosum.

Apart from casual UV-exposure through sunlight, UV is therapeutically used to treat inflammatory and neoplastic skin diseases like psoriasis and atopic dermatitis or cutaneous T-cell lymphoma. It can be produced by artificial lamps or ample filters and usually needs regular and repetitive visits (3–5 per week, 20–30 treatments) of practice rooms to apply (Zamberk et al. 2010). UVB narrowband (311 nm) is recommended as it represents the biologically active wave length of UVB avoiding unwanted effects of neighboring wave lengths. UVB may be used in adolescents, but should be very critically used in children (Nguyen et al. 2009). UVA monotherapy will only show minor anti-inflammatory effects but will accelerate skin aging as well as induce skin malignancy. Combination with psoralen either orally or in bath water or cream to increase the UV sensibility (PUVA) is regularly and successfully used in adults but should be avoided in children and adolescents (Eisert et al. 2019b).

13 Systemic Treatment

Effective and well-tolerated systemic treatment for chronic skin diseases is increasingly available and used in adults (Nast et al. 2015, 2018). Limited evidence for children and adolescents, however, will result in critical individual discussion of therapeutic options on one side, should, however, on the other not withhold ample and effective treatment of those affected (Eisert et al. 2019b; Posso-De Los Rios et al. 2014; van Geel et al. 2015; Napolitano et al. 2016). Whereas treatment goals and algorithms for psoriasis have been defined for adults and may cautiously be transferred to children, they are missing for other chronic inflammatory skin disorders. Recently, a German S2k guideline was published on the therapy of psoriasis in children and adolescents, the first one available on this issue (Eisert et al. 2019a, b). While summarizing the relevant systemic treatment options in the following chapter, local and national regulations regarding reimbursement, licensing, and drug monitoring as well as other recommendations and guidelines should be taken into account.

14 Systemic Corticosteroids

Though systemic corticosteroids are still widely used for the treatment of plaque psoriasis, general expert consensus is that they should be avoided for skin manifestations (Nast et al. 2018; Eisert et al. 2019b). Despite their immediate, reliable, and effective responses, continued and repetitive use will result in a number of severe unwanted effects which are especially relevant for children. Systemic corticosteroids may in single cases be used short-term for highly inflammatory skin manifestations, for acute arthritis or generalized pustular psoriasis and should be rapidly substituted by other immunomodulatory agents. Initial doses should be 0.5–1 mg/kg body weight prednisolone or equivalent. If administered for a few days, no tapering will be necessary.

15 Methotrexate

Methotrexate (MTX) is probably the most frequently used immunomodulatory agent in childhood (Eisert et al. 2019b; Posso-De Los Rios et al. 2014). As folic acid antagonist is exerts immunomodulatory activity on T-cells and cells of innate immunity. It is generally well-tolerated in childhood as limiting effects of lifestyle drugs relevant for adults (e.g. alcohol) as well as concomitant medication are mostly absent. Nevertheless, there is no official label for MTX use in children. It may be used for psoriasis arthritis, pustular psoriasis, severe manifestations of plaque psoriasis and guttate psoriasis. Maximal clinical effects may take up to 3 months to appear. Therefore, initial dosing should be 10–15 mg per square meter body surface once per week and may be increased every 4–8 weeks by 2.5 mg. With respect to gastrointestinal tolerance, the oral dose may be divided into a morning and evening dose; alternatively subcutaneous application should be used. The following day, 5 mg of folic acid should be administered to improve tolerability. After maximal clinical improvement, MTX doses should be slowly decreased again by 2.5 mg every 4–8 weeks; long-term and continuous application is reasonable and often necessary in individual cases. Blood count, liver enzymes, and renal parameters, preferentially creatinine, should be controlled after 1 and 6 weeks, thereafter every 6–12 weeks.

16 Ciclosporin

Ciclosporin (CSA) is an inhibitor of intracellular calcineurin resulting in the downregulation of various inflammatory cytokines, especially IL-2 by T-cells. Compared to methotrexate, clinical effects are evident after 4–8 weeks already; on the other side, continuous use longer than 6 months is critical with regard to nephrotoxic symptoms and possible arterial hypertension (Eisert et al. 2019b; Di Lernia et al. 2016; Pereira et al. 2006). Dosing ranges between 2.5 and 5 mg/kg body weight divided in two daily doses. It may be started with 2.5–3 mg, and increased when clinical effects are small or missing, or alternatively started with 4–5 mg/kg body weight for severe disease. After clinical improvement, daily dosing can be reduced by 0.5 mg/kg body weight every month. Blood monitoring should include blood count, liver enzymes, serum electrolytes, and creatinine before treatment, after 4, 8, and 12 weeks, and every 3 months thereafter. CSA may be combined with any topical treatment, not, however, with UV treatment.

17 Fumarates

Fumaric acid esters or fumarates are a mixture of three compounds that have been licensed in Germany for the treatment of adult plaque psoriasis since 1994, the single substance dimethyl fumarate (DMF) in Europe since 2017. Available data from case reports, retrospective studies, and a controlled study not published yet suggest both good efficacy and tolerability in children and adolescents (Reich et al. 2016; Balak et al. 2013; van Geel et al. 2016; Eisert et al. 2019b). Dosing is increased over weeks similar to adult dosing, and efficacy is monitored by month 3. Full clinical effects may take more than 3 to 6 months to appear. Monitoring should include blood count, liver enzymes, and creatinine before treatment, initially every 4 weeks and from month 4 on every 8 weeks.

18 Retinoids

Vitamin A derivatives have been used over decades for hyperkeratotic diseases and diseases of sebaceous glands. Currently acitretin and isotretinoin are available (Kopp et al. 2004). The latter is preferably used for acne in adolescents and is less effective in hyperkeratosis yet better tolerated and less critical with respect to pregnancy: both agents need a monthly negative pregnancy test to start and continue, yet women should not become pregnant at least 3 years after stopping acitretin but only 4–12 weeks after stopping isotretinoin. This aspect becomes relevant for adolescent girls. Though no clinical studies on acitretin are available for childhood, numerous case reports and retrospective chart reviews suggest good effectivity and tolerance especially for pustular psoriasis and erythroderma, however, with relapses after stopping the treatment. Reassuring data on long-term efficacy and tolerability are available for various forms of ichthyosis. Combination with narrowband UVB may increase clinical improvement in psoriasis which usually takes 2–3 months. No effects are seen on psoriasis arthritis. Initial dosing should be 0.3–0.5 mg/kg body weight and may be increased stepwise up to 1 mg/kg body weight. Upon improvement, the doses should be slowly tapered to around 0.2 mg/kg body weight. The German guideline recommends acitretin for moderate to severe pustular psoriasis of girls and boys before puberty and for male adolescents (Eisert et al. 2019b; Guenther et al. 2017; Chen et al. 2018). Unwanted effects are dryness of skin and mucous membranes which may limit the treatment in childhood, alopecia, and bone as well as muscle pain. Effects on bone development of spine and long bones should be clinically monitored and evaluated by X-ray if necessary. Laboratory monitoring includes blood count, liver enzymes, triglycerides, cholesterol and HDL, creatinine, and urea before treatment, initially every 4 weeks and every 12 weeks from month three on. A monthly negative pregnancy test is mandatory if relevant.

19 Biologics

Biologics have dramatically changed our therapeutic options of adult psoriasis in the last decades. These fusion proteins or monoclonal antibodies specifically inhibit the pathogenetically relevant inflammatory cytokines tumor necrosis factor alpha (TNFα), IL-12/IL-23, IL-17, and IL-23 with very good efficacy and tolerability. Using the recently licensed anti-IL-23 agents, PASI 90 improvements of more than 70% can be achieved. However, only few of these agents are evaluated and licensed for childhood psoriasis. A number of case reports on the use of biologics in childhood psoriasis are available, including pustular disease (Eisert et al. 2019b; Wright et al. 2010; Saikaly and Mattes 2016).

20 TNF-Blockers

Two TNF-blockers are available for subcutaneous application in children, the fusion protein etanercept from the age of 6 years and the monoclonal antibody adalimumab for children from 4 years and older.

21 Adalimumab

The monoclonal anti-TNF antibody was licensed in 2008 for children above the age of 4 suffering from severe plaque psoriasis who have responded insufficiently to topical and UV therapy (Braun et al. 2018; Wright et al. 2010). The German guideline recommends adalimumab for moderate to severe psoriasis in childhood with a 71% consensus (Eisert et al. 2019b). Five of seven experts preferred methotrexate. There is no license for juvenile psoriasis arthritis nor axial or ankylosing spondylarthritis. At a body weight up to 30 kg, adalimumab is started with 20 mg once a week for 2 weeks, thereafter 20 mg every 2 weeks, similarly at a body weight above 30 kg with 40 mg. Clinical evaluation and decision for continued treatment should be done at week 16. Initial laboratory monitoring includes differential blood count, liver enzymes, hepatitis B/C, and HIV serology with differential blood count and liver enzymes after 4 and 12 weeks, thereafter every 3 months. The German guideline recommends initial tuberculin skin test in children younger and quantiferon test in children older than 5 years. Chest X-ray should only be done with clear clinical suspicion. Annual Tb screening is not necessary with low Tb risk and initially negative Tb tests.

22 Etanercept

Etanercept is licensed for chronic severe psoriasis in children from 6 years and older who have not responded to or have not tolerated at least one conventional systemic agent or UV therapy, in addition to psoriasis arthritis above the age of 12 in children who have not responded to or not tolerated methotrexate. The German guideline recommends etanercept only when adalimumab or methotrexate failed. The dosing is individually adapted to body weight, with 0.8 mg/kg up to 50 mg per doses, above the weight of 62.5 kg with 50 mg as prefilled syringe or pen. Clinical evaluation and decision for continued treatment should be done at week 12. The initial and continuous laboratory monitoring including Tb screening is identical to adalimumab.

23 IL-12/IL-23 Blocker Ustekinumab

The monoclonal antibody ustekinumab is directed against the p40 unit shared by IL-12 and IL-23 and is licensed for children from the age of 12. It is applied at weeks 0 and 4 and every 3 months thereafter. Dosing is 40 mg at a body weight between 60 and 100 kg, 90 mg above 100 kg. Below 60 kg the recommended dose is 0.75 mg/kg body weight which can be drawn individually from a 45 mg glass vial. Clinical evaluation and decision for continued treatment should be done at week 28. Initial and continuous laboratory monitoring including Tb screening is identical to adalimumab.

24 Biosimilars

Biosimilars have become available after patent expired for adalimumab and etanercept. Regulations demand comparability to the original agents with respect to efficacy and safety which have to be proven in a least one licensed adult indication. Transfer of such data to children is critical, and biosimilar effects should be examined in juvenile patients in well-controlled clinical studies. Therefore, the use of both agents as biosimilars in children should be individually decided (Nast et al. 2018; Braun et al. 2018; Eisert et al. 2019b).

25 Novel Agents

The oral phosphodiesterase 4 (PDE-4) inhibitor apremilast has been licensed for adult plaque psoriasis and psoriasis arthritis in the USA in 2014 and in EU and Switzerland in 2015. Controlled clinical studies in children are ongoing and licensing for children may be expected soon. Several other clinical phase 2 and 3 studies are ongoing for adult psoriasis including novel monoclonal antibodies and oral inhibitors of Janus kinase (JAK) and phosphodiesterase 4 (PDE-4). Current regulatory procedures demand early initiation of clinical studies in juvenile patients.

References

Albrecht L, Bourcier M, Ashkenas J et al (2011) Topical psoriasis therapy in the age of biologics: evidence-based treatment recommendations. J Cutan Med Surg 15:309–321

Augustin M, Glaeske G, Radtke MA, Christophers E, Reich K, Schafer I (2010) Epidemiology and comorbidity of psoriasis in children. Br J Dermatol 162:633–636

Balak DM, Oostveen AM, Bousema MT, Venema AW, Arnold WP, Seyger MM et al (2013) Effectiveness and safety of fumaric acid esters in children with psoriasis: a retrospective analysis of 14 patients from The Netherlands. Br J Dermatol 168:1343–1347

Beattie PE, Lewis-Jones MS (2006) A comparative study of impairment of quality of life in children with skin disease and children with other chronic childhood diseases. Br J Dermatol 155:145–151

Benoit S, Hamm H (2007) Childhood psoriasis. Clin Dermatol 25:555–562

Braun J, Lorenz HM, Muller-Ladner U, Schneider M, Schulze-Koops H, Specker C et al (2018) Revised version of the statement by the DGRh on biosimilars-update 2017. Z Rheumatol 77:81–90

Brune A, Miller DW, Lin P, Cotrim-Russi D, Paller AS (2007) Tacrolimus ointment is effective for psoriasis on the face and intertriginous areas in pediatric patients. Pediatr Dermatol 24:76–80

Bruner CR, Feldman SR, Ventrapragada M, Fleischer AB Jr (2003) A systematic review of adverse effects associated with topical treatments for psoriasis. Dermatol Online J 9:2

Castellsague J, Kuiper JG, Pottegard A, Anveden Berglind I, Dedman D, Gutierrez L et al (2018) A cohort study on the risk of lymphoma and skin cancer in users of topical tacrolimus, pimecrolimus, and corticosteroids (Joint European Longitudinal Lymphoma and Skin Cancer Evaluation – JOELLE study). Clin Epidemiol 10:299–310

Celleno L (2018) Topical urea in skincare: a review. Dermatol Ther 31:e12690

Cellucci T, Guzman J, Petty RE, Batthish M, Benseler SM, Ellsworth JE et al (2016) Management of Juvenile Idiopathic Arthritis 2015: a position statement from the Pediatric Committee of the Canadian Rheumatology Association. J Rheumatol 43:1773–1776

Chen P, Li C, Xue R, Chen H, Tian X, Zeng K et al (2018) Efficacy and safety of acitretin monotherapy in children with pustular psoriasis: results from 15 cases and a literature review. J Dermatolog Treat 29:353–363

Chiam LY, de Jager ME, Giam YC, de Jong EM, van de Kerkhof PC, Seyger MM (2011) Juvenile psoriasis in European and Asian children: similarities and differences. Br J Dermatol 164:1101–1103

Cortés H, Del Prado-Audelo ML, Urbán-Morlán Z, Alcalá-Alcalá S, González-Torres M, Reyes-Hernández OD, González-Del Carmen M, Leyva-Gómez G (2019) Pharmacological treatments for cutaneous manifestations of inherited ichthyoses. Arch Dermatol Res. https://doi.org/10.1007/s00403-019-01994-x. [Epub ahead of print]

de Jager ME, de Jong EM, van de Kerkhof PC, Seyger MM (2010) Efficacy and safety of treatments for childhood psoriasis: a systematic literature review. J Eur Acad Dermatol Venereol 62:1013–1030

de Oliveira ST, Maragno L, Arnone M, Fonseca Takahashi MD, Romiti R (2010) Generalized pustular psoriasis in childhood. Pediatr Dermatol 27:349–354

Di Lernia V, Stingeni L, Boccaletti V, Calzavara Pinton PG, Guarneri C, Belloni Fortina A et al (2016) Effectiveness and safety of cyclosporine in pediatric plaque psoriasis: a multicentric retrospective analysis. J Dermatol Treatment 27:395–398

Dogan B, Karabudak O, Harmanyeri Y (2008) Antistreptococcal treatment of guttate psoriasis: a controlled study. Int J Dermatol 47:950–952

Eichenfield LF, Lucky AW, Boguniewicz M, Langley RG, Cherill R, Marshall K, Bush C, Graeber M (2002) Safety and efficacy of pimecrolimus (ASM 981) cream 1% in the treatment of mild and moderate atopic dermatitis in children and adolescents. J Am Acad Dermatol 46:495–504

Eisert L, Augustin M, Bach S, Dittmann M, Eiler R, Fölster-Holst R, Gerdes S, Hamm H, Höger P, Horneff G, von Kiedrowski R, Philipp S, Pleimes M, Schläger M, Schuster V, Staubach P,

Weberschock T, Werner RN, Nast A, Sticherling M (2019a) S2k guidelines for the treatment of psoriasis in children and adolescents – Short version part 1. J Dtsch Dermatol Ges 17:856–870
Eisert L, Augustin M, Bach S, Dittmann M, Eiler R, Fölster-Holst R, Gerdes S, Hamm H, Höger P, Horneff G, von Kiedrowski R, Philipp S, Pleimes M, Schlaeger M, Schuster V, Staubach P, Weberschock T, Werner RN, Nast A, Sticherling M (2019b) S2k guidelines for the treatment of psoriasis in children and adolescents – Short version part 2. J Dtsch Dermatol Ges 17:959–973
Finlay AY (2005) Current severe psoriasis and the rule of tens. Br J Dermatol 152:861–867
Finlay AY, Khan GK (1994) Dermatology life quality index (DLQI) – a simple practical measure for routine clinical use. Clin Exp Dermatol 19:210–216
Fluhr JW, Pfisterer S, Gloor M (2000) Direct comparison of skin physiology in children and adults with bioengineering methods. Pediatr Dermatol 17:436–439
Fredriksson T, Pettersson U (1978) Severe psoriasis: oral therapy with a new retinoid. Dermatologica 157:238–244
Friedman AJ, von Grote EC, Meckfessel MH (2016) Urea: a clinically oriented overview from bench to bedside. J Drugs Dermatol 15:633–639
Gelmetti C (2009) Therapeutic moisturizers as adjuvant therapy for psoriasis patients. Am J Clin Dermatol 10(Suppl 1):7–12
Groot N, Heijstek MW, Wulffraat NM (2015) Vaccinations in paediatric rheumatology: an update on current developments. Curr Rheumatol Rep 17:46
Guenther L, van de Kerkhof PC, Snellmann E et al (2002) Efficacy and safety of a new combination of calcipotriol and betamethasone dipropionate (once or twice daily) compared to calcipotriol (twice daily) in the treatment of psoriasis vulgaris: a randomized double-blind, vehicle-controlled clinical trial. Br J Dermatol 147:316–323
Guenther LC, Kunynetz R, Lynde CW, Sibbald RG, Toole J, Vender R, Zip C (2017) Acitretin use in dermatology. J Cutan Med Surg 21(3_suppl):2S–12S
Gunes AT, Fetil E, Akarsu S, Ozbagcivan O, Babayeva L (2015) Possible triggering effect of influenza vaccination on psoriasis. J Immunol Res 2015:258430
Heijstek MW, Ott de Bruin LM, Bijl M, Borrow R, van der Klis F, Kone-Paut I et al (2011) EULAR recommendations for vaccination in paediatric patients with rheumatic diseases. Ann Rheum Dis 70:1704–1712
Horton DB, Scott FI, Haynes K, Putt ME, Rose CD, Lewis JD et al (2016) Antibiotic exposure, infection, and the development of pediatric psoriasis: a nested case-control study. JAMA Dermatol 152:191–199
Kara T, Topkarci Z, Yilmaz S, Akaltun I, Erdogan B (2019) Pediatric patients with psoriasis and psychiatric disorders: premorbidity and comorbidity in a case-control study. SO – J Dermatolog Treat 30:129–134
Kokolakis GP, Ioannidou D, Cholongitas E, Kruger-Krasagakis S (2010) Guttate psoriasis occurring on varicella lesions. J Dermatol 37:857–859
Kopp T, Karlhofer F, Szepfalusi Z, Schneeberger A, Stingl G, Tanew A (2004) Successful use of acitretin in conjunction with narrowband ultraviolet B phototherapy in a child with severe pustular psoriasis, von Zumbusch type. Br J Dermatol 151:912–916
Körber A, Wilsmann-Theis D, Augustin M, von Kiedrowski R, Mrowietz U, Rosenbach T, Meller S, Pinter A, Sticherling M, Gerdes S, PsoNet Förderverein (2019) Topische Therapie bei Psoriasis vulgaris – ein Behandlungspfad. J Dtsch Dermatol Ges 17(Suppl 4):3–14
Kortuem KR, Davis MD, Witman PM, McEvoy MT, Farmer SA (2010) Results of Goeckerman treatment for psoriasis in children: a 21-year retrospective review. Pediatr Dermatol 27:518–524
Kragballe J, Gjertsen BT, De Hoop D et al (1991) Double blind, right-left comparison of calcipotriol and betamethasone valerate in treatment of psoriasis vulgaris. Lancet 337:193–196
Kragballe K, Austad J, Barnes L et al (2006) A 52-week randomized safety study of calcipotriol/betamethasone dipropionate two-compound product in the treatment of psoriasis. Br J Dermatol 154:1150–1160

Langley RG, Ellis CN (2004) Evaluating psoriasis with psoriasis area and severity index, psoriasis global assessment, and lattice system physician's global assessment. J Am Acad Dermatol 51:563–569

Lewis-Jones MS, Finlay AY (1995) The children's dermatology life quality index (CDLQI): initial validation and practical use. Br J Dermatol 132:942–949

Liao PB, Rubinson R, Howard R, Sanchez G, Frieden IJ (2002) Annular pustular psoriasis – most common form of pustular psoriasis in children: report of three cases and review of the literature. Pediatr Dermatol 19:19–25

Lindh JD, Bradley M (2015) Clinical effectiveness of moisturizers in atopic dermatitis and related disorders: a systematic review. Am J Clin Dermatol 16:341–359

Lowes MA, Bowcock AM, Krueger JG (2007) Pathogenesis and therapy of psoriasis. Nature 445:866–873

Madan RK, Levitt J (2014) A review of toxicity from topical salicylic acid preparations. J Am Acad Dermatol 70:788–792

Malecic C, Young H (2016) Tacrolimus for the management of psoriasis: clinical utility and place in therapy. Psoriasis 6:153–163

Mason AR, Mason J, Cork M, Dooley G, Hancock H (2013) Topical treatments for chronic plaque psoriasis. Cochrane Database Syst Rev. (3):CD005028. https://doi.org/10.1002/14651858.CD005028.pub3.

Mazereeuw-Hautier J, Vahlquist A, Traupe H, Bygum A, Amaro C, Aldwin M, Audouze A, Bodemer C, Bourrat E, Diociaiuti A, Dolenc-Voljc M, Dreyfus I, El Hachem M, Fischer J, Gånemo A, Gouveia C, Gruber R, Hadj-Rabia S, Hohl D, Jonca N, Ezzedine K, Maier D, Malhotra R, Rodriguez M, Ott H, Paige DG, Pietrzak A, Poot F, Schmuth M, Sitek JC, Steijlen P, Wehr G, Moreen M, O'Toole EA, Oji V, Hernandez-Martin A (2019a) Management of congenital ichthyoses: European guidelines of care, part one. Br J Dermatol 180:272–281

Mazereeuw-Hautier J, Hernández-Martín A, O'Toole EA, Bygum A, Amaro C, Aldwin M, Audouze A, Bodemer C, Bourrat E, Diociaiuti A, Dolenc-Voljč M, Dreyfus I, El Hachem M, Fischer J, Ganemo A, Gouveia C, Gruber R, Hadj-Rabia S, Hohl D, Jonca N, Ezzedine K, Maier D, Malhotra R, Rodriguez M, Ott H, Paige DG, Pietrzak A, Poot F, Schmuth M, Sitek JC, Steijlen P, Wehr G, Moreen M, Vahlquist A, Traupe H, Oji V (2019b) Management of congenital ichthyoses: European guidelines of care, part two. Br J Dermatol 180:484–495

Mrowietz U, Kragballe K, Reich K, Spuls P, Griffiths CE, Nast A et al (2011) Definition of treatment goals for moderate to severe psoriasis: a European consensus. Arch Dermatol Res 303:1–10

Napolitano M, Megna M, Balato A, Ayala F, Lembo S, Villani A et al (2016) Systemic treatment of pediatric psoriasis: a review. Dermatol Ther (Heidelberg) 6:125–142

Nast A, Gisondi P, Ormerod AD, Saiag P, Smith C, Spuls PI, Arenberger P, Bachelez H, Barker J, Dauden E, de Jong EM, Feist E, Jacobs A, Jobling R, Kemény L, Maccarone M, Mrowietz U, Papp KA, Paul C, Reich K, Rosumeck S, Talme T, Thio HB, van de Kerkhof P, Werner RN, Yawalkar N (2015) European S3-guidelines on the systemic treatment of psoriasis vulgaris – update 2015 – Short version – EDF in cooperation with EADV and IPC. J Eur Acad Dermatol Venereol 29:2277–2294

Nast A, Amelunxen L, Augustin M, Boehncke WH, Dressler C, Gaskins M, Härle P, Hoffstadt B, Klaus J, Koza J, Mrowietz U, Ockenfels HM, Philipp S, Reich K, Rosenbach T, Rzany B, Schlaeger M, Schmid-Ott G, Sebastian M, von Kiedrowski R, Weberschock T (2018) S3 Guideline for the treatment of psoriasis vulgaris, update - short version part 1 - systemic treatment. J Dtsch Dermatol Ges 16:645–669

Nguyen T, Gattu S, Pugashetti R, Koo J (2009) Practice of phototherapy in the treatment of moderate-to-severe psoriasis. Curr Probl Dermatol 38:59–78

Osier E, Wang AS, Tollefson MM, Cordoro KM, Daniels SR, Eichenfield A et al (2017) Pediatric psoriasis comorbidity screening guidelines. JAMA Dermatol 153:698–704

Owen CM, Chalmers RJ, O'Sullivan T, Griffiths CE (2001) A systematic review of anti-streptococcal interventions for guttate and chronic plaque psoriasis. Br J Dermatol 145:886–890

Paghdal KV, Schwartz RA (2009) Topical tar: back to the future. J Am Acad Dermatol 61:294–302
Pan M, Heinecke G, Bernardo S, Tsui C, Levitt J (2013) Urea: a comprehensive review of the clinical literature. Dermatol Online J 19:20392
Park SB, Suh DH, Youn JI (1999) A pilot study to assess the safety and efficacy of topical calcipotriol treatment in childhood psoriasis. Pediatr Dermatol 16:321–325
Pereira TM, Vieira AP, Fernandes JC, Sousa-Basto A (2006) Cyclosporin A treatment in severe childhood psoriasis. J Eur Acad Dermatol Venereol 20:651–656
Peter Rout D, Nair A, Gupta A, Kumar P (2019) Epidermolytic hyperkeratosis: clinical update. Clin Cosmet Investig Dermatol 12:333–344
Posso-De Los Rios CJ, Pope E, Lara-Corrales I (2014) A systematic review of systemic medications for pustular psoriasis in pediatrics. Pediatr Dermatol 31:430–439
Pourchot D, Bodemer C, Phan A, Bursztejn AC, Hadj-Rabia S, Boralevi F et al (2017) Nail psoriasis: a systematic evaluation in 313 children with psoriasis. Pediatr Dermatol 34:58–63
Rachakonda TD, Dhillon JS, Florek AG, Armstrong AW (2015) Effect of tonsillectomy on psoriasis: a systematic review. J Am Acad Dermatol 72:261–275
Reich K, Hartl C, Gambichler T, Zschocke I (2016) Retrospective data collection of psoriasis treatment with fumaric acid esters in children and adolescents in Germany (KIDS FUTURE study). J Dtsch Dermatol Ges 14:50–58
Ringold S, Weiss PF, Beukelman T, DeWitt EM, Ilowite NT, Kimura Y et al (2013) 2013 update of the 2011 American College of Rheumatology recommendations for the treatment of juvenile idiopathic arthritis: recommendations for the medical therapy of children with systemic juvenile idiopathic arthritis and tuberculosis screening among children receiving biologic medications. Arthritis Rheum 65:2499–2512
Ruiz-Maldonado R, Zapata G, Lourdes R, Robles C (1982) Cushing's syndrome after topical application of corticosteroids. Am J Dis Child 136:274–275
Saikaly SK, Mattes M (2016) Biologics and pediatric generalized pustular psoriasis: an emerging therapeutic trend. Cureus 8:e652
Saraswat A, Agarwal R, Katare OP, Kaur I, Kumar B (2007) A randomized, double-blind, vehicle-controlled study of a novel liposomal dithranol formulation in psoriasis. J Dermatolog Treat 18:40–45
Sekhon S, Jeon C, Nakamura M, Afifi L, Yan D, Wu JJ et al (2018) Review of the mechanism of action of coal tar in psoriasis. J Dermatol Treat 29:230–232
Skinner AC, Perrin EM, Moss LA, Skelton JA (2015) Cardiometabolic risks and severity of obesity in children and young adults. N Engl J Med 373:1307–1317
Ståhle M, Atakan N, Boehncke WH, Chimenti S, Daudén E, Giannetti A, Hoeger P, Joly P, Katsambas A, Kragballe K, Lambert J, Ortonne JP, Prinz JC, Puig L, Seyger M, Strohal R, Van De Kerkhoff P, Sterry W (2010) Juvenile psoriasis and its clinical management: a European expert group consensus. J Dtsch Dermatol Ges 8:812–818
Steele JA, Choi C, Kwong PC (2005) Topical tacrolimus in the treatment of inverse psoriasis in children. J Am Acad Dermatol 53:713–716
Stein Gold LF (2016) Topical therapies for psoriasis: improving management strategies and patient adherence. Semin Cutan Med Surg 35(2 Suppl 2):S36–S44. quiz S45
Sticherling M, Augustin M, Boehncke WH, Christophers E, Domm S, Gollnick H, Reich K, Mrowietz U (2011) Therapy of psoriasis in childhood and adolescence – a German expert consensus. J Dtsch Dermatol Ges 9:815–823
Svendsen MT, Jeyabalan J, Andersen KE, Andersen F, Johannessen H (2016) Worldwide utilization of topical remedies in treatment of psoriasis: a systematic review. J Dermatolog Treat 13:1–10
Swanbeck G, Inerot A, Martinsson T, Wahlstrom J, Enerback C, Enlund F et al (1995) Age at onset and different types of psoriasis. Br J Dermatol 133:768–773
Takeichi T, Akiyama M (2016) Inherited ichthyosis: non-syndromic forms. J Dermatol 43:242–251

Thorleifsdottir RH, Eysteinsdottir JH, Olafsson JH, Sigurdsson MI, Johnston A, Valdimarsson H et al (2016) Throat infections are associated with exacerbation in a substantial proportion of patients with chronic plaque psoriasis. Acta Derm Venereol 96:788–791

Thorleifsdottir RH, Sigurdardottir SL, Sigurgeirsson B, Olafsson JH, Sigurdsson MI, Petersen H et al (2017) Patient-reported outcomes and clinical response in patients with moderate-to-severe plaque psoriasis treated with tonsillectomy: a randomized controlled trial. Acta Derm Venereol 97:340–345

Tollefson MM, Van Houten HK, Asante D, Yao X, Maradit KH (2018) Association of psoriasis with comorbidity development in children with psoriasis. JAMA Dermatol 154:286–292

van de Kerkhof PC (2015) An update on topical therapies for mild-moderate psoriasis. Dermatol Clin 33:73–77

van de Kerkhof PC, Werfel T, Haustein UF et al (2002) Tacalcitol ointment in the treatment of psoriasis vulgaris: a multicentre, placebo-controlled, double-blind study on efficacy and safety. Br J Dermatol 135:758–765

van Geel MJ, Mul K, de Jager ME, van de Kerkhof PC, de Jong EM, Seyger MM (2015) Systemic treatments in paediatric psoriasis: a systematic evidence-based update. J Eur Acad Dermatol Venereol 29:425–437

van Geel MJ, van de Kerkhof PC, Oostveen AM, de Jong EM, Seyger MM (2016) Fumaric acid esters in recalcitrant pediatric psoriasis: a prospective, daily clinical practice case series. J Dermatolog Treat 27:214–220

van Geel MJ, Otero ME, de Jong EM, van de Kerkhof PC, Seyger MM (2017) Validation of the simplified psoriasis index in Dutch children and adolescents with plaque psoriasis. Br J Ddermatol 176:771–776

Weindl G, Roeder A, Schafer-Korting M, Schaller M, Korting HC (2006) Receptor-selective retinoids for psoriasis: focus on tazarotene. Am J Clin Dermatol 7:85–97

Weinstein GD, Koo JY, Krueger GG et al (2003) Tazarotene cream in the treatment of psoriasis: two multicenter, double-blind, randomized, vehicle-controlled studies of the safety and efficacy of tazarotene creams 0.05% and 0.1% applied once daily for 12 weeks. J Am Acad Dermatol 48:760–767

Wright NA, Piggott CD, Eichenfield LF (2010) The role of biologics and other systemic agents in the treatment of pediatric psoriasis. Semin Cutan Med Surg 29:20–27

Yoneda K (2016) Inherited ichthyosis: syndromic forms. J Dermatol 43:252–263

Zamberk P, Velazquez D, Campos M, Hernanz JM, Lazaro P (2010) Paediatric psoriasis – narrowband UVB treatment. J Eur Acad Dermatol Venereol 24:415–419

Zhu TH, Nakamura M, Farahnik B, Abrouk M, Singh RK, Lee KM, Hulse S, Koo J, Bhutani T, Liao W (2016) The patient's guide to psoriasis treatment. Part 4: Goeckerman therapy. Dermatol Ther (Heidelb) 6:333–339

Pharmacological Heart Failure Therapy in Children: Focus on Inotropic Support

Dietmar Schranz

Contents

Abstract

Pediatric heart failure is a clinical syndrome, which needs to be distinctly defined and the pathophysiological consequences considered. Pharmacological treatment depends on the disease- and age-specific myocardial characteristics. Acute and chronic low cardiac output is the result of an inadequate heart rate (rhythm), myocardial contractility, preload and afterload, and also ventriculo-ventricular interaction, synchrony, atrio-ventricular and ventricular-arterial coupling. The treatment of choice is curing the cause of heart failure, if possible.

Acute HF therapy is still based to the use of catecholamines and inodilators. The cornerstone of chronic HF treatment consists of blocking the endogenous, neuro-humoral axis, in particular the adrenergic and renin-angiotensin-aldosterone system.

Before neprilysin inhibitors are used in young children, their potential side-effect for inducing Alzheimer disease needs to be clarified. The focus of the current review is put on the differential use of the inotropic drugs as epinephrine, norepinephrine, dopamine and dobutamine, and also the inodilators milrinone and levosimendan. Considering effects and side-effects of any cardiac stimulating

D. Schranz (✉)
Pediatric Heart Center, Johann Wolfgang Goethe University Clinic, Frankfurt, Germany
e-mail: dietmar.schranz@paediat.med.uni-giessen.de

W. Kiess et al. (eds.), *Pediatric Pharmacotherapy*,
Handbook of Experimental Pharmacology 261, https://doi.org/10.1007/164_2019_267

treatment strategy, co-medication with ß-blockers, angiotensin converting inhibitors (ACEIs), angiotensin blockers (ARBs) and mineralocorticoid receptor antagonists (MRAs) is not a contradiction, but a senseful measure, even still during the acute inotropic treatment.

Missing sophisticated clinical trials using accurate entry criteria and clinically relevant endpoints, there is especially in cardiovascular diagnosis and treatment of young children a compromise of evidence-based versus pathophysiology-based procedures. But based on the pharmacological and pathophysiological knowledge a hypothesis-driven individualized treatment is already currently possible and therefore indicated.

Keywords
Children · Heart failure · Inotrops · Pharmacology

1 Definition and Pathophysiology of Heart Failure

Pediatric heart failure (HF) is defined as a clinical syndrome (Kirk et al. 2014; Braunwald 2013). Cardiac output (CO) and systemic blood flow (SBF) are acute or chronically reduced, whether at rest or only during exercise. Therefore, HF is also characterized by a general mismatch of blood supply and demand independent whether caused by ventricular dysfunction, pressure or volume overload, or arrhythmias. From the pathophysiological point of view, low CO might be caused by the sum of all components but even any single component of either inadequate heart rate (rhythm), myocardial contractility, preload and afterload or loss of ventriculo-ventricular interaction, synchronized contractility, or atrioventricular and ventricular-arterial coupling.

Neurohumoral and molecular abnormalities are related to the severity of HF and independent if caused by pump or over-circulation failure. Over-circulation can also be related to a normal or even hypercontractile myocardium. Causes of pump failing might be associated with congenital or acquired diseases. Therefore, the treatment of choice of any heart failure is correction of the cause of the disease, whenever such is possible.

2 Pharmacological Therapy of Pediatric Heart Failure (PHF)

Medical HF therapy of adult patients with chronic heart failure led to a significant improvement in survival (Braunwald 2013). While acute HF therapy is still related to the use of catecholamines and inodilators, the cornerstone of chronic HF treatment consists of blocking the endogenous, neurohumoral axis, in particular the adrenergic and renin-angiotensin-aldosterone system (Yancy et al. 2017). Since decades, ß-blockers (BB), angiotensin-converting enzyme inhibitors (ACEIs), angiotensin II receptor blockers (ARBs), and mineralocorticoid receptor antagonists (MRAs) are successfully used in adults with a safe, but highly effective, treatment profile (Yancy et al. 2017). Meanwhile, novel agents, which combined blocking of neprilysin enzyme and angiotensin receptors (sacubitril, Entresto®), are approved for HF therapy in adults (McMurray et al. 2014). However, that does not mean neprilysin enzyme inhibitors have to be used in children; at first, there is not a need for utilizing inhibitors of the enzyme neprilysin as long as the current available anti-congestive cardiovascular drugs are not fully exhausted in terms of the drug-specific pharmacological profile and tailored to the disease. Furthermore, the theoretical side effects of neprilysin inhibitors inducing Alzheimer disease need fully be excluded. Neprilysin is an important cerebral transmitter for avoiding plaque formation (Yasojima et al. 2001; Farris et al. 2007; El-Amouri et al. 2008). Nevertheless, considering the success story in treating adult HF, the question arises: what did run wrong over the last decades treating pediatric patients with HF? Especially, considering patients with a high cardiac regeneration potential, which inverse correlates to the patient's age (Mollovaa et al. 2013). Still today, the pediatric heart failure therapy is based on the triple *D* strategy (Kreidberg et al. 1963; Engle et al. 1978; Digitalis Investigation Group (DIG) 1997; Rodriguez et al. 2008; Kantor et al. 2013), *d*iuretics, *d*igoxin, and *d*iet (fluid restriction). Diuretics are used as first-line heart failure drugs, oftentimes independent on their need and the pathophysiological condition with any signs of systemic or pulmonary vein congestion, only based on the diagnosis "heart failure," neglecting that HF is a "syndrome" in consequence of multiple possible diseases (Schranz and Voelkel 2016). The MR-antagonist spironolactone is usually utilized by pediatricians as a diuretic drug, instead of a low dosage with a significant impact on myocardial fibrosis as it could demonstrated in adults (Pitt et al. 1999) and even in children (Masutani et al. 2013).

Digoxin is though recommended but in modern pediatric guidelines remarked with a questionable effectiveness (Kantor et al. 2013). ACEIs and BB are recommended for functional class I and II but still less used (Kantor et al. 2013; Masutani et al. 2013), not to mention their use, tailored on the specific pediatric disease (Rodriguez et al. 2008; Schranz and Voelkel 2016). Still in 2006, only 5% of pediatric HF patients received BB in the USA (Towbin et al. 2006), since then there is only a slight tendency for increasing utilization (Frobel et al. 2009). Additionally, there is not only a low pediatric experience treating chronic heart failure with BB but further without any differential use regarding the specific drug profiles in consideration of the cause of HF (Masarone et al. 2017). It might be a crucial reason that "negative" results of the few studies labeled as evidence-based because of its double-blind, randomized, placebo-controlled multicenter study design led to the worldwide opinion of pediatricians and also pediatric cardiologists that ß-blockers are questionable for treating infants and children with HF (Kantor et al. 2013; Shaddy et al. 2007; Pasquali Sara et al. 2008; Rossano and Shaddy 2014). These results of "evidence-based" studies had a dramatic impact on the current chronic therapy of HF in children. Considering the lack of "evidence-based" studies, the chance arises that pediatric heart failure therapy will become earlier individualized by pharmacological and pathophysiological knowledge in context of the molecular specifics of pediatric cardiovascular diseases (Noori and Seri 2015).

3 Acute Heart Failure Therapy

Regarding HF caused by myocardial dysfunction, the goal of acute medical therapy consists of life-saving measures to transfer the acute dysfunctional heart back to normal or chronic livable condition. In affluent countries, patients with irreversible myocardial injuries are bridged for heart transplantation (HTx) in part with utilizing an assist device (Towbin et al. 2006); young children with left-sided dilated cardiomyopathy (DCM) and preserved right ventricular function are also back to a functional regeneration (Schranz et al. 2013, 2018).

4 Inotropic Drugs

4.1 Considerations Before Utilizing Inotropic Drugs

4.1.1 Receptor: Physiological Aspects

Adrenergic receptors (ARs) are involved in the regulation of cardiovascular, bronchial, and gastrointestinal smooth muscle tone. In principle, three AR types are differentiated, alpha-, beta (ß)-, and dopaminergic receptors; endogenous AR agonists are available as sympathetic transmitter and neurohumoral agents (Lefkowitz and Caron 1985).

Alpha-1 (a,b,c)-adrenergic and alpha-2 (a,b,c) receptors are differentiated (Han et al. 1987); alpha-1 agonists cause phosphatidylinositol-dependent cellular calcium influx; postsynaptic alpha-1 AR stimulation leads to vasoconstriction, positive-inotropic, and negative-chronotropic myocardial effects. Presynaptic alpha-2 AR stimulation counteracts via adenyl cyclase pathway the alpha-1 AR activation; one important effect is the inhibition of norepinephrine release from the synaptic vesicles. The central alpha-2 stimulation inhibits via reflex circuit within the locus coeruleus and leads to peripheral vasodilation and heart rate decrease. Stimulation of postsynaptic alpha-2 AR is associated with an arteriolar vasoconstriction (Brodde 1991). The main ARs of the heart are ß1- and ß2-receptors (Bristow 1989); the role of also cloned ß3-ARs concerning its sinoatrial effects is still not fully understood (Emorine et al. 1989).

Non-failing adult hearts have ß1/ß2 ratio of almost 80 to 20, respectively (Brodde 1991; Bristow 1989). The affinity of ß2-AR to the adenylate cyclase (AC) seems to be higher; both ß-ARs transmit positive-inotropic and positive-chronotropic activity. A failing adult heart is characterized by almost unchanged ß2-AR density, contrary to downregulated ß1-receptors; the resulting ratio changes to a ratio of almost 60 to 40, respectively. Additionally, AR subsensitivity due to uncoupling of ß-AR is described (Brodde 1991). More recently published studies analyzing harvested hearts of adult and pediatric patients with dilative cardiomyopathy (DCM) confirmed the known AR pathophysiology of failing adult hearts but also demonstrate differences to pediatric DCM patients. Pediatric DCM patients showed both ß1- and ß2-AR downregulation (Miyamoto et al. 2014). Considering the pathways of ß1- and ß2-ARs, coupling to intracellular signaling responsible for contractility and remodeling are different and even though more complex. Chronic ß1-receptor stimulation might be associated with cardiotoxic properties (apoptosis, necrosis), whereas the ß2-receptor stimulation seems to be "cardioprotective" (Bristow 1989; Miyamoto et al. 2014; Lakatta 1993; Xiao et al. 2004; Bernstein et al. 2011). Hence, therapeutic strategies were developed in advanced heart failure patients by blocking selectively the ß1-AR combined with simultaneous ß2-AR stimulation (Navaratnarajah et al. 2014). Patients with myocarditis and DCM (Narula et al. 1996; Collucci 1998) but also children after cardiopulmonary bypass with cardiac arrest seem to have endogenous, norepinephrine-related myocardial injury by excessive ß1-stimulation recognizable by ß1-selective desensitization followed by AR downregulation (Schranz et al. 1993). The mechanism of AR desensitization is caused by AR phosphorylation by a protein kinase and ß-adreno-kinase (Bristow 1989). Regarding coronary vessels, alpha-receptors dominate epicardial coronary vessels, whereas ß-receptors preferring endocardial coronaries (Young et al. 1990). Activation of alpha-receptors led to vasoconstriction. Therefore, newborns with hypoplastic left heart syndrome with an associated small (1–2 mm) ascending aorta are jeopardized by vasoconstriction and consecutive additional ischemic arrest if resuscitated by too high dosages of epi- or norepinephrine. Coronaries and the peripheral vessel system react on ß-AR, in particular of ß2-stimulation with vasodilation as well as the bronchial and gastrointestinal smooth muscle system. Nephrogenic renin release is in particular related to ß1-AR stimulation (Atlas 2007).

4.1.2 Neonatal Myocardial Aspects

Inotropic treatment needs to be reflected in context of the physiologic less compliant myocardium of neonates and in particular premature babies (Teitel et al. 2008; Borg et al. 1984; Jonker et al. 1985; Sperelakis and Pappano 1983). Contrary to highly compliant adult hearts, there is a quite lower ratio of contractile elements to the nutritive interstitial tissue (Teitel et al. 2008; Borg et al. 1984; Sperelakis and Pappano 1983; Li et al. 1996). Only severely injured neonatal hearts (i.e., myocarditis, congenital DCM) might be effectively treated by inotropic agents (Norris et al. 2008) but only in terms of an acute HF treatment. Inotropes are clinically best indicated, when the heart rate does not or increase only slightly during or despite continuous infusion of catecholamines (Norris et al. 2008). Additionally, neonates have an imbalanced cardiac autonomous innervation with vagal preference (Borg et al. 1984), one reason for hypoxia-induced bradycardia or even a systolic reaction of infants compared to tachycardic reactions or ventricular fibrillation as usually seen in adult patients. Despite less matured sympathetic innervation, the cardiac ß-receptors are already fully developed (Atlas 2007; Jonker et al. 1985). Further, the myocardial calcium-dependent contraction as well as relaxation differs between children and adults (Sperelakis and Pappano 1983; Li et al. 1996). Contraction is dependent on the binding of calcium to the myofilaments. But calcium is also important to regulate cardiomyocyte growth, differentiation, and development as well as gene expression (Sperelakis and Pappano 1983). Cardiac myocytes contract by a rapid elevation of calcium of the cytoplasmatic calcium concentration. Adult myocytes open L-type calcium channels during action potential triggering release of sarcoplasmic stored calcium via ryanodine receptors leading to an approximate tenfold increase of free cytosolic calcium concentrations (Sperelakis and Pappano 1983; Li et al. 1996). Cardiac contraction in premature and term neonates depends mainly on a transmembrane myocardial calcium influx and calcium removal from the cells via Na^{+}/Ca^{2+}exchanger (NCX) receptors. Further, the function of the sarcoplasmatic reticulum is inversely developed to the age (Teitel et al. 2008; Jonker et al. 1985). Considering the physiological conditions of the neonatal heart, calcium is in principle a strong and effective inotropic substance; low calcium levels (< 0.9 mmol/l ionized calcium) have to be avoided in any, especially young, dysfunctional hearts. Further, inotropic properties of digoxin based on NCX blocking properties are also inversely related to the patient's age (Schranz 1993; Louch et al. 2015). However, the less compliant neonatal myocardium and especially of premature hearts contradicts oftentimes an effective use of digoxin as an inotropic drug, but not as a negative chronotropic agent.

4.2 Digoxin

It can be assumed that digoxin is still the most commonly used oral inotropic drug treating pediatric HF in the world. Digoxin is traditionally used despite its very narrow therapeutic range and the lack of trial evidence (Schranz 1993; Louch et al. 2015). In adults, digoxin improved quality of life, but not the survival rate (Seguchi et al. 1999). Digoxin is mostly unsuitable for acute HF treatment especially in the setting of renal failure and acute myocarditis and in combination of amiodarone or even carvedilol, all favoring digoxin toxicity (Digitalis Investigation Group 1997; Ratnapalan et al. 2003); in any case, electrolyte imbalances (low serum levels of potassium and magnesium) should be corrected before therapy with digoxin is started.

For chronic HF therapy, digoxin might be indicated as a fourth-line drug in patients with a pure systolic dysfunctional heart, when ß-blocker, ACEI, and mineralocorticoid inhibitors are already applied, but the heart is still beating too fast and the patient's age is young (Schranz and Voelkel 2016; Hussey and Weintraub 2016). Digoxin should be avoided in HF with a restrictive cardiac physiology and because of its vasoconstrictive properties in patients with a need for a low systemic vascular resistance. The observation of some beneficial effects of digoxin in HLHS during the interstage after Norwood surgery (Oster et al. 2016) might be related to its heart rate-reducing effects and consecutive increased diastolic time interval, which might be related to an improved diastolic inflow counteracting probably a digoxin-dependent increase of systemic vascular resistance.

Targeting digoxin serum concentrations from 0.5 to 0.9 ng/ml is achievable by a maintenance dosage of 10 μg/kg/day.

4.3 Characterization of Catecholamines, PDE-III-Inhibitors and Calcium Sensitizers

Epinephrine and its biosynthetic precursor norepinephrine are endogenous catecholamines. Epinephrine with its ß1-, ß2-, and alpha-adrenoreceptor (AR) stimulation and norepinephrine with ß1- and alpha-AR agonistic properties are worldwide still the most utilized catecholamines (Furchgott 1959). Epinephrine is the drug of choice to resuscitate pediatric patients suffering cardiac arrest; the dose efficacy correlates inversely to the patient's age (Clutter et al. 1980). The hemodynamic effectiveness of epinephrine correlates to its serum concentrations (Shavit et al. 1989). The basal level in adults ranged between 24 and 74 pg/ml. Serum levels between 75 and 125 pg/ml increase the heart rate (ß-stimulation). The diastolic blood pressure might decrease via ß2-stimulation with serum levels of 150–200 pg/ml. Higher serum levels cause vasoconstriction by dominant alpha-receptor stimulation. Depending on the utilized (resuscitation) dosages, coronary and cerebral perfusion pressure should be re-established by vasoconstriction with consecutive increase of systemic vascular resistance (Rs); contractility and heart rate can additionally improve in lower dosages, when myocardial perfusion pressure is re-established and adequate. Contrary to other catecholamines (dobutamine, dopamine), epinephrine has the advantage of a remaining effectiveness also during acidosis. Epinephrine is like isoprenaline a "full AR agonist"; its high affinity to the ß1- and ß2-ARs guarantees effective action also during a dobutamine refractory cardiovascular state (Barber and Wyckoff 2006). The value of the myocardial alpha-receptor stimulation during acute and in particular young patients with decompensated cardiovascular shock is still not fully understood. However, alpha-mimetic stimulation might be inversely preserved to the patient's age; it seems that neonatal myocytes react more pronounced to alpha-AR stimulation compared to adult hearts as well as the troponin C-calcium affinity (Mullett et al. 1992). Considering pharmacological and pathophysiological conditions, the main indication for treating patients with epinephrine is a combined risk of reduced myocardial contractility with endangered coronary perfusion pressure. Epinephrine is usually used by continuous infusion in a wide range of dosages of 0.001–0.01 – 0.1–1 – (5) µg/kg/min depending on the therapeutic aims. The drug is in particular suitable, when the patient's cardiovascular condition is changing in short time intervals. Low dosages, in children even in a dosage of 0.01–0.3 µg/kg/min, outweigh ß-mimetic effects. Regarding special myocardial conditions with a high risk of endogenous induced (norepinephrine release) myocardial apoptosis and necrosis like in infants with DCM, there is a need and not a contradiction utilizing a ß1-receptor blocker (oral bisoprolol or intravenously landiolol, metoprolol or esmolol) together with continuously infused epinephrine (Recla et al. 2013). Highly specific ß1-receptor blockers favor myocardial contractility via ß2-agonistic effects, avoiding further myocardial injury by additional exogenous ß1-stimulation, and do allow alpha-mimetic stimulation, if needed (Wyckoff et al. 2015). Apart from cardiovascular shock, inappropriate epinephrine application needs always, almost continuously excluded; oxygen debt, inadequate vasoconstriction (intravascular volume deficit), disturbance of microcirculation are well-known side effects. Epinephrine stimulates even the renal renin release and activity via renal ß1-receptor stimulation as well as by vasoconstriction, if not counteracted by an improved cardiac output and consecutive renal blood flow. Positive effects of epinephrine on the respiratory tract might even be attractive (side effects) in cardiovascular-compromised patients. Beneficial effects of epinephrine in low dosage of 0.001 μg/kg/min mediated by ß(2)-receptors are expected in particular to treat young children and infants by its bronchodilative properties and inhibitory effects on mast cell degranulation. Metabolic effects of applied epinephrine correspond to endogenous stress reactions as gluconeogenesis and insulin resistance but also to low potassium serum level related to proarrhythmic effects (ß2-mediated). Alkaline medium inactivates epinephrine; hence combined application with bicarbonate has to be avoided.

Norepinephrine serum levels correlate with the severity of heart failure (Ross et al. 1987). Considering an *age-dependent changes in the beta-adrenoceptor–G protein(s)–adenylyl cyclase system* (Brodde et al. 1995), norepinephrine acts as a positive inotrope as the precursor of epinephrine and as neurotransmitter via ß1- and perhaps alpha-AR mimetic properties. The alpha-mimetic effects constrict veins and arteries; ß2-mimetic effects are not applicable. Norepinephrine continuously infused in a low dosage of 0.01 μg/kg/min stimulates preferentially ß1-receptors; slightly higher dosages of 0.05–0.1 μg/kg/min have mixed ß1- and alpha-mimetic effects; in high dosages, above 0.1 (−5) μg/kg/min, alpha-receptor-related effects are dominant. The main indication of norepinephrine is restoring or maintaining an adequate coronary or myocardial perfusion pressure. The norepinephrine dosage is used by its effects; therefore, therapy counteracting measures as intravascular volume depletion have to be excluded avoiding inadequate high norepinephrine dosages with consecutive myocardial apoptosis followed by necrosis. Volume-resistant cardiovascular conditions with loss of peripheral precapillary vascular tone (sepsis, anaphylactic reaction, post-cardiopulmonary bypass) indicate the use of norepinephrine. Intravascular volume depletion excluded, norepinephrine infusion in relative low dosages of 0.05–0.1 (max0.3) μg/kg/min is highly effective with less side-effects in particular, as on renal and pulmonary vascular system; considering the ratio of effects and side effects, norepinephrine is almost always to prefer dopamine in high (alpha-mimetic) dosage. Side effects of dopamine are tachycardia, pulmonary vasoconstriction, high myocardial oxygen consumption as well as TRH and prolactin inhibiting effects. The option to add dopamine in low dosages (2 μg/kg/min) remains open. An important indication of norepinephrine is "right" heart failure associated with high right ventricular end-diastolic pressures (RVEDP), independent if caused by cardiac or pulmonary diseases. Low myocardial perfusion pressure (difference of systemic diastolic blood pressure and RVEDP or right atrial pressure (RAP)/coronary sinus pressure) needs often be treated by continuous norepinephrine infusion but even by immediate bolus injection in acute cardiovascular-compromised conditions. Myocardia performance is related to the adequacy of coronary perfusion; therefore, an additional ß1-blockade to avoid ß1-related tachycardia is not a contraindication but a highly effective measure (myocardial necrosis, diastolic time!). Clinical conditions with no chance to reduce pulmonary vascular resistance (Rp) can be effectively treated by increasing systemic vascular resistance (Rs) (Vlahakes et al. 1981).

Dopamine, a precursor of norepinephrine, acts as an endogenous peripheral and central neurotransmitter. Dopamine is a partial AR agonist by dose-dependent stimulation of ß1-, ß2-, alpha-, and dopaminergic (DA) receptors (Lokhandwala and Barrett 1982; Seri 1995; Barrington et al. 1995; Noori and Seri 2012; Liet et al. 2002); opposite to other catecholamines, dopamine's activity is almost 50% related to norepinephrine release from vesicles of sympathetic nerve endings (DA-2 receptor stimulation). Therefore, the inotropic effect of dopamine is limited in newborns and heart-transplanted patients with an imbalanced sympathetic and vagal nerve system and in chronic heart failure with myocardial norepinephrine depletion. Beyond any additional questionable indications for dopamine treating acute pediatric heart failure, the norepinephrine release by dopamine might especially be problematic in patients with myocarditis and dilated cardiomyopathy; apoptosis and necrosis are already induced in the highest degree of ß1-stimulation in consequence of myocardial norepinephrine release. Norepinephrine-related ß1-desensitization is already observed after cardiopulmonary bypass surgery with cardiac arrest (Schranz et al. 1993), which further underlines a problematic use of dopamine as a postsurgical inotropic drug; in addition to its toxicity profile, dopamine specific side effects like low T3 syndrome have to be considered particularly in treating premature patients rarely with a real need for inotropic support. Dopamine is usually used by continuous infusion in variable dosages, in neonates by a dose response based on the patient effect (Dempsey and Barrington 2007); further, the clearance of dopamine is dependent on gestational age and severity of the disease (Seri et al. 1993; Padbury et al. 1987). Low dosages in a range of 1–2 (4) µg/kg/min stimulate preferentially DA-1 and DA-2 receptors with vasodilative effects on renal, mesenteric, and cerebral vessels. Improved renal perfusion and sodium reabsorptive effects at proximal renal tubules induce saluretic effects; DA receptors at the zona glomerulosa of the adrenal cortex inhibit aldosterone release. The dopamine-related inhibition of TSH (low T3 syndrome) and prolactin (immune-modulating) might be forcing infection diseases (Noori et al. 2003). Dopamine dosages of 5–10 µg/kg/min lead to dominated ß-AR-related effects but, as already mentioned, by releasing stored norepinephrine. Contrary to norepinephrine, dopamine acts unpredictable in high alpha-mimetic dosages of 10 µg/kg/min. Dopamine constricts the venous, pulmonary, as well as systemic vascular system mostly associated with a non-opportune tachycardia or even tachyarrhythmia. Animal studies have shown that norepinephrine has a 20 times higher systemic vs pulmonary vasoconstrictive effect (Schindler et al. 2004); therefore, norepinephrine can be used more effective with less side effects than dopamine treating hypotension in context of a pulmonary hypertension.

In summary, the relative uncritical use of dopamine treating in particular premature and term neonates should be considered in terms of effect and possible side effects including currently unknown neurological consequences; a historical familiarity should not play a role utilizing dopamine especially on neonatal intensive care.

Dobutamine is a synthetically prepared catecholamine with preferential ß1- and ß2-agonistic properties (Sonnenblick et al. 1979). Dobutamine is utilized as a racemic mixture of (+) and (−) isomers. The isomeric mixture is responsible for ß-AR activity but concerning the alpha-receptors with its neutralizing effects. The inotropic activity of dobutamine is preferentially based on stimulation of ß1-AR. Following its synthetic manufacturing in the 1970s, it was even immediately used treating pediatric myocardial diseases (Driscoll et al. 1979; Schranz et al. 1982). The inotropic effect of dobutamine can clinically best monitored by the patient's heart rate response. Dobutamine has been shown to increase cardiac output, by its augmenting effects on stroke volume and/or increase of heart rate. In case of a preferential increase of the cardiac stroke volume, the heart rate remains stable, decreases, or does only slightly increase. Therefore, an inappropriate use of dobutamine is reciprocated by an inadequate increase of the heart rate; only patients with a sinus bradycardia (i.e., patients after heart transplantation, sick sinus syndrome) might benefit from the heart rate increasing ß1- and ß2-effects. Considering the ß-AD agonist dobutamine, systemic and pulmonary vascular resistance (opposite to dopamine) decrease when intravascular volume depletion is excluded and inadequate increase of the heart rate (diastolic filling time) is avoided. In context of a possible mismatch of myocardial oxygen supply and consumption and its ß-adrenergic stimulating effects, tachycardia and tachyarrhythmias need to be permanently considered, as long as dobutamine is used, in particular, if inadequately used or overdosed in relation to the myocardial disease (Roeleveld and de Klerk 2018; Ergenekon et al. 2017). Since phosphodiesterase type III inhibitors are preferentially used in pediatric heart failure patients, dobutamine, even in combination with continuous infusion of low-dose nitroglycerine, is more and more less indicated and applied. Dobutamine is usually utilized in dosages of (2.5) 5–(10) μg/kg/min, which leads to dominated ß-AR-related effects. Dobutamine in high dosage above 10 μg/kg/min is mostly not convincing in relation to positive (inotropic) and negative (chronotropic, antiarrhythmic) effects (HR, myocardial consumption). In cardiogenic shock with associated metabolic acidosis, the partial ß-AR agonist dobutamine is not further indicated, but instead epinephrine is preferentially used.

Milrinone is currently the most used phosphodiesterase type III inhibitor (PDE III inhibitor) treating children with HF (Ferrer-Barba et al. 2016). The bipyridine derivative amrinone and imidazole derivative enoximone were the first PDE III inhibitors used also in children (Dage et al. 1987; Schranz et al. 1989; Allen-Webb et al. 1994). PDE III inhibitors are characterized by blocking the isoenzyme IIIc of phosphodiesterases localized predominantly in heart muscle and vascular smooth muscle cells. The delayed breakdown of cAMP influences also the intracellular calcium homeostasis with an increase of slow calcium influx of the myocardial cells and augmented storage of releasable calcium from the sarcoplasmatic reticulum. The mechanism is related to an increase of contractility. The cAMP increase of the smooth muscle cells improves the calcium efflux and led consecutively to smooth muscle relaxation (Barton et al. 1996). Regarding the positive-inotropic and vasodilative properties, PDE III inhibitors are grouped into inodilators. The inodilative effect of PDE III inhibitors was evidenced by adult and pediatric patients (Hoffman et al. 2003). However, compared to shorter and stronger acting milrinone, they were affected with too many side effects which include handling problems (central line occlusion) and less control considering a too long half-life but even thrombocytopenic reaction in particular related to the use of amrinone. Proarrhythmic potentials have been seen by the use of all PDE III inhibitors, but heart failure symptoms improve in pediatric patients without an increased incidence of sudden death which have been seen in adult patients treated with PDE III inhibitors (Burkhardt et al. 2015). Considering the receptor and adenylate cyclase-mediated cAMP increase, ß-receptor agonist and PDE III inhibitors have additive, and maybe synergistic, effects. Therefore, low cAMP levels in heart failure seem not to be related to increased PDE activity, but more likely to decrease adenylate cyclase activity associated with downregulation and desensitization of the ß-adrenergic receptor in HF. Important age-related differences in phosphodiesterase activity and effects of chronic PDE III inhibition were observed in idiopathic dilated cardiomyopathy patients (Nakano et al. 2015). Tachyphylaxis or tolerance is described with chronic PDE III inhibitors in adults. Chronic therapy with the PDE III inhibitor milrinone in children led to elevated cAMP and higher downstream phospholamban phosphorylation contributing to sustained hemodynamic benefits in pediatric DCM patients. In contrast, higher total PDE and PDE III activities in adult DCM patients during PDE III inhibitor treatment may perpetuate lower myocardial cAMP and phospholamban phosphorylation levels, limiting the potential benefits of PDE III inhibitors in adults. Therefore, milrinone is effectively used to prevent or treat low cardiac output syndrome (LCOS) in children undergoing heart surgery. It is used for stabilization decompensating heart failure as associated with dilated cardiomyopathy (Nakano et al. 2017; Curley et al. 2017) and even in heart failure with a single ventricle physiology (Curley et al. 2017). The substance is used for bridging to transplant, but even to recovery (Schranz and Voelkel 2016).

Milrinone is used in continuous infusion in dosages ranging between 0.3 and 1 μg/kg/min.

Levosimendan is a further inodilator (Rognoni et al. 2011); it exerts inotropic and vasodilating effects based on myocardial calcium-sensitizing properties opening up vascular ATP-dependent potassium channels. The pharmacological profile of levosimendan makes this drug very attractive in myocardial HF of neonates and infants considering their endogenous myocardial calcium handling (Veldman et al. 2006). Less proarrhythmic and reversal effects of toxic dosages of ß-blockers expand the indication of the use of levosimendan; postoperative low cardiac output or intermittent treatment in infants and young children with DCM even as an accompanying drug are currently the most indicated pediatric cardiovascular conditions (Angadi et al. 2013). Levosimendan is mostly applied in a continuous infusion of 24 h in a dosage of 0.1 or 0.2 μg/kg/min with or without a loading dose for 10–15 min.

Like PDE III inhibitors, hypotension can mostly be avoided if the treated patients have no intravascular volume depletion as very often is observed by overtreatment of diuretics or other reasons of volume loss.

4.3.1 Conclusion

Pharmacological support of the failing pediatric heart remains a challenging task. The first therapeutic goal is resuscitating or maintaining cardiac output, which is vital for sufficient end-organ perfusion. The second aim, however, should be cardiac restoration and regeneration; accepting a chronic heart failure or organ replacement should be the last exit. The regenerative potentials are enormous, the younger the patient is. However, the unique biochemical and structure properties of the neonatal non-failing and especially failing heart do not necessarily allow to extrapolate results of adult's studies to young children. Already the mismatch of noncontractile tissue mass to the contractile myocardium, the differences in intracellular myocardial calcium handling but in particular varieties of receptor physiologies between a failing adult and pediatric heart need to be considered for an adequate cardiac therapy. Missing evidence-based data treating pediatric HF should not be led to therapeutic nihilism; it needs a differentiated, hypothesis-driven therapeutic strategy based on the pharmacological drug profile, pathophysiological condition, and the molecular features. In this context, the pediatric HF is characterized by a lower beta adrenergic agents responsiveness and a heart rate dependent cardiac output; both, limiting the ability to increase stroke volume, favor therefore the use of inodilators of the Ca++-senitizer and PDE-III-inhibitor family. Regenerative strategies with mobilizing endogenous potentials to exogenous supported by exogenous stem cell therapy and gene therapy offer perspectives for future restoration of the failing neonatal and young patients' hearts.

References

Allen-Webb EM, Ross MP, Pappas JB, McGough EC, Banner W Jr (1994) Age-related amrinone pharmacokinetics in a pediatric population. Crit Care Med 22(6):1016–1024

Angadi U, Westrope C, Chowdhry MF (2013) Is levosimendan effective in pediatric heart failure and post-cardiac surgeries? Interact Cardiovasc Thorac Surg 17:710e4

Atlas SA (2007) The renin-angiotensin aldosterone system: pathophysiological role and pharmacologic inhibition. J Manag Care Pharm 13:9–20

Barber CA, Wyckoff MH (2006) Use and efficacy of endotracheal versus intravenous epinephrine during neonatal cardiopulmonary resuscitation in the delivery room. Pediatrics 118:1028–1034

Barrington KJ, Finer NN, Chan W (1995) A blind, randomized comparison of the circulatory effects of dopamine and epinephrine infusions in the newborn piglet during normoxia and hypoxia. Crit Care Med 23:740–748

Barton P, Garcia J, Kouatli A, Kitchen L, Zorka A, Lindsay C, Lawless S, Giroir B (1996) Hemodynamic effects of i.v. milrinone lactate in pediatric patients with septic shock. A prospective, double-blinded, randomized, placebo-controlled, interventional study. Chest 109 (5):1302–1312

Bernstein D, Fajardo G, Zhao M (2011) The role of β-adrenergic Receptors in heart failure: differential regulation of cardiotoxicity and cardioprotection. Prog Pediatr Cardiol 31(1):35–38

Borg TK, Rubin K, Lundgren E, Borg K, Obrink B (1984) Recognition of extracellular matrix components by neonatal and adult cardiac myocytes. Dev Biol 104(1):86–96
Braunwald E (2013) Heart failure. JACC Heart Fail 1:1–20
Bristow MR (1989) Mol Pharmacol 35:295–303
Brodde O-E (1991) ß1and ß2-adrenoceptors in the human heart: properties, function, and alterations in chronic heart failure. Pharmacol Rev 43:203–242
Brodde OE, Zerkowski HR, Schranz D et al (1995) Age-dependent changes in the beta-adrenoceptor–G protein(s)–adenylyl cyclase system in human right atrium. J Cardiovasc Pharmacol 26:20–26
Burkhardt BE, Rucker G, Stiller B (2015) Prophylactic milrinone for the prevention of low cardiac output syndrome and mortality in children undergoing surgery for congenital heart disease. Cochrane Database Syst Rev (3):CD009515. Circ Heart Fail 2015; 8(1): 57–63
Clutter WE, Bier DM, Shah SD, Cryer PE (1980) Epinephrine plasma metabolic clearance rates and physiologic thresholds for metabolic and hemodynamic actions in man. J Clin Invest 66:94
Collucci WS (1998) The effects of norepinephrine on myocardial biology:Implications fort he therapy of heart failure. Clin Cardiol 21(Suppl 1):20–24
Curley M, Liebers J, Maynard R (2017) Continuous intravenous milrinone therapy in pediatric outpatients. J Infus Nurs 40(2):92–96
Dage RC, Kariya T, Hsieh CP, Roebel LE, Cheng HC, Schnettler RA, Grisar JM (1987) Pharmacology of enoximone. Am J Cardiol 60(5):10C–14C
Dempsey EM, Barrington KJ (2007) Treating hypotension in the preterm infant: when and with what: a critical and systematic review. J Perinatol 27:469–478
Digitalis Investigation Group (1997) The effect of digoxin on mortality and morbidity in patients with heart failure. N Engl J Med 336:525–533
Digitalis Investigation Group (DIG) (1997) The effect of digoxin in mortality and morbidity in patients with heart failure. N Engl J Med 306:525–533
Driscoll DJ, Gillette PC, Duff DF, Nihill MR, Gutgesell HP, Vargo TA, Mullins CE, McNamara DG (1979) Hemodynamic effects of dobutamine in children. Am J Cardiol 43 (3):581–585
El-Amouri SS, Zhu H, Yu J, Marr R, Verma IM (2008) Kindy MS neprilysin: an enzyme candidate to slow the progression of Alzheimer's disease. Am J Pathol 172:1342–1354
Emorine LJ, Marullo S, Briend-Sutren MM, Patey G, Tate K, Delavier-Klutchko C, Strosberg AD (1989) Molecular characterization of the human beta 3-adrenergic receptor. Science 245 (4922):1118–1121
Engle MA, Lewy JE, Lewy PR, Metcoff J (1978) The use of furosemide in the treatment of edema in infants and children. Pediatrics 62:811–818
Ergenekon E, Rojas-Anaya H, Bravo MC, Kotidis C, Mahoney L, Rabe H (2017) Cardiovascular drug therapy for human newborn: review of pharmacodynamic data. Curr Pharm Des 23 (38):5850–5860
Farris W, Schutz SG, Cirrito JR, Shankar GM, Sun X, George A, Leissring MA, Walsh DM, Qiu WQ, Holtzman DM, Selkoe DJ (2007) Loss of neprilysin function promotes amyloid plaque formation and causes cerebral amyloid angiopathy. Am J Pathol 171:241–251
Ferrer-Barba A, Gonzalez-Rivera I, Bautista-Hernandez V (2016) Inodilators in the management of low cardiac output syndrome after pediatric cardiac surgery. Curr Vasc Pharmacol 14(1):48–57
Frobel A-K, Hulpke-Wette M, Schmidt KG, Läer S (2009) Beta-blockers for congestive heart failure in children. In: Cochrane database of systematic reviews [Internet]. Wiley, New York. http://onlinelibrary.wiley.com. https://doi.org/10.1002/14651858.CD007037.pub2/abstract
Furchgott RF (1959) The receptors for epinephrine and norepinephrine (adrenergic receptors). Pharmacol Rev 11:429–441
Han C, Abel PW, Minneman KP (1987) Alpha1Adrenoceptor subtypes linked to different mechanisms for increasing intracellular Ca2+ in smooth muscle. Nature 329:333–335

Hoffman TM, Wernovsky G, Atz AM et al (2003) Efficacy and safety of milrinone in preventing low cardiac output syndrome in infants and children after corrective surgery for congenital heart disease. Circulation 107(7):996–1002

Hussey AD, Weintraub RG (2016) Drug treatment of heart failure in children: focus on recent recommendations from the ISHLT guidelines for the management of pediatric heart failure. Paediatr Drugs 18:89e99

Jonker SS, Zhang L, Louey S, Giraud GD, Thornburg KL, Faber JJ (1985) Myocyte enlargement, differentiation, and proliferation kinetics in the fetal sheep heart. J Appl Physiol 102:1130–1142

Kantor PF, Lougheed J, Dancea A, McGillion M, Barbosa N, Chan C et al (2013) Presentation, diagnosis, and medical management of heart failure in children: Canadian Cardiovascular Society guidelines. Can J Cardiol 29(12):1535–1552

Kirk R, Dipchand AI, Rosenthal DN, Addonizio L, Burch M, Chrisant M, Dubin A, Everitt M, Gajarski R, Mertens L et al (2014) The international society of heart and lung transplantation guidelines for the management of pediatric heart failure: executive summary. J Heart Lung Transplant 33:888–909

Kreidberg MB, Chernoff HL, Lopez WL (1963) Treatment of cardiac failure in infancy and childhood. N Engl J Med 268:23–30

Lakatta EG (1993) β_1-adrenoceptor stimulation and β_2-adrenoceptor stimulation differ in their effects on contraction, cytosolic Ca^{2+}, and Ca^{2+} current in single rat ventricular cells. Circ Res 73:286–300

Lefkowitz RJ, Caron MG (1985) Adrenergic-receptors: molecular mechanisms of clinically relevant regulation. Clin Res 33:395–406

Li F, Wang X, Capasso JM, Gerdes AM (1996) Rapid transition of cardiac myocytes from hyperplasia to hypertrophy during postnatal development. J Mol Cell Cardiol 28:1737–1746

Liet JM, Boscher C, Gras-Leguen C, Gournay V, Debillon T, Rozé JC (2002) Dopamine effects on pulmonary artery pressure in hypotensive preterm infants with patent ductus arteriosus. J Pediatr 140:373–375

Lokhandwala MF, Barrett RJ (1982) Cardiovascular dopamine receptors: physiological, pharmacological and therapeutic implications. J Auton Pharmacol 2(3):189–215

Louch WE, Koivumäki JT, Tavi P (2015) Calcium signaling in developing cardiomyocytes: implications for model systems and disease. J Physiol 593(5):1047–1063

Masarone D, Valente F, Rubino M, Vastarella R, Gravino R, Rea A, Russo MG, Pacileo G, Limongelli G (2017) Pediatric heart failure: a practical guide to diagnosis and management. Pediatr Neonatol 58(4):303–312

Masutani S, Saiki H, Kurishima C, Ishido H, Tamura M, Senzaki H (2013) Heart failure with preserved ejection fraction in children. Hormonal imbalance between aldosterone and brain natriuretic peptide. Circ J 77:2375–2382

McMurray JJ, Packer M, Desai AS et al (2014) Angiotensin-neprilysin inhibition versus enalapril in heart failure. N Engl J Med 371:993–1004

Miyamoto SD, Stauffer BL, Nakano S, Sobus R, Nunley K, Nelson P et al (2014) Beta-adrenergic adaptation in pediatric idiopathic dilated cardiomyopathy. Eur Heart J 35(1):33–41

Mollovaa M, Bersella K, Walsha S, Savlaa S, Tanmoy Dasa L, Park S-Y, Silbersteine SL, dos Remediosg DG, Grahama D, Colana D, Kühn B (2013) Cardiomyocyte proliferation contributes to heart growth in young humans. Proc Natl Acad Sci U S A 110:1446–1451

Mullett CJ, Kong JQ, Romano JT, Polak MJ (1992) Age-related changes in pulmonary venous epinephrine concentration, and pulmonary vascular response after intratracheal epinephrine. Pediatr Res 31:458–461

Nakano SJ, Miyamoto SD, Movsesian M, Nelson P, Stauffer BL, Sucharov CC (2015) Age-related differences in phosphodiesterase activity and effects of chronic phosphodiesterase inhibition in idiopathic dilated cardiomyopathy. Circ Heart Fail 8(1):57–63

Nakano SJ, Sucharov J, van Dusen R, Cecil M, Nunley K, Wickers S, Karimpur-Fard A, Stauffer BL, Miyamoto SD, Sucharov CC (2017) Cardiac adenylyl cyclase and phosphodiesterase

expression profiles vary by age, disease, and chronic phosphodiesterase inhibitor treatment. J Card Fail 23(1):72–80
Narula J, Haider N, Virmani R, DiSalvo TG, Kolodgie FD, Hajjar RJ, Schmidt U, Semigran MJ, Dec GW, Khaw BA (1996) Apoptosis in myocytes in end-stage heart failure. N Engl J Med 335 (16):1182–1189
Navaratnarajah M, Siedlecka U, Ibrahim M, van Doorn C, Soppa G, Gandhi A et al (2014) Impact of combined clenbuterol and metoprolol therapy on reverse remodelling during mechanical unloading. PLoS One 9(9):e92909
Noori S, Seri I (2012) Neonatal blood pressure support: the use of inotropes, luisitropes, and other vasopressor agents. Clin Perinatol 39:221–238
Noori S, Seri I (2015) Evidence-based versus pathophysiology-based approach to diagnosis and treatment of neonatal cardiovascular compromise. Semin Fetal Neonatal Med 20(4):238–245
Noori S, Freidlich P, Seri I (2003) Developmentally regulated cardiovascular, renal and neuroendocrine effects of dopamine. NeoReviews 4:e283–e288. https://doi.org/10.1542/neo.4-10-e283
Norris RA, Borg TK, Butcher JT, Baudino TA, Banerjee I, Markwald RR (2008) Neonatal and adult cardiovascular pathophysiological remodeling and repair: developmental role of periostin. Ann N Y Acad Sci 1123:30–40
Oster ME, Kelleman M, McCracken C, Ohye RG, Mahle WT (2016) Association of digoxin with interstage mortality: results from the pediatric heart network single ventricle reconstruction trial public use dataset. J Am Heart Assoc 5(1):e002566
Padbury JF, Agata Y, Baylen BG, Ludlow JK, Polk DH, Goldblatt E et al (1987) Dopamine pharmacokinetics in critically ill newborninfants. J Pediatr 110:293–298
Pasquali Sara K, Matthew H, Slonim Anthony D, Jenkins Kathy J, Marino Bradley S, Cohen Meryl S et al (2008) Off-label use of cardiovascular medications in children hospitalized with congenital and acquired heart disease. Circ Cardiovasc Qual Outcomes 1(2):74–83
Pitt B, Zannad F, Remme WJ, Cody R, Castaigne A, Perez A, Palensky J, Wittes J (1999) The effect of spironolactone on morbidity and mortality in patients with severe heart failure. N Engl J Med 341:709–717
Ratnapalan S, Griffiths K, Costei AM, Benson L, Koren G (2003) Digoxin-carvedilol interactions in children. J Pediatr 142:572–574
Recla S, Steinbrenner B, Schranz D (2013) Medical therapy in dilated cardiomyopathy and pulmonary arterial banding in children. J Heart Lung Transplant 32(10):1045–1046
Rodriguez W, Selen A, Avant D, Chaurasia C, Crescenzi T, Gieser G et al (2008) Improving pediatric dosing through pediatric initiatives: what we have learned. Pediatrics 121(3):530–539
Roeleveld PP, de Klerk JCA (2018) The Perspective of the intensivist on inotropes and postoperative care following pediatric heart surgery: an international survey and systematic review of the literature. World J Pediatr Congenit Heart Surg 9(1):10–21
Rognoni A, Lupi A, Lazzero M, Bongo AS, Rognoni G (2011) Levosimendan: from basic science to clinical trials. Recent Pat Cardiovasc Drug Discov 6:9e15
Ross RD, Daniels SR, Schwartz DC, Hannon DW, Shukla R, Kaplan S (1987) Plasma norepinephrine levels in infants and children with congestive heart failure. Am J Cardiol 59:911–914
Rossano JW, Shaddy RE (2014) Update on pharmacological heart failure therapies in children: do adult medications work in children and if not, why not? Circulation 129:607–612
Schindler MB, Hislop AA, Haworth SG (2004) Postnatal changes in response to norepinephrine in the normal and pulmonary hypertensive lung. Am J Respir Crit Care Med 170(6):641–646
Schranz D (1993) Kardiovaskuläre Erkrankungen. In: Pädiatrische Intensivmedizin. 2. Auflage Gustav Fischer Verlag Stuttgart Jena
Schranz D, Voelkel NF (2016) "Nihilism" of chronic heart failure therapy in children and why effective therapy is withheld. Eur J Pediatr 175:445–455
Schranz D, Stopfkuchen H, Jüngst BK, Clemens R, Emmrich P (1982) Hemodynamic effects of dobutamine in children with cardiovascular failure. Eur J Pediatr 139(1):4–7

Schranz D, Huth R, Dahm M, Iversen S, Hein E, Stopfkuchen H, Jüngst BK (1989) Acute hemodynamic response to intravenous enoximone: an animal study and preliminary report in infants after cardiac surgery. J Cardiovasc Pharmacol 14(Suppl 1):S62–S68

Schranz D, Droege A, Broede A, Brodermann G, Schafer E, Oelert H, Brodde OE (1993) Uncoupling of human cardiac adrenoceptors during cardiopulmonary bypass with cardioplegic cardiac arrest. Circulation 87:422–426

Schranz D, Rupp S, Müller M, Schmidt D, Bauer A, Valeske K et al (2013) Pulmonary artery banding in infants and young children with left ventricular dilated cardiomyopathy: a novel therapeutic strategy before heart transplantation. J Heart Lung Transplant 32(5):475–481

Schranz D, Akintuerk H, Bailey L (2018) Pulmonary artery banding for functional regeneration of end-stage dilated cardiomyopathy in young children: world network report. Circulation 137 (13):1410–1412

Seguchi M, Nakazawa M, Momma K (1999) Further evidence suggesting a limited role of digitalis in infants with circulatory congestion secondary to large ventricular septal defect. Am J Cardiol 83:1408–1411

Seri I (1995) Cardiovascular, renal, and endocrine actions of dopamine in neonates and children. J Pediatr 126:333–344

Seri I, Rudas G, Bors Z, Kanyicksa B, Tulassay T (1993) Effects of low dose dopamine infusions in cardiovascular and renal functions, cerebral blood flow and plasma catecholamine levels in sick preterm neonates. Pediatr Res 34:742–749

Shaddy RE, Boucek MM, Hsu DT et al (2007) Carvedilol for children and adolescents with heart failure: a randomized controlled trial. JAMA 298(117):1–9

Shavit G, Sagy M, Nadler E, Vidne BA, Gitter S (1989) Myocardial response to alpha-agonist (phenylephrine) in relation to age. Crit Care Med 17(12):1324–1327

Sonnenblick EH, Frishman WH, LeJemtel TH (1979) Dobutamine: a new synthetic cardioactive sympathetic amine. N Engl J Med 300(1):17–22

Sperelakis N, Pappano AJ (1983) Physiology and pharmacology of developing heart cells. Pharmacol Ther 22:1–39

Teitel DF, Cassidy SC, Fineman JR (2008) Circulation physiology. In: Moss AJ, Allen HD (eds) Moss and Adams' heart disease in infants, children, and adolescents: including the fetus and young adult. Wolters Kluwer Health/Lippincott Williams & Wilkins, Philadelphia

Towbin JA, Lowe AM, Colan SD et al (2006) Incidence, causes, and outcomes of dilated cardiomyopathy in children. JAMA 296:1867–1876

Veldman A, Rupp S, Schranz D (2006) New inotropic pharmacologic strategies targeting the failing myocardium in the newborn and infant. Mini Rev Med Chem 6(7):785–792

Vlahakes GJ, Turley K, Hoffman JI (1981) The pathophysiology of failure in acute right ventricular hypertension: hemodynamic and biochemical correlations. Circulation 63(1):87–95

Wyckoff MH, Aziz K, Escobedo MB, Kapadia VS, Kattwinkel J, Perlman JM, Simon WM, Weiner GM, Zaichkin JG (2015) Part 13: neonatal resuscitation: 2015 American heart association guidelines update for cardiopulmonary resuscitation and emergency cardiovascular care. Circulation (132):S543–S560

Xiao R-P, Zhu W, Zheng M, Chakir K, Bond R, Lakatta EG et al (2004) Subtype-specific β-adrenoceptor signaling pathways in the heart and their potential clinical implications. Trends Pharmacol Sci 25(7):358–365

Yancy CW, Jessup M, Bozkurt B, Butler J, Casey DE, Colvin MM et al (2017) 2017 ACC/AHA/HFSA focused update of the 2013 ACCF/AHA guideline for the management of heart failure: a report of the American College of Cardiology/American Heart Association Task Force on Clinical Practice Guidelines and the Heart Failure Society of America. J Am Coll Cardiol 28:236

Yasojima K, McGeer EG, McGeer PL (2001) Relationship between beta amyloid peptide generating molecules and neprilysin in Alzheimer disease and normal brain. Brain Res 919:115–121

Young MA, Vatner DE, Vatner SF (1990) Alpha- and beta-adrenergic control of large coronary arteries in conscious calves. Basic Res Cardiol (85 Suppl 1):97–109

Arterial Hypertension in Children

Wolfgang Rascher and Christian Paech

Contents

Abstract

Pharmacological treatment of arterial hypertension in children is mainly based on individual experience, but there is evidence that blocking the angiotensin system reduces systolic and diastolic blood when compared to placebo, and these drugs are safe to use for a short duration, also in children under 6 years of age. Blocking the angiotensin system either by angiotensin-converting enzyme inhibitors or by antagonizing the angiotensin 1 receptor is effective,

W. Rascher (✉)
Department of Pediatrics and Adolescent Medicine, Friedrich-Alexander – University Erlangen-Nürnberg, Erlangen, Germany
e-mail: wolfgang.rascher@uk-erlangen.de

C. Paech
Department for Pediatric Cardiology, University of Leipzig – Heart Center, Leipzig, Germany
e-mail: christian.paech@medizin.uni-leipzig.de

W. Kiess et al. (eds.), *Pediatric Pharmacotherapy*,
Handbook of Experimental Pharmacology 261, https://doi.org/10.1007/164_2020_359

but did not display a consistent dose-response relationship with escalating doses, but the effective doses are known. Calcium channel antagonists are effective antihypertensives in children, but the evidence is limited. Based on small-sized studies, beta-blockers modestly reduce systolic blood pressure, but have no significant effect on diastolic blood pressure compared to placebo. They act in combination to antagonize reflex tachycardia induced by vasodilators. The most commonly used antihypertensive agents are safe to use in short-term studies.

Keywords

Antihypertensives · Arterial hypertension · Clinical trials · Pediatrics

1 Definition, Diagnosis, and Classification

Criteria for the diagnosis of hypertension in adults are not applicable to children. A value of 140/90 mmHg for random (casual) blood pressure and 135/85 mmHg for daytime ambulatory blood pressure has been generally accepted as the upper limit of normal in adults, and this might also be true for older adolescents. The range of "normal" blood pressure in children and adolescents is uncertain, but European guidelines recommended that normal blood pressure is values below the 90th percentile and high-normal blood pressure values range between the 90th and 95th percentile (Lurbe et al. 2016) (Table 1).

Thus, arterial hypertension in children is defined as the persistence of blood pressure above the 95th percentile. Values above this, if confirmed by two further examinations, are compatible with the diagnosis of hypertension. Various reference tables for normal blood pressure centiles of children and adolescents have been published; the most valid for casual office blood pressure measurement by auscultation was published by the International Pediatric Nephrology Association (IPNA 2011). If blood pressure were taken by an oscillometric device, centiles of the German KiGGS Study are helpful (Neuhauser et al. 2011).

Table 1 Definition and classification of hypertension in children and adolescents

Category	SBP and/or DBP percentile (0–15 years)	SBP and/or DBP values (16 years and older)
Normal	<90th percentile	<130/85 mmHg
High-normal	≥90th to <95th percentile	130–139/85–89 mmHg
Hypertension	≥95th percentile	≥140/90 mmHg
Stage 1 hypertension	95th to the 99th percentile plus 5 mmHg	140–159/90–99 mmHg
Stage 2 hypertension	>99th percentile plus 5 mmHg	160–179/100–109 mmHg
Isolated systolic hypertension	SBP ≥ 95th percentile and DBP < 90th percentile	≥140/<90 mmHg

SBP systolic blood pressure, *DBP* diastolic blood pressure; from Lurbe et al. (2016)

2 Treatment Options

In primary hypertension, non-pharmacological treatment should be initiated (e.g., reduction of dietary sodium chloride intake, reduction of body weight in obese children and adolescents, and dynamic exercises), although the therapeutic success of non-pharmacological intervention is so far not sufficiently established. Drug treatment should be carefully considered after non-pharmacological intervention has failed. Factors other than blood pressure that influence the decision to begin drug treatment include a family history of early complications of hypertension (renal failure, stroke, heart disease), target organ involvement (cardiac enlargement, left ventricular hypertrophy, retinal vascular changes), and the presence of other risk factors for coronary heart disease.

Secondary hypertension, mainly caused by renal diseases in children, required early and sufficient drug treatment. Chronic renal failure has been evaluated in a large prospective trial with valid end points (50% decline in glomerular filtration rate (GFR) or progression to end-stage renal disease (ESRD) over a period of 5 years) (ESCAPE Trial Group 2009). Strict control of blood pressure is able to slow the progression of renal failure. In this trial, 29.9% of the patients in the intensified blood pressure control with ramipril reached the end point (50% GFR loss or progression to ESRD) compared to 41.7% of patients with a conventional blood pressure target.

In children with underlying chronic kidney disease, target blood pressure should be below the 75th percentile in children without and in those with proteinuria below the 50th percentile (Lurbe et al. 2016). This 50th percentile is also the goal for children with diabetes mellitus type 1. The corresponding targets for adolescents and adults are 130/80 mmHg with a renal disease without proteinuria and a target blood pressure below 120/75 mmHg in case of proteinuria. In general, blood pressure should be lowered below the 90th age-, sex-, and height-specific percentile in children with arterial hypertension.

In rare cases, surgical intervention is the treatment of choice (coarctation of the aorta, pheochromocytoma, neuroblastoma, or renovascular hypertension). Following surgery, it often takes weeks or months before the blood pressure becomes completely normal after discontinuation of antihypertensive therapy.

3 Antihypertensive Agents

Historically pharmacological treatment of hypertension in children was based on individual experience. The legislation changes in the United States to promote clinical trials to improve pediatric drug treatment (Food and Drug Administration Modernization Act, 1997; Best Pharmaceuticals for Children Act, 2002) have led to clinical trials with antihypertensive agents in children and to approval of some of these drugs (Chu et al. 2014). The EU Regulation of Medicinal Products for Paediatric Use (EU Regulation 1901/2006/EC) has further stimulated clinical trials using appropriate evidence-based methodology with antihypertensive drugs in the pediatric population. The number of adequate dose recommendations based on careful dose-finding studies in various age groups of pediatric patients with arterial hypertension has been increased as well as age-appropriate drug formulations and safety aspects (Chu et al. 2014; Lurbe et al. 2016; Meyers and Siu 2011; Rascher 2016). However, due to a limited number of patients and the short duration of clinical trials in children with arterial hypertension, the evidence is still limited (Chaturvedi et al. 2014).

There have been five trials comparing the antihypertensive agent directly against placebo, and the majority of clinical studies were dose-finding and included three trials of angiotensin-converting enzyme inhibitors (enalapril, fosinopril, lisinopril), seven trials of angiotensin receptor antagonists (candesartan, irbesartan, losartan, olmesartan, valsartan), and one trial of a calcium channel antagonist (amlodipine) (Chaturvedi et al. 2014). Furthermore, an excellent outcome study was published with ramipril (ESCAPE Trial Group 2009).

Observational and randomized clinical trials with antihypertensive agents in children and adolescents have been excellently reviewed (Meyers and Siu 2011; Chu et al. 2014). A clear dose relationship for only three drugs (enalapril, lisinopril, losartan) has been shown (Benjamin et al. 2008). Dose and safety aspects have been recently reviewed (Siddiqi and Shatat 2019).

Dosages of antihypertensive agents in childhood based on clinical trials, summary of product characteristics and published experience are shown in Table 2.

3.1 Angiotensin-Converting Enzyme Inhibitors

The most powerful target for treating high blood pressure is blocking the renin-angiotensin-aldosterone system (RAAS). Angiotensin-converting enzyme (ACE) converts angiotensin I to angiotensin II, a potent vasoconstrictor peptide that also stimulates aldosterone production. ACE inhibitors lower blood pressure by decreasing angiotensin II.

In children and adolescents, ACE inhibitors are the most commonly prescribed antihypertensive for both primary and secondary hypertension (Snauwaert et al. 2017; Yoon et al. 2012; Welch et al. 2012). ACE inhibitors also have anti-proteinuric effects, which is beneficial in children with chronic kidney disease (Seeman et al. 2004; Simonetti et al. 2007; Soergel et al. 2000; Van den Belt et al. 2018; Wühl et al. 2004). Similar as in adult trials, pediatric trials provide evidence that some ACE inhibitors may be less efficacious in blacks (Menon et al. 2006).

Captopril was the first ACE inhibitor and the first used successfully in children with severe renal hypertension (Mirkin and Newman 1985). However, in newborns and small infants, cerebral and renal complications have been reported, which occurred if the initial dose was too high. This age group requires substantially lower doses per unit body surface than older infants and children for the control of hypertension. In order to prevent a rapid decrease in blood pressure following the first dose of captopril, a low dose of 0.2 mg/kg (in newborns, 0.05 mg/kg) should be given. If this dose is tolerated, the dose can be increased rapidly, to 1–2 mg/kg per day if necessary. Long-term treatment should not exceed 2–3 mg/kg per day

Table 2 Dosage of oral antihypertensive agents in children and adolescents

	Age group	Initial dose	Maximum dose	Dosage interval	Pediatric label for hypertension (EU) (Germany)	Pediatric label for hypertension (USA)
Angiotensin-converting enzyme inhibitors						
Captopril	Premature to > term ≤7 days	0.01 mg/kg/dose	0.5 mg/kg/day	8–12 h		
	Term neonates > 7 days	0.05–0.1 mg/kg/dose	0.5 mg/kg/day	8–12 h		
	Infants	0.15–0.3 mg/kg/dose	6 mg/kg/day	8–12 h	Yes	
	Children	0.3–0.5 mg/kg/dose	6 mg/kg/day	8–12 h		
	Older children	6.25–12.5 mg/dose	6 mg/kg/day	8–12 h		
	Adolescents	12.5–25 mg/dose	450 mg/day	8–12 h		
Enalapril	Neonates	0.1 mg/kg/day	0.5 mg/kg/day	24 h		
	Infants and children	0.1 mg/kg/day	0.5 mg/kg/day	24 h	>6 years	6–16 years
	Adolescents	2.5–5 mg/day	40 mg/day	24 h		
Lisinopril	Infants and children <6 years	0.1 mg/kg/dose	0.5 mg/kg/day	24 h		
	≥6 years	0.07 mg/kg/dose (max. 5 mg/dose)	>0.61 mg/kg or 40 mg/day	24 h	>6 years	≥6 years
Fosinopril	>50 kg	5–10 mg/day	40 mg/day	24 h		6–16 years
Ramipril	>3 years	1,25 mg/m^2/day	6 mg/m^2/day	24 h		
Angiotensin II receptor antagonists						
Losartan	≥6 years	0.7 mg/kg/dose or 50 mg/day	100 mg/day	24 h	>6 years	≥6 years
Valsartan	≥6 years	1.3 mg/kg/dose or 40 mg/day	160 mg/day	24 h	>6 years	6–16 years

(continued)

Table 2 (continued)

	Age group	Initial dose	Maximum dose	Dosage interval	Pediatric label for hypertension (EU) (Germany)	Pediatric label for hypertension (USA)
Candesartan	1–5 years	0.2 mg/kg/day	0.4 mg/kg/day	12–24 h		1–16 years
	6–17 years, <50 kg	4–8 mg/day	16 mg/day	12–24 h	>6 years	
	6–17 years, >50 kg	8–16 mg/day	32 mg/day	12–24 h		
Olmesartan	1–5 years, ≥50	0.3 mg/kg/day	0.6 mg/kg/day	24 h		
	6–16 years, 20–35 kg	10 mg/day	20 mg/day	24 h	>6 years	6–12 years
	≥35 kg	20 mg/day	40 mg/day	24 h		
Calcium channel antagonists						
Amlodipine	6–17 years	2.5 mg/day	10 mg/day	24 h	>6 years	≥6 years
Nifedipine extended release	Children	0.25–0.5 mg/kg/day	3 mg/kg/day up to 120 mg/day	8–12 h		No
	Adolescent	30 mg/day	120 mg/day			
Beta-receptor antagonists						
Propranolol	1–17 years	1 mg/kg/day	4 mg/kg/day up to 640 mg/day	8–12 h	Licensed only in cardiac arrhythmia	Yes
Metoprolol immediate release	1–17 years	1 mg/kg/day	6 mg/kg/day up to 200 mg/day	12 h		≥6 years
Metoprolol extended release	≥6 years	1 mg/kg/day	2 mg/kg/day or 200 mg/day	24 h		
Metoprolol extended release		23.75 mg/day	95 mg/day	24 h	>6 years	
Diuretics						
Hydrochlorothiazide		0.25 mg/kg/day	1 mg/kg/day	24 h	No	No

Chlorthalidone	5–12 years	0.5 mg/kg/48 h	1.7 mg/kg/48 h	24–48 h	No	No
	12–18 years	25 mg/day	50 mg/day	24–48 h		
Furosemide		0.5 mg/kg/day	5 mg/kg/day	8–12 h	Licensed only for edema treatment	No
Torasemide	>12 years	2.5 mg/day	5 mg/day	24 h	>12 years	
Others						
Clonidine	Children	0.005 mg/kg/day	0.3 mg/kg/day	8–12 h	No	No
Hydralazine	Children	1 mg/kg/day	10 mg/kg/day	12 h	No	No
Minoxidil	Children < 12 years	0.1–0.2 mg/kg/day	50 mg/day	12 h	Yes	Yes
	Adolescents > 12 years	5 mg/day	100 mg/day	12 h	Yes	Yes
Only emergency						
Nifedipine	Acute hypertensive emergency	0.25 mg/kg/day	0.5 mg/kg			
Urapidil	Acute hypertensive emergency	1 mg/kg/day				
Diazoxide	Only for treatment of acute hypertensive emergencies	2 mg/kg single dose	6 mg/kg			
Nitroprusside sodium	Only for treatment of refractory hypertensive emergencies	0.5 μg/kg per min	8 μg/kg per min			

or 150 mg in adolescents, although higher doses have been recommended. Because of multiple dosing per day, captopril is no longer the drug of choice.

Enalapril is a prodrug that must be metabolically converted to enalaprilat. Peak serum concentration occurred at 3–4 h after oral administration. The longer plasma half-life of 12 h is an advantage to improve compliance. Since enalapril is excreted by the kidneys, dosage should be reduced in patients with renal failure. As with captopril, approximately one-third of enalaprilat is cleared during hemodialysis.

Ramipril has also been used in children (Soergel et al. 2000), but studies failed to demonstrate a reliable dose-response relationship in children. On the other hand, excellent outcome data are available in children with renal failure (ESCAPE Trial Group 2009), and the drug is therefore used extensively in children with renal hypertension and progressive renal failure. A clear dose relationship has been shown for enalapril and lisinopril (Benjamin et al. 2008). Overall, increasing an effective dose of an ACE inhibitor will often not result in a better blood pressure response. Therefore, early combination therapy is required instead of multiple-dose escalation.

Fosinopril also reduced systolic and diastolic blood pressure in three dose levels (0.1, 0.3, and 0.6 mg/kg). During the dose-response phase, all three doses were equally effective in lowering systolic blood pressure (Li et al. 2004). During the placebo withdrawal phase, there was an adjusted mean systolic blood pressure increase of 5.2 mmHg for the placebo group and 1.5 mmHg for the fosinopril group, a net withdrawal effect of 3.7 mmHg. The lack of a clear dose response in the cohort can be explained either by using high doses, by a narrow dose range, or by a true absence of a dose response.

Lisinopril demonstrated a dose-response reduction in systolic and diastolic blood pressure between the lowest and each of the higher doses used (Soffer et al. 2003). Blood pressure in the placebo group increased after withdrawal of lisinopril. The dose-response relationship was consistent across all subgroups (e.g., age, Tanner stage, ethnicity, gender). Pharmacokinetics of lisinopril in hypertensive infants and children are relatively consistent across age groups and consistent with data in healthy adults (Hogg et al. 2007).

3.2 Angiotensin II Receptor Type 1 Antagonists

Angiotensin II receptor type 1 antagonists (AR antagonists) inhibit the final step of the RAAS on the heart, kidney, blood vessels, and adrenal glands and inhibit vasoconstriction and lower blood pressure (Burnier 2001). AR antagonists are effective at reducing proteinuria secondary to diabetes and may be particularly useful in patients with chronic kidney disease (Webb et al. 2010). Antagonizing the angiotensin II receptor 1 is highly effective to lower blood pressure in children with arterial hypertension, and a variety of AR antagonists have been studied in children.

Losartan was the first AR antagonist studied in children. The drug reduced systolic and diastolic pressure in a dose-dependent manner (Shahinfar et al. 2005).

It was also studied in a clinical trial focused on reduction of proteinuria in hypertensive (*n*: 60) and normotensive (*n*: 246) children with chronic kidney disease (Webb et al. 2010). Losartan reduced proteinuria by 35.9% and was superior to both placebo (normotensive cohort) and amlodipine (hypertensive cohort).

Valsartan reduced systolic and diastolic pressure in a dose-dependent manner (10, 20 mg for children <35 kg and 20, 40 mg for children ≥35 kg), but a statistically significant difference in blood pressure response between the low- and medium-dose groups could not be demonstrated (Wells et al. 2011). Valsartan was also studied in hypertensive children aged between 1 and 5 years, tested in three dose regimes (Flynn et al. 2008). All three dosing groups achieved a statistically significant reduction in systolic blood pressure but failed to demonstrate a linear dose-response between the three groups.

Candesartan lowered significantly systolic and diastolic blood pressure compared to placebo, but did not yield a clear dose-response relationship in all dose levels. The lack of dose response was attributed to a narrow dose range studied (Trachtman et al. 2008). In children aged 1–5 years, systolic and diastolic blood pressure fell in all three dosing groups (Schaefer et al. 2010), and a statistically significant, dose-related, 57% median decline in proteinuria was found with candesartan at 4 weeks follow-up.

Olmesartan showed a dose-dependent, statistically significant reduction in systolic and diastolic blood pressure (Hazan et al. 2010). Mean blood pressure reductions were smaller in black adolescents. The olmesartan dose response remained statistically significant when adjusted for body weight. In a second period, blood pressure rose in those patients switching to placebo, whereas patients continuing to receive olmesartan therapy maintained consistent blood pressure reduction. Olmesartan demonstrated a pharmacokinetic profile in pediatric patients similar to that of adults when adjusted for body size (Wells et al. 2012).

3.3 Calcium Antagonists

Calcium channel blockers of the dihydropyridine type, e.g., amlodipine, felodipine, or nifedipine, are highly selective for vascular smooth muscle and are commonly prescribed for pediatric hypertension (Yoon et al. 2012; Welch et al. 2012).

Amlodipine demonstrated a dose-response reduction in systolic and diastolic blood pressure beginning at doses of 0.06 mg/kg per day or higher (Flynn et al. 2004). The underlying cause of hypertension had no effect on the response to amlodipine. Systolic blood pressure response equal or lower to the 95th percentile was achieved in 34.6% of subjects with systolic hypertension.

Nifedipine has been shown to reduce blood pressure effectively and safely in pediatric hypertensive emergencies. The doses used range between 0.25 and 0.5 mg/kg as single or repeated oral dose, when blood pressure response is insufficient. Slow-release preparations of nifedipine have been used as vasodilators to treat sustained renal hypertension in children in Germany, although this experience has not yet been reported in print. The dose used ranges between

0.5 and 2.0 mg/kg per day. The drug has been replaced by amlodipine (0.06–0.3 mg/kg/day), which is licensed in children over 6 years.

3.4 Beta-Adrenergic Blockers

Based on two small-sized studies, beta-blockers modestly reduce systolic blood pressure by 4 mmHg, but have no significant effect on diastolic blood pressure compared to placebo. Otherwise they lower blood pressure in combination with vasodilators by blocking reflex tachycardia. They have their role when two or more antihypertensive drugs are required and reflex tachycardia has to be antagonized to lower blood pressure.

Propranolol is effective and safe in doses from 1 to 4 mg/kg per day, but only case series and retrospective experience have been published. Occasionally higher doses, up to 16 mg/kg per day, are tolerated without significant side effects. It is not clearly established whether an increase in dosage to >5 mg/kg per day has any further blood pressure-lowering effects, although this might be possible, since bioavailability varies between 20% and 50% due to a high first-pass metabolism in the liver.

Atenolol is eliminated via the kidney and has a longer half-life than propranolol; a single morning dose appeared to be sufficient. Only retrospective reports are available for atenolol as antihypertensive agent in children.

Metoprolol significantly reduced systolic blood pressure compared to placebo, but with no dose-response effect (Batisky et al. 2007). Only high doses of extended released metoprolol (2 mg/kg) demonstrated significant reductions in diastolic blood pressure compared to placebo. At the end of the dose-ranging study, the response rate for metoprolol was 46%.

3.5 Diuretics

Diuretics represent an important principle of antihypertensive agents. They can be broadly divided into three categories, thiazide diuretics, loop diuretics, and potassium-sparing diuretics. All three classes target different parts of the nephron to decrease sodium and water reabsorption, thereby creating a natriuretic effect that decreases extracellular volume and reduces blood pressure.

Hydrochlorothiazide belongs to the group of thiazide diuretics and is extensively studied and used to treat arterial hypertension in adults. Thiazide diuretics block sodium-chloride co-transporters at the distal convoluted tubule to decrease sodium reabsorption. It is not known whether this acute action is solely responsible for reducing peripheral resistance and chronically lower blood pressure in hypertensive patients. Pediatric experience has been reported with hydrochlorothiazide in abstract form more than 40 years ago (Mirkin et al. 1977). Increasing the dose of thiazides affects blood pressure only marginally but may be associated with increased incidence and severity of side effects such as hypokalemia, hyperuricaemia, impairment of glucose tolerance, and disturbances of lipid metabolism.

Chlorthalidone has a longer half-life than hydrochlorothiazide, and the dose interval is 24 or 48 h. Only limited experience in children with arterial hypertension has been communicated with the drug (Bachmann 1984).

Furosemide as a loop diuretic is essential in children with advanced heart failure and chronic renal failure when thiazides often are not effective. It has its role in reducing sodium and water retention in various diseased states and age categories. There are no data supporting the efficacy of furosemide to reduce blood pressure in children compared to placebo. When prescribed alone, loop diuretics lower blood pressure acutely, but not chronically because the activated RAAS will compensate for the lost fluid volume. Loop diuretics inhibit the sodium-potassium-chloride transporter (Na-K-2Cl transporter) on the thick ascending loop of Henle to decrease the osmotic gradient producing a potent natriuretic effect.

Torasemide is loop diuretic with a longer half-life compared to furosemide. It is indicated in chronic heart failure and arterial hypertension in adults and adolescents 12 years of age or older.

3.6 Other Drugs

Hydralazine and *minoxidil* have been used as vasodilators but have limited use. *Clonidine* lowers sympathetic outflow via central alpha-2 adrenergic stimulation. Clonidine is indicated if beta-blockers are contraindicated and blocking reflex tachycardia is required.

The alpha-1 adrenergic blocker *prazosin* does not affect presynaptic alpha-1 adrenergic receptors, as do *phentolamine* and *phenoxybenzamine*. The alpha blockers are highly needed pre- and perioperatively in patients with pheochromocytoma.

4 Specific Treatment Aspects

4.1 Safety Aspects

The antihypertensive agents used in children have been shown in short-term studies to be well tolerated and safe. This is particularly true for ACE inhibitors and AR antagonists. Knowing the right dose for treating a hypertensive child on the basis of randomized controlled studies is a major advantage for safe application. Despite using drugs for decades, data regarding safety of antihypertensive agents in children remain limited. Also, in adults, side effects from lifelong treatment can be observed sometimes after 40 years of treatment.

Pharmacoepidemiological studies have shown an increased risk of nonmelanoma skin cancer (NMSC) [basal cell carcinoma (basalioma), squamous cell carcinoma of the skin (spinalioma)] when exposed to increasing cumulative doses of hydrochlorothiazide (Pedersen et al. 2018; Pottegard et al. 2017). The photosensitizing effect of hydrochlorothiazide may be responsible as a possible mechanism for the development of tumors. The Pharmacovigilance Risk Assessment

Committee (PRAC) of the European Medicines Agency (EMA) has evaluated the available data sources and considered there was a biologically plausible mechanistic model supporting the increased risk of nonmelanoma skin cancer following higher cumulative doses of hydrochlorothiazide (Pharmacovigilance Risk Assessment Committee 2018). Therefore, the EMA recommended to include the new information in the summary of product characteristics of hydrochlorothiazide-containing products. The long-term use of the drug in children should be considered, particularly since alternative drugs are available. If necessary, high doses should be avoided.

Since the renin system is important in the later pregnancy for fetal kidney formation, blocking the RAAS by ACE inhibitors or angiotensin II receptor antagonists in the second and third trimester may cause fetal renal dysfunction with postpartum oligo- or anhydramnios, which can be irreversible or temporary (ACE inhibitor or angiotensin II receptor antagonist fetopathy). Other possible characteristic symptoms include contractures of the extremities, hypoplasia of the skull, pulmonary hypoplasia, and very seldom thrombosis of the inferior vena cava (Cooper et al. 2006; Hünseler et al. 2011). Severe fetopathy can lead to stillbirth or death in the newborn period. The highly critical period for fetopathy symptoms begins at week 20 of pregnancy. Therefore, agents blocking the renin system should be should be discontinued as soon as pregnancy is detected and have to be replaced by other antihypertensive drugs.

Specific indications, contraindications, and side effects are listed in Table 3.

4.2 Approach to Treat Children with Antihypertensive Agents

The management of children with chronically elevated blood pressure starts with low doses of a given drug and rapidly increased to a recommended therapeutic dose. Treatment should be started with ACE inhibitors. High-dose monotherapy should be avoided because of side effects and lack of efficacy. Often blood pressure response is insufficient when escalating the dose. Therefore, early combination of two or more antihypertensive drugs should be used initially. Combination therapy should follow a rational approach (Table 4). In some patients, in whom treatment is accompanied by an effective blood pressure control for an extended period, it may be possible to reduce the number and dose of drugs.

4.3 Hypertensive Emergencies

Hypertensive emergencies with clinical signs of hypertensive encephalopathy or of pulmonary edema require immediate therapy (Seeman et al. 2019). Randomized controlled studies with acute hypertension are lacking; only case reports and retrospective data are available. Many drugs have been tried and are recommended (Seeman et al. 2019).

Oral nifedipine at a dose of 0.25–0.5 mg/kg is efficient (Yiu et al. 2004). If there is insufficient response within 15 min, marked tachycardia may occur, which points to

Table 3 Indications, contraindications, and side effects of antihypertensive agents

Drug class	Indication	Contraindication	Side effects
Angiotensin-converting enzyme inhibitors	Diabetes mellitus, progressive renal disease	Renal artery stenosis, GFR increase, pregnancy	Skin rashes, taste disturbances, cough, hyperkalemia, fetopathy
Angiotensin II receptor antagonists	Diabetes mellitus, progressive renal disease	Renal artery stenosis, GFR increase, pregnancy	Skin rashes, taste disturbances, angioedema, hyperkalemia, fetopathy
Beta-adrenergic antagonists	Reflex tachycardia	Asthma, concurrent diabetes mellitus	Bradycardia and bronchoconstriction
Calcium channel blockers			Gastrointestinal disturbances, constipation, edema of the legs, gingival hyperplasia
Centrally acting alpha-adrenergic antagonists (clonidine)	Reflex tachycardia		Sedation, bradycardia
Loop diuretics (furosemide, torasemide)	Only when GFR <30 mL/min/m^2 and fluid overload		Hypokalemia, hypercalciuria
Thiazide diuretics (hydrochlorothiazide)	Only in combination therapy	GFR $<$ 30 mL/min/m^2	Hypokalemia, hyperuricemia, impairment of glucose tolerance, disturbances of lipid metabolism, increased risk of some types of skin and lip cancer (nonmelanoma skin cancer)
Vasodilators (minoxidil, hydralazine)	Only in combination therapy		Induce tachycardia, salt and water retention, hypertrichosis

Table 4 Rational combination of antihypertensive drugs

Two drugs	ACE inhibitor or AR antagonist + diuretic
	ACE inhibitor or AR antagonist + calcium channel antagonist
	Diuretic + ACE inhibitor or AR antagonist
Three drugs	ACE inhibitor or AR antagonist + diuretic + beta-blocker
	ACE inhibitor or AR antagonist + diuretic + calcium channel antagonist
	ACE inhibitor or AR antagonist + diuretic + clonidine
	Diuretic + beta-blocker + vasodilator (ACE inhibitor or AR antagonist or calcium channel antagonist or hydralazine or minoxidil)
	Diuretic + clonidine + vasodilator (ACE inhibitor or AR antagonist or calcium channel antagonist or hydralazine or minoxidil)

ACE Angiotensin Converting Enzyme, *AR* angiotensin II receptor sympathetic stimulation, and therefore clonidine in a dose of 2–6 µg/kg is indicated, given either subcutaneously, intramuscularly, or slowly intravenously.

Urapidil is an alpha-1 adrenergic receptor antagonist. It acts primarily on arteries to dilate the vessels (vasodilating) and is mainly used for acute increases in blood pressure. The published experience is the pediatric population which is limited (Schöber et al. 1984).

The use of diazoxide (2–6 mg/kg) is established in childhood hypertension, but no longer recommended as a first-line drug, since bolus injection may be associated with a precipitous reduction in blood pressure to hypotensive levels. In states of fluid retention, furosemide (2–7 mg/kg intravenously) should be combined. If there is no satisfactory response to the drugs discussed above, sodium nitroprusside (0.5–8 µg/kg per min) should be administered as a continuous infusion with the patient under constant surveillance. The infusion rate must be continuously adjusted to the changes in blood pressure. Thiocyanate levels should be monitored. In terminal renal failure, fluid removal by dialysis may be the only way to control hypertension.

References

Bachmann H (1984) Propranolol versus chlorthalidone – a prospective therapeutic trial in children with chronic hypertension. Helv Paediatr Acta 39:55–61

Batisky DL, Sorof JM, Sugg J et al (2007) Efficacy and safety of extended release metoprolol succinate in hypertensive children 6 to 16 years of age: a clinical trial experience. J Pediatr 150:134–139

Benjamin DK Jr, Smith PB, Jadhav P et al (2008) Pediatric antihypertensive trial failures: analysis of end points and dose range. Hypertension 51:834–840

Burnier M (2001) Angiotensin II type 1 receptor blockers. Circulation 103:904–912

Chaturvedi S, Lipszyc DH, Licht C et al (2014) Pharmacological interventions for hypertension in children. Cochrane Database Syst Rev 2:CD008117

Chu PY, Campbell MJ, Miller SG, Hill KD (2014) Anti-hypertensive drugs in children and adolescents. World J Cardiol 6:234–244

Cooper WO, Hernandez-Diaz S, Arbogast PG et al (2006) Major congenital malformations after first-trimester exposure to ACE inhibitors. N Engl J Med 354:2443–2451

ESCAPE Trial Group, Wühl E, Trivelli A, Picca S et al (2009) Strict blood-pressure control and progression of renal failure in children. N Engl J Med 361:1639–1650

Flynn JT, Newburger JW, Daniels SR et al (2004) A randomized, placebo-controlled trial of amlodipine in children with hypertension. J Pediatr 145:353–359

Flynn JT, Meyers KE, Neto JP, Pediatric Valsartan Study Group et al (2008) Efficacy and safety of the angiotensin receptor blocker valsartan in children with hypertension aged 1 to 5 years. Hypertension 52:222–228

Hazan L, Hernández Rodriguez OA, Bhorat AE et al (2010) A double-blind, dose-response study of the efficacy and safety of olmesartan medoxomil in children and adolescents with hypertension. Hypertension 55:1323–1330

Hogg RJ, Delucchi A, Sakihara G et al (2007) A multicenter study of the pharmacokinetics of lisinopril in pediatric patients with hypertension. Pediatr Nephrol 22:695–701

Hünseler C, Paneitz A, Friedrich D et al (2011) Angiotensin II receptor blocker induced fetopathy: 7 cases. Klin Padiatr 223:5–9

International Pediatric Nephrology Association (IPNA) (2011) (updated January 2012) (http://www.iphapediatrichypertension.org/wp-core/wp-content/uploads/BPLimitsChart0112.pdf). Accessed 8 Feb 2020

Li JS, Berezny K, Kilaru R et al (2004) Is the extrapolated adult dose of fosinopril safe and effective in treating hypertensive children? Hypertension 44:289–293

Lurbe E, Agabiti-Rosei E, Cruickshank JK et al (2016) 2016 European Society of Hypertension guidelines for the management of high blood pressure in children and adolescents. J Hypertens 34(10):1887–1920

Menon S, Berezny KY, Kilaru R et al (2006) Racial differences are seen in blood pressure response to fosinopril in hypertensive children. Am Heart J 152:394–399

Meyers RS, Siu A (2011) Pharmacotherapy review of chronic pediatric hypertension. Clin Ther 33:1331–1356

Mirkin BL, Newman TJ (1985) Efficacy and safety of captopril in the treatment of severe childhood hypertension: report of the International Collaborative Study Group. Pediatrics 75:1091–1100

Mirkin BL, Sinaiko AR, Cooper M, Anders M (1977) Hydrochlorothiazide therapy in hypertensive and renal insufficient children: elimination kinetics and metabolic effects. Pediatr Res 11:418

Neuhauser HK, Thamm M, Ellert U et al (2011) Blood pressure percentiles by age and height from nonoverweight children and adolescents in Germany. Pediatrics 127:e978–e988

Pedersen SA, Gaist D, Schmidt SAJ et al (2018) Hydrochlorothiazide use and risk of nonmelanoma skin cancer: a nationwide casecontral study fram Denmark. J Am Acad Dermatol 78:673–681

Pharmacovigilance Risk Assessment Committee (PRAC) (2018) PRAC recommendations on signals. EMA/PRAC/595691/2018 https://www.ema.europa.eu/documents/prac-recommendation/prac-recommendations-signals-adopted-3-6-september-2018-prac-meeting_en-0.pdf. Accessed 10 Feb 2020

Pottegard A, Hallas J, Diesen M et al (2017) Hydrochlorothiazide use is strongly associated with risk of lip cancer. J Intern Med 282:322–331

Rascher W (2016) Treatment of hypertension in children. In: Turner N, Lameire N, Goldsmith DJ et al (eds) Textbook of clinical nephrology, 4th edn. Oxford University Press, Oxford, pp 1825–1830

Schaefer F, Van de Walle J, Zurowska A, Candesartan in Children with Hypertension Investigators et al (2010) Efficacy, safety and pharmacokinetics of candesartan cilexetil in hypertensive children from 1 to less than 6 years of age. J Hypertens 28:1083–1090

Schöber JG, Pilossoff W, Bühlmeyer K (1984) Urapidil therapy for acute hypertensive crises in infants and children. Eur J Pediatr 143:87–91

Seeman T, Dusek J, Vondrák K et al (2004) Ramipril in the treatment of hypertension and proteinuria in children with chronic kidney diseases. Am J Hypertens 17:415–420

Seeman T, Hamdani G, Mitsnefes M (2019) Hypertensive crisis in children and adolescents. Pediatr Nephrol 34(12):2523–2537

Shahinfar S, Cano F, Soffer BA et al (2005) A double-blind, dose-response study of losartan in hypertensive children. Am J Hypertens 18:183–190

Siddiqi N, Shatat IF (2019) Antihypertensive agents: a long way to safe drug prescribing in children. Pediatr Nephrol. https://doi.org/10.1007/s00467-019-04314-7

Simonetti GD, Rizzi M, Donadini R, Bianchetti MG (2007) Effects of antihypertensive drugs on blood pressure and proteinuria in childhood. J Hypertens 25:2370–2376

Snauwaert E, Vande Walle J, De Bruyne P (2017) Therapeutic efficacy and safety of ACE inhibitors in the hypertensive paediatric population: a review. Arch Dis Child 102:63–71

Soergel M, Verho M, Wühl E et al (2000) Effect of ramipril on ambulatory blood pressure and albuminuria in renal hypertension. Pediatr Nephrol 15:113–118

Soffer B, Zhang Z, Miller K et al (2003) A double blind, placebo-controlled, dose-response study of the effectiveness and safety of lisinopril for children with hypertension. Am J Hypertens 16:795–800

Trachtman H, Hainer JW, Sugg J et al (2008) Efficacy, safety, and pharmacokinetics of candesartan cilexetil in children aged 6 to 17 years. J Clin Hypertens 10:743–750

Van den Belt SM, Heerspink HJ, Gracchi V, ESCAPE Trial Group et al (2018) Early proteinuria lowering by angiotensin-converting enzyme inhibition predicts renal survival in children with CKD. J Am Soc Nephrol 29:2225–2233
Webb NJ, Lam C, Loeys T et al (2010) Randomized, double-blind, controlled study of losartan in children with proteinuria. Clin J Am Soc Nephrol 5:417–424
Welch WP, Yang W, Taylor-Zapata P, Flynn JT (2012) Antihypertensive drug use by children: are the drugs labeled and indicated? J Clin Hypertens 14:388–395
Wells T, Blumer J, Meyers KE et al (2011) Effectiveness and safety of valsartan in children aged 6 to 16 years with hypertension. J Clin Hypertens 13:357–365
Wells TG, Blowey DL, Sullivan JE et al (2012) Pharmacokinetics of olmesartan medoxomil in pediatric patients with hypertension. Paediatr Drugs 14:401–409
Wühl E, Mehls O, Schaefer F, ESCAPE Trial Group (2004) Antihypertensive and antiproteinuric efficacy of ramipril in children with chronic renal failure. Kidney Int 66:768–776
Yiu V, Orrbine E, Rosychuk RJ et al (2004) The safety and use of short-acting nifedipine in hospitalized hypertensive children. Pediatr Nephrol 19:644–650
Yoon EY, Cohn L, Rocchini A et al (2012) Antihypertensive prescribing patterns for adolescents with primary hypertension. Pediatrics 129:e1–e8

Understanding the Effects of Kidney Disease and Dialysis Treatment on Pharmacotherapy in Children

Verena Gotta, Olivera Marsenic, and Marc Pfister

Contents

Abstract

Chronic kidney disease (CKD) and acute kidney injury (AKI) requiring renal replacement therapy (RRT) by dialysis are rare conditions in pediatric patients. In pediatric patients with CKD, dialysis is mainly performed using peritoneal dialysis (PD) or intermittent hemodialysis (HD). In patients with AKI, continuous renal replacement therapy (CRRT) using hemofiltration, hemodialysis, or both techniques can be used. This chapter reviews (1) physiology and epidemiology of kidney disease and dialysis in children and (2) pharmacokinetic principles to be

V. Gotta (✉) · M. Pfister
Pediatric Pharmacology and Pharmacometrics, University of Basel Children's Hospital, Basel, Switzerland
e-mail: verena.gotta@ukbb.ch

O. Marsenic
Pediatric Nephrology, Yale University School of Medicine, New Haven, CT, USA

W. Kiess et al. (eds.), *Pediatric Pharmacotherapy*,
Handbook of Experimental Pharmacology 261, https://doi.org/10.1007/164_2019_224

considered for developing pediatric dose recommendations under different dialysis modalities. Methods for both calculating and predicting dialysis drug clearance are reviewed; scaling approaches for predicting dialysis clearance in pediatric patients from data obtained in adults are discussed.

Keywords
Acute kidney injury · Chronic kidney disease · Modeling · Pediatrics · Pharmacokinetics · Pharmacometrics · Renal dialysis

1 Introduction

Dose recommendations for patients with kidney disease requiring dialysis have been found to be incomplete and inconsistent, and sometimes lack scientific quantitative evidence (Vidal et al. 2005; Khanal et al. 2014). In pediatric patients with kidney disease, the situation is further complicated by the fact that pediatric dose recommendations per se are already heterogeneous, in particular for drugs used off-label, both on national and international levels (Cella et al. 2010; Metsvaht et al. 2015). Regulatory guidance (Center for Drug Evaluation and Research (CDER) 2010; Committee for Medicinal Products for Human use (CHMP) 2015) has increased pharmacokinetic studies of new drugs in adult patients on chronic hemodialysis (Matzke et al. 2016). Due to the rarity of kidney disease and dialysis in children however, the pediatric population remains under investigated.

Pathophysiology, epidemiology, and dialysis prescriptions can further differ between pediatric and adult dialysis patients (*reviewed in* Sects. 2 and 3 *of this chapter*), which has to be considered when translating pharmacokinetic findings from adults to pediatric patients and developing dose recommendations (Sect. 4 *of this chapter*).

2 Definition and Epidemiology of Kidney Disease in Children

2.1 Acute Kidney Injury

Acute kidney injury (AKI) is defined as an abrupt reduction in kidney function as measured by a rapid decline in glomerular filtration rate (GFR) (Andreoli 2004, 2009) and is reported to occur in 5% of noncritically ill children and in 27% of critically ill children (Kwiatkowski and Sutherland 2017). AKI is largely caused by systemic illnesses, multiorgan injury, and disease-related therapies rather than primary renal diseases (Kwiatkowski and Sutherland 2017). Advances in management of pediatric diseases such as bone marrow and solid organ transplantations, congenital heart disease surgery, and the care of very low birth weight infants contribute to AKI incidence. AKI is characterized by impairment of nitrogenous waste product excretion and inability to regulate water, electrolyte and acid–base homeostasis due to functional or structural changes in the kidney. AKI can be categorized as prerenal (reduced effective renal blood flow), renal (intrinsic renal disorder), or postrenal (mainly urinary tract obstruction). That is, any process that interferes with the structure or function of the renal vasculature, glomeruli, renal tubules, interstitium, or urinary tract can result in AKI. Similar to RIFLE criteria in adults, pediatric (p) RIFLE criteria help stratify AKI and project its course in children. pRIFLE criteria (Akcan-Arikan et al. 2007) stands for: R – risk for renal dysfunction, I – injury to the kidney, F – failure of kidney function, L – loss of kidney function, and E – end stage renal disease. Pathophysiologic processes commonly responsible for renal injury are hypovolemia, decrease in effective blood volume, nephrotoxicity, acute tubular necrosis, acute interstitial nephritis, glomerulonephritis, and renal vein thrombosis. Drugs most commonly implicated in renal injury include various antibiotics (i.e., vancomycin and gentamicin), lithium, nonsteroidal anti-inflammatory drugs, and diuretics (Bunchman and Ferris 2011; Ulinski et al. 2012; Kwiatkowski and Sutherland 2017).

AKI is diagnosed by an increase in serum creatinine concentration, which reflects a decrease in the glomerular filtration rate (GFR). It is now recognized that serum creatinine identifies AKI with some delay, and therefore biomarkers that allow its earlier recognition have been identified (serum neutrophil gelatinase-associated lipocalin (NGAL) and cystatin C; urinary NGAL, interleukin-18 and kidney injury molecule-1 (KIM-1)) (Akcan-Arikan et al. 2007). Some of those markers may be used for improved prediction of renal drug clearance (Brou et al. 2015; Downes et al. 2017). Cystatin C and KIM-1 are also accepted biomarkers for monitoring of drug-induced kidney toxicity in preclinical development and partly clinical trials (Griffin et al. 2018).

Management of AKI (Andreoli 2004, 2009; Benfield and Bunchman 2004; Marsenic and Baluarte 2011) entails correction of hypovolemia, electrolyte, and acid–base abnormalities. Decreased renal blood flow can be improved by drugs such as dopamine and fenoldopam (Knoderer et al. 2008). When known, the drug suspected to have caused AKI should be discontinued. Hypertension that can occur in AKI is related to volume overload due to oliguria/anuria or to alterations in vascular tone (i.e., renin-mediated) and its initial therapy is with diuretics and antihypertensives. Renal replacement therapy by dialysis is used if AKI is severe, and its complications are resistant to medical management.

2.2 Chronic Kidney Disease

Chronic kidney disease (CKD) is a state of irreversible kidney damage which leads to decrease in kidney function. The median incidence of CKD in children younger than 19 years worldwide is reported to be nine cases (range 4–18) per million of the age-related population, with congenital anomalies of the urinary tract (CAKUT) being the predominant disorder in younger patients, and glomerulonephritis the leading cause of CKD in adolescents (Rees et al. 2017). The stages of CKD are based on estimated glomerular filtration rate (GFR) (mL/min per 1.73 m^2) most commonly from serum creatinine using the Schwartz equations (Marsenic and

Baluarte 2011; KDIGO (Kidney Disease: Improving Global Outcomes) CKD Work Group 2013): Stage 1: ≥90, Stage 2: 60–89, Stage 3a: 45–59, Stage 3b: 30–44, Stage 4: 15–29, Stage 5: <15 (i.e., end stage renal disease (ESRD)). CKD stages and GFR serve to monitor CKD progression and allow timely planning for RRT, as well as to guide medication dosing throughout CKD based on estimated GFR (Veltri et al. 2004). Once CKD is in ESRD stage, RRT therapy by kidney transplantation or maintenance dialysis is necessary (Chua and Warady 2017).

3 Physiology of Various Dialysis Modalities

Renal replacement therapy (RRT) by dialysis is performed for decreased kidney function in AKI or CKD. The common indications for RRT are fluid and solute removal in various settings such as fluid overload, hyperkalemia, acidosis, hyperphosphatemia, uremia, ingestions of dialyzable toxins/medications, and/or hyperammonemia. RRT is performed via several dialysis modalities. Intermittent hemodialysis (HD) and continuous renal replacement therapy (CRRT) use extracorporeal blood flow and dialysis filters for blood purification, while peritoneal dialysis (PD) requires a catheter placed between the two layers of the peritoneal membrane which serves as a filter for blood clearance (Brophy 2008; Walters et al. 2009). Solute removal is achieved by processes of diffusion and convection. Solute diffusion is dependent on concentration gradient between blood and dialysate and is the main mechanism for clearance of small molecules (size <500 Da). Convection removes solutes via solvent "drag," i.e., solutes move with fluid, and is mainly responsible for removal of larger molecules, known as middle molecules (size 500–60,000 Da) (Duranton et al. 2012). Fluid removal, also known as ultrafiltration (UF), is achieved by transmembrane pressure (TMP) gradient and osmosis. TMP is a modifiable HD device setting that allows controlling fluid removal rate. Osmosis, a process of fluid movement from lower to higher osmotic environment, is a process that is the main fluid removal mechanism in PD, with less prominent effect in HD modalities (Golper et al. 2014; Rees et al. 2017).

All dialysis modalities may result in increased drug clearance causing reduced effective dose of medications and requiring drug level monitoring with more frequent or higher drug doses. Factors that influence dialysis clearance are discussed below in more detail (Veltri et al. 2004). Briefly, molecules that easily pass through dialysis filters have small molecular weight, high water solubility, low protein binding, and small volume of distribution, while the opposite is true for molecules that are highly protein bound and have high lipid solubility (see Sect. 4.1).

3.1 Continuous Renal Replacement Therapy

CRRT is indicated in critically ill and hemodynamically unstable children in whom abrupt changes in solute concentrations and extracellular fluid volume are not well tolerated. CRRT is based on pump-driven veno-venous access. Its advantages include gradual and continuous removal of solutes and modification of extracellular fluid volume, as well as more efficient clearance of higher molecular weight solutes (Brophy 2008; Walters et al. 2009; Sutherland and Alexander 2012). There are several types of CRRT (Sutherland and Alexander 2012): (1) continuous veno-venous hemofiltration (CVVH): uses only convective clearance with high ultrafiltration rate and replacement of ultrafiltrate with replacement fluid that contains electrolytes; (2) continuous veno-venous hemodialysis (CVVHD): uses mainly diffusive clearance with use of dialysate countercurrent to the blood in the hemofilter; (3) continuous veno-venous hemodiafiltration (CVVHDF): uses both convective and diffusive clearance and uses both replacement and dialysate fluids during the treatment. All CRRT modalities require pediatric size-appropriate vascular access, adequate blood flow, a dialysis filter, and anticoagulation via heparin (systemic) or citrate (regional). Depending on modality, dialysis fluid and/or replacement fluid is needed. Dosing of all CVVH components in children is weight or body surface area based. For example, CVVHDF prescription for an adolescent would resemble the following: Blood flow (Q_B) 200 mL/min, dialysate flow (Q_D) 1,000 mL/1.73m^2/h and flow of replacement fluid (Q_{rf}) 1,000 mL/1.73m^2/h (typical values for 50 kg are summarized in Table 1). Complications are mainly related to anticoagulation, excessive fluid removal, temperature instability, dialysis membrane reactions, and unintentional electrolyte and amino-acid losses.

3.2 Intermittent Hemodialysis

Intermittent HD (IHD) is especially useful for rapid removal of small-size molecules such as in toxic ingestions, hyperammonemia and for electrolyte disturbances (Benfield and Bunchman 2004; Brophy 2008; Walters et al. 2009; Bunchman and Ferris 2011; Auron and Brophy 2012). Different dialysis fluid compositions allow more or less efficient treatment of electrolyte abnormalities. IHD is also the modality of choice for maintenance hemodialysis in ESRD. In comparison to CVVH (Brophy 2008; Walters et al. 2009; Murray and Liu 2011; Sutherland and Alexander 2012; Golper et al. 2014), HD membranes have smaller pore size and are less permeable to larger molecules which makes this therapy less efficient in removing larger and protein-bound toxins. Low-flux membranes further have smaller pore size than high-flux membranes. Membranes used are also not as permeable to water, and therefore IHD does not require replacement fluid. To maximize efficiency of therapy in short amount of time, IHD uses faster blood flow rates and higher dialysate flow rates. IHD provides rapid removal of solutes, while desired fluid removal is performed in a single session over a few hours, and therefore IHD can only be considered for patients who are hemodynamically stable and can tolerate rapid solute and fluid shifts. Anticoagulation is mainly systemic with heparin. A typical IHD would be performed thrice weekly. Vascular access is provided via size-appropriate tunnelled central line. Components of IHD prescription in children are weight and body surface area based. A typical IHD prescription in an adolescent would include Q_B 300 mL/min, Q_D 600 mL/min, size-appropriate dialysis filter, and duration of 3 h

Table 1 Examples of typical dialysis prescription parameters for a 50-kg adolescent

	Intermittent hemodialysis (IHD)	Peritoneal dialysis (PD)	Continuous veno-venous hemofiltration (CVVH)	Continuous veno-venous hemodialysis (CVVHD)	Continuous veno-venous hemodiafiltration (CVVHDF)
Blood flow, Q_B (mL/min)	300	(≈1,200[a])	200	200	200
Dialysate flow, Q_D (mL/min)	600	≈(7–)33[b]	*Not used*	17(–34)	17
Ultrafiltration, Q_{UF} (mL/min)	<11[c]	(0.7–)2[d]	≈17[e]	≈5[e]	≈13[e]
Duration (h) per day	3 (3×/week)	8(–24)[f]	24	24	24
Clearance limiting factor	Q_B	Q_D (mainly achieved by modifying fill volume)	Q_{UF}	Q_D	Q_D and Q_{UF}

Numbers can vary for a given patient according to tolerability and clinical indication
[a]Splanchnic blood flow (Paton et al. 1985)
[b]Calculated as dialysate volume/dwell time (=2,000 mL/60 min for eight overnight cycles at 1 h in automated PD; lower in continuous ambulatory PD with 2,500 mL/6 h for four manual exchanges as given in brackets)
[c]Corresponding to ≤13 mL/kg/min (Gotta et al. 2019b)
[d]Assuming an ultrafiltration volume of 1 L over 8 h (eight overnight cycles at 1 h) in automated PD, and over 24 h in continuous ambulatory PD (given in brackets), respectively
[e]Ultrafiltration rate (Q_{UF}) usually greater than or equal to replacement fluid (Q_{rf}), rate prescribed as clinically indicated, example rates taken from Mehta (1999)
[f]8 h overnight in automated PD, 24 h in continuous ambulatory PD (given in brackets)

(typical values for 50 kg are summarized in Table 1). If IHD is planned to continue chronically, native AV fistula is created for vascular access to avoid chronic use of central lines and to decrease the risk of blood stream infection. IHD is most commonly performed in-center, but with appropriate training it can be performed by the patient and caregiver at home (home-HD) (Chua and Warady 2017; Rees et al. 2017). Common complications include hypotension due to rapid fluid removal from intravascular space, bleeding due to systemic anticoagulation, and membrane reactions. Dialysis disequilibrium syndrome is represented by neurologic symptoms of varying severity due to cerebral edema as a result of rapid change in solute concentration (rapid drop in serum osmolarity) in central nervous system (CNS) (Zepeda-Orozco and Quigley 2012). This may occur in first HD treatment in a very uremic patient and can be prevented by using mannitol and prescribing less efficient dialysis for the first three treatments, with the aim to gradually reduce blood urea nitrogen (BUN) (Benfield and Bunchman 2004; Brophy 2008; Walters et al. 2009).

3.3 Peritoneal Dialysis

PD is the preferred dialysis modality in children <5 years of age (Verrina et al. 2009) as blood vessel anatomy in young children makes long-term vascular access difficult and associated with a number of complications. PD requires insertion of the peritoneal catheter into the peritoneal cavity between the parietal and visceral peritoneal membranes. The barrier for solute and fluid transfer in PD is comprised of capillary endothelium, endothelial basement membrane, and interstitium and mesothelium of the peritoneal membrane. The peritoneal surface area approximately equals body surface area (1.8 m^2 for 70 kg weight and 172 height), or even the surface area of glomerular capillaries (1.5–4.5 m^2 for two kidneys of 150 g) (Paton et al. 1985). Dialysis fluid is inserted into the peritoneal cavity and left to dwell for one to several hours. During the dwell time solute and fluid removal occur by diffusion and osmosis, respectively (Warady et al. 2004; Clarkson et al. 2010). Most types of peritoneal dialysis fluid contain dextrose that creates an osmotic gradient for fluid removal. PD efficiency is dependent on volume, duration, and frequency of dialysis fluid exchanges (Warady et al. 2004; Clarkson et al. 2010; Bunchman and Ferris 2011). It can be performed in any child whose peritoneal cavity is intact and will admit sufficient volume of peritoneal dialysis fluid (Benfield and Bunchman 2004; Warady et al. 2004; Brophy 2008; Walters et al. 2009). A typical pediatric PD prescription in an adolescent varies based on patient's characteristics (i.e., size and peritoneal membrane properties), but an example of continuous PD would be eight overnight cycles, 1 h dwell time, fill volume 2,000 mL, last fill 1,000 mL, net UF goal 1,000 mL/day, with therapy performed 7 days a week at home (Table 1). In comparison to blood-based therapies (IHD and CVVH), PD is advantageous in avoidance of vascular access and need for anticoagulation, and it can be used in patients with hemodynamic instability as it provides gradual and continuous solute and fluid removal. However, it is least efficient in rapid solute and toxin removal and does not allow for dynamic adjustments in solute and fluid removal rates. It is therefore not a modality of choice where rapid corrections of fluid and solutes/toxins removal are needed (Warady et al. 2004; Brophy 2008; Walters et al. 2009). Complications (Brophy 2008; Clarkson et al. 2010) of PD include peritonitis, which can alter membrane permeability, PD catheter exit-site infection, leak around PD catheter, hydrothorax due to dialysis fluid leak into pleural space, and hyperglycemia due to dextrose absorption from the dialysis fluid.

4 Developing Personalized Dose Recommendations

4.1 General Considerations

Whether dose adjustment is required in a patient with kidney disease on dialysis depends mainly on drug-specific factors, and also patient- and dialysis-treatment-related factors need to be considered (Fig. 1).

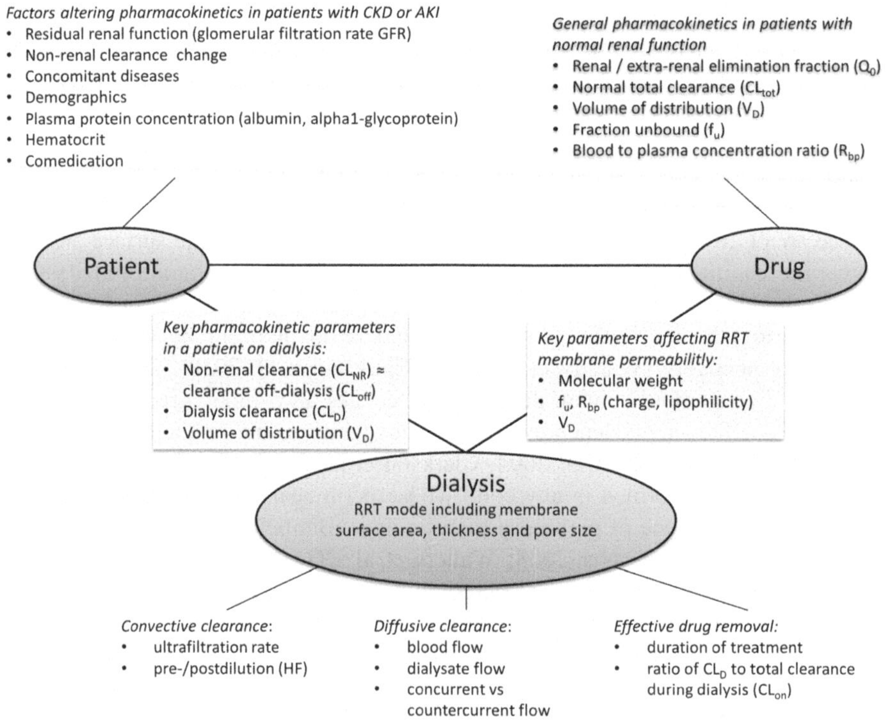

Fig. 1 Illustration of drug-, patient- and dialysis-related factors influencing pharmacokinetics in patients with acute or chronic kidney disease on continuous or intermittent dialysis. *CKD* chronic kidney disease, *AKI* acute kidney injury, *RRT* renal replacement therapy by dialysis, *HF* hemofiltration

Drug-specific factors include physicochemical and pharmacokinetic characteristics of the drug determining total clearance (CL_{tot}), volume of distribution (V_D) and fraction unbound (f_u) in a patient with renal insufficiency (Fig. 1), and possibly additional dialytic clearance (CL_D, Fig. 2). Dose adjustment in CKD or AKI is frequently needed if the drug is >30% renally excreted in the healthy reference population (Center for Drug Evaluation and Research (CDER) 2010). It is frequently not considered necessary for extra-renally excreted drugs, but significantly altered nonrenal clearance has been reported in patients with CKD and AKI (Nolin et al. 2008; Matzke et al. 2016; Dao et al. 2017). For example, reduced nonrenal clearance of vancomycin, imipenem, and meropenem has been reported in ESRD and AKI compared to healthy patients, while nonrenal clearance was higher in AKI compared to ESRD patients (Vilay et al. 2008). Prior dose adjustment and dose individualization by therapeutic drug monitoring is especially important for drugs with a narrow therapeutic range (e.g., oncology drugs and some psychotropic agents) and drugs with well-defined pharmacokinetic-pharmacodynamic relationships (e.g., many anti-infectives). It is less important for drugs whose dosing is best guided by clinical dose titration or alternative treatment monitoring (e.g., blood pressure monitoring).

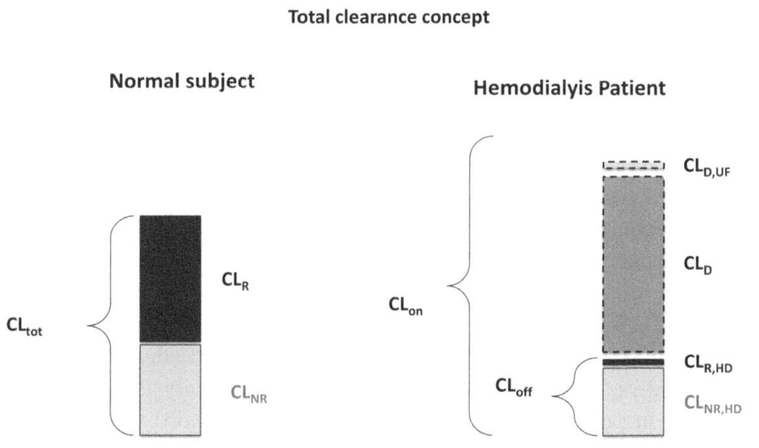

$$CL_{tot} = CL_{NR} + CL_R$$

$$CL_{on} \approx CL_{NR,HD} + CL_D$$

$$CL_{off} \approx CL_{NR,HD}$$

Fig. 2 Conceptual illustration of total drug clearance (CL_{tot}) in a normal subject (*left*) and a patient on intermittent hemodialysis (HD) (*right*). In a normal patient CL_{tot} is the sum of nonrenal and renal clearance (CL_{NR} + CL_R). The hemodialysis (HD) patient has two drug clearances: on- and off-dialysis (CL_{on} and CL_{off}). CL_{off} approximately equals nonrenal clearance of the hemodialysis patient ($CL_{NR,HD}$) assuming residual renal function to be negligible. Note that $CL_{NR,HD}$ may be lower than in a patient with normal kidney function ($CL_{NR,HD} \leq CL_{NR}$). CL_{on} is approximately the sum of nonrenal ($CL_{NR,HD}$) and dialysis clearance (CL_D); convective clearance by ultrafiltration ($CL_{D,UF}$) is most frequently negligible but can be more important in patients on CRRT

Patient-related factors that need to be considered include obviously state of kidney disease and residual renal function (estimated or measured GFR), which is usually assumed to be proportional to renal clearance (CL_R). Like for any other situation demographic characteristics (age and weight) and concomitant diseases, including nutrition status, can also be associated with pharmacokinetic alterations. Pharmacokinetics in acutely sick patients with AKI may be altered by multiorgan dysfunction, fluid overload, or dehydration (altering non-renal clearance CL_{NR}, V_D, f_u). Concomitant diseases in CKD are likely to differ between pediatric and adult patients with CKD with congenital diseases being the major cause for RRT compared to diabetes in adults. Plasma protein binding can be altered by disease-related changes in albumin (frequently low in CKD) and α-acid glycoprotein (frequently elevated in CKD). Total plasma exposure may hence be altered without necessarily altered free drug concentration. The blood-to-plasma concentration ratio of a drug (R_{bp}) may be altered by anemia (measured as low hematocrit), which is relevant for the prediction of plasma dialysis clearance from blood flow (see below), since only unbound drug in the plasma is dialyzed (Matzke et al. 2011; Gotta et al. 2017).

Whether dialytic clearance (CL_D) is significant (frequently defined as >30% of drug dose eliminated by dialysis, or as $CL_D > 30\%$ of total clearance (Atkinson and Umans 2009)) depends on the modality of RRT, intensity of prescription (lowest flow rate is clearance limiting, Table 1), and duration of therapy (Veltri et al. 2004; Gotta et al. 2017). Figure 3 illustrates the relative amount of diffusive and convective clearance for different RRT modalities discussed above.

All the above-mentioned factors are relevant for both adult and pediatric patients with kidney disease. In the pediatric population however, the pharmacokinetics in the healthy reference population may be less well defined, and pediatric particularities of dialysis prescription may need to be taken into account. Supplemental dose recommendations may hence need to be re-evaluated for pediatric patients. For example, intensity of chronic hemodialysis appears to be weight-dependent, and it has been shown to be the most intensified in pediatric and young adult patients of 25–50 kg body weight (median dialysis dose in terms of spKt/V_{urea}: 1.71, with K: urea dialyzer clearance, t: treatment duration, V: distribution volume of urea, sp.: single pool urea distribution model). Lowest dialysis dose delivery has been observed in patients >100 kg (median spKt/V_{urea}: 1.35) (Gotta et al. 2018). Also UF rates are higher in pediatric compared to adult hemodialysis patients (Gotta et al. 2019b). Additionally, it needs to be considered that some dose recommendations for patients undergoing RRT issued before 2000 are potentially insufficient due to increased efficiency of RRT technology and prescription, especially with the introduction of high-flux filters (Mueller and Smoyer 2009; Matzke et al. 2011).

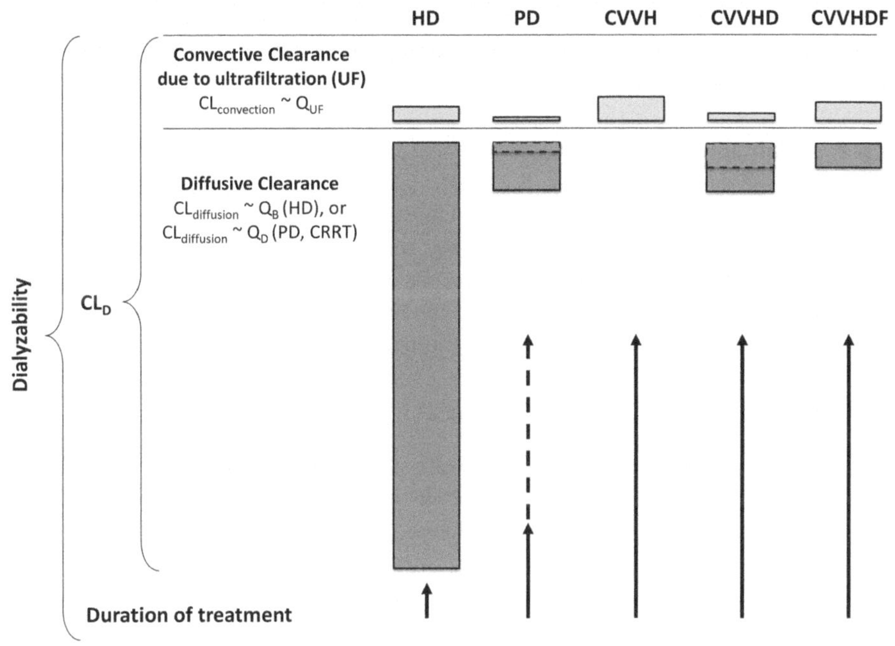

Fig. 3 Comparison of total dialysis clearance ($CL_D = CL_{convection}$ (*light gray bars*) + $CL_{diffusion}$ (*dark gray bars*)) and relative treatment duration (*arrow lengths*) for different renal replacement therapies (for numbers: see Table 1). Dialyzability is determined by both CL_D and treatment duration. *HD* intermittent hemodialysis, *PD* peritoneal dialysis, *CVVH* continuous veno-venous hemofiltration, *CVVHD* continuous veno-venous hemodialysis, *CVVHDF* continuous veno-venous hemodiafiltration

4.2 Principles of Dose Adjustment

4.2.1 Loading Dose

If the drug's half-life is significantly increased in the patient with impaired kidney function, a loading dose (D_L) may be useful to quickly achieve therapeutic target concentrations (C_{target}).

$$D_L = C_{target} \cdot V_D \tag{1a}$$

The estimate of the patient's volume of distribution (V_D) may be easily verified by measuring pre-dose (C_{trough}) and peak plasma concentration (C_{max}) for a drug that quickly distributes homogenously into body tissues (as demonstrated by one-compartment distribution kinetics), when given as i.v. bolus:

$$V_D = D\,(\text{i.v.})/\left(C_{max} - C_{trough}\right) \tag{1b}$$

Note that for drugs with multicompartmental distribution kinetics more plasma samples in the elimination phase will be necessary to reliably estimate corresponding peripheral and central volumes of distribution. Also note that the apparent volume of distribution (V_D/F) estimated after extravascular administration can be altered by changes in the bioavailability (F).

4.2.2 Maintenance Dose

Changes in the daily maintenance dose ($D_{M,24h}$) in the absence of dialysis treatment are mainly proposed with the goal to achieve equal daily area under the curve ($AUC_{24h,patient} = AUC_{24h,normal}$). The extra-renal elimination fraction in patients with normal renal function (Q_0) is frequently used to estimate the required dose adjustment (Dettli 1976), assuming equal bioavailability and nonrenal clearance in patients with and without impaired kidney function:

$$D_{M,24h} = (D_{normal,24h} \cdot Q_0) + \left(D_{normal,24h} \cdot (1 - Q_0) \cdot GFR_{patient}/GFR_{normal}\right) \quad (2)$$

with $D_{normal,24h}$ being the normal daily reference dose and GFR_{normal} the GFR of patient with normal kidney function (in adults ≈ 100–120 mL/min = 6–7.2 L/h).

For some drugs it is important to achieve C_{trough} within the therapeutic range (e.g., vancomycin) or to achieve C_{max} (e.g., aminoglycosides). For such drugs it may be appropriate to alter also the normal dosing frequency of the drug in addition to the total daily dose. Such optimal dosing regimens are usually derived from pharmacometric modeling and simulation.

4.2.3 Supplemental Dose

To evaluate the need of a supplemental dose ($D_{supplement}$), the amount of drug removed ($A_{removed}$) has to be measured directly or estimated from dialysis clearance (CL_D) and the fraction of drug removed by dialysis (f_{el}):

$$D_{supplement} = A_{removed} = A_{pre} \cdot f_{el} \quad (3a)$$

$$A_{pre} = C_{pre} \cdot V_D \quad (3b)$$

$$f_{el} = f_{tot,on} \cdot f_{HD} \quad (3c)$$

$$f_{tot,on} = 1 - \exp(-(CL_D + CL_{off})/V_D \cdot time) \quad (3d)$$

$$f_{HD} = CL_D/(CL_D + CL_{off}) = CL_D/CL_{tot,on} \quad (3e)$$

with A_{pre} being the amount of drug in the body before the start of dialysis, which can be calculated from the pre-dialysis concentration C_{pre} and V_D.

$f_{tot,on}$ is the total drug fraction lost from body during dialysis, f_{HD} is the fraction of elimination imputable to dialysis. CL_D is not to be confounded with total drug clearance *during* dialysis ($CL_{tot,on} = CL_D + CL_{off}$, see Fig. 2) and f_{el} not with fraction of drug removed *during* dialysis ($f_{tot,on}$, frequently reported as "reduction ratio" = $1 - C_{post\text{-}HD}/C_{pre\text{-}HD}$). The reduction ratio can additionally be a misleading indicator of drug removal during dialysis for drugs with multicompartmental distribution kinetics, as indicated by a post-dialysis rebound in drug concentrations.

4.3 Calculation, Prediction and Scaling of Dialysis Clearance

Guidance has been published to evaluate A_{removed} and CL_D for patients on CRRT, IHD, and PD, and regulatory guidance is available for new chemical entities, which mainly relates to IHD (see below: "further guidance"). Main aspects applying to all three RRT modalities are summarized in the following. A_{removed} and CL_D are best calculated using the "recovery method," a gold-standard method that is also used to determine renal clearance (Atkinson and Umans 2009). More mechanistic approaches to predict or scale CL_D can be used in a complementary manner, or when the recovery method is not feasible. Guidance about optimal scaling of dialysis clearance is limited; some potential useful approaches are discussed in the following.

4.3.1 Intermittent Hemodialysis

Calculation of A_{removed} and CL_D using the "recovery method" requires collection of the total dialysate volume (V_{dial}) as well as measurement of the drug's concentration in the dialysate (C_{dial}):

$$A_{\text{removed}} = C_{\text{dial}} \cdot V_{\text{dial}} \tag{4a}$$

Hemodialysis clearance ($\text{CL}_{D,\text{HD}}$) can then be calculated from the area under the curve of plasmatic concentrations during dialysis ($\text{AUC}_{0\text{-}t}$) over the dialysis duration (time t). Alternatively, the average plasma concentration (C_{av}) entering the dialyzer over time may be used (Gotta et al. 2017):

$$\text{CL}_{D,\text{HD}} = \frac{A_{\text{removed}}}{\text{AUC}_{0\text{-}t}} = \frac{A_{\text{removed}}}{C_{\text{av}} \cdot t} \tag{4b}$$

A limiting factor in praxis can be however that the V_{dial} is too large to be collected, and that C_{dial} is that low that it cannot be well quantified by analytical methods. In rare cases adsorption or metabolism at the dialysis membrane may further lead to underestimation of CL_D by this method (Shiraishi et al. 2012).

Alternatively, the "AV-difference method" can be applied to first estimate CL_D and then predict A_{removed}. Therefore, one or several paired pre- and post-dialyzer plasma concentration samples ($C_{\text{pre-filter}}$ and $C_{\text{post-filter}} = C_{\text{Arterial}}$ and C_{Venous}) are collected during dialysis to calculate the extraction ratio (ER) of the drug:

$$\text{ER} = \frac{C_A - C_V}{C_A} = \frac{C_{\text{pre-filter}} - C_{\text{post-filter}}}{C_{\text{pre-filter}}} \tag{5a}$$

Since blood flow (Q_B) is slower than Q_D in chronic HD, Q_B becomes the limiting factor for dialysis clearance ($\text{CL}_{D,\text{blood}} \leq Q_B$). In most instances pharmacokinetic parameters relate to plasma rather than whole blood, and hence the plasma flow through the dialyzer (Q_P) needs to be predicted from the drug's blood-to-plasma concentration ratio (R_{bp}) (Atkinson and Susla 2012):

$$Q_P = Q_B \cdot R_{\text{b:p}} \tag{5b}$$

$$\text{CL}_{D,\text{HD}} = Q_P \cdot \text{ER} \tag{5c}$$

Assuming that the maximum ER that can be achieved equals the unbound fraction (f_u) of the drug (i.e., all unbound drug molecules are cleared during their passage through the filter), Eq. (5c) simplifies to (Gotta et al. 2017):

$$\text{Maximum CL}_{D,\text{HD}} = Q_P \cdot f_u \tag{5d}$$

Clearance rate for a small molecule like urea ($R_{\text{bp}} = 1$) (Odeh et al. 1993) is around 250–275 mL/min under a blood flow of 300–400 mL/min (resulting ER = 0.68–0.83) (Gotta et al. 2018).

One may assume that scaling of dialysis clearance calculated in adults ($Q_B \approx 400$ mL/min) may be achieved by replacing Q_B by pediatric blood flow rates (Q_B ranging from ≈70 to 350 mL/min in infants and adolescents (Gotta et al. 2018)) in Eq. (5c), when ER has been reported in adults. However, in this case it needs to be considered that the ER is likely to be altered pediatric patients due to several factors: (1) different surface area and associated mass-transfer area coefficient (KoA) for various solutes (KoA for urea in mL/min/kg tends to be higher in lower weight patients), (2) frequent use of low-flux filters in children compared to adolescents and adults, (3) higher dialysis to blood flow ratios prescribed ($Q_D/Q_B \approx 1.5$ in adults versus a range of ≈4.7 to ≈2 in infants and adolescents (Gotta et al. 2018)), which increases the concentration gradient between blood and dialysis fluid, and hence the efficiency of dialysis.

Hence, a better scaling approach would be to account for those factors, using a mechanistic equation derived for this purpose, developed for countercurrent flow (Michaels 1966) (Fig. 4):

$$\text{CL}_{D,\text{blood}} = Q_B \cdot \frac{e^{(z)} - 1}{\left(e^z - \frac{Q_B}{Q_D}\right)}, \quad \text{with} \quad z = \frac{\text{koA}}{Q_D} \cdot \left(1 - \frac{Q_B}{Q_D}\right) \tag{6a}$$

This equation has been successfully used to scale dabigatran dialysis clearance over a blood flow range of 200–400 mL/min in adults (Liesenfeld et al. 2013), after the estimation of dabigatran filter KoA in vivo. Indeed, this equation could explain why dialysis clearance only increases by 30% when increasing blood flow by 100% (doubling from 200 to 400 mL/min).

Although KoA is assumed to be a constant, it can be filter-specific, lower in low- versus high-flux filters, and increase in vivo with high dialysate to blood flow ratios, as used in infants. For urea, the following correction equation allowed to obtain nonbiased urea dialysis clearance prediction over a large age and weight range (Gotta et al. 2019a):

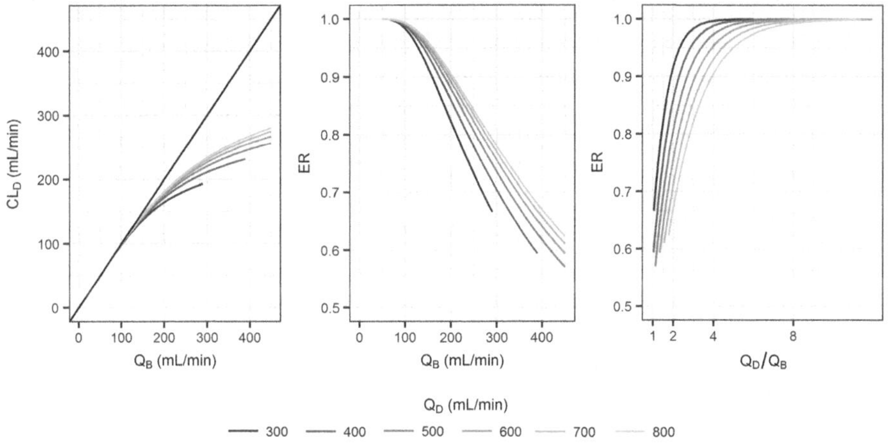

Fig. 4 Illustration of mechanistically derived nonlinear relationship between increase in blood flow (Q_B) and dialysis clearance (CL_D) (*left*), corresponding decline in the extraction ratio ($ER = CL_D/Q_B$) (*middle*), and dependence of the ER on Q_D/Q_B ratio (*right*) (Michaels 1966). Simulations were made using a mass-transfer area coefficient (KoA) of 560 mL/min

$$\mathrm{KoA}_c = \mathrm{KoA} \cdot f_{c,\,\mathrm{KoA}} \tag{6b}$$

$$f_{c,\,\mathrm{KoA}} = 1 \cdot \left(\frac{Q_D}{Q_B}/1.5\right)^{0.625} \cdot (0.883 \quad \text{if lowflux}) \tag{6c}$$

where KoA_c is the corrected KoA value, and $f_{c,\mathrm{KoA}}$ is the in vivo correction factor.

Increasing blood flow in adults may further result in a sub-proportional increase in dialysis clearance because actual blood flow does not increase linearly with the prescribed flow. A correction equation has been proposed for this purpose (Depner et al. 2004):

$$\begin{aligned} Q_{(B,\mathrm{true})} &= Q_B - 0.0122 \cdot Q_B \cdot ((Q_B - 200)/100)^{2.37}, \quad \text{for } Q_B > 200\,\mathrm{mL/min} \\ Q_{(B,\mathrm{true})} &= Q_B, \quad \text{for } Q_B \leq 200\,\mathrm{mL/min} \end{aligned} \tag{7}$$

4.3.2 Peritoneal Dialysis

In line with Eqs. (4a) and (4b) also peritoneal dialysis clearance (CL_{PD}) is best calculated using the recovery method (Paton et al. 1985; Blowey 2004):

$$CL_{D,\mathrm{PD}} = \frac{A_{\mathrm{removed}}}{\mathrm{AUC}_{0\text{-}t}} = \frac{C_{\mathrm{dial}} \cdot V_{\mathrm{PD,\,drain}}}{\mathrm{AUC}_{0\text{-}t}} = \frac{C_{\mathrm{dial}} \cdot V_{\mathrm{PD,\,drain}}}{C_{\mathrm{av,\,plasma}} \cdot t} \tag{8a}$$

where $V_{\mathrm{PD,drain}}$ is the drain volume (sum of fill volume and ultrafiltrate), C_{dial} is the drug concentration in the dialysate, $C_{\mathrm{av,plasma}}$ is the average drug plasma concentration, and t is the dwelling time. Small molecules like urea rapidly equilibrate (within ≈120 min) (Madhukar and Ramesh 2018; Roychowdhury and Talpaz 2011) with the dialysate ($C_{\mathrm{dial}}/C_{\mathrm{plasma}} \rightarrow 1$), and Eq. (8a) can then be approximated by

$CL_{CAPD} \approx V_{PD,drain}/t \approx Q_{D,PD}$. The clearance rate of small molecules like urea is ≈10 mL/min, and thus small compared to intermittent HD (Matzke et al. 2011). In line with that, also drug peritoneal clearance for many hydrophilic antibiotics has been reported mainly ≤10 mL/min in continuous ambulatory PD (Paton et al. 1985). However, the fraction of dose eliminated can still be significant for hydrophilic drugs poorly bound to plasma proteins like amikacin ($f_{el} = 50\%$) (Keller et al. 1990). It should also be considered that patients on PD may have more frequently residual renal function than patients on intermittent HD, and that dialysate instilled into the peritoneal cavity can be a significant part of total V_D of a drug.

In the absence of pharmacokinetic data and assuming that CL_D in peritoneal dialysis is limited by the dialysate outflow rate ($Q_{D,PD} = V_{PD,drain}/\text{time} << $ splanchnic blood flow) and that all unbound drug is eliminated ($f_{tot,on} \approx f_u$), the fraction of dose eliminated by peritoneal dialysis can be approximated by (Keller et al. 1990):

$$f_{el} \approx Q_{D,PD}/\left(Q_{D,PD} + CL_{off}\right) \cdot f_u \tag{8b}$$

This equation has been shown for example to yield good predictions of f_{el} for amikacin (hydrophilic molecule distributing mainly into extracellular body water with V_D of ≈0.28 L/kg, and low protein binding with $f_u \geq 0.9$). For larger molecules like vancomycin (MW = 1,448 g/mol) however, dwell time may be insufficient to reach equilibrium during a dwell period, leading to overestimation of f_{el} by Eq. (8b) (Keller et al. 1990).

4.3.3 Continuous Renal Replacement Therapies (CRRT)

As illustrated in Fig. 2, diffusive clearance during CRRT is lower than in intermittent HD, while convective clearance can be increased due to higher ultrafiltration, which is compensated by adding replacement fluid before or after the filter. As for HD (Eqs. 4a and 4b), the "recovery method" is also used as gold standard for all CRRT techniques for clearance calculation (Atkinson and Susla 2012):

$$CL_{D,CRRT} = \frac{C_{effluent} \cdot V_{effluent}}{AUC_{0\text{-}t}} = \frac{C_{effluent} \cdot V_{effluent}}{C_{av,plasma} \cdot t} \tag{9a}$$

where $C_{effluent}$ is the drug concentration in the dialysate ($=C_{Dial}$) in CVVHD, the drug concentration in the ultrafiltrate ($=C_{UF}$) in CVVHF, or the concentration in the effluent containing both dialysate and ultrafiltrate in CVVHDF (Mueller and Golper 2019). $V_{effluent}$ is the volume of effluent collected (dialysate, ultrafiltrate, or both) over a given time interval (time t).

Assuming that the ratio of $C_{effluent}$ to C_{plasma} is constant throughout the treatment, and given that the ratio of $V_{effluent}/t$ equals the effluent rate $Q_{effluent}$ ($=Q_D$ in CVVHD, $=Q_{UF}$ in CVVHF, and $=Q_D + Q_{UF}$ in CVVHDF, respectively), a simple estimate of dialysis clearance can be obtained by (Veltri et al. 2004):

$$CL_{D,\mathrm{CRRT}} = Q_{\mathrm{effluent}} \cdot \frac{C_{\mathrm{effluent}}}{C_{\mathrm{plasma}}} = Q_{\mathrm{effluent}} \cdot \frac{C_{\mathrm{effluent}}}{(C_A - C_V)/2} \approx Q_{\mathrm{effluent}} \cdot f_u \tag{9b}$$

Note that in CVVHD, CL_D is limited by Q_D – in contrast to Q_B in chronic HD. While the ratio $C_{\mathrm{effluent}}/C_{\mathrm{plasma}}$ is called dialysate saturation coefficient (SD) in CVVHD and CVVHDF, the ratio $C_{\mathrm{UF}}/C_{\mathrm{plasma}}$ is called sieving coefficient (SC) in CVVH (Atkinson and Susla 2012; Mueller and Golper 2019). SD in fact depends on the Q_B/Q_D ratio, and hence $CL_{D,\mathrm{CRRT}}$ will not increase linearly with increasing Q_D, especially for larger molecules. At slow dialysate flow rates SD will be close to SC as there is enough time for equilibration. CL_D in CVVHDF may be lower than the sum of convective and diffusive clearance obtained under equivalent CVVH and CVVHD prescriptions, since convection can decrease the concentration gradient driving diffusion (Mueller and Golper 2019). The SC in CVVH frequently equals f_u of a drug (Blowey 2004; Pea et al. 2007). Care has to be taken, when f_u is significantly altered in a patient, or when drug adsorption to the hemofilter occurs.

In contrast to HD, replacement fluid is given in CVVH and CVVHDF, which can be added before or after the filter (pre- or postdilution mode). For the postdilution mode (Pea et al. 2007) Eq. (9b) applies (simplified presentation):

$$CL_{D(\mathrm{postdilution})} = Q_{\mathrm{effluent}} \cdot \mathrm{SC} \tag{9c}$$

In the predilution model, plasma is diluted by the substitution fluid before entering the filter, and drug clearance will hence be lower, which can be expressed as a dilution factor (DF) (Pea et al. 2007):

$$\begin{aligned} CL_{D(\mathrm{predilution})} &= Q_{\mathrm{effluent}} \cdot \mathrm{SC} \cdot \mathrm{DF} \\ \mathrm{DF} &= Q_B/(Q_B + Q_{\mathrm{UF}}) \end{aligned} \tag{9d}$$

Q_B should be further corrected for red blood cell distribution (see Eq. 5b) to obtain an estimate of plasmatic DF (Mueller and Golper 2019).

4.4 Further Guidance and Role of Pharmacometric Modeling and Simulation

Besides regulatory guidance (Center for Drug Evaluation and Research (CDER) 2010; Committee for Medicinal Products for Human use (CHMP) 2015), clinically oriented recommendations are available for pharmacokinetic assessment, dose individualization strategies, and transparent reporting of pharmacokinetics in patients on dialysis due to poisoning and chronic or acute renal failure (Matzke et al. 2011; Lavergne et al. 2014; Nolin et al. 2015; Gotta et al. 2017). Key parameters to be determined include CL_D, CL_{off}, or CL_{NR} and V_D in the dialysis patient (Fig. 1), and it can be advised to measure f_u to re-evaluate total target concentrations.

In combination with pharmacokinetic calculations cited above, pharmacometric modeling and simulation is recognized as a useful tool to develop optimal and personalized dose recommendations for patients with kidney disease (Zhang et al.

2014; Rodieux et al. 2015; Gotta et al. 2017). Many drug labels have been enhanced by such pharmacometric approaches, as, e.g., demonstrated for saxagliptin (Zhang et al. 2012). Depending on the study and sampling design, such methods allow for example: estimation or integration of multicompartmental distribution kinetics, which is important to account for a potential rebound in drug concentration after IHD; estimation or integration of changes in the apparent volume of distribution; incorporation of relevant literature or in vitro data; and inter- or extrapolation of pharmacokinetics to new patient populations, such as patients of different age, weight, and kidney function (Zhang et al. 2012) or on different dialysis prescription (Liesenfeld et al. 2013).

References

Akcan-Arikan A, Zappitelli M, Loftis LL et al (2007) Modified RIFLE criteria in critically ill children with acute kidney injury. Kidney Int 71:1028–1035

Andreoli S (2004) Acute renal failure: clinical evaluation and management. In: Avner E, Harmon W, Niaudet P (eds) Pediatric nephrology. Lippincott Williams & Wilkins, Philadelphia, pp 1233–1251

Andreoli SP (2009) Acute kidney injury in children. Pediatr Nephrol 24:253–263

Atkinson AJ, Susla GM (2012) Pharmacokinetics in patients requiring renal replacement therapy. In: Huang S-M, Lertora J, Atkinson A (eds) Principles of clinical pharmacology, 3rd edn. Elsevier, San Diego, pp 65–79

Atkinson AJ, Umans JG (2009) Pharmacokinetic studies in hemodialysis patients. Clin Pharmacol Ther 86:548–552

Auron A, Brophy PD (2012) Hyperammonemia in review: pathophysiology, diagnosis, and treatment. Pediatr Nephrol 27:207–222

Benfield M, Bunchman T (2004) Management of acute renal failure. In: Pediatric nephrology. Lippincott Williams & Wilkins, Philadelphia, pp 1253–1266

Blowey D (2004) Principles of drug administration in children receiving renal replacement therapy. In: Warady B, Schaefer F, Fine R, Alexander S (eds) Pediatric dialysis. Springer, Dordrecht, pp 545–565

Brophy PD (2008) Renal supportive therapy for pediatric acute kidney injury in the setting of multiorgan dysfunction syndrome/sepsis. Semin Nephrol 28:457–469

Brou NA, Jacqz-Aigrain E, Zhao W (2015) Cystatin C as a potential biomarker for dosing of renally excreted drugs. Br J Clin Pharmacol 80:20–27

Bunchman TE, Ferris ME (2011) Management of toxic ingestions with the use of renal replacement therapy. Pediatr Nephrol 26:535–541

Cella M, Knibbe C, Danhof M, Della Pasqua O (2010) What is the right dose for children? Br J Clin Pharmacol 70:597–603

Center for Drug Evaluation and Research (CDER) (2010) Guidance for industry pharmacokinetics in patients with impaired renal function – study design, data analysis, and impact on dosing and labeling. CDER, Rockville

Chua AN, Warady BA (2017) Care of the pediatric patient on chronic dialysis. Adv Chronic Kidney Dis 24:388–397

Clarkson M, Magee C, Brenner B (2010) Peritoneal dialysis. In: Clarkson M, Magee C, Brenner B (eds) Pocket companion to Brenner & Rector's the kidney. Elsevier, Philadelphia, pp 730–752

Committee for Medicinal Products for Human use (CHMP) (2015) Guideline on the evaluation of the pharmacokinetics of medicinal products in patients with decreased renal function. CHMP, London

Dao K, Chtioui H, Lu Y et al (2017) Pharmacokinetics of pomalidomide in a patient receiving hemodialysis using a high-cutoff filter. Am J Kidney Dis 69:553–554

Depner TA, Greene T, Daugirdas JT et al (2004) Dialyzer performance in the HEMO study: in vivo K0A and true blood flow determined from a model of cross-dialyzer urea extraction. ASAIO J 50:85–93

Dettli L (1976) Drug dosage in renal disease. Clin Pharmacokinet 1:126–134

Downes KJ, Dong M, Fukuda T et al (2017) Urinary kidney injury biomarkers and tobramycin clearance among children and young adults with cystic fibrosis: a population pharmacokinetic analysis. J Antimicrob Chemother 72:254–260

Duranton F, Cohen G, De Smet R et al (2012) Normal and pathologic concentrations of uremic toxins. J Am Soc Nephrol 23:1258–1270

Golper TA, Fissell R, Fissell WH et al (2014) Hemodialysis: core curriculum 2014. Am J Kidney Dis 63:153–163

Gotta V, Dao K, Rodieux F et al (2017) Guidance to develop individual dose recommendations for patients on chronic hemodialysis. Expert Rev Clin Pharmacol 10:737–752

Gotta V, Marsenic O, Pfister M (2018) Age- and weight-based differences in haemodialysis prescription and delivery in children, adolescents and young adults. Nephrol Dial Transplant 33:1649–1660

Gotta V, Marsenic O, Pfister M (2019a) Understanding urea kinetic factors that enhance personalized hemodialysis prescription in children. ASAIO J. https://doi.org/10.1097/MAT.0000000000000941

Gotta V, Pfister M, Marsenic O (2019b) Ultrafiltration rates in children on chronic hemodialysis routinely exceed weight based adult limit. Hemodial Int 23:126–128

Griffin BR, Faubel S, Edelstein CL (2018) Biomarkers of drug-induced kidney toxicity. Ther Drug Monit 41:213–226

KDIGO (Kidney Disease: Improving Global Outcomes) CKD Work Group (2013) KDIGO 2012 clinical practice guideline for the evaluation and management of chronic kidney disease – Kidney International Supplements. J Int Soc Nephrol 3:1–150

Keller E, Reetze P, Schollmeyer P (1990) Drug therapy in patients undergoing continuous ambulatory peritoneal dialysis. Clin Pharmacokinet 18:104–117

Khanal A, Castelino RL, Peterson GM, Jose MD (2014) Dose adjustment guidelines for medications in patients with renal impairment: how consistent are drug information sources? Intern Med J 44:77–85

Knoderer CA, Leiser JD, Nailescu C et al (2008) Fenoldopam for acute kidney injury in children. Pediatr Nephrol 23:495–498

Kwiatkowski DM, Sutherland SM (2017) Acute kidney injury in pediatric patients. Best Pract Res Clin Anaesthesiol 31:427–439

Lavergne V, Ouellet G, Bouchard J et al (2014) Guidelines for reporting case studies on extracorporeal treatments in poisonings: methodology. Semin Dial 27:407–414

Liesenfeld KH, Staab A, Härtter S et al (2013) Pharmacometric characterization of dabigatran hemodialysis. Clin Pharmacokinet 52:453–462

Madhukar M, Ramesh K (2018) Mechanisms of solute clearance and ultrafiltration in peritoneal dialysis. www.uptodate.com. Accessed 1 Feb 2019

Marsenic O, Baluarte H (2011) Acute and chronic renal failure. In: Florin T, Ludwig S, Aronson P, Werner H (eds) Netter's pediatrics. Elsevier, Philadelphia, pp 397–407

Matzke GR, Aronoff GR, Atkinson AJ et al (2011) Drug dosing consideration in patients with acute and chronic kidney disease – a clinical update from Kidney Disease: Improving Global Outcomes (KDIGO). Kidney Int 80:1122–1137

Matzke GR, Dowling TC, Marks SA, Murphy JE (2016) Influence of kidney disease on drug disposition: an assessment of industry studies submitted to the FDA for new chemical entities 1999-2010. J Clin Pharmacol 56:390–398

Mehta RL (1999) Supportive therapies: intermittent hemodialysis, continuous renal replacement therapies, and peritoneal dialysis. In: Schrier RW (ed) Atlas of diseases of the kidney, vol 1, online edn. Wiley-Blackwell, Philadelphia, pp 19.1–19.16. www.kidneyatlas.org

Metsvaht T, Nellis G, Varendi H et al (2015) High variability in the dosing of commonly used antibiotics revealed by a Europe-wide point prevalence study: implications for research and dissemination. BMC Pediatr 15:14

Michaels AS (1966) Operating parameters and performance criteria for hemodialyzers and other membrane-separation devices. Trans Am Soc Artif Intern Organs 12:387–392

Mueller BA, Golper TA (2019) Drug removal in continuous renal replacement therapy. In: UpToDate. www.uptodate.com. Accessed 1 Feb 2019

Mueller BA, Smoyer WE (2009) Challenges in developing evidence-based drug dosing guidelines for adults and children receiving renal replacement therapy. Clin Pharmacol Ther 86:479–482

Murray P, Liu K (2011) Management of renal replacement therapy in acute kidney injury. Nephrol Self Assess Program 10:242–246

Nolin TD, Naud J, Leblond FA, Pichette V (2008) Emerging evidence of the impact of kidney disease on drug metabolism and transport. Clin Pharmacol Ther 83:898–903

Nolin TD, Aronoff GR, Fissell WH et al (2015) Pharmacokinetic assessment in patients receiving continuous RRT: perspectives from the kidney health initiative. Clin J Am Soc Nephrol 10:159–164

Odeh YK, Wang Z, Ruo TI et al (1993) Simultaneous analysis of inulin and 15N2-urea kinetics in humans. Clin Pharmacol Ther 53:419–425

Paton TW, Cornish WR, Manuel MA, Hardy BG (1985) Drug therapy in patients undergoing peritoneal dialysis clinical pharmacokinetic considerations. Clin Pharmacokinet 10:404–426

Pea F, Viale P, Pavan F, Furlanut M (2007) Pharmacokinetic considerations for antimicrobial therapy in patients receiving renal replacement therapy. Clin Pharmacokinet 46:997–1038

Rees L, Schaefer F, Schmitt CP et al (2017) Chronic dialysis in children and adolescents: challenges and outcomes. Lancet Child Adolesc Health 1:68–77

Rodieux F, Wilbaux M, van den Anker JN, Pfister M (2015) Effect of kidney function on drug kinetics and dosing in neonates, infants, and children. Clin Pharmacokinet 54:1183–1204

Roychowdhury S, Talpaz M (2011) Managing resistance in chronic myeloid leukemia. Blood Rev 25:279–290

Shiraishi Y, Okajima M, Sai Y et al (2012) Elimination of teicoplanin by adsorption to the filter membrane during haemodiafiltration: screening experiments for linezolid, teicoplanin and vancomycin followed by in vitro haemodiafiltration models for teicoplanin. Anaesth Intensive Care 40:442–449

Sutherland SM, Alexander SR (2012) Continuous renal replacement therapy in children. Pediatr Nephrol 27:2007–2016

Ulinski T, Sellier-Leclerc A-L, Tudorache E et al (2012) Acute tubulointerstitial nephritis. Pediatr Nephrol 27:1051–1057

Veltri MA, Neu AM, Fivush BA et al (2004) Drug dosing during intermittent hemodialysis and continuous renal replacement therapy: special considerations in pediatric patients. Paediatr Drugs 6:45–65

Verrina E, Cappelli V, Perfumo F (2009) Selection of modalities, prescription, and technical issues in children on peritoneal dialysis. Pediatr Nephrol 24:1453–1464

Vidal L, Shavit M, Fraser A et al (2005) Systematic comparison of four sources of drug information regarding adjustment of dose for renal function. Br Med J 331:263–266

Vilay AM, Churchwell MD, Mueller BA (2008) Clinical review: drug metabolism and nonrenal clearance in acute kidney injury. Crit Care 12:235

Walters S, Porter C, Brophy PD (2009) Dialysis and pediatric acute kidney injury: choice of renal support modality. Pediatr Nephrol 24:37–48

Warady B, Morgenstern B, Alexander S (2004) Peritoneal dialysis. In: Avner E, Harmon W, Niaudet P (eds) Pediatric nephrology. Lippincott Williams & Wilkins, Philadelphia, pp 1375–1394

Zepeda-Orozco D, Quigley R (2012) Dialysis disequilibrium syndrome. Pediatr Nephrol 27:2205–2211

Zhang L, Boulton DW, Pfister M (2012) A pharmacometric approach to quantify the impact of chronic kidney disease and hemodialysis on systemic drug exposure: application to saxagliptin. J Clin Pharmacol 52:126S–133S

Zhang L, Roy A, Pfister M (2014) Pharmacometrics in chronic kidney disease. In: Crommelin DJA, Lipper RA (eds) Applied pharmacometrics. American Association of Pharmaceutical Scientists 2014. Springer, New York, pp 109–137

Pharmacokinetics and Pharmacodynamics of Drugs in Obese Pediatric Patients: How to Map Uncharted Clinical Territories

Elke H. J. Krekels and Catherijne A. J. Knibbe

Contents

Abstract

Clinicians are increasingly faced with challenges regarding the pharmacological treatment of obese pediatric patients. To provide guidance for these treatments, a better understanding of the impact of obesity on pharmacological processes in children is needed. Results on pharmacological studies in adults show however ambiguous patterns regarding the impact of obesity on ADME processes or on drug pharmacodynamics. Additionally, based on the limited research performed

E. H. J. Krekels
Division of Systems Biomedicine and Pharmacology, Leiden Academic Centre for Drug Research, Leiden University, Leiden, The Netherlands

C. A. J. Knibbe (✉)
Division of Systems Biomedicine and Pharmacology, Leiden Academic Centre for Drug Research, Leiden University, Leiden, The Netherlands

Department of Clinical Pharmacy, St. Antonius Hospital, Nieuwegein, The Netherlands
e-mail: c.knibbe@antoniusziekenhuis.nl

W. Kiess et al. (eds.), *Pediatric Pharmacotherapy*,
Handbook of Experimental Pharmacology 261, https://doi.org/10.1007/164_2019_250

in obese pediatric patients, it becomes clear that findings from obese adults cannot be expected to always translate directly to similar findings in obese children. To improve knowledge on drug pharmacology in obese pediatric patients, studies should focus on quantifying the impact of maturation, obesity, and other relevant variables on primary pharmacological parameters and on disentangling systemic (renal and/or hepatic) and presystemic (gut and/or first-pass hepatic) clearance. For this, data is required from well-designed clinical trials that include patients with not only a wide range in age but also a range in excess body weight, upon oral and intravenous dosing. Population modelling approaches are ideally suitable for this purpose and can also be used to link the pharmacokinetics to pharmacodynamics and to derive drug dosing regimens. Generalizability of research findings can be achieved by including mechanistic aspects in the data analysis, for instance, using either extrapolation approaches in population modelling or by applying physiologically based modelling principles. It is imperative that more and smarter studies are performed in obese pediatric patients to provide safe and effective treatment for this special patient population.

Keywords

ADME · Obesity · Pediatrics · Pharmacodynamics · Pharmacokinetics · Physiologically based modelling · Population modelling

1 Introduction

Around the world, the body weight of both adult and pediatric populations is generally increasing (Abarca-Gómez et al. 2017), and as a result, clinicians are increasingly faced with pharmacological treatment challenges for overweight and obese patients. In children, a global definition of overweight or obesity is lacking, but most definitions are based on a comparison of body mass index (BMI; the ratio of body weight in kg and the square of the length in m) to age- and sex-specific values, although there is evidence that using BMI to define obesity may lead to underestimation of the problem (Reilly et al. 2018). The CDC, for instance, defines overweight and obesity in children and adolescents as BMI above the 85th or 95th percentile of age- and sex-specific values in their growth charts, respectively. In 2013 an extensive survey found 23.8% of boys and 22.6% of girls to be either overweight or obese in developed countries, while in developing countries these numbers were 12.9% and 13.4%, respectively (Ng et al. 2014).

Obesity leads to physiological changes to the extent that the American Medical Association has officially classified obesity as a disease in 2013. Both adipose tissue and lean body weight are increased in obesity, with the ratio of fat and lean body mass being higher than in non-obese individuals. It is now also widely believed that both obese adult and obese pediatric patients are in a chronic state of low-grade inflammation (Wellen and Hotamisligil 2003; Rainone et al. 2016), which may impact the expression of metabolic enzymes, drug transporters, and plasma proteins (Ulvestad et al. 2013; Blouin et al. 1987). These and other changes may impact processes underlying the pharmacokinetics and pharmacodynamics of drugs, resulting in increased variability in drug pharmacology. The impact of these changes needs to be understood, to be able to provide guidance on safe and effective drug dosing in obese (pediatric) patients.

This paper provides an overview of current knowledge on the impact of overweight and obesity on the pharmacokinetics and pharmacodynamics of drugs. Specific focus is on pediatric patients; however, as the amount of information in this special population is very limited, findings in the adult population are also reviewed to assess whether generalizations from this population can be derived. Subsequently, guidance will be provided on how to perform future studies on drug pharmacology in obese children.

2 Drug Pharmacology in Obese Adults

Drug exposure is dependent on processes related to absorption, distribution, metabolism, and excretion (ADME), which together results in pharmacokinetic profiles of drugs. The impact of obesity on ADME processes of different drugs has to a certain extent been studied in adults. However, findings from studies on different drugs, even when metabolized by the same pathway, are sometimes counterintuitive or may appear contradictory, making it difficult to derive generalizable dosing recommendations, even for adults.

Drug responses are dependent on both pharmacokinetics and pharmacodynamics, meaning that both drug exposure and the exposure-response relationships will result in desired and undesired drug effects. A small number of adult studies have shown that not just drug pharmacokinetics, but also drug pharmacodynamics may be altered with obesity.

2.1 Absorption in Obese Adults

The most common route for drug administration is oral. Factors that may impact the absorption rate and/or the bioavailability of orally administered drugs in obese patients include an increase in gastric emptying and intestinal motility (Xing and Chen 2004; Cardoso-Júnior et al. 2007), increased permeability of the gut due to loss of tight junction function and resulting increases in paracellular transport, which was observed both in adults and in children (Rainone et al. 2016; Teixeira et al. 2012), decreased expression of CYP enzymes in the gut and liver, which was found to increase with BMI in adults (Ulvestad et al. 2013), and increased splanchnic blood flow, which may carry drugs away faster from the metabolic enzymes in the gut wall (Alexander et al. 1962–1963).

Interestingly, for trazodone (Greenblatt et al. 1987), cyclosporine (Flechner et al. 1989), dexfenfluramine (Cheymol et al. 1995), and moxifloxacin (Kees et al. 2011), obesity was found to not impact bioavailability, despite the aforementioned physiological changes in obese patients. For propranolol a trend toward higher bioavailability in obese patients compared to non-obese patients was found, based on similar systemic clearance values in both groups upon intravenous dosing but smaller oral apparent clearance values in the obese upon oral dosing (Bowman et al. 1986). Similar trends in oral apparent clearance have been observed for alprazolam and triazolam, which for triazolam even reached statistical significance (Abernethy et al. 1984). However, in the absence of data upon intravenous dosing, it cannot be established whether these differences indeed arise from differences in bioavailability, from differences in clearance, or a combination of both. The same limitation applies to a study on vortioxetine, in which based on similar areas under the concentration-time curve (AUC) and steady-state concentrations (Greenblatt et al. 2018a), the bioavailability for vortioxetine can be assumed to be similar between obese and non-obese patients, while another possible explanation for the presented observations is that bioavailability and clearance change with similar magnitudes. For midazolam, one study did not find a difference in the bioavailability between obese and non-obese patients (Greenblatt et al. 1984), while a later study did find an increased bioavailability for midazolam in morbidly obese patients (Brill et al. 2014a). These differences in findings can potentially be attributed to differences in study design and data analysis, but another possible explanation could be that the latter study included patients with much higher body weights, which could imply that differences in bioavailability for midazolam only become apparent with extreme obesity, which may or may not also be linked to the duration a patient has been obese.

For midazolam, the absorption rate was found to be reduced in obese patients (Brill et al. 2014a). Studies using time to maximum concentration (Tmax) as a proxy for absorption rate suggest decreases in absorption rate of paracetamol (Lee et al. 1981) and levothyroxine (Michalaki et al. 2011) and unaltered absorption rate values for morphine (Lloret-Linares et al. 2014). It should, however, be noted that Tmax is impacted by parameters other than absorption rate and can therefore not be regarded as a pure proxy of absorption rate.

2.2 Distribution Volume in Obese Adults

Drug distribution is impacted by system-specific as well as drug-specific properties. With respect to system-specific changes in obesity, increases in the physical size of the body will increase blood and tissue volumes, additionally cardiac output and tissue perfusion might change (Alexander et al. 1962–1963; Lemmens et al. 2006), and all may be expected to impact drug distribution rates and distribution volume. Moreover, lipophilicity, a drug-specific property, may theoretically lead to increased partitioning into fat tissue, thereby increasing distribution volume for these drugs in the obese. However, specific and non-specific drug binding to blood or tissue constituents, the presence of blood constituents competing for plasma protein binding, as well as the presence of drug transporter proteins on tissue membranes may either further increase or decrease tissue partitioning and as a result lipophilicity is generally not a good predictor of distribution volume (Jain et al. 2011; Knibbe et al. 2015).

For drugs that are hydrophilic or only weakly or moderately lipophilic, partitioning into fat tissue is generally limited. It seems obesity mostly leads to at best moderate increases in distribution volume, as was seen for methylxanthines, aminoglycosides, beta-blockers, ibuprofen, phenazone, certain benzodiazepines, ranitidine, and heparin (Morgan and Bray 1994; Davis et al. 1990; Cheymol et al. 1997; Smit et al. 2019). For the hydrophilic drug vancomycin, however, both moderate and large increases in distribution volume values have been reported in the obese (Adane et al. 2015; Blouin et al. 1982).

Due to the impact of aforementioned mechanisms that may impact drug partitioning into fat, the expected increase in distribution volume of lipophilic compounds in the obese is in fact found to be highly variable. For posaconazole (Greenblatt et al. 2018b), lipophilic benzodiazepines such as midazolam (Brill et al. 2014a), thiopental sodium, phenytoin, verapamil, and lidocaine (Morgan and Bray 1994), distribution volume was found to be greatly increased in the obese, while the distribution volume for propofol, digoxin, cyclosporine, and prednisolone was found to remain constant in the obese (Morgan and Bray 1994; van Kralingen et al. 2011a; Abernethy et al. 1981).

By reducing the unbound drug fraction, plasma protein binding may limit the distribution of drugs into peripheral tissue, as only unbound drug is believed to be able to diffuse into tissue. Results regarding potential changes in concentrations of serum albumin and α1-acid glycoprotein in the obese are contradictory but generally indicated only relatively small changes (Benedek et al. 1983; Cheymol et al. 1987; Pai et al. 2007). Increases in triglycerides that may compete with drugs for plasma protein binding (Benedek et al. 1983) may increase the unbound fraction of some drugs. A decrease in unbound drug fraction has been reported for propranolol, while unbound fractions of phenytoin, alprazolam, cefazolin, daptomycin, and various benzodiazepines have been reported to remain unchanged (Abernethy et al. 1984; Greenblatt et al. 1984; Benedek et al. 1983; Cheymol et al. 1987; Pai et al. 2007; Brill et al. 2014b). It should be noted that decreased unbound drug fractions will proportionally reduce the total clearance of drugs with a low or intermediate extraction ratio, which result in unaltered unbound drug concentrations in the obese.

In addition to changes in distribution volume, it also has to be kept in mind that tissue penetration of drugs may be reduced in obese patients. For cefazolin, subcutaneous tissue concentrations were found to be considerably reduced in obese patients, while systemic exposure to this drug was similar to values in non-obese patients. Such reduced local exposure may reduce the apparent efficacy of prophylactic treatments of postoperative wound infections with this antibiotic (Brill et al. 2014b).

2.3 Metabolism in Obese Adults

Drug metabolism mainly occurs in the liver. Due to abnormal fat disposition and the low-grade chronic inflammation, nonalcoholic fatty liver disease, ranging from steatosis to nonalcoholic steatohepatitis (NASH), is common in obese individuals (Harnois et al. 2006; Machado et al. 2006). Potential other changes including changes in plasma protein binding, liver blood flow and perfusion, expression of transporters on hepatocytes, and metabolic enzymes in the hepatocytes may all further impact hepatic metabolic drug clearance. How these changes impact the hepatic metabolism of drugs depends to a large extent on the extraction ratio.

For drugs with a low or intermediate extraction ratio, plasma protein binding may be a limiting factor for hepatic metabolism; however, generally no large changes in protein binding are observed in obesity (Benedek et al. 1983; Cheymol et al. 1987; Pai et al. 2007) as mentioned before. For these drugs, the intrinsic clearance, which is impacted by the expression and activity of metabolic enzymes, is likely the most limiting factor for hepatic metabolism in the obese. Generally, clearance of CYP3A4 substrates is reduced with obesity, although statistical significance of findings is not always reached in trials (Brill et al. 2012). This trend is in line with observations of reduced CYP3A4 activity in adult and pediatric patients with nonalcoholic fatty liver disease or inflammation (Woolsey et al. 2015; Kolwankar et al. 2007; Brussee et al. 2018). For caffeine and theophylline, both substrates for CYP1A2, no changes in clearance were observed with obesity (Caraco et al. 1995; Jusko et al. 1979), although for the latter a trend toward increased clearance was observed after correcting for confounding factors. The clearance of substrates for other CYP enzymes, including CYP2C9, CYP2C19, CYP2D6, and CYP2E1, also appears to be increased to various extents in obese patients (Brill et al. 2012; Emery et al. 2003; van Rongen et al. 2016), although especially for CYP2C19 and CYP2D6 the impact of polymorphisms on inter-individual differences in clearance seems to be more pronounced than the impact of obesity.

Remarkably, a drug-drug interaction study seems to suggest that compared to non-obese patients, the relative impact of CYP3A inhibition by posaconazole on oral exposure to lurasidone is less pronounced in obese, but that the effect of the inhibition does persist longer (Greenblatt et al. 2018b). It has to be mentioned however that at least 66% of this difference was reported to be attributable to the reduced oral exposure to posaconazole in obese patients in combination with a prolonged washout of this drug in the obese. The authors attribute the difference in the exposure of posaconazole, which is mainly metabolized by UGT enzymes, to increased clearance and distribution volume in the obese. In addition to posaconazole, the glucuronidation of paracetamol, lorazepam, oxazepam, and garenoxacin has been reported to be increased with obesity (van Rongen et al. 2016; Abernethy et al. 1982, 1983; Van Wart et al. 2004), although the finding for garenoxacin may have been confounded by an underestimation of creatinine clearance in the obese. Interestingly, UGT2B15 has been shown to be present in adipose tissue, which has been proposed to cause the reduced plasma levels for testosterone in obese men (Tchernof et al. 1999); it is however unknown whether this is also responsible for increased glucuronidation of drug substrates in obese patients.

For drugs with a high extraction ratio, hepatic blood flow and perfusion are the main rate limiting factors for hepatic metabolism. Fatty liver disease has been suggested to reduce sinusoidal perfusion (Farrell et al. 2008), which could reduce hepatic clearance, while an increased cardiac output in obese patients might overall direct more blood to the liver, which could increase hepatic clearance for drug with a high extraction ratio. For propofol, clearance was consistently found to be increased in obese adults (van Kralingen et al. 2011a; Dong et al. 2016; Diepstraten et al. 2013; Cortínez et al. 2010). Findings for sufentanil and paclitaxel also indicate a trend toward increased clearance in obese patients (Schwartz et al. 1991; Sparreboom et al. 2007). A tendency toward increased hepatic blood flow in obese patients is further supported by findings for midazolam and fentanyl, which are mainly metabolized by CYP3A4 metabolism and have an intermediate to high extraction ratio. Clearance for these drugs has been reported to be the same or even increased in obese versus non-obese individuals (Greenblatt et al. 1984; Brill et al. 2014a; Shibutani et al. 2004), which could be interpreted as that reduced CYP3A4 activity in obese individuals is compensated by increases in hepatic blood flow and perfusion. Findings for the clearance of morphine do however not fit this narrative. Morphine is mainly cleared through glucuronidation and has an intermediate to high extraction ratio; both factors are believed to yield increased clearance with obesity, yet in a clinical study the clearance of morphine in obese patients was found to be similar to the clearance in non-obese patients (de Hoogd et al. 2017); this could suggest a role for obesity-related changes in transporter expression or activity.

Influx or efflux transporters on hepatocytes may, respectively, increase or decrease the presentation of drugs to metabolic enzymes in the hepatocytes and can thereby impact hepatic metabolic clearance. The impact of hepatic drug transporters on drug clearance has hitherto remained largely understudied in most patient populations. Rodent studies do suggest that expression or functionality of hepatic transporters may be changed in models for NASH (Dzierlenga et al. 2015; Fisher et al. 2009). Human studies also found expression of transporters in obese patients to be altered, even to the extent that it can in some cases impact drug clearance (Ulvestad et al. 2013). The directionality of these transporters and the differences in their increased or decreased expression and functionality may result in enhanced or reduced hepatic metabolic clearance for various drugs in obese patients.

2.4 Excretion Clearance in Obese Adults

The kidneys are the primary drug excretion organs. As for the liver, kidney blood flow and perfusion may be altered in obesity, and as only unbound drug can be filtered in the glomeruli, potential changes in plasma protein binding can also impact excretion clearance of drugs. The biggest impact of altered excretion clearance in the obese and overweight is, however, likely the result of reported increases in glomerular filtration rate (GFR), which is believed to result from changed kidney function (Ribstein et al. 1995; Chagnac et al. 2008; Park et al. 2012). This may explain the increases in renal clearance observed in obese patient for drugs that are exclusively renally cleared including vancomycin, gentamycin, amikacin, and tobramycin (Adane et al. 2015; Blouin et al. 1982; Brill et al. 2012; Bauer et al. 1983, 1998). Interestingly, the excretion of morphine metabolites was found to be decreased in obese patients (de Hoogd et al. 2017). Although in animals these metabolites were found to be mainly excreted by the kidneys, one possible explanation provided by the authors is that in humans biliary excretion of morphine metabolites might be more relevant than renal excretion.

In addition to GFR, active tubular secretion facilitated by drug transporters is also believed to be increased in obese patients, which may further add to the increased renal excretion of drugs like oseltamivir and its active metabolite, procainamide, ciprofloxacin, and cisplatin in the obese (Sparreboom et al. 2007; Chairat et al. 2016; Christoff et al. 1983; Allard et al. 1993). Recently a more prominent role for obesity-related induction of OCT2 has been suggested to play a role in the increase in metformin clearance (van Rongen et al. 2018a) and gentamicin clearance (Smit et al. 2019), but not tobramycin clearance (Smit et al. 2019).

Less is known about tubular reabsorption of drugs in the obese. One study, for instance, found the clearance of lithium to be increased with obesity, which was attributed to impaired reuptake (Reiss et al. 1994). Another study, however, found the excretion of lithium to be reduced in those obese with an increased filtration fraction, as this increased filtration fraction increases the oncotic pressure, which in turn increases reabsorption (Chagnac et al. 2008).

2.5 Pharmacodynamics in Obese Adults

For a limited number of drugs, differences in pharmacodynamics between obese and non-obese patients have been studied. A recent Chinese study, for instance, found for propofol that the EC50 (i.e., the concentration at which half the maximum effect is obtained) was reduced in morbidly obese patients compared to non-obese controls. Such an increase in drug potency suggests that a similar effect can be obtained at lower plasma concentrations (Dong et al. 2016). A previous study performed in Europe did, however, not find differences in the efficacy or potency of propofol between morbidly obese and non-obese patients (van Kralingen et al. 2011a).

For atracurium, a study reported no differences in the distribution volume and clearance between obese and non-obese patients. As atracurium in this study was dosed based on body weight, the concentrations in obese patients were systematically higher than in non-obese patients, yet no difference was observed in the time of recovery from neuromuscular blockade, from which the authors concluded that the efficacy of this drug may be reduced in obese patients (Varin et al. 1990). Another study found, however, that when atracurium is dosed based on ideal body weight, predictable efficacy profiles in terms of train-of-four (TOF) ratios, intubation conditions, and need for antagonism with neostigmine can be expected between individual morbidly obese patients (van Kralingen et al. 2011b). Unfortunately plasma concentrations were not obtained, but it is expected that dosing based on ideal body weight in the morbidly obese yields similar exposure than non-obese patients, which would suggest that there are in fact no differences in efficacy between these populations. From these studies it can therefore not be concluded if there truly is a difference in the relationship between concentration and effect of atracurium for obese and non-obese adults.

Reduced insulin sensitivity and type 2 diabetes are commonly encountered in obese patients, which is likely the result of the low-grade chronic inflammation in these patients. The reduced insulin sensitivity will also impact the sensitivity to exogenous insulin used in the pharmacological treatment of these patients.

For infectious diseases it is often believed that similar target exposures between patient subpopulations will yield similar efficacy, as the microorganisms that a drug is treating do generally not differ between these populations. However, as the immune response and immune cell differentiation and activity are dysregulated in obesity, anti-infective drugs may appear to be less effective in the obese as the hosts' immune system is less efficient in clearing an infection (Huttunen and Syrjänen 2013). Similarly, the efficacy of other treatments that are based on interactions with the hosts' immune response may be expected to be altered in obesity. In this respect immunogenicity in obese patients has been shown to be increased for the flu vaccine, while for hepatitis B no difference in the immune response between obese and non-obese patients has been observed (Xiong et al. 2017).

Reduced tissue penetration of antimicrobial drugs in obese patients, which has, for instance, been shown for cefazolin as mentioned before (Brill et al. 2014b), will cause a shift toward reduced efficacy when assessing the relationships between systemic drug exposure (e.g., blood concentrations) and observed efficacy. Although this presents itself as an apparent difference in drug pharmacodynamics, this should not be interpreted as such, because the underlying mechanism that is driving the observed differences is drug distribution to the site of action, which is a pharmacokinetics process.

3 Drug Pharmacology in Obese Pediatric Patients

Table 1 provides an overview of the changes in drug pharmacological parameters associated with obesity in the adult population, for the various drugs discussed above. In obese adults, multiple physiological changes occur, including increase in body size and volume of fat tissue and increase in cardiac output and altered organ perfusion; altered enzyme and transporter expression and functionality, intestinal, hepatic, and renal dysfunction; and altered plasma protein binding. The dynamics of these changes may differ depending on the underlying mechanism, and the impact of each change on the pharmacokinetics and/or pharmacodynamics of a drug may in some cases depend on drug properties. Additionally, some of the changes may have opposing effects on pharmacological parameters.

In children, growth and maturation are additional dynamic factors that may impact the pharmacokinetics and/or pharmacodynamics of drug. In obese children these changes occur in conjunction with the physiological changes induced by obesity. Moreover, the off-label and/or unlicensed use of drugs in the pediatric population is still relatively high, and as a result optimized drug dosing recommendations may not be available for a large number of drugs even in

Table 1 Overview of reported changes in pharmacological parameters for different drugs in obese individuals compared to non-obese peers

	Adults									Children	
	Primary PK				Secondary PK				PD		
Drug	ka	*F*	*V*	CL	AUC	Tmax	*t*½	fu	EC50	CL	Reference
Alprazolam				↓[a]				↔			Abernethy et al. (1984)
Amikacin				↑							Bauer et al. (1983)
Atracurium			↔	↔					↓/↔		Varin et al. (1990) and van Kralingen et al. (2011b)
Busulfan				↑[a]						↑	Bartelink et al. (2012) and Gibbs et al. (1999)
Caffeine				↔							Caraco et al. (1995)
Cefazolin								↔			Brill et al. (2014b)
Ciprofloxacin				↑							Allard et al. (1993)
Cisplatin				↑							Sparreboom et al. (2007)
Cyclosporine		↔	↔								Flechner et al. (1989) and Morgan and Bray (1994)
Daptomycin											Pai et al. (2007)
Dexfenfluramine		↔									Cheymol et al. (1995)
Digoxin			↔								Abernethy et al. (1981)
Fentanyl				↑							Shibutani et al. (2004)
Gentamycin				↑							Bauer et al. (1983)
Heparin			↔/↑								Morgan and Bray (1994)
Ibuprofen			↔/↑								Morgan and Bray (1994)
Levothyroxine						↓					Michalaki et al. (2011)
Lidocaine			↑								Morgan and Bray (1994)
Lorazepam				↑							Abernethy et al. (1983)
Lithium				↑							Reiss et al. (1994)
Metformin				↑						↑	van Rongen et al. (2018a) and Bardin et al. (2012)
Midazolam	↓	↔ (O) ↑ (MO)	↑	↔				↔		↑	Greenblatt et al. (1984), Brill et al. (2014a) and van Rongen et al. (2018b)

Morphine				↔		↔					Lloret-Linares et al. (2014) and de Hoogd et al. (2017)
Moxifloxacin		↔									Kees et al. (2011)
Oxazepam				↑							Abernethy et al. (1983)
Oseltamivir				↑							Chairat et al. (2016)
Paclitaxel				↑							Sparreboom et al. (2007)
Paracetamol/ acetaminophen				↑		↓					Lee et al. (1981), van Rongen et al. (2016) and Abernethy et al. (1982, 1983)
Phenazone			↔/↑								Morgan and Bray (1994)
Phenytoin			↑					↔			Morgan and Bray (1994) and Benedek et al. (1983)
Posaconazole			↑	↑							Greenblatt et al. (2018b)
Prednisolone			↔								Morgan and Bray (1994)
Procainamide				↑							Christoff et al. (1983)
Propofol			↔	↑					↑/↔	↑	van Kralingen et al. (2011a), Dong et al. (2016), Diepstraten et al. (2013) and Cortínez et al. (2010)
Propranolol		↑		↔ ↓[a]				↓			Bowman et al. (1986) and Cheymol et al. (1987)
Ranitidine			↔/↑								Davis et al. (1990)
Sufentanil				↑							Schwartz et al. (1991)
Theophylline				↔							Jusko et al. (1979)
Thiopental sodium				↑							Morgan and Bray (1994)
Trazodone		↔									Greenblatt et al. (1987)
Triazolam				↓[a]							Abernethy et al. (1984)
Tobramycin				↑							Bauer et al. (1983)
Vancomycin			↑	↑							Adane et al. (2015), Blouin et al. (1982) and Bauer et al. (1998)

(continued)

Table 1 (continued)

	Adults									Children	
	Primary PK				Secondary PK				PD		
Drug	ka	*F*	*V*	CL	AUC	Tmax	*t*½	fu	EC50	CL	Reference
Verapamil			↑								Morgan and Bray (1994)
Vortioxetine					↔						Greenblatt et al. (2018a)

PK pharmacokinetics, *PD* pharmacodynamics, *ka* absorption rate constant, *F* oral bioavailability, *V* volume of distribution, *CL* systemic clearance, *AUC* area under the curve/exposure, *Tmax* time of peak concentration, sometimes used as proxy for ka, *t*½ elimination half-life, sometimes used as a proxy for CL, *fu* fraction unbound, *EC50* potency, concentration at which half the maximum effect occurs, *O* obese, *MO* morbidly obese

↑ indicates increase, ↓ indicates decrease, ↔ indicates no change

[a]Indicates apparent oral clearance

non-obese pediatric patients. For those drugs for which dedicated pediatric studies have been performed, body weight is often found as a predictive descriptor of the impact of changes in both body size and maturation on pharmacokinetic parameters. Whether the pediatric dosing recommendations based on body weight that are derived from such studies should be maintained in obese pediatric patients is essential to know in order to develop rational dosing guidelines for the growing number of obese pediatric patients, because inconsistent dosing strategies are currently being adopted in clinical practice for these patients (Gade et al. 2018).

Unfortunately, the number of studies that assess the relationship between size or age descriptors and pharmacological parameters in obese pediatric patients is much more limited than in adults. In this case it may be tempting to extrapolate findings from obese adult populations to children. However, also for this, findings between different drugs and between obese adults and obese children are sometimes counterintuitive or may appear contradictory, making it difficult to derived generalizable dosing recommendations or approaches for extrapolations of findings between adults and children.

3.1 Similarities and Differences in Drug Clearance Between Obese Adults and Children

As drug clearance is the main driver of drug exposure at steady state and therefore of required maintenance doses, we focus on this parameter in this section.

When analyzing the pharmacokinetics of propofol in obese and non-obese adults, adolescents, and children simultaneously, a relationship was found between total body weight and clearance, with decreased values in young adults, adolescents, and children (Diepstraten et al. 2013). In this case obese adolescents with the same body weight as obese adults had lower clearance values than these adults, but their clearance values could be higher than those of non-obese adults with lower body weights.

For busulfan, the covariate relationship that defined the impact of maturation on clearance in non-obese individuals across a wide pediatric age range was based on body weight. It was found that this weight-based relationship could also be used to define clearance in obese pediatric individuals (Bartelink et al. 2012). This means that for two children of the same age, total clearance will be higher in the obese child compared to the non-obese child and, alternatively, that total clearance is the same in an obese child, compared to a non-obese child of the same weight (that is inevitably older than the obese child). Others have found that busulfan clearance per kilogram body weight is lower in children with a BMI higher than the 85th percentile of their age, compared to children with a lower BMI (Browning et al. 2011). Although the results of these studies cannot be directly compared due to the different parameterizations of the impact of weight and age on clearance, the results could point in the same direction. This is because to obtain total clearance, the clearance per kilogram is multiplied by more kilograms in obese children compared to non-obese children. It cannot, however, be excluded that in terms of total values, there are differences between obese and non-obese children for the clearance of busulfan. In adults it has, for instance, also been observed that for busulfan, the apparent oral clearance per kilogram body weight is lower in obese and even lower in morbidly obese patients compared to non-obese and underweight patients, while in terms of total apparent oral clearance values, this translated into elevated values in obese adults and even further elevated values in morbidly obese adults (Gibbs et al. 1999). For absolute clearance values obtained upon intravenous administration of busulfan in adults, values expressed per kilogram were also found to decrease with severity of obesity, but it was not reported how this translated into total absolute clearance values (Nguyen et al. 2006).

Findings on the pharmacokinetics of metformin in overweight and obese adolescents were in line with the findings above for propofol and busulfan, in that clearance increases with increasing age, which was parameterized in this study as weight-for-age-and-length (van Rongen et al. 2018a). On top of this first function, a second function was identified describing the linear increase in metformin clearance with excess body weight in this adolescent population (van Rongen et al. 2018a), which is also in line with findings for propofol and busulfan. Compared to values reported in literature, the clearance values in the obese adolescents were found to be comparable to values in non-obese adults and showed a tendency to be lower compared to clearance in obese adults. Most interestingly, however, a study on metformin in obese adults showed that lean body weight was the best size descriptor for inter-individual differences in clearance (Bardin et al. 2012), which suggest a much more limited impact of excess body weight on the clearance of metformin in the obese adult population, compared to the obese adolescent population.

Correlations between a reduced metabolic clearance by CYP3A isoenzymes and both decreasing age in children and increasing inflammation and organ failure have been reported (Woolsey et al. 2015; Kolwankar et al. 2007; Brussee et al. 2018). In adults, obesity was found to generally reduce the apparent oral clearance of CYP3A substrates (Brill et al. 2012), while studies in morbidly obese adults with midazolam, which is predominantly metabolized by CYP3A, showed systemic clearance not to be impacted by obesity, potentially due to compensations by increasing blood flow (Brill et al. 2014a). Interestingly, and quite unexpectedly, a dedicated pharmacokinetic study for midazolam in overweight and obese adolescents showed the systemic clearance in these adolescents to be substantially higher than the systemic clearance in the morbidly obese adults (van Rongen et al. 2018b). In fact, the clearance values in the obese adolescents were more in line with clearance values obtained in the same morbidly obese patients described above, 1 year after bariatric surgery and after considerable weight loss (Brill et al. 2015). The clearance values of obese adults after weight loss were found to be higher than their clearance values before weight loss surgery. Potentially these findings can be explained by recovery of CYP3A activity in the liver after substantial weight loss. The differences between obese adolescents and obese adults can possibly be explained by the hypothesis that in obesity suppression of the CYP3A activity increases with the duration of the disease and therefore takes time to fully manifest, while the increase in cardiac output and hepatic blood flow is more closely linked to the increase in excess body weight. This was further confirmed by the finding that within the population of obese adolescents, midazolam clearance was found to increase with weight, which may in its turn be related to an increased liver blood flow. As described above, an increasing impact of obesity with increased duration of this disease has also been suggested as a possible explanation for the fact that bioavailability of midazolam in the morbidly obese adults was increased compared to non-obese adults, while in obese patients that have not reached the state of morbid obesity, the bioavailability is not (yet) impacted (Greenblatt et al. 1984; Brill et al. 2014a).

Table 1 also summarizes the findings regarding the impact of obesity on drug clearance in the pediatric population for the drugs discussed in this section. The examples above illustrate that generalizable conclusions on how to translate findings regarding the impact of obesity from adults to children are not obvious. Findings for propofol are in line with the expectation that, due to maturation, clearance in children is lower than clearance in adults and indeed show that clearance in obese children is lower than clearance on obese adults. Additionally, total clearance increased with excess body weight, meaning that obese adolescents with body weights higher than non-obese adults can have higher propofol clearance values than the non-obese adults. Similar trends are seen in both adult and pediatric patients for busulfan in which obesity or excess body weight increases the clearance. Findings for metformin are in line with propofol and busulfan in adolescents, as excess body weight increases clearance in this population as well, but clearance values in adolescents do not appear to increase far beyond values in non-obese adults, nor do clearance values in obese adults increase far beyond the values in non-obese adults, suggesting that the impact of excess body weight on the clearance of metformin diminishes when patients reach adulthood. In adults there is – unexpectedly – also no difference in the clearance of midazolam between obese and non-obese individuals, potentially because the reduced CYP3A activity that may be anticipated in the obese is compensated by increased blood flow. Yet in adolescents, midazolam clearance is in fact increasing with obesity. If these observations for midazolam can indeed be attributed to the duration of obesity as influencer on CYP3A activity, as hypothesized, the generalizability of findings in any study, whether in the adult or pediatric population, is limited without taking disease duration into account.

In summary, the highlighted examples show that there may or may not be contradictions in terms of the absence or presence of differences in drug clearance between obese and non-obese individuals of the adult or pediatric population. Moreover, the directionality of the impact of obesity on drug clearance cannot be presumed to follow the same pattern in adults and children.

4 How to Study Drug Pharmacology in Obese Children

Although research efforts are increasing, generally the pharmacokinetics and pharmacodynamics of drugs in children remain understudied. Studies in obese pediatric patients are even more limited. As generic scaling cannot be derived based on body weight (as proxy for maturation) nor on results described in current literature, further research efforts are required on drug pharmacology in obese children. For this research several considerations should be taken into account.

4.1 Focus on Primary Pharmacological Parameters with Population Modelling

Pharmacokinetic studies are ideally focused on quantifying primary pharmacokinetic parameters like absorption rate, bioavailability, clearance, and distribution volume, rather than descriptive metrics like C_{max}, t_{max}, and observed AUC. This has the advantage that findings can be more directly linked to physiological mechanisms underlying drug pharmacokinetics, which will increase our understanding of the impact of obesity-related physiological changes, which may in turn aid in the definition of generalizable conclusions.

In pediatric patients, the population approach, also known as non-linear mixed effects modelling, is the preferred method to quantify primary pharmacological parameters (De Cock et al. 2011). In this approach, observed data on pharmacological outcome measures of all individuals in a study are analyzed simultaneously while still taking into account that different observations come from different individuals. This method can handle dense, sparse, and unbalanced data that are obtained during routine clinical practice or in multiple studies with different designs. Since this method can separate inter-individual variability from residual unexplained variability, it is ideally suitable for the establishment of covariate relationships that define correlations between patient or treatment characteristics and inter-individual variability in model parameters. Defined covariate relationships (related to obesity or other patient-related variables) on primary parameters can be directly used as the basis for drug dosing recommendations. Clearance is, for instance, the only determinant for steady-state concentration and drives through concentrations and is therefore important for the establishment of maintenance doses and dosing intervals. Distribution volume, on the other hand, drives peak concentrations and time-to-steady-state and is therefore important for peak concentrations and loading doses and the dosing of drugs that are driven by peak concentrations.

4.1.1 Disentangle Presystemic and Systemic Processes Impacting Exposure

Both presystemic (gut and/or first-pass hepatic) and systemic (renal and/or hepatic) clearance impact the overall exposure, quantified as AUC, of orally administered drugs. The parameters quantifying these processes are bioavailability and clearance, respectively. When only data upon oral drug administration is available, bioavailability cannot be quantified and obtained values for clearance, as well as distribution volume is indicated as apparent parameter values or "parameter over F," meaning that the true values of these parameters change proportionally with bioavailability. To enable a physiological interpretation of observed differences in AUC between obese and non-obese patients of orally administered drugs, it would be beneficial to study the pharmacokinetics of these drugs both after intravenous and oral administration. Ideally, this is performed in the same patient at the same time, to exclude the impact of inter-individual and inter-occasion differences. Different approaches are available to achieve this experimentally. In a semi-simultaneous approach proposed by Brill et al., patients receive an oral drug dose first, followed by an intravenous dose a few hours later, with blood sampling to measure drug concentrations following both administrations (Brill et al. 2014a). With microdosing designs truly simultaneous oral and intravenous administration can be achieved. By having therapeutic intravenous drug administration and simultaneous administration of an oral microdose of the isotopically labeled drug and measuring the concentration-time profiles of both labeled and unlabeled drug, systemic and presystemic clearance can be quantified with low experimental variability (Hohmann et al. 2015). Proof-of-principle studies have confirmed that microdose studies are also suitable throughout the pediatric population (Mooij et al. 2014).

4.1.2 Inclusion Criterion in Pediatric Clinical Trials

Body weight is often identified as most predictive descriptor for the impact of maturational changes on pharmacokinetic parameters in populations of children with age-appropriate body weights, but how such findings should be extrapolated to obese children is generally unknown. An important question in obese children is how weight related to obesity versus weight related to maturation or growth adds to changes in the pharmacokinetics or pharmacodynamics of drugs. Proposed approaches to disentangle the impact of maturation and obesity in obese pediatric patients are focused on defining sex, length, and age-appropriate body weights for normal weight children as descriptor of maturation and quantifying excess weight as descriptor of obesity (van Rongen et al. 2018a). To enable the disentanglement of age- and obesity-induced changes in body size in the data analysis process, patient inclusion of the clinical study should ascertain inclusion of not just a wide range in body weight per se but also in a wide range in deviations from appropriate body weights or excess body weight.

Also, given that disease duration has been suggested to drive to what extent the impact of obesity on processes underlying drug pharmacology manifests for some parameters, but not for others, it may be prudent to record disease duration in future studies on the impact of obesity on drug pharmacology. This may be true for both the adult and pediatric population, particularly when predictions based on obese adults to obese adolescents are foreseen.

Finally, it has to be noted that the pediatric population is already relatively small and as a result the absolute amount of obese pediatric patients is small. Consequently, inclusion of a sufficient number of obese pediatric patients in clinical trials may be challenging (Tamborlane et al. 2016). Therefore, instead of RCTs, alternative designs for studies in this special patient population should be explored. For this the *Learning Healthcare System* may offer relevant insights (http://www.learninghealthcareproject.org/section/background/learning-healthcare-system).

4.1.3 Linking Pharmacokinetics to Pharmacodynamics

In developing evidence-based drug dosing regimens, it should be remembered that the efficacy and safety of drugs are based on both the pharmacokinetics and pharmacodynamics of these drugs and it is possible for changes in one to (partially) counteract or enhance the change in the other. It may not be necessary to perform dedicated pediatric pharmacodynamics studies for all drugs. The pediatric decision tree from the FDA, for instance, defines when pediatric pharmacokinetic studies to develop dosing regimen that yield the same exposure in adults and children suffice (https://www.fda.gov/media/71277/download). However for a large number of drugs that do not meet the required criteria, age-appropriate target exposures are not known for children in general and, also in this case, even less is known about obese children. Regarding the obese pediatric subpopulation, priority should be given in this regard to pharmacodynamics studies on drugs for disease conditions that result from or are common with obesity, including, for instance, type 2 diabetes. Additionally, due to the low-grade systemic inflammation in obesity, pediatric pharmacodynamics studies on drugs that act on or with the immune system are imperative.

4.1.4 Generalization of Findings

Population modelling approaches are ideally suitable to study the impact of obesity in conjunction with maturation on the pharmacokinetics and pharmacodynamics of drugs. A drawback of this method is, however, that it would require dedicated studies for all relevant drugs in obese patients of all ages which would require an unrealistic amount of resources. Therefore, research efforts should also be directed toward gaining a deeper understanding of how obesity-related physiological changes in processes underlying drug pharmacokinetics and pharmacodynamics translate into changes in pharmacokinetic and pharmacodynamics parameters, both in adults and in children. Methods that combine population approaches with physiological insight would contribute to the generalizability of findings (Knibbe et al. 2011).

In pediatric patients with age-appropriate body weights, the between-drug extrapolation of covariate relationships for clearance for drugs sharing an elimination route has, for instance, been explored (Krekels et al. 2012a; De Cock et al. 2014; Calvier et al. 2018a). In this approach, pharmacological parameters are considered to reflect system-specific properties, drug-specific properties, or a combination of both. Methods that can derive and retain information on system-specific aspects of drug pharmacokinetics and use this in the translation of findings to drugs with different drug-specific properties should also be explored for both adult and pediatric obese patients.

4.1.5 Physiologically Based Pharmacokinetic Models

Another way to advance our knowledge would be a more extensive use of physiologically based pharmacokinetic (PBPK) models, where system-specific parameters truly reflect physiological or anatomical measures, in order to predict how drugs with specific physicochemical properties interact with the system (Johnson and Rostami-Hodjegan 2011). Although these models require a vast amount of data on changes in system-specific properties for specific patient subpopulations, the information that can be derived from this will be generalizable. An improved understanding of how, on top of maturational changes, physiological and anatomical parameters change with obesity will truly allow us to predict for all types of drugs how pharmacokinetic parameters will change in obese children of all ages. Although, contrary to population pharmacokinetic models, PBPK models cannot serve as a direct basis for drug dosing algorithms, information needed for the development of these algorithms can be derived from them. With appropriate PBPK models, we do not need to study every drug in every subpopulation separately anymore.

Application of PBPK approaches requires large amounts of data and specialized software or personnel. Therefore, simplified scaling methods to derive pharmacokinetic parameters for special patient populations are always sought after. Calvier et al. have illustrated how PBPK models can form the basis for the systematic evaluation of simplified scaling methods, to establish criteria required for accurate scaling with simplified methods (Calvier et al. 2017, 2018a). This concept was illustrated for pediatric populations with age-appropriate weights but could easily be extended to other populations for which PBPK parameters are known.

Another interesting application of PBPK modelling approaches is that these models can be used to assess the impact of changes in physiological or anatomical parameters in isolation. As such, it can be used for hypothesis testing, to establish which changes or combination of changes in the underlying physiology are likely to explain differences in observed primary pharmacokinetic parameters. This concept has been introduced for pediatric populations with age-appropriate weights (Krekels et al. 2012b) and could also be extended to other populations even when not all parameters are known in this population.

Finally, combinations of population pharmacokinetic modelling and PBPK modelling concepts can be used to quantify physiological or anatomical parameter from pharmacokinetic data, when direct measures of these parameters are not possible. Using such an approach has been successfully used to derive intrinsic clearance values for midazolam in the liver and gut wall in obese patients and patients after weight loss surgery (Brill et al. 2016), which allowed for the disentanglement of presystemic and systemic clearance of this drug. It has even be illustrated how optimal design principles in population modelling can be used to optimize the design of the clinical study to ascertain *a priory* that data obtained with a specific study design will indeed allow for precise and accurate estimation of the parameters of interest (Calvier et al. 2018b).

5 Conclusion

Although pharmacological studies in obese adults are increasingly being performed, they have not yet yielded a thorough understanding of the exact physiological changes with this disease and how these impact processes underlying drug pharmacokinetics and pharmacodynamics. This prevents the generalizability of findings. In obese pediatric patients, pharmacological studies are much more limited, but a number of these have shown that observations in adult patients cannot always be directly extrapolated to this younger population. Given the increased incidence of pediatric obesity worldwide, it is absolutely imperative that we perform more and smarter studies in this subpopulation, to increase our knowledge on the impact of this disease in combination with maturational changes on drug pharmacology, which is needed to provide safe and effective treatment for these children as well.

References

Abarca-Gómez L, Abdeen ZA, Hamid ZA, Abu-Rmeileh NM, Acosta-Cazares B, Acuin C et al (2017) Worldwide trends in body-mass index, underweight, overweight, and obesity from 1975 to 2016: a pooled analysis of 2416 population-based measurement studies in 128·9 million children, adolescents, and adults. Lancet 390(10113):2627–2642

Abernethy DR, Greenblatt DJ, Smith TW (1981) Digoxin disposition in obesity: clinical pharmacokinetic investigation. Am Heart J 102(4):740–744

Abernethy DR, Divoll M, Greenblatt DJ, Ameer B (1982) Obesity, sex, and acetaminophen disposition. Clin Pharmacol Ther 31(6):783–790

Abernethy DR, Greenblatt DJ, Divoll M, Shader RI (1983) Enhanced glucuronide conjugation of drugs in obesity: studies of lorazepam, oxazepam, and acetaminophen. J Lab Clin Med 101 (6):873–880

Abernethy DR, Greenblatt DJ, Divoll M, Smith RB, Shader RI (1984) The influence of obesity on the pharmacokinetics of oral alprazolam and triazolam. Clin Pharmacokinet 9(2):177–183

Adane ED, Herald M, Koura F (2015) Pharmacokinetics of vancomycin in extremely obese patients with suspected or confirmed Staphylococcus aureus infections. Pharmacotherapy 35 (2):127–139

Alexander JK, Dennis EW, Smith WG, Amad KH, Duncan WC, Austin RC (1962–1963) Blood volume, cardiac output, and distribution of systemic blood flow in extreme obesity. Cardiovasc Res Cent Bull 1:39–44

Allard S, Kinzig M, Boivin G, Sörgel F, LeBel M (1993) Intravenous ciprofloxacin disposition in obesity. Clin Pharmacol Ther 54(4):368–373

Bardin C, Nobecourt E, Larger E, Chast F, Treluyer J-M, Urien S (2012) Population pharmacokinetics of metformin in obese and non-obese patients with type 2 diabetes mellitus. Eur J Clin Pharmacol 68(6):961–968

Bartelink IH, van Kesteren C, Boelens JJ, Egberts TCG, Bierings MB, Cuvelier GDE et al (2012) Predictive performance of a busulfan pharmacokinetic model in children and young adults. Ther Drug Monit 34(5):574–583

Bauer LA, Edwards WA, Dellinger EP, Simonowitz DA (1983) Influence of weight on aminoglycoside pharmacokinetics in normal weight and morbidly obese patients. Eur J Clin Pharmacol 24(5):643–647

Bauer LA, Black DJ, Lill JS (1998) Vancomycin dosing in morbidly obese patients. Eur J Clin Pharmacol 54(8):621–625

Benedek IH, Fiske WD, Griffen WO, Bell RM, Blouin RA, McNamara PJ (1983) Serum alpha 1-acid glycoprotein and the binding of drugs in obesity. Br J Clin Pharmacol 16(6):751–754

Blouin RA, Bauer LA, Miller DD, Record KE, Griffen WO (1982) Vancomycin pharmacokinetics in normal and morbidly obese subjects. Antimicrob Agents Chemother 21(4):575–580

Blouin RA, Kolpek JH, Mann HJ (1987) Influence of obesity on drug disposition. Clin Pharm 6 (9):706–714

Bowman SL, Hudson SA, Simpson G, Munro JF, Clements JA (1986) A comparison of the pharmacokinetics of propranolol in obese and normal volunteers. Br J Clin Pharmacol 21 (5):529–532

Brill MJE, Diepstraten J, van Rongen A, van Kralingen S, van den Anker JN, Knibbe CAJ (2012) Impact of obesity on drug metabolism and elimination in adults and children. Clin Pharmacokinet 51(5):277–304

Brill MJE, van Rongen A, Houwink API, Burggraaf J, van Ramshorst B, Wiezer RJ et al (2014a) Midazolam pharmacokinetics in morbidly obese patients following semi-simultaneous oral and intravenous administration: a comparison with healthy volunteers. Clin Pharmacokinet 53 (10):931–941

Brill MJE, Houwink API, Schmidt S, Van Dongen EPA, Hazebroek EJ, van Ramshorst B et al (2014b) Reduced subcutaneous tissue distribution of cefazolin in morbidly obese versus non-obese patients determined using clinical microdialysis. J Antimicrob Chemother 69 (3):715–723

Brill MJ, van Rongen A, van Dongen EP, van Ramshorst B, Hazebroek EJ, Darwich AS et al (2015) The pharmacokinetics of the CYP3A substrate midazolam in morbidly obese patients before and one year after bariatric surgery. Pharm Res 32(12):3927–3936

Brill MJE, Välitalo PAJ, Darwich AS, van Ramshorst B, van Dongen HPA, Rostami-Hodjegan A et al (2016) Semiphysiologically based pharmacokinetic model for midazolam and CYP3A mediated metabolite 1-OH-midazolam in morbidly obese and weight loss surgery patients. CPT Pharmacometrics Syst Pharmacol 5(1):20–30

Browning B, Thormann K, Donaldson A, Halverson T, Shinkle M, Kletzel M (2011) Busulfan dosing in children with BMIs $\geq$ 85% undergoing HSCT: a new optimal strategy. Biol Blood Marrow Transplant 17(9):1383–1388

Brussee JM, Vet NJ, Krekels EHJ, Valkenburg AJ, Jacqz-Aigrain E, van Gerven JMA et al (2018) Predicting CYP3A-mediated midazolam metabolism in critically ill neonates, infants, children and adults with inflammation and organ failure. Br J Clin Pharmacol 84(2):358–368

Calvier EAM, Krekels EHJ, Välitalo PAJ, Rostami-Hodjegan A, Tibboel D, Danhof M et al (2017) Allometric scaling of clearance in paediatric patients: when does the magic of 0.75 fade? Clin Pharmacokinet 56(3):273–285

Calvier EAM, Krekels EHJ, Yu H, Välitalo PAJ, Johnson TN, Rostami-Hodjegan A et al (2018a) Drugs being eliminated via the same pathway will not always require similar pediatric dose adjustments. CPT Pharmacometrics Syst Pharmacol 7(3):175–185

Calvier EAM, Nguyen TT, Johnson TN, Rostami-Hodjegan A, Tibboel D, Krekels EHJ et al (2018b) Can population modelling principles be used to identify key PBPK parameters for paediatric clearance predictions? An innovative application of optimal design theory. Pharm Res 35(11):209

Caraco Y, Zylber-Katz E, Berry EM, Levy M (1995) Caffeine pharmacokinetics in obesity and following significant weight reduction. Int J Obes Relat Metab Disord 19(4):234–239

Cardoso-Júnior A, Coelho LGV, Savassi-Rocha PR, Vignolo MC, Abrantes MM, de Almeida AM et al (2007) Gastric emptying of solids and semi-solids in morbidly obese and non-obese subjects: an assessment using the 13C-octanoic acid and 13C-acetic acid breath tests. Obes Surg 17(2):236–241

Chagnac A, Herman M, Zingerman B, Erman A, Rozen-Zvi B, Hirsh J et al (2008) Obesity-induced glomerular hyperfiltration: its involvement in the pathogenesis of tubular sodium reabsorption. Nephrol Dial Transplant 23(12):3946–3952

Chairat K, Jittamala P, Hanpithakpong W, Day NPJ, White NJ, Pukrittayakamee S et al (2016) Population pharmacokinetics of oseltamivir and oseltamivir carboxylate in obese and non-obese volunteers. Br J Clin Pharmacol 81(6):1103–1112

Cheymol G, Poirier JM, Barre J, Pradalier A, Dry J (1987) Comparative pharmacokinetics of intravenous propranolol in obese and normal volunteers. J Clin Pharmacol 27(11):874–879

Cheymol G, Weissenburger J, Poirier JM, Gellee C (1995) The pharmacokinetics of dexfenfluramine in obese and non-obese subjects. Br J Clin Pharmacol 39(6):684–687

Cheymol G, Poirier JM, Carrupt PA, Testa B, Weissenburger J, Levron JC et al (1997) Pharmacokinetics of beta-adrenoceptor blockers in obese and normal volunteers. Br J Clin Pharmacol 43 (6):563–570

Christoff PB, Conti DR, Naylor C, Jusko WJ (1983) Procainamide disposition in obesity. Drug Intell Clin Pharm 17(7–8):516–522

Cortínez LI, Anderson BJ, Penna A, Olivares L, Muñoz HR, Holford NHG et al (2010) Influence of obesity on propofol pharmacokinetics: derivation of a pharmacokinetic model. Br J Anaesth 105 (4):448–456

Davis RL, Quenzer RW, Bozigian HP, Warner CW (1990) Pharmacokinetics of ranitidine in morbidly obese women. DICP 24(11):1040–1043

De Cock RFW, Piana C, Krekels EHJ, Danhof M, Allegaert K, Knibbe CAJ (2011) The role of population PK-PD modelling in paediatric clinical research. Eur J Clin Pharmacol 67(Suppl. 1):5–16

De Cock RFW, Allegaert K, Sherwin CMT, Nielsen EI, de Hoog M, van den Anker JN et al (2014) A neonatal amikacin covariate model can be used to predict ontogeny of other drugs eliminated through glomerular filtration in neonates. Pharm Res 31(3):754–767

de Hoogd S, Välitalo PAJ, Dahan A, van Kralingen S, Coughtrie MMW, van Dongen EPA et al (2017) Influence of morbid obesity on the pharmacokinetics of morphine, morphine-3-glucuronide, and morphine-6-glucuronide. Clin Pharmacokinet 56(12):1577–1587

Diepstraten J, Chidambaran V, Sadhasivam S, Blussé van Oud-Alblas HJ, Inge T, van Ramshorst B et al (2013) An integrated population pharmacokinetic meta-analysis of propofol in morbidly obese and nonobese adults, adolescents, and children. CPT Pharmacometrics Syst Pharmacol 2 (9):e73

Dong D, Peng X, Liu J, Qian H, Li J, Wu B (2016) Morbid obesity alters both pharmacokinetics and pharmacodynamics of propofol: dosing recommendation for anesthesia induction. Drug Metab Dispos 44(10):1579–1583

Dzierlenga AL, Clarke JD, Hargraves TL, Ainslie GR, Vanderah TW, Paine MF et al (2015) Mechanistic basis of altered morphine disposition in nonalcoholic steatohepatitis. J Pharmacol Exp Ther 352(3):462–470

Emery M, Fisher JM, Chien JY, Kharasch ED, Dellinger EP, Kowdley KV et al (2003) CYP2E1 activity before and after weight loss in morbidly obese subjects with nonalcoholic fatty liver disease. Hepatology 38(2):428–435

Farrell GC, Teoh NC, Mccuskey RS (2008) Hepatic microcirculation in fatty liver disease. Anat Rec Adv Integr Anat Evol Biol 291(6):684–692

Fisher CD, Lickteig AJ, Augustine LM, Oude Elferink RPJ, Besselsen DG, Erickson RP et al (2009) Experimental non-alcoholic fatty liver disease results in decreased hepatic uptake transporter expression and function in rats. Eur J Pharmacol 613(1–3):119–127

Flechner SM, Kolbeinsson ME, Tam J, Lum B (1989) The impact of body weight on cyclosporine pharmacokinetics in renal transplant recipients. Transplantation 47(5):806–810

Gade C, Christensen HR, Dalhoff KP, Holm JC, Holst H (2018) Inconsistencies in dosage practice in children with overweight or obesity: a retrospective cohort study. Pharmacol Res Perspect 6 (3):e00398

Gibbs JP, Gooley T, Corneau B, Murray G, Stewart P, Appelbaum FR et al (1999) The impact of obesity and disease on busulfan oral clearance in adults. Blood 93(12):4436–4440

Greenblatt DJ, Abernethy DR, Locniskar A, Harmatz JS, Limjuco RA, Shader RI (1984) Effect of age, gender, and obesity on midazolam kinetics. Anesthesiology 61(1):27–35

Greenblatt DJ, Friedman H, Burstein ES, Scavone JM, Blyden GT, Ochs HR et al (1987) Trazodone kinetics: effect of age, gender, and obesity. Clin Pharmacol Ther 42(2):193–200

Greenblatt DJ, Harmatz JS, Chow CR (2018a) Vortioxetine disposition in obesity. J Clin Psychopharmacol 38(3):172–179

Greenblatt DJ, Harmatz JS, Ryan MJ, Chow CR (2018b) Sustained impairment of lurasidone clearance after discontinuation of posaconazole. J Clin Psychopharmacol 38(4):289–295

Harnois F, Msika S, Sabaté J-M, Mechler C, Jouet P, Barge J et al (2006) Prevalence and predictive factors of non-alcoholic steatohepatitis (NASH) in morbidly obese patients undergoing bariatric surgery. Obes Surg 16(2):183–188

Hohmann N, Kocheise F, Carls A, Burhenne J, Haefeli WE, Mikus G (2015) Midazolam microdose to determine systemic and pre-systemic metabolic CYP3A activity in humans. Br J Clin Pharmacol 79(2):278–285

Huttunen R, Syrjänen J (2013) Obesity and the risk and outcome of infection. Int J Obes 37 (3):333–340

Jain R, Chung SM, Jain L, Khurana M, Lau SWJ, Lee JE et al (2011) Implications of obesity for drug therapy: limitations and challenges. Clin Pharmacol Ther 90(1):77–89

Johnson TN, Rostami-Hodjegan A (2011) Resurgence in the use of physiologically based pharmacokinetic models in pediatric clinical pharmacology: parallel shift in incorporating the knowledge of biological elements and increased applicability to drug development and clinical practice. Paediatr Anaesth 21(3):291–301

Jusko WJ, Gardner MJ, Mangione A, Schentag JJ, Koup JR, Vance JW (1979) Factors affecting theophylline clearances: age, tobacco, marijuana, cirrhosis, congestive heart failure, obesity, oral contraceptives, benzodiazepines, barbiturates, and ethanol. J Pharm Sci 68(11):1358–1366

Kees MG, Weber S, Kees F, Horbach T (2011) Pharmacokinetics of moxifloxacin in plasma and tissue of morbidly obese patients. J Antimicrob Chemother 66(10):2330–2335

Knibbe CAJ, Krekels EHJ, Danhof M (2011) Advances in paediatric pharmacokinetics. Expert Opin Drug Metab Toxicol 7(1):1–8

Knibbe CAJ, Brill MJE, van Rongen A, Diepstraten J, van der Graaf PH, Danhof M (2015) Drug disposition in obesity: toward evidence-based dosing. Annu Rev Pharmacol Toxicol 55 (1):149–167

Kolwankar D, Vuppalanchi R, Ethell B, Jones DR, Wrighton SA, Hall SD et al (2007) Association between nonalcoholic hepatic steatosis and hepatic cytochrome P-450 3A activity. Clin Gastroenterol Hepatol 5(3):388–393

Krekels EHJ, Neely M, Panoilia E, Tibboel D, Capparelli E, Danhof M et al (2012a) From pediatric covariate model to semiphysiological function for maturation: part I – extrapolation of a covariate model from morphine to zidovudine. CPT Pharmacometrics Syst Pharmacol 1(10):e9

Krekels EHJ, Johnson TN, den Hoedt SM, Rostami-Hodjegan A, Danhof M, Tibboel D et al (2012b) From pediatric covariate model to semiphysiological function for maturation: part II – sensitivity to physiological and physicochemical properties. CPT Pharmacometrics Syst Pharmacol 1:e10

Lee WH, Kramer WG, Granville GE (1981) The effect of obesity on acetaminophen pharmacokinetics in man. J Clin Pharmacol 21(7):284–287

Lemmens H, Bernstein D, Brodsky J (2006) Estimating blood volume in obese and morbidly obese patients. Obes Surg 16(6):773–776

Lloret-Linares C, Hirt D, Bardin C, Bouillot J-L, Oppert J-M, Poitou C et al (2014) Effect of a Roux-en-Y gastric bypass on the pharmacokinetics of oral morphine using a population approach. Clin Pharmacokinet 53(10):919–930

Machado M, Marques-Vidal P, Cortez-Pinto H (2006) Hepatic histology in obese patients undergoing bariatric surgery. J Hepatol 45(4):600–606

Michalaki MA, Gkotsina MI, Mamali I, Markantes GK, Faltaka A, Kalfarentzos F et al (2011) Impaired pharmacokinetics of levothyroxine in severely obese volunteers. Thyroid 21 (5):477–481

Mooij MG, van Duijn E, Knibbe CAJ, Windhorst AD, Hendrikse NH, Vaes WHJ et al (2014) Pediatric microdose study of [14C]paracetamol to study drug metabolism using accelerated mass spectrometry: proof of concept. Clin Pharmacokinet 53(11):1045–1051

Morgan DJ, Bray KM (1994) Lean body mass as a predictor of drug dosage. Implications for drug therapy. Clin Pharmacokinet 26(4):292–307

Ng M, Fleming T, Robinson M, Thomson B, Graetz N, Margono C et al (2014) Global, regional, and national prevalence of overweight and obesity in children and adults during 1980-2013: a systematic analysis for the Global Burden of Disease Study 2013. Lancet 384(9945):766–781

Nguyen L, Leger F, Lennon S, Puozzo C (2006) Intravenous busulfan in adults prior to haematopoietic stem cell transplantation: a population pharmacokinetic study. Cancer Chemother Pharmacol 57(2):191–198

Pai MP, Norenberg JP, Anderson T, Goade DW, Rodvold KA, Telepak RA et al (2007) Influence of morbid obesity on the single-dose pharmacokinetics of daptomycin. Antimicrob Agents Chemother 51(8):2741–2747

Park EJ, Pai MP, Dong T, Zhang J, Ko C-W, Lawrence J et al (2012) The influence of body size descriptors on the estimation of kidney function in normal weight, overweight, obese, and morbidly obese adults. Ann Pharmacother 46(3):317–328

Rainone V, Schneider L, Saulle I, Ricci C, Biasin M, Al-Daghri NM et al (2016) Upregulation of inflammasome activity and increased gut permeability are associated with obesity in children and adolescents. Int J Obes 40(6):1026–1033

Reilly JJ, El-Hamdouchi A, Diouf A, Monyeki A, Somda SA (2018) Determining the worldwide prevalence of obesity. Lancet 391(10132):1773–1774

Reiss RA, Haas CE, Karki SD, Gumbiner B, Welle SL, Carson SW (1994) Lithium pharmacokinetics in the obese. Clin Pharmacol Ther 55(4):392–398

Ribstein J, du Cailar G, Mimran A (1995) Combined renal effects of overweight and hypertension. Hypertension 26(4):610–615

Schwartz AE, Matteo RS, Ornstein E, Young WL, Myers KJ (1991) Pharmacokinetics of sufentanil in obese patients. Anesth Analg 73(6):790–793

Shibutani K, Inchiosa MA, Sawada K, Bairamian M (2004) Accuracy of pharmacokinetic models for predicting plasma fentanyl concentrations in lean and obese surgical patients: derivation of dosing weight ("pharmacokinetic mass"). Anesthesiology 101(3):603–613

Smit C, Wasmann RE, Goulooze SC, Hazebroek EJ, Van Dongen EPA, Burgers DMT et al (2019) A prospective clinical study characterizing the influence of morbid obesity on the pharmacokinetics of gentamicin: towards individualized dosing in obese patients. Clin Pharmacokinet. https://doi.org/10.1007/s40262-019-00762-4

Smit C, Wasmann RE, Wiezer MJ, van Dongen HPA, Mouton JW, Brüggemann RJM, Knibbe CAJ (2019) Tobramycin clearance is best described by renal function estimates in obese and non-obese individuals: results of a prospective rich sampling pharmacokinetic study. Pharm Res 36(8):112. https://doi.org/10.1007/s11095-019-2651-2

Sparreboom A, Wolff AC, Mathijssen RHJ, Chatelut E, Rowinsky EK, Verweij J et al (2007) Evaluation of alternate size descriptors for dose calculation of anticancer drugs in the obese. J Clin Oncol 25(30):4707–4713

Tamborlane WV, Haymond MW, Dunger D, Shankar R, Gubitosi-Klug R, Bethin K et al (2016) Expanding treatment options for youth with type 2 diabetes: current problems and proposed solutions. Diabetes Care 39(3):323–329

Tchernof A, Lévesque E, Beaulieu M, Couture P, Després JP, Hum DW et al (1999) Expression of the androgen metabolizing enzyme UGT2B15 in adipose tissue and relative expression measurement using a competitive RT-PCR method. Clin Endocrinol 50(5):637–642

Teixeira TFS, Souza NCS, Chiarello PG, Franceschini SCC, Bressan J, Ferreira CLLF et al (2012) Intestinal permeability parameters in obese patients are correlated with metabolic syndrome risk factors. Clin Nutr 31(5):735–740

Ulvestad M, Skottheim IB, Jakobsen GS, Bremer S, Molden E, Åsberg A et al (2013) Impact of OATP1B1, MDR1, and CYP3A4 expression in liver and intestine on interpatient pharmacokinetic variability of atorvastatin in obese subjects. Clin Pharmacol Ther 93(3):275–282

van Kralingen S, Diepstraten J, Peeters MYM, Deneer VHM, van Ramshorst B, Wiezer RJ et al (2011a) Population pharmacokinetics and pharmacodynamics of propofol in morbidly obese patients. Clin Pharmacokinet 50(11):739–750

van Kralingen S, van de Garde EMW, Knibbe CAJ, Diepstraten J, Wiezer MJ, van Ramshorst B et al (2011b) Comparative evaluation of atracurium dosed on ideal body weight vs. total body weight in morbidly obese patients. Br J Clin Pharmacol 71(1):34–40 van Rongen A, Välitalo PAJ, Peeters MYM, Boerma D, Huisman FW, van Ramshorst B et al (2016) Morbidly obese patients exhibit increased CYP2E1-mediated oxidation of acetaminophen. Clin Pharmacokinet 55(7):833–847

van Rongen A, van der Aa MP, Matic M, van Schaik RHN, Deneer VHM, van der Vorst MM et al (2018a) Increased metformin clearance in overweight and obese adolescents: a pharmacokinetic substudy of a randomized controlled trial. Pediatr Drugs 20(4):365–374

van Rongen A, Brill MJE, Vaughns JD, Välitalo PAJ, van Dongen EPA, van Ramshorst B et al (2018b) Higher midazolam clearance in obese adolescents compared with morbidly obese adults. Clin Pharmacokinet 57(5):601–611

Van Wart S, Phillips L, Ludwig EA, Russo R, Gajjar DA, Bello A et al (2004) Population pharmacokinetics and pharmacodynamics of garenoxacin in patients with community-acquired respiratory tract infections. Antimicrob Agents Chemother 48(12):4766–4777

Varin F, Ducharme J, Théorêt Y, Besner JG, Bevan DR, Donati F (1990) Influence of extreme obesity on the body disposition and neuromuscular blocking effect of atracurium. Clin Pharmacol Ther 48(1):18–25

Wellen KE, Hotamisligil GS (2003) Obesity-induced inflammatory changes in adipose tissue. J Clin Invest 112(12):1785–1788

Woolsey SJ, Mansell SE, Kim RB, Tirona RG, Beaton MD (2015) CYP3A activity and expression in nonalcoholic fatty liver disease. Drug Metab Dispos 43(10):1484–1490

Xing J, Chen JDZ (2004) Alterations of gastrointestinal motility in obesity. Obes Res 12 (11):1723–1732

Xiong Y, Fukuda T, Knibbe CAJ, Vinks AA (2017) Drug dosing in obese children. Pediatr Clin N Am 64(6):1417–1438

Medicinal Uses of Hematopoietic Growth Factors in Neonatal Medicine

Robert D. Christensen

Contents

Abstract

This review focuses on certain hematopoietic growth factors that are used as medications in clinical neonatology. It is important to note at the chapter onset that although all of the pharmacological agents mentioned in this review have been approved by the US Food and Drug administration for use in humans, none have been granted a specific FDA indication for neonates. Thus, in a sense, all of the agents mentioned in this chapter could be considered experimental, when

R. D. Christensen (✉)
Divisions of Neonatology and Hematology/Oncology, Department of Pediatrics, University of Utah, Salt Lake City, UT, USA

Intermountain Healthcare, Salt Lake City, UT, USA
e-mail: Robert.christensen@hsc.utah

W. Kiess et al. (eds.), *Pediatric Pharmacotherapy*,
Handbook of Experimental Pharmacology 261, https://doi.org/10.1007/164_2019_261

used in neonates. However, a great many of the pharmacological agents utilized routinely in neonatology practice do not have a specific FDA indication for this population of patients. Consequently, many of the agents reviewed in this chapter are considered by some practitioners to be nonexperimental and are used when they judge such use to be "best practice" for the disorders under treatment.

The medicinal uses of the agents in this chapter vary considerably, between geographic locations, and sometimes even within an institutions. "Consistent approaches" aimed at using these agents in uniform ways in the practice of neonatology are encouraged. Indeed some healthcare systems, and some individual NICUs, have developed written guidelines for using these agents within the practice group. Some such guidelines are provided in this review. It should be noted that these guidelines, or "consistent approaches," must be viewed as dynamic and changing, requiring adjustment and refinement as additional evidence accrues.

Keywords
Darbepoetin · Erythropoietin · G-CSF · Neutropenia · Thrombopoietin

1 Recombinant Human G-CSF

1.1 Neonatal Neutropenia

Neutrophils are crucial to antibacterial host defense (Kobayashi et al. 2018). People who lack neutrophils, whether because of a congenital or an acquired defect, typically have repeated local and systemic infections and sometimes untimely death (Donadieu et al. 2017; Dale and Makaryan 2018). Severe chronic neutropenia (SCN) is a cluster of diagnoses bearing the common feature of very low circulating neutrophil concentrations from birth (Dale and Makaryan 2018; Christensen and Calhoun 2004). The advent of recombinant granulocyte colony-stimulating factor (rG-CSF) dramatically improved the lives of patients with SCN, in most cases elevating their circulating neutrophil concentrations to "safe" levels, reducing infectious illnesses, and extending their life expectancy (Welte and Zeidler 2009).

Rarely, patients with SCN are diagnosed as neonates, or even as patients in neonatal intensive care units (Zeidler et al. 2000; Calhoun and Christensen 1997). However, the majority of patients with SCN are not diagnosed until several months of age, after infectious episodes have prompted an evaluation into immunological deficiencies. When SCN is diagnosed in a neonate, that patient should receive the benefit of rG-CSF treatment (Kobayashi et al. 2018; Donadieu et al. 2017; Dale and Makaryan 2018; Christensen and Calhoun 2004; Welte and Zeidler 2009). Whether neonates who have other varieties of neutropenia, distinct from SCN, benefit from rG-CSF treatment is far less certain (Christensen and Calhoun 2004).

Neutropenia can be defined statistically as a blood neutrophil concentration below the 5th percentile of the reference range population. For neonates, this definition is complicated because the reference range varies by several situations including gestational age, postnatal age, gender, type of delivery (vaginal delivery vs. cesarean

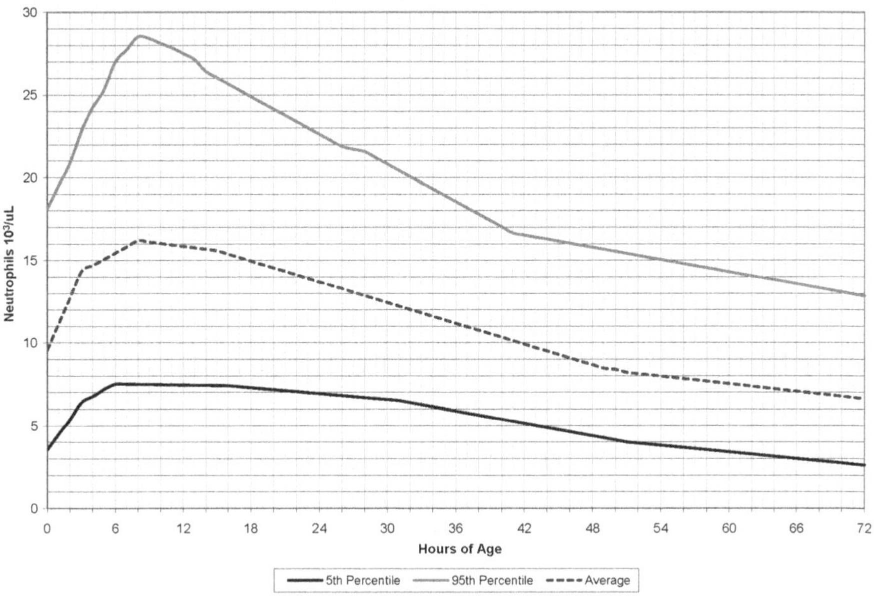

Fig. 1 Reference range for blood neutrophil concentrations during the first 72 h after birth of term and late preterm neonates. A total of 12,149 values were used in this analysis. The 5th percentile, mean, and 95th percentile values are shown. From Schmutz et al. (2008)

section), and altitude (meters above sea level) (Schmutz et al. 2008). Figure 1 shows the 5th and 95th percentile limits for blood neutrophil counts during the first 72 h after birth of term and late preterm neonates among neonates in the Intermountain Healthcare hospitals in the Western United States (Schmutz et al. 2008). Reference ranges for blood neutrophil counts at altitudes of 4,000–5,000 ft. above sea level have a wider range of values than do those at sea level. This is illustrated in Fig. 2, which shows the reference range at sea level and at high-altitude superimposed. The dots on the graph show counts of neonates at Intermountain Healthcare hospitals who would have been judged to have an elevated neutrophil count if the sea level range was used, but who are seen to have a normal count when the appropriate reference range is used (Lambert et al. 2009). The largest altitude-dependent discrepancy is in the 95th percentile reference interval value. The definition of neutropenia is very similar in the sea level (Manroe et al. 1979; Mouzinho et al. 1992) and the high-altitude (Schmutz et al. 2008; Lambert et al. 2009) reference ranges (Fig. 2).

A much simpler approach to defining neutropenia in a neonate is to use a neutrophil concentration <1,000/μL and to define *severe* neutropenia by a count persistently <500/μL (Christensen and Calhoun 2004; Welte and Zeidler 2009). Although this approach lacks the accuracy of the data-derived reference range approach, it has the advantages that it is easy to remember and is in keeping with standard definitions used in pediatric and adult medicine (Furutani et al. 2018). Furthermore, it is not clear whether blood neutrophil counts labeled as "low" by the

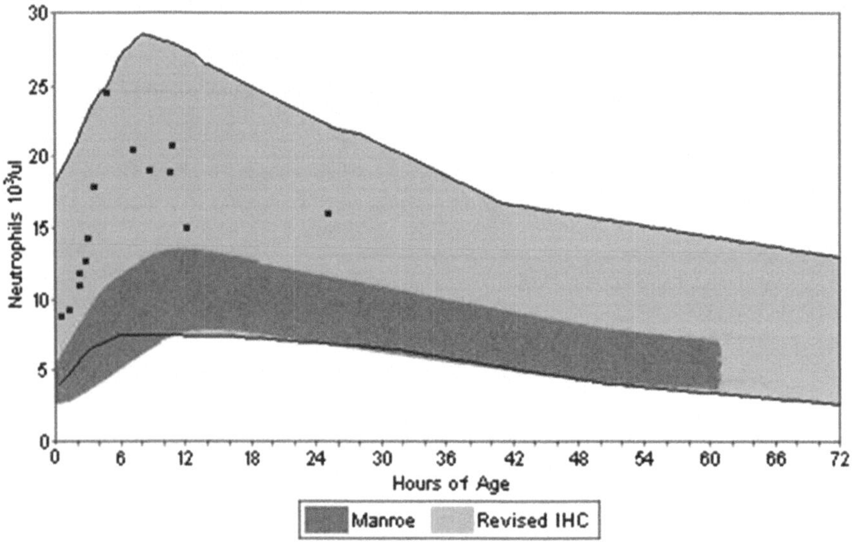

Fig. 2 Reference range for blood neutrophil concentrations, superimposing the Monroe (Dallas, Texas) and the Schmutz (Intermountain Healthcare) curves. The dots represent neonates in Utah that would have been regarded as having an elevated neutrophil count using the sea level (Dallas) curve, but fell within the high-altitude (Intermountain) Schmutz curve. From Lambert et al. (2009)

Table 1 Varieties of neutropenia among neonates that are generally considered "Severe Chronic Neutropenia"

Kostmann syndrome autosomal recessive type
Severe congenital neutropenia autosomal dominant type
Shwachman-Diamond syndrome
Barth syndrome
Cartilage-hair hypoplasia
Cyclic neutropenia
Glycogen storage disease type 1b
Severe neonatal immune-mediated neutropenias

reference range approach actually convey a host-defense deficiency, unless the count is $<1{,}000/\mu L$.

1.2 Severe Chronic Neutropenia in a Neonate

Kostmann Syndrome (Including Autosomal Recessive Severe Congenital Neutropenia [MIM #610738] and Autosomal Dominant Severe Congenital Neutropenia [MIM #202700]) Table 1 lists varieties of neutropenia that are generally considered as part of the SCN syndrome. The prototype for SCN is Kostmann syndrome, initially described in 1956 in a kindred in Northern Sweden (Kostmann 1956; Carlsson and Fasth 2001; Aprikyan et al. 2004; Khincha and Savage 2016). Patients with this variety of SCN generally have circulating neutrophil concentrations <200/μL and a marrow aspirate or biopsy with a "maturation arrest" where few neutrophilic cells are seen beyond the promyelocyte stage. The original family had what appeared to be an autosomal recessive disorder, but most kindreds subsequently reported seem to have an autosomal dominant inheritance. The condition is the result of mutations in the ELA2 (neutrophil elastase) gene (Donadieu et al. 2017; Dale and Makaryan 2018; Welte and Zeidler 2009; Khincha and Savage 2016). rG-CSF treatment is almost always effective in increasing blood neutrophil concentrations and reducing febrile illnesses; however it does not usually correct the gingivitis that is a prominent feature of this condition in some families. This is probably because rG-CSF does not increase the natural antimicrobial peptide (LL-37) deficiency in these patients (Zetterstrom 2002; Carlsson et al. 2006).

Shwachman-Diamond Syndrome (MIM #260400) This variety of severe chronic neutropenia is generally diagnosed after manifestations of exocrine pancreatic insufficiency, with diarrhea and failure to thrive. It is generally inherited as an autosomal recessive marrow failure and cancer predisposition syndrome. Patients with this condition are generally compound heterozygotes or homozygotes for mutations in the Shwachman-Bodian-Diamond syndrome gene at 7q11, but the molecular function of the affected protein product remains unclear (Alter 2017). Some children with this syndrome respond favorably to rG-CSF, while others progress to bone marrow failure and require bone marrow transplantation (Alter 2017; Bezzerri and Cipolli 2018).

Barth Syndrome (MIM #302060) These patients are generally males with dilated cardiomyopathy, organic aciduria, growth failure, muscle weakness, feeding problems, and neutropenia (Steward et al. 2019). The underlying genetic abnormality involves mutations in the tafazzin gene (TAZ) at Xq28. The condition is characterized by defective remodeling of phospholipid side chains in mitochondrial membranes. G-CSF can be helpful in patients as an adjunct to treating infections, or as a preventive measure if their neutropenia is severe.

Cartilage-Hair Hypoplasia (MIM #250250) This is an autosomal recessive form of short-limbed dwarfism caused by mutations in the untranslated portions of the *RMRP* gene, which forms the RNA subunit of the RNase MRP complex. This complex is involved in ribosome assembly. The severity-degree of the phenotype appears to correlate with the effect of the mutation on RNase MRP functioning. The condition is associated with neutropenia and frequent infections. These patients have short pudgy hands, redundant skin, and hyperextensible joints in the hands and feet and flexor contractions at the elbow. Neutropenia occurs in some of these patients, and those cases have been reported to benefit from rG-CSF administration (Thiel and Rauch 2011).

Cyclic Hematopoiesis (MIM #162800) This condition is caused by mutation in the ELA2 (neutrophil elastase) gene, mapping to 19p13.3. The disorder is characterized by regular 21-day cyclic fluctuations in the blood concentration of neutrophils, monocytes, eosinophils, lymphocytes, platelets, and reticulocytes. The neutropenia can be severe, leading to serious infections (Donadieu et al. 2017; Dale and Makaryan 2018). Because it generally takes several cycles before the diagnosis is considered, most cases are not discovered as neonates. rG-CSF administration is useful in preventing the very low nadir neutrophil counts and in preventing infectious complications (Donadieu et al. 2017; Dale and Makaryan 2018; Alter 2017).

Glycogen Storage Disease Type 1b (MIM #232220) von Gierke disease is an autosomal recessive disorder caused by a deficiency of the enzyme glucose 6-phosphate translocase, which transports glucose 6-phosphate into the endoplasmic reticulum for further metabolism. In GSD-1b, glucose 6-phosphate accumulates intracellularly. Affected neonates present with hypoglycemia, hepatomegaly, growth failure, and neutropenia. Patients with GSD-1b have recurrent bacterial infections, oral ulcers, and inflammatory bowel disease. The gene causing GSD-1b is located on chromosome 11q23 (Pierre et al. 2008). rG-CSF can help these patients avoid the recurrent bacterial infections that are otherwise a problematic part of this condition.

Severe Immune-Mediated Neonatal Neutropenia Most of the very severe and prolonged immune-mediated neonatal neutropenias are alloimmune (Lewin and Bussel 2015; Dale 2017). However, a few severe and prolonged cases have been found to be autoimmune (maternal autoimmune disease), and a few have been found to be autoimmune neutropenia of infancy (a primary isolated autoimmune phenomenon in neonates) (Farruggia et al. 2017).

Alloimmune neonatal neutropenia is a relatively common condition where the mother develops antibodies to antigens present on paternal and fetal neutrophils. Antineutrophil antibodies have been found in the serum of as many as 20% of randomly surveyed pregnant and postpartum women. Most such antibodies cause little problem to the fetus and neonate, but up to 2% of consecutively sampled neonates have neutropenia on this basis. This variety of neutropenia can be severe and prolonged, with a median duration of neutropenia of about 7 weeks, but a range up to 6 months. Repeated infections can occur in these patients until their severe neutropenia remits. Delayed separation of the umbilical cord and skin infections are the most common infectious complications, but serious and life-threatening infections can occur. The mortality rate in this condition, due to overwhelming infection, is reported to be 5%. Severe cases have been successfully treated with rG-CSF (Maheshwari et al. 2002; Makeshwari et al. 2002; Calhoun et al. 2001). Unlike patients with other varieties of SCN, the neutropenia in this condition will remit spontaneously, and the rG-CSF treatment can be stopped. Remission occurs when maternal antineutrophil antibody in the neonate has dropped significantly (Table 2).

Neonatal autoimmune neutropenia occurs when mothers have autoimmune diseases, and their antineutrophil antibodies cross the placenta and bind to fetal neutrophils. Clinical features are generally much milder than in alloimmune neonatal neutropenia, and it is rare that a patient with this variety of neonatal neutropenia

Table 2 Varieties of neutropenia among neonates that are NOT classified as "Severe Chronic Neutropenia"

Pregnancy-induced hypertension
Severe intrauterine growth restriction
The twin-twin transfusion syndrome
Rh hemolytic disease
Bacterial infection
Fungal infection
Necrotizing enterocolitis
Chronic idiopathic neutropenia of prematurity

needs rG-CSF treatment (Farruggia et al. 2017; Maheshwari et al. 2002; Makeshwari et al. 2002; Calhoun et al. 2001).

Autoimmune neutropenia of infancy is an unusual disorder where the fetus, and subsequently the neonate, has a primary isolated autoimmune phenomenon. Neutrophil-specific antibodies are found in the neonate's serum, reactive against his/her own neutrophils, but no antibodies are found in the mother's serum. Most cases occur in children between 3 and 30 months of age, with a reported incidence of 1:100,000 children. Affected children present with minor infections. Bux reported 240 cases, and reported that 12% presented with severe infections, including pneumonia, sepsis, or meningitis (Bux 2008; Bux et al. 1998). The neutropenia in this condition generally persists much longer than in cases of alloimmune neutropenia, with a median duration of about 30 months and a range from 6 to 60 months. This variety of neonatal neutropenia can be severe, with blood neutrophil concentrations often <500/μL. rG-CSF administration can increase the neutrophil count and reduce infectious complications.

1.3 Neonatal Neutropenia NOT Categorized as Severe Chronic Neutropenia

Pregnancy-Induced Hypertension (PIH) Neutropenia due to PIH is the most common variety of neutropenia seen in the NICU (Koenig and Christensen 1989a, 1991). Perhaps 50% of neonates born to mothers with PIH have this variety of neutropenia. The ANC can be very low, frequently <500/μL, but generally rises spontaneously within the first days and is almost always >1,000/μL by day 3. Usually no leukocyte "left shift" is seen, and no toxic granulation, Dohle bodies, or vacuolization are present in the neutrophils. It is not clear whether this variety of neutropenia predisposes neonates to acquire bacterial infections. Usually the condition is so transient that such a predisposition seems very unlikely. The condition is probably caused by an inhibitor of neutrophil production of placental origin that depresses G-CSF production (Koenig and Christensen 1991; Tsao et al. 1999; Doron et al. 1994).

In a multicentered study from Brazil involving over 900 VLBW neonates (300 born to women with PIH), no increases were observed in rates of early or late neonatal sepsis in the PIH group. Logistic regression indicated that neutropenia significantly increased the odds of early-onset sepsis but not late-onset sepsis. In addition, neutropenia was much more common in those who died. It was neutropenia, not PIH, which carried an association with poor outcome; PIH itself was not a risk factor either for sepsis or for death (Procianoy et al. 2010). Similarly, in a retrospective analysis by Teng et al., VLBW neonates with early neutropenia associated with PIH did not have increased odds of developing late-onset bacterial infection (Teng et al. 2009).

Several clinical trials have tested administering rG-CSF prophylactically to neonates with neutropenia, most of which had neutropenia associated with PIH. Kocherlakota found a protective effect of rG-CSF administration toward early infections (Kocherlakota and La Gamma 1998), and Miura found a protective effect late-onset infections (Miura et al. 2001). In a large multicentered, randomized, placebo-controlled trial in France ($n = 200$), the rG-CSF recipients had only a transient (2-week) period of fewer infections, but did not have an overall significant improvement in infection-free survival (Kuhn et al. 2009).

GM-CSF administration was tested as a means of prophylaxing very preterm neonates against infections. Treatment was not associated with improved or more adverse neurodevelopmental, general, health, or educational outcomes at 2 years and at 5 years (Marlow et al. 2015).

Neutropenia Associated with Severe Intrauterine Growth Restriction This variety of neonatal neutropenia seems to be mechanistically identical to that associated with PIH. We found no difference in the onset, duration, or severity of neutropenia in SGA neonates vs. neonates born after PIH (Christensen et al. 2006a). In a recent analysis of 3,650 SGA neonates, we found that neutropenia was not independently associated with maternal hypertensive disorders, over and above the effect of SGA (Christensen et al. 2015). Thus, we maintain that the neutropenia of PIH is more properly termed the neutropenia of SGA and that it is transient with few clinical consequences and with no clear benefit of rG-CSF administration (Christensen et al. 2015).

The Twin-Twin Transfusion Syndrome The donor in a twin-twin transfusion is generally neutropenic, but the recipient can also have neutropenia, although usually not as severe (Koenig et al. 1991). As with the varieties of neutropenia accompanying PIH and SGA, there is generally no leukocyte “left shift” nor are there neutrophil morphological abnormalities. This condition is also transient, with the ANC generally spontaneously rising to >1,000/uL by 2 or 3 days, and, thus, no rG-CSF administration is warranted.

Rh Hemolytic Disease Neonates with anemia from Rh hemolytic disease are usually neutropenic on the first day of life (Koenig and Christensen 1989b). This variety of neutropenia is similar to that of PIH/SGA and donors in a twin-twin transfusion and is likely due to reduced neutrophil production. The neutropenia is transient, is not accompanied by a leukocyte left shift, and generally resolves in a day or two; thus, no specific treatment is generally required.

Bacterial Infection Two strategies have been proposed for rG-CSF usage during neonatal infections. Since neutropenia commonly accompanies overwhelming septic shock in neonates, perhaps rG-CSF might be a reasonable adjunct to antibiotics and intensive care treatment. Second, since neutrophil function, particularly chemotaxis, is immature among neonates, perhaps rG-CSF administration might be a reasonable way to prevent nosocomial infections among high-risk neonatal patients. Animal models for both potential uses of rG-CSF were established and supported these hypotheses. In a Cochrane review, Carr et al. examined both potential uses (Carr et al. 2003). They located 7 studies (involving 257 neonates) where infected neonates were treated with rG-CSF vs. placebo (Carr et al. 2003; Ahmad et al. 2002; Bedford-Russell et al. 2001; Bilgin et al. 2001; Drossou-Agakidou et al. 1998; Schibler et al. 1998; Gillan et al. 1994). They located 3 studies (359 neonates) where rG-CSF vs. placebo was used as prophylaxis against infections (Cairo et al. 1995, 1999; Carr et al. 1999). They found no evidence that the addition of rG-CSF or rGM-CSF to antibiotic therapy in preterm infants with suspected systemic infection reduces immediate all-cause mortality. No significant survival advantage was seen at 14 days from the start of therapy [typical RR 0.71 (95% CI 0.38, 1.33); typical RD −0.05 (95% CI −0.14, 0.04)]. They conducted a subgroup analysis of 97 infants from three of the studies who, in addition to systemic infection, had a low neutrophil count (<1,700/uL) at trial entry. This subgroup did show a significant reduction in mortality by day 14 [RR 0.34 (95% CI 0.12, 0.92); RD −0.18 (95% CI −0.33, −0.03); NNT 6 (95% CI 3–33)].

The three prophylaxis studies did not show a significant reduction in mortality in neonates receiving rGM-CSF [RR 0.59 (95% CI 0.24, 1.44); RD −0.03 (95% CI −0.08, 0.02)]. The identification of sepsis as the primary outcome of prophylaxis studies has been hampered by inadequately stringent definitions of systemic infection. Carr et al. concluded that there is currently insufficient evidence to support the introduction of either rG-CSF or rGM-CSF into neonatal practice, either as treatment of established systemic infection to reduce resulting mortality or as prophylaxis to prevent systemic infection in high-risk neonates (Carr et al. 2003).

Fungal Infection Thrombocytopenia is known to accompany fungal infection in the NICU, but neutropenia can also accompany such infections. No studies have specifically focused on using rG-CSF among neutropenic neonates with fungal infection.

Necrotizing Enterocolitis Neutropenia is relatively common among severe cases of NEC. Some cases are transient and resemble the neutropenia following endotoxin (Kling and Hutter 2003). No studies have focused on using rG-CSF among neutropenic neonates with NEC.

Chronic Idiopathic Neutropenia of Prematurity Certain preterm neonates develop neutropenia when 4 to 10 weeks old. This variety of neutropenia is often associated with a patient's spontaneous recovery from the anemia of prematurity.

Neutrophil counts are generally <1,000/μL but rarely <500/μL (Juul et al. 1998a; Juul and Christensen 2003; Chirico et al. 2002). The condition is transient, lasting a few weeks to perhaps a month or more. It appears to be a hyporegenerative neutropenia, because it is not accompanied by a leukocyte "left shift" nor morphological abnormalities of the neutrophils. Patients with this condition have a "rG-CSF mobilizable neutrophil reserve," meaning that if rG-CSF is given, their neutrophil count increases within hours. This fact has been taken as evidence that these patients do not have a significant host-defense deficiency, as in theory they can supply neutrophils to tissues when needed (Juul and Christensen 2003). Thus, although these patients are neutropenic, this condition is likely benign and needs no treatment.

1.4 Other Proposed Uses for rG-CSF in the NICU

rG-CSF has been tested as a neuroprotectant in a rodent model of neonatal hypoxic-ischemic brain damage. Subcutaneous G-CSF administration, beginning 1 h after the injury, prevented brain atrophy, preserved reflexes, and improved motor coordination and memory. In addition, animals treated with G-CSF had better somatic growth (Fathali et al. 2010).

G-CSF is found in amniotic fluid, which is swallowed by the fetus in large quantities, up to 200 mL/k/day. The G-CSF swallowed binds to receptors on enterocytes and conveys antiapoptotic actions (Gersting et al. 2004). A sterile, isotonic, simulated amniotic fluid containing rG-CSF has been administered to NICU patients who are otherwise NPO (nil per os) with the hypothesis that such will prevent disuse atrophy of the intestinal villi that otherwise occurs during the NPO period. Safety and early efficacy studies of this approach seem promising (Sullivan et al. 2002; Christensen et al. 2005; Barney et al. 2007).

rG-CSF and rGM-CSF have both been examined as means of prophylaxis against nosocomial infections in VLBW neonates. A large multicentered, randomized trial by Carr et al. (2009) involved 280 neonates ≤31 weeks gestation, and <10th percentile for birth weight were randomized within 72 h of birth to receive GM-CSF 10 μg/k/day subcutaneously for 5 days or standard management. The primary outcome was sepsis-free survival 14 days from trial entry. They observed a significant increase in blood neutrophil count in the GM-CSF recipients, but no difference in sepsis-free short-term survival.

Aktas et al. from Istanbul reported a randomized trial of G-CSF plus antibiotics vs. antibiotics alone among 56 neutropenic preterm infants with proven or suspected sepsis. The neutrophil count was significantly higher on the second and third study day in the G-CSF recipients, but the mortality rate was unaffected (Aktaş et al. 2015).

The current consensus is that rG-CSF and rGM-CSF should not be used routinely in NICUs for prophylaxis against nosocomial infections because the evidence for such usage is at best very weak.

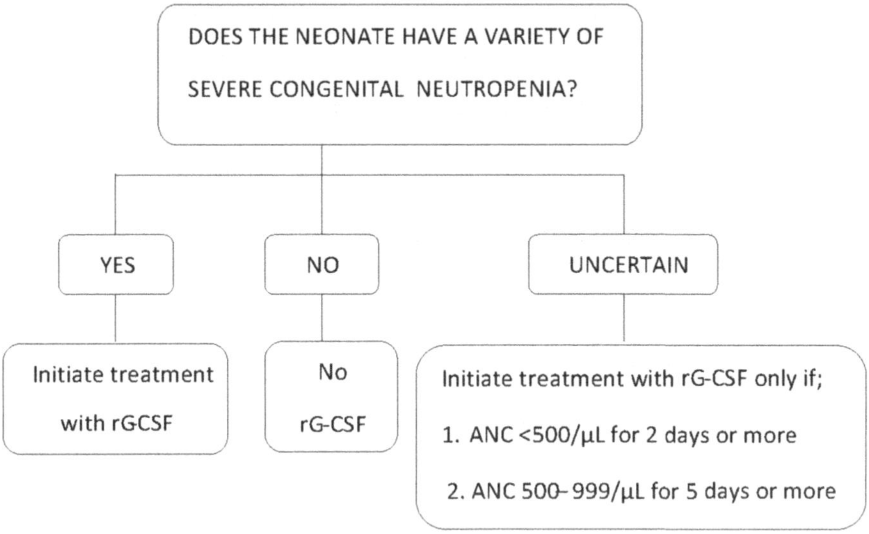

Fig. 3 Guidelines for assisting in the decision regarding which neutropenic NICU patients should be treated with rG-CSF, based on the variety of neutropenia. Modified from Calhoun et al. (2000)

1.5 Pharmacologic Considerations

In the USA rG-CSF is marketed by Amgen (Thousand Oaks, CA) under the generic name *filgrastim* and the brand name Neupogen®. It is administered by subcutaneous injection or IV. An approved indication is severe chronic neutropenia where it is intended to reduce the incidence and duration of the sequelae of severe neutropenia, namely, fever, infections, and oropharyngeal ulcers. The proposed dosing (see next section) in neonates with severe chronic neutropenia is 10 μg/kg subcutaneously once per day for 3 consecutive days, then reevaluation. Dosing is aimed at keeping the blood neutrophil count above 500/μL. This can sometimes be accomplished with dosing every 7–10 days.

1.6 A Proposed Consistent Approach to the Use of rG-CSF in the NICU

The following proposal was introduced as a guideline to serve until sufficient data is accumulated for conducting an evidence-based assessment of the risks and benefits of rG-CSF use in each of the neutropenic conditions in the NICU (Calhoun et al. 2000). Briefly (Fig. 3), we propose if a neonatal patient has neutropenia, and that variety of neutropenia is known to be a variety of SCN, the patient should be referred to pediatric hematology and treated with rG-CSF.

We propose beginning treatment with a dose of 10 μg/kg subcutaneously, once per day for 3 consecutive days. Thereafter doses are given as needed to titrate the

ANC to around 1,000/μL. We propose if a neonatal patient has neutropenia, and the variety of neutropenia is NOT one of the varieties of SCN, rG-CSF treatment should not be used. We propose if a neonatal patient has neutropenia, and the variety of neutropenia is NOT known (and therefore might be a SCN variety), while evaluating the variety of neutropenia, rG-CSF treatment could be instituted if the ANC was <500/μL for 2 days or more, or <1,000/μL for 5–7 days or more.

We did not include criteria for administering rGM-CSF, as we found insufficient evidence for its use in the NICU. If one follows this schema (Fig. 2), it will result in little use of rG-CSF in any given NICU. However, the schema should focus the rG-CSF usage on those patients with the most to gain and least to lose by its application. As additional pertinent investigative work is published, these guidelines should be modified accordingly.

2 Recombinant Human Erythropoiesis Stimulating Agents

2.1 Erythropoietin and Darbepoetin

During human fetal and neonatal development, erythropoietin has critical erythropoietic and non-erythropoietic actions (McPherson and Juul 2010; Shiou et al. 2011). Although initially described by, and principally known for, its actions on erythroid progenitors, erythropoietin is also an important physiological growth factor for fetal small intestinal villous enterocytes and neurons (Arsenault et al. 2010; Juul 2000).

Human amniotic fluid contains erythropoietin in concentrations of 25–40 mU/mL. In the third trimester, a fetus swallows 200–300 mL of amniotic fluid per kilogram body weight per day and thus swallows 10–15 U of erythropoietin/kg/day (Juul 2000). In humans, erythropoietin does not cross the placenta from the maternal to the fetal circulation, and it appears that the source of the erythropoietin in amniotic fluid is not the maternal circulation. In the second and third trimesters, amniotic fluid is largely derived from fetal urine, with minor constituents from fetal tracheal effluent and the placenta and fetal membranes. However, erythropoietin in amniotic fluid does not appear to come from fetal urine. The fetal kidney makes little erythropoietin before delivery, studies using in situ hybridization and immunohistochemistry indicate that the source of erythropoietin in amniotic fluid is largely placental: from mesenchymal and endothelial cells in the deciduae and from the amnion (Brace et al. 2006).

Erythropoietin is present in human colostrum and breast milk in concentrations of 10–20 mU/mL (Arsenault et al. 2010; Juul 2000). Erythropoietin concentrations in mother's milk do not correlate with erythropoietin concentrations in her blood. In fact, over the first weeks of lactation, maternal serum erythropoietin concentrations fall, whereas milk erythropoietin concentrations increase, reaching the highest concentrations in women breast-feeding for a year or more. The source of erythropoietin in breast milk appears to be mammary gland epithelium (Juul 2000).

Erythropoietin in human amniotic fluid, colostrum, and breast milk is relatively protected from proteolytic digestion in the fetal and neonatal gastrointestinal tract.

Rather than being absorbed from the gastrointestinal tract into the blood, the erythropoietin swallowed by the fetus and neonate binds to erythropoietin receptors on the luminal surface of villous enterocytes, where it serves topically as a growth and development factor. Indeed, experimental animals artificially fed formulas devoid of erythropoietin have retarded villous development, a condition that can be remedied by enteral recombinant erythropoietin and blocked by anti-erythropoietin antibody.

Erythropoietin is produced by cells in the developing central nervous system and is present in relatively high concentrations in fetal cerebrospinal fluid (CSF) (Juul et al. 1997, 1998b, 1999; Dame et al. 2001). Among newborn infants, the highest concentrations of erythropoietin in the CSF are seen in the most premature neonates, and by several years of age, CSF erythropoietin concentrations are generally below 1 mU/mL. Erythropoietin receptors are expressed on human fetal neurons, and at least small quantities of recombinant erythropoietin, administered intravenously, cross the blood-brain barrier and appear in the cerebrospinal fluid (Wu et al. 2012). Erythropoietin in the central nervous system is a neuroprotectant from hypoxia. Erythropoietin production increases rapidly in the brain during hypoxia, and when erythropoietin binds to receptors on neurons, antiapoptotic activity is induced. The clinical utility of recombinant erythropoietin as a neuroprotectant is a topic of recent and ongoing studies (Wu et al. 2012; Ohls et al. 2013, 2014, 2016a; Juul and Pet 2015; Natalucci et al. 2016; Fischer et al. 2017; Juul et al. 2018).

The liver is the primary site of erythropoietin production in the fetus. The kidney does not become the primary site until several months after birth. In the human fetus, the kidney produces about 5% of the total erythropoietin during mid-gestation. The developmental mechanisms regulating the switch in erythropoietin production from the liver to the kidney are not completely known but may involve developmental expression of transcription activators such as hypoxia-inducible factor and hepatic nuclear factor 4, or developmental methylation of promoter and enhancer regions. Alternatively, the switch might involve the GATA transcription factors, particularly GATA-2 and GATA-3, which are negative regulators of erythropoietin gene transcription.

Erythropoietin ameliorates experimental damage to the placenta and fetal liver induced by lipopolysaccharide (Dijkstra et al. 2010). Elevated concentrations of erythropoietin in fetal blood and/or amniotic fluid may indicate fetal hypoxia, and although erythropoietin may have a protective role for some fetal cells, such as neurons, placental, hepatic, and intestinal villous cells, it might be a marker for poor neurodevelopmental outcome based on severe or chronic hypoxia (Bhandari et al. 2011; Christensen et al. 2014a).

Darbepoetin alfa (Darbe; trade name Aranesp) is a hyperglycosylated analogue of recombinant human erythropoietin (Epo) with two additional N-linked carbohydrate chains, introduced into the primary Epo sequence using site-directed mutagenesis (Fig. 4). Although Darbe stimulates erythropoiesis by the same mechanism as endogenous Epo, its increased carbohydrate content provides Darbe with lower clearance, longer half-life, and more sustained erythropoietic effects than Epo.

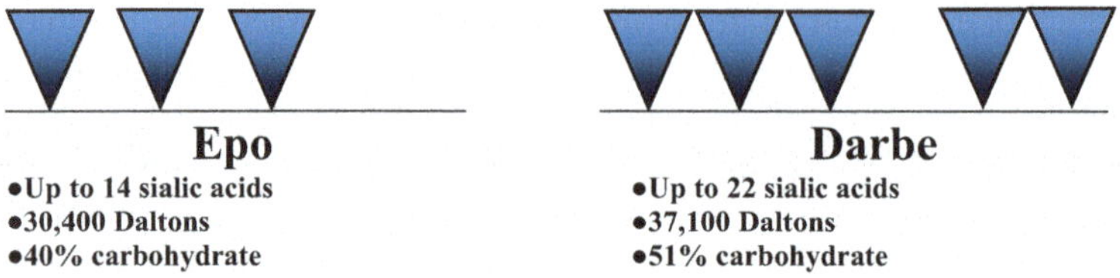

Fig. 4 Schematic diagram showing the difference between recombinant erythropoietin (Epo) and Darbepoetin alfa (Darbe). The additional carbohydrate chains in Darbe result in more biological activity and longer serum half-life

This feature permits a reduction in the frequency of Darbe administration compared to Epo (Patel and Ohls 2015; Ohls et al. 2016b).

2.2 Transfusion Avoidance with ESAs

Elements to avoid erythrocyte transfusion in neonates include delayed clamping of the umbilical cord, or cord milking, at birth, obtaining the initial blood for laboratory testing using otherwise discarded fetal blood in the umbilical cord after birth, efforts to reduce the volume and frequency of phlebotomy for laboratory testing, and use of erythropoiesis stimulating agents (ESAs), such as erythropoietin and darbepoetin (Christensen et al. 2014b; Henry et al. 2015). Randomized placebo-controlled studies aimed at avoiding transfusions indicate a small reduction if ESAs are used (Ohlsson and Aher 2017). Early ESAs were associated with decreased rates of IVH, PVL, and NEC. Studies on neurodevelopmental outcomes are ongoing, but in one completed trial, ESAs were associated with better short- and long-term neurodevelopment (Ohls et al. 2014, 2016a).

2.3 Pharmacological Considerations

Somewhat limited pharmacological studies have been reported on neonates treated with erythropoietin (Epo) or darbepoetin (Darbe) (Saleh et al. 2013; Roberts et al. 2015; An et al. 2017). Both Epo and Darbe are primarily cleared by binding to erythropoietin receptors. Relevant and generalizable findings include (1) the Iowa group reported that preterm infants, when stimulated with rEpo, have a marked capacity to produce additional erythrocytes (sevenfold increase) that could result in a decrease need for red blood cell transfusions (Saleh et al. 2013). (2) The Utah group reported that darbepoetin administered to neonates with hypoxemic ischemic encephalopathy and treated with hypothermia was best described with a 1-compartment model. They found a clearance of 0.015 L/h/kg and a volume of distribution of 0.51/kg. They also found that increasing gestational age was associated with decreased clearance (Roberts et al. 2015). (3) The Iowa group reported studies of preterm neonates who received single doses of Darbe and found that, like adult subjects, preterm neonate's kinetics were best described by a two-compartment model. In contrast to the pharmacokinetic parameters in adults, Darbe in neonates was more rapidly cleared (0.03–0.05 L/h/kg), and the volume of distribution was much greater (0.84 L/kg) (An et al. 2017).

3 Thrombopoietic Stimulating Agents

3.1 Neonatal Thrombocytopenia

Platelet transfusions were introduced into clinical medicine about 60 years ago, when they were shown to reduce the mortality rate of patients with leukemia that were bleeding secondary to hyporegenerative thrombocytopenia. In modern neonatology units, platelet transfusions are integral and indeed are lifesaving for some neonates. However the great majority of platelet transfusions currently administered in NICUs are not given in the original paradigm, to treat thrombocytopenic hemorrhage, but instead are administered prophylactically with the hope that they will reduce the risk of spontaneous bleeding. Weighting the risks and benefits of platelet transfusion, although this task is imprecise, should be attempted each time a platelet transfusion is ordered. Adopting guidelines specific for platelet transfusion will improve consistency of care and will generally reduce transfusion usage, thereby reducing costs and conserving valuable blood bank resources. Initiating specific programs to improve compliance with transfusion guidelines can further improve NICU transfusion practice.

The Reference Range Concept in Neonatal Hematology The term "thrombocytopenia" indicates a low concentration of platelets in the blood. For decades the definition of thrombocytopenia, among patients of all ages, has been a platelet count <150,000/μL (Roberts et al. 2008; Ferrer-Marin et al. 2010). However, a more accurate method to define any abnormal clinical laboratory test is to identify values that fall outside the appropriate "reference range." Reference ranges are particularly applicable to neonatology because "normal ranges" for laboratory tests are not available for neonates. This is because blood is not drawn on healthy neonates for the purpose of establishing normal ranges, as is generally done with adults. Instead, "reference ranges" are used, which consist of the 5th–95th percentile values assembled from very large numbers of neonates with minimal pathology or with pathology not thought to be relevant to the laboratory parameter under study. Using this approach, it is clear that among preterm infants, the long-held definition of thrombocytopenia (platelet count <150,000/μL) is overly simplistic, inaccurate, and sometimes quite misleading.

Defining the Reference Ranges for Platelet Count and Mean Platelet Volume in Preterm and Term Neonates Using Large Multihospital Databases Reference ranges for blood concentrations of platelets in preterm and term infants, on the day of birth, are shown in Fig. 5a (Wiedmeier et al. 2009). For

Panel A. Initial platelet counts.

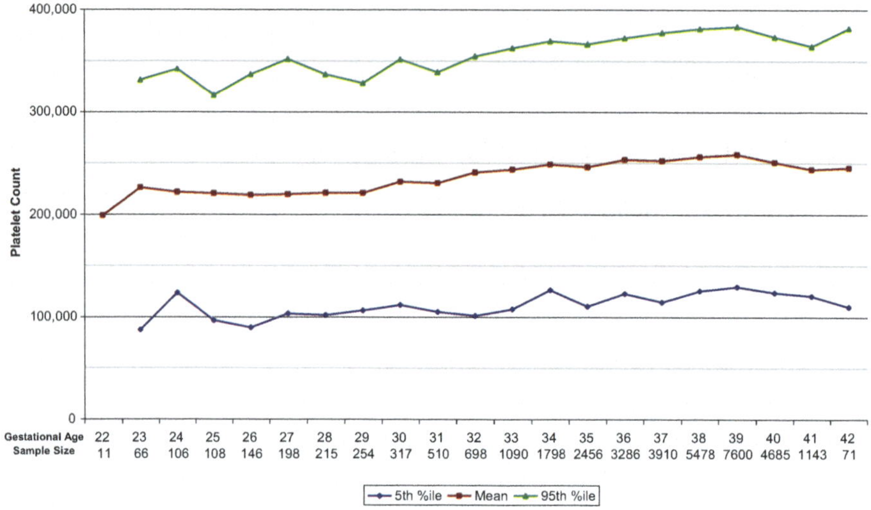

Panel B. Initial MPV measurements.

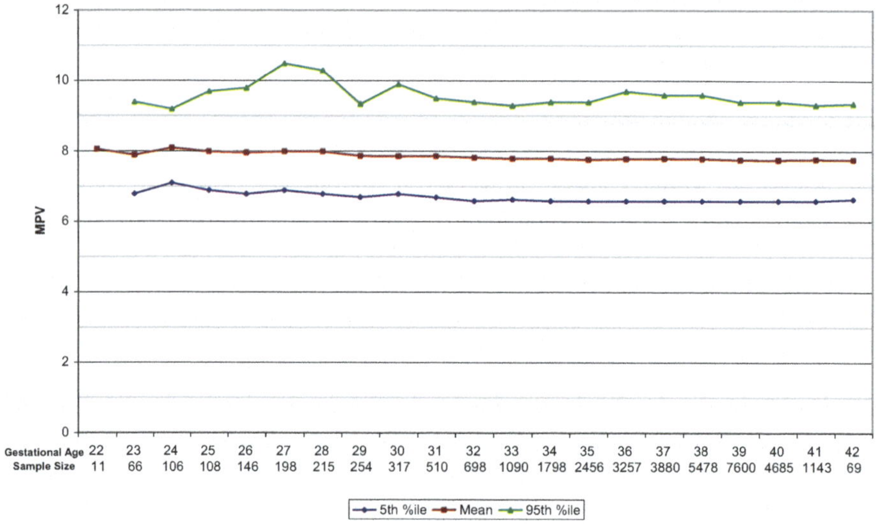

Fig. 5 The first recorded platelet counts (Panel **a**) and mean platelet volume (MPV) determinations (Panel **b**) obtained in the first 3 days after birth are shown for neonates of 22–42 weeks gestation. Mean values are given by the middle line, and the 5th and 95th percentiles are given by the lower and upper lines. (Panel **a**) Initial platelet counts. (Panel **b**) Initial MPV measurements

neonates below 33 weeks gestation, the 5th percentile value is approximately 100,000/μL. Thus platelet counts in the range of 100,000–150,000/μL, previously termed "mild thrombocytopenia," should be recognized as within the reference range and therefore not abnormal. Although the reference ranges for platelet count increase gradually from 23 to 40 weeks gestation, the mean platelet volume stays the same during this period (Fig. 5b) (Wiedmeier et al. 2009).

Platelet counts are expected to gradually rise during the first 2 weeks following birth. As shown in Fig. 6, counts at 14–21 days of age are generally 50% higher than they were at birth. This increase is likely the result of a physiological surge of thrombopoietin at birth (Ferrer-Marin et al. 2010; Wiedmeier et al. 2009; Murray et al. 2000; Sola et al. 1999; Kline et al. 2008). Thrombopoietin is the primary physiological regulator of platelet production. Similarly, the MPV increases over the first 14 days following birth, likely indicative of accelerated platelet production. When the reference range concept is applied to preterm and term neonates, the definitions of thrombocytosis and thrombocytopenia are both seen to be highly dependent on postnatal age (Wiedmeier et al. 2009).

Relationships Between Maternal and Fetal Platelet Counts Discovering thrombocytopenia in a pregnant woman can be concerning to families and physicians, including the pediatricians and/or neonatologists planning to provide care for the neonate. The reference range for platelet counts during pregnancy changes by trimester (Fig. 7a) (Jensen et al. 2011). Largely the result of dilution of mother's blood by her expanding plasma volume, her platelet counts gradually fall as pregnancy progresses, however her MPV does not change (Fig. 7b). The lower reference range for platelet count during the third trimester is about 115,000/μL; thus maternal platelet counts in the range of 115,000–150,000/μL, previously termed "mild

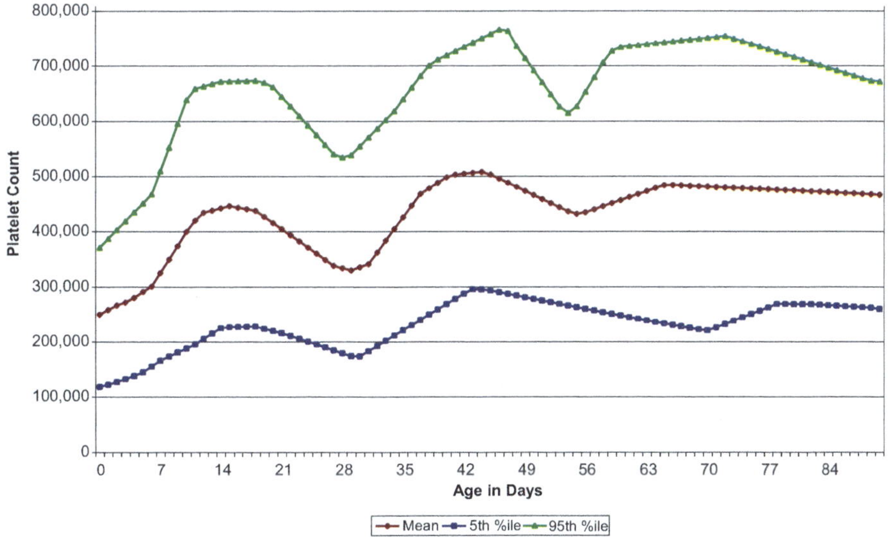

Fig. 6 The effect of advancing postnatal age on platelet counts during the first 90 days following birth. Mean values are given by the middle line, and the 5th and 95th percentile are given by the lower and upper lines, respectively

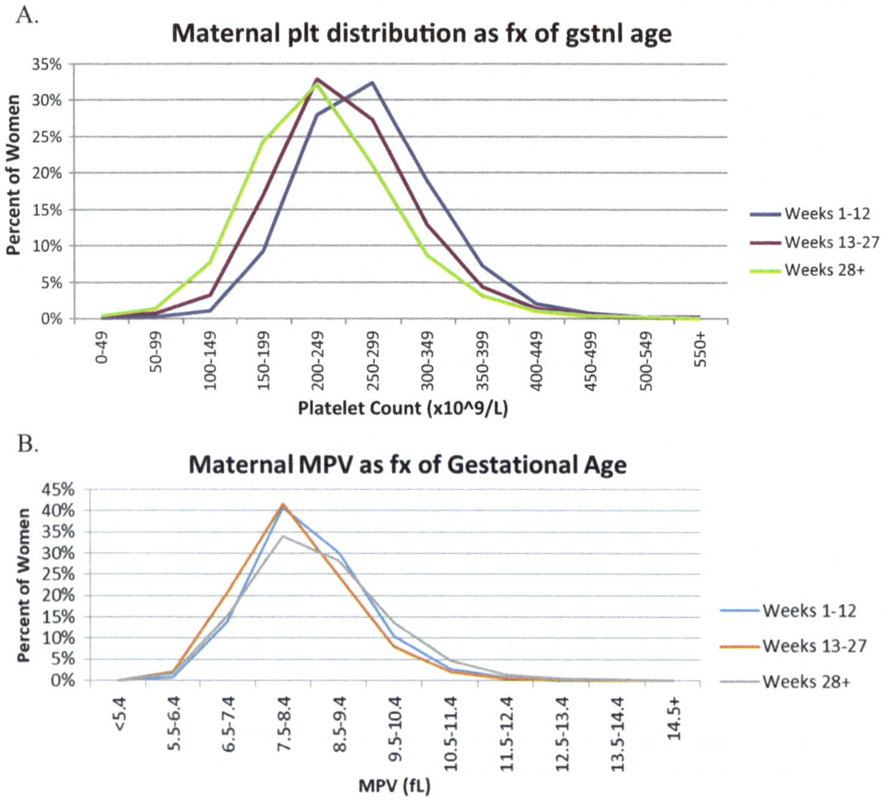

Fig. 7 Platelet counts ($n = 92{,}518$) obtained on pregnant women ($n = 41{,}887$) according to trimester; first ($n = 28{,}266$), second ($n = 24{,}573$), and third ($n = 39{,}679$). Panel (**a**) displays blood concentrations of platelets ($\times 10^9$/L), and Panel (**b**) displays mean platelet volume (fL)

thrombocytopenia," are in fact within the reference range and thus should not be considered abnormal.

Pregnant women with a platelet count <50,000/μL most likely have hematopathology such as ITP or HELLP syndrome, but a variety of causes are identified, and perhaps 20–25% of these women have no recognized etiology for their thrombocytopenia. If a women's platelet count is >75,000/μL at delivery, it is unlikely that her neonate with have thrombocytopenia, because in this population of patients, there is no correlation between maternal and fetal platelet count (Jensen et al. 2011). However if her platelet count is <50,000/μL at delivery, the relative risk of severe thrombocytopenia in her neonate is increased by about eightfold. On that basis, we advise measuring the neonate's platelet count when the mother's count is found to be <50,000/μL.

Cause of Severe Thrombocytopenia in NICU Patients Most cases of thrombocytopenia identified in the NICU are not severe. However, perhaps 25% of cases have a count that falls below 50,000/μL, a threshold where the condition is generally termed "severe neonatal thrombocytopenia" (Christensen et al. 2006b; Baer et al. 2009; Stanworth et al. 2009). The majority of cases of severe neonatal thrombocytopenia are recognized at birth or shortly thereafter. This is the case among extremely low birth weight neonates (ELBW, <1,000 g) and is also the case when all NICU patients are studied, regardless of gestational age. Clearly, thrombocytopenia at any time during the NICU stay is more common in the smallest patients, with a prevalence exceeding 80% of those weight less than 600 g at birth (Christensen et al. 2006b), compared with about 1% of those weighing over 2,000 g at birth. Biological differences have been observed between fetal, neonatal, and adult megakaryocytes, and these are likely involved in the marked susceptibility of ELWB neonates to develop thrombocytopenia (Hu et al. 2010).

While alloimmune neonatal thrombocytopenia is common among thrombocytopenic, otherwise healthy appearing, term neonates (Bussel and Sola-Visner 2009; Bussel and Primiani 2008; Murphy and Bussel 2007), a wide variety of causes and associations are seen among ELBW neonates. Unfortunately, the largest etiologic category for thrombocytopenia among ELBW neonates is "unknown or idiopathic" (Christensen et al. 2006b). When an association or cause is known, the most common explanations are maternal hypertension, SGA status, DIC, bacterial or fungal infection, or necrotizing enterocolitis.

3.2 Risks and Benefits of Platelet Transfusion in the NICU

Platelet transfusions can be lifesaving, but they also carry risks. Some such risks are at least partly defined, such as a risk of bacterial contamination of the donor platelets (Baer et al. 2011). Other risks are poorly defined but still quantifiable. Figure 8 is typical of several reports showing a positive association between the number of platelet transfusion received and the mortality rate (Baer et al. 2007, 2011; Garcia et al. 2001; Del Vecchio et al. 2001). This relationship is multifactorial and complex, but analyses indicate the very high likelihood that the multiple transfusions themselves are involved in the elevated mortality rate.

It is not possible to precisely evaluate and contrast the risks vs. benefits each time a platelet transfusion is considered in the NICU. Although imprecise, this process of attempting to weigh the risks and benefits is important before any platelet transfusion is ordered. Benefits are more likely in cases of thrombocytopenic hemorrhage than in cases where the platelets are given prophylactically. Unfortunately, some platelet transfusions are given in situations where the potential benefits are nil. Surveys indicate some clinicians give prophylactic platelet transfusions to stable neonates with platelet counts in the range 100,000–150,000/μL (Josephson et al. 2009; Cremer et al. 2011). Since the bleeding time is not prolonged in this platelet count range (Del Vecchio et al. 2008), and since these platelet counts are within the reference range

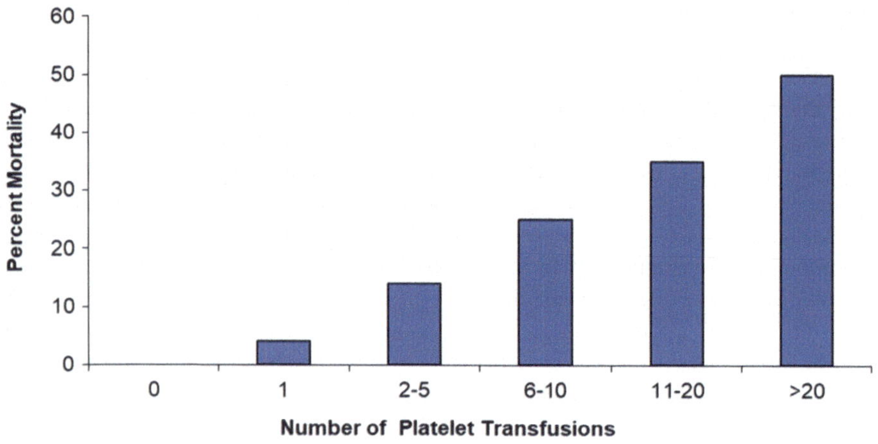

Fig. 8 Mortality rate of NICU patients with severe thrombocytopenia is displayed according to the number of platelet transfusions received

(Wiedmeier et al. 2009), it is very unlikely that any benefit is provided by a platelet transfusion. Thus, when well-appearing neonates receive prophylactic platelet transfusions because of a platelet count in the 100,000–150,000/μL range, they are being subjected to risk unbalanced by any known benefit (Fig. 8).

Curley et al. reported a large, multicentered randomized trial assessing outcomes of preterm infants who received platelet transfusions at a "trigger" level of 50,000/μL vs. 25,000/μL. Randomizing 660 neonates, they found that specific adverse outcomes (death or new major bleeding) were more common on those in the high-threshold group. Moreover, adverse events such as chronic lung disease were more frequent in the high-threshold group. On that basis, many NICUs have decided that prophylactic platelet transfusions to preterm infants should NOT be administered at a trigger level of 50,000/μL and have moved the transfusion level down considerably, to perhaps 25,000–30,000/μL (Curley et al. 2018).

3.3 Thrombopoietin Mimetics

In 1994 thrombopoietin (Tpo) was identified, and the recombinant molecule became available for study (Metcalf 1994). Trials with Tpo and a pegylated form of Tpo were promising until some patients developed anti-Tpo antibodies, leading to aplastic anemia, which led to the cessation of development of this potential approach to treat thrombocytopenia. Subsequent studies focused on means of stimulating the Tpo receptor using molecules that have no homology with Tpo. Two such products have been approved by the US FDA, Eltrombopag (Glaxo, Smith, Klein) and Romiplostim (Amgen).

Few neonates have been treated with either agent. No consistent approach or consensus for treatment with either agent has been developed for thrombocytopenic neonates, but caution has been issued for each. Tpo receptors are expressed on various non-hematopoietic cells including cells in the brain, and non-thrombopoietic actions during the neonatal period have not been defined. Eltrombopag is a powerful chelator of iron (Vlachodimitropoulou et al. 2017). It crosses the blood-brain barrier and impairs iron-dependent hippocampal neuron dendrite development (Bastian et al. 2017). Moreover, neonatal mice have a rather poor response to these agonists compared with adult mice (Sparger et al. 2018).

References

Ahmad A, Laborada G, Bussel J, Nesin M (2002) Comparison of recombinant G-CSF, recombinant human GM-CSF and placebo for treatment of septic preterm infants. Pediatr Infect Dis J 21:1061–1065

Aktaş D, Demirel B, Gürsoy T, Ovalı F (2015) A randomized case-controlled study of recombinant human granulocyte colony stimulating factor for the treatment of sepsis in preterm neutropenic infants. Pediatr Neonatol 56:171–175

Alter BP (2017) Inherited bone marrow failure syndromes: considerations pre- and posttransplant. Hematology Am Soc Hematol Educ Program 2017(1):88–95

An G, Ohls RK, Christensen RD, Widness JA, Mock DM, Veng-Pedersen P (2017) Population pharmacokinetics of darbepoetin in infants following single intravenous and subcutaneous dosing. J Pharm Sci 106:1644–1649

Aprikyan AA, Carlsson G, Stein S, Oganesian A, Fadeel B, Dale DC, Palmblad J, Henter JI (2004) Neutrophil elastase mutations in severe congenital neutropenia patients of the original Kostmann family. Blood 103:389

Arsenault JE, Webb AL, Koulinska IN, Aboud S, Fawzi WW, Villamor E (2010) Association between breast milk erythropoietin and reduced risk of mother-to-child transmission of HIV. J Infect Dis 202:370–373

Baer VL, Lambert DK, Henry E, Snow GL, Sola-Visner MC, Christensen RD (2007) Do platelet transfusions in the NICU adversely affect survival? Analysis of 1600 thrombocytopenic neonates in a multihospital healthcare system. J Perinatol 27:790–796

Baer VL, Lambert DK, Henry E, Christensen RD (2009) Severe thrombocytopenia in the NICU. Pediatrics 124:e1095–e1100

Baer VL, Lambert DK, Henry E, Snow GL, Butler A, Christensen RD (2011) Among very-low-birth-weight neonates is red blood cell transfusion an independent risk factor for subsequently developing a severe intraventricular hemorrhage? Transfusion 51:1170–1178

Barney CK, Lambert DK, Alder SC, Scoffield SH, Schmutz N, Christensen RD (2007) Treating feeding intolerance with an enteral solution patterned after human amniotic fluid: a randomized, controlled, masked trial. J Perinatol 27:28–31

Bastian TW, Duck KA, Michalopoulos GC, Chen MJ, Liu ZJ, Connor JR, Lanier LM, Sola-Visner MC, Georgieff MK (2017) Eltrombopag, a thrombopoietin mimetic, crosses the blood-brain barrier and impairs iron-dependent hippocampal neuron dendrite development. J Thromb Haemost 15:565–574

Bedford-Russell AR, Emmerson AJB, Wilkinson N, Chant T, Sweet DG, Halliday HL, Holland B, Davies EG (2001) A trial of recombinant human granulocyte colony stimulating factor for the treatment of very low birthweight infants with presumed sepsis and neutropenia. Arch Dis Child Fetal Neonatal Ed 84:F172–F176

Bezzerri V, Cipolli M (2018) Shwachman-diamond syndrome: molecular mechanisms and current perspectives. Mol Diagn Ther 23:281–290. https://doi.org/10.1007/s40291-018-0368-2

Bhandari V, Buhimschi CS, Han CS, Lee SY, Pettker CM, Campbell KH et al (2011) Cord blood erythropoietin and interleukin-6 for prediction of intraventricular hemorrhage in the preterm neonate. J Matern Fetal Neonatal Med 24(5):673–679

Bilgin K, Yaramis A, Haspolat K, Tas A, Gunbey S, Derman O (2001) A randomized trial of granulocyte-macrophage colony-stimulating factor in neonates with sepsis and neutropenia. Pediatrics 107:36–41

Brace RA, Cheung CY, Davis LE, Gagnon R, Harding R, Widness JA (2006) Sources of amniotic fluid erythropoietin during normoxia and hypoxia in fetal sheep. Am J Obstet Gynecol 195:246–225

Bussel JB, Primiani A (2008) Fetal and neonatal alloimmune thrombocytopenia: progress and ongoing debates. Blood Rev 22:33–52

Bussel JB, Sola-Visner M (2009) Current approaches to the evaluation and management of the fetus and neonate with immune thrombocytopenia. Semin Perinatol 33:35–42

Bux J (2008) Human neutrophil alloantigens. Vox Sang 94:277–285

Bux J, Behrens G, Jaeger G, Welte K (1998) Diagnosis and clinical course of autoimmune neutropenia in infancy; analysis of 240 cases. Blood 91:181–186

Cairo MS, Christensen RD, Sender LS, Ellis R, Rosenthal J, van de Ven C, Worcester C, Agosti JM (1995) Results of a phase I/II trial of recombinant human granulocyte-macrophage colony-stimulating factor in very low birthweight neonates: significant induction of circulatory neutrophils, monocytes, platelets, and bone marrow neutrophils. Blood 86:2509–2515

Cairo MS, Agosti J, Ellis R, Laver JJ, Puppala B, DeLemos R, Givner L, Nesin M, Wheeler G, Seth T, van de Ven C, Fanaroff A (1999) A randomised double-blind placebo-controlled trial of prophylactic recombinant human GM-CSF to reduce nosocomial infection in very low birthweight neonates. J Pediatr 134:64–70

Calhoun DA, Christensen RD (1997) The occurrence of Kostmann syndrome in preterm neonates. Pediatrics 99:259–261

Calhoun DA, Christensen RD, Edstrom CS, Juul SE, Ohls RK, Schibler KR, Sola MC, Sullivan SE (2000) Consistent approaches to procedures and practices in neonatal hematology. Clin Perinatol 27:733–753

Calhoun DA, Rimsza LM, Burchfield DJ, Millsaps M, Christensen RD, Budania J, McCullough J (2001) Congenital autoimmune neutropenia in two premature neonates. Pediatrics 108:181–184

Carlsson G, Fasth A (2001) Infantile genetic agranulocytosis, morbus Kostmann: presentation of six cases from the original "Kostmann family" and a review. Acta Paediatr 90:757–764

Carlsson G, Wahlin YB, Johansson A, Olsson A, Eriksson T, Claesson R, Hanstrom L, Henter JI (2006) Periodontal disease in patients from the original Kostmann family with severe congenital neutropenia. J Periodontol 77:744–751

Carr R, Modi N, Doré CJ, El-Rifai R, Lindo D (1999) A randomised controlled trial of prophylactic GM-CSF in human newborns less than 32 weeks gestation. Pediatrics 103:796–802

Carr R, Modi N, Dore C (2003) G-CSF and GM-CSF for treating or preventing neonatal infections. Cochrane Database Syst Rev 3:CD003066

Carr R, Brocklehurst P, Doré CJ, Modi N (2009) Granulocyte-macrophage colony stimulating factor administered as prophylaxis for reduction of sepsis in extremely preterm, small for gestational age neonates (the PROGRAMS trial): a single-blind, multicentre, randomised controlled trial. Lancet 373:226–233

Chirico G, Motta M, Villani P, Cavazza A, Cardone ML (2002) Late-onset neutropenia in very low birthweight infants. Acta Paediatr Suppl 91:104–108

Christensen RD, Calhoun DA (2004) Congenital neutropenia. Clin Perinatol 31:29–38

Christensen RD, Havranek T, Gerstmann DR, Calhoun DA (2005) Enteral administration of a simulated amniotic fluid to very low birth weight neonates. J Perinatol 25:380–385

Christensen RD, Henry E, Wiedmeier SE, Stoddard RA, Lambert DK (2006a) Low blood neutrophil concentrations among extremely low birth weight neonates: data from a multihospital health-care system. J Perinatol 26:682–687

Christensen RD, Henry E, Wiedmeier SE, Stoddard RA, Sola-Visner MC, Lambert DK, Kiehn TI, Ainsworth S (2006b) Thrombocytopenia among extremely low birth weight neonates: data from a multihospital healthcare system. J Perinatol 26:348–353

Christensen RD, Lambert DK, Richards DS (2014a) Estimating the nucleated red blood cell 'emergence time' in neonates. J Perinatol 34:116–119

Christensen RD, Carroll PD, Josephson CD (2014b) Evidence-based advances in transfusion practice in neonatal intensive care units. Neonatology 106:245–253

Christensen RD, Yoder BA, Baer VL, Snow GL, Butler A (2015) Early-onset neutropenia in small-for-gestational-age infants. Pediatrics 136:e1259–e1267

Cremer M, Sola-Visner M, Roll S, Josephson CD, Yilmaz Z, Bührer C, Dame C (2011) Platelet transfusions in neonates: practices in the United States vary significantly from those in Austria, Germany, and Switzerland. Transfusion 51(12):2634–2641

Curley A, Stanworth SJ, Willoughby K, Fustolo-Gunnink SF, Venkatesh V, Hudson C, Deary A, Hodge R, Hopkins V, Lopez Santamaria B, Mora A, Llewelyn C, D'Amore A, Khan R, Onland W, Lopriore E, Fijnvandraat K, New H, Clarke P, Watts T, PlaNeT2 MATISSE Collaborators (2018) Randomized trial of platelet-transfusion thresholds in neonates. N Engl J Med. https://doi.org/10.1056/NEJMoa1807320

Dale DC (2017) How I manage children with neutropenia. Br J Haematol 178(3):351–363

Dale DC, Makaryan V (2018) ELANE-related neutropenia. In: Adam MP et al (eds) GeneReviews. University of Washington, Seattle

Dame C, Juul SE, Christensen RD (2001) The biology of erythropoietin in the central nervous system and its neurotrophic and neuroprotective potential. Biol Neonate 79:228–235

Del Vecchio A, Sola MC, Theriaque DW, Hutson AD, Kao KJ, Wright D, Garcia MG, Pollock BH, Christensen RD (2001) Platelet transfusions in the neonatal intensive care unit: factors predicting which patients will require multiple transfusions. Transfusion 41:803–808

Del Vecchio A, Latini G, Henry E, Christensen RD (2008) Template bleeding times of 240 neonates born at 24 to 41 weeks gestation. J Perinatol 28:427–431

Dijkstra F, Jozwiak M, de Matteo R, Duncan J, Hale N, Harding R et al (2010) Erythropoietin ameliorates damage to the placenta and fetal liver induced by exposure to lipopolysaccharide. Placenta 31(4):282–288

Donadieu J, Beaupain B, Fenneteau O, Bellanné-Chantelot C (2017) Congenital neutropenia in the era of genomics. Br J Haematol 179:557–574

Doron MW, Makhlouf RA, Katz VL, Lawson EE, Stiles AD (1994) Increased incidence of sepsis at birth in neutropenic infants of mothers with preeclampsia. J Pediatr 125:452–458

Drossou-Agakidou V, Kanakoudi-Tsakalidou F, Taparkou A, Tzimouli V, Tsandali H, Kremenopoulos G (1998) Administration of recombinant human granulocyte-colony stimulating factor to septic neonates induces neutrophilia and enhances the neutrophil respiratory burst and beta2 integrin expression results of a randomized controlled trial. Eur J Pediatr 157:583–588

Farruggia P, Puccio G, Fioredda F, Lanza T, Porretti L, Ramenghi U, Barone A, Bonanomi S, Finocchi A, Ghilardi R, Ladogana S, Marra N, Martire B, Notarangelo LD, Onofrillo D, Pillon M, Russo G, Lo Valvo L, Serafinelli J, Tucci F, Zunica F, Verzegnassi F, Dufour C (2017) Autoimmune neutropenia of childhood secondary to other autoimmune disorders: data from the Italian neutropenia registry. Am J Hematol 92(9):E546–E549

Fathali N, Lekic T, Zhang JH, Tang J (2010) Long-term evaluation of granulocyte-colony stimulating factor on hypoxic-ischemic brain damage in infant rats. Intensive Care Med 36:1602–1608

Ferrer-Marin F, Liu ZJ, Gutti R, Sola-Visner M (2010) Neonatal thrombocytopenia and megakaryocytopoiesis. Semin Hematol 47:281–288

Fischer HS, Reibel NJ, Bührer C, Dame C (2017) Prophylactic early erythropoietin for neuroprotection in preterm infants: a meta-analysis. Pediatrics 139:e20164317

Furutani E, Newburger PE, Shimamura A (2018) Neutropenia in the age of genetic testing: advances and challenges. Am J Hematol 94:384–393. https://doi.org/10.1002/ajh.25374

Garcia MG, Duenas E, Sola MC, Hutson AD, Theriaque D, Christensen RD (2001) Epidemiologic and outcome studies of patients who received platelet transfusions in the neonatal intensive care unit. J Perinatol 21:415–420
Gersting JA, Christensen RD, Calhoun DA (2004) Effects of enterally administering granulocyte colony-stimulating factor to suckling mice. Pediatr Res 55:802–806
Gillan ER, Christensen RD, Suen Y et al (1994) A randomized, placebo-controlled trial of recombinant human granulocyte colony-stimulating factor administration in newborn infants with presumed sepsis: significant induction of peripheral and bone marrow neutrophilia. Blood 84:1427–1433
Henry E, Christensen RD, Sheffield MJ, Eggert LD, Carroll PD, Minton SD, Lambert DK, Ilstrup SJ (2015) Why do four NICUs using identical RBC transfusion guidelines have different gestational age-adjusted RBC transfusion rates? J Perinatol 35:132–136
Hu A, Slayton WB, Rimsza LM, Bailey M, Sallmon H, Sola-Visner MC (2010) Differences between newborn and adult mice in their response to immune thrombocytopenia. Neonatology 98:100–108
Jensen J, Wiedmeier SE, Henry E, Silver RM, Christensen RD (2011) Linking maternal platelet counts with neonatal platelet counts and outcomes using the data repositories of a multihospital healthcare system. Am J Perinatol 28:597–604
Josephson CD, Su LL, Christensen RD, Hillyer CD, Castillejo MI, Emory MR, Lin Y, Hume H, Easley K, Poterjoy B, Sola-Visner M (2009) Platelet transfusion practices among neonatologists in the United States and Canada: results of a survey. Pediatrics 123:278–285
Juul SE (2000) Nonerythropoietic roles of erythropoietin in the fetus and neonate. Clin Perinatol 27:527–541
Juul SE, Christensen RD (2003) Effect of recombinant granulocyte colony-stimulating factor on blood neutrophil concentrations among patients with "idiopathic neonatal neutropenia": a randomized, placebo-controlled trial. J Perinatol 23:493–497
Juul SE, Pet GC (2015) Erythropoietin and neonatal neuroprotection. Clin Perinatol 42:469–481
Juul SJ, Harcum J, Li Y, Christensen RD (1997) Erythropoietin is present in the cerebrospinal fluid of neonates. J Pediatr 130:428–430
Juul SE, Calhoun DA, Christensen RD (1998a) "Idiopathic neutropenia" in very low birthweight infants. Acta Paediatr 87:963–968
Juul SE, Yachnis AT, Christensen RD (1998b) Tissue distribution of erythropoietin and erythropoietin receptor in the developing human fetus. Early Hum Dev 52:235–249
Juul SE, Stallings SA, Christensen RD (1999) Erythropoietin in the cerebrospinal fluid of neonates who sustained CNS injury. Pediatr Res 46:543–547
Juul SE, Comstock BA, Heagerty PJ, Mayock DE, Goodman AM, Hauge S, Gonzalez F, Wu YW (2018) High-dose erythropoietin for asphyxia and encephalopathy (HEAL): a randomized controlled trial - background, aims, and study protocol. Neonatology 113:331–338
Khincha PP, Savage SA (2016) Neonatal manifestations of inherited bone marrow failure syndromes. Semin Fetal Neonatal Med 21:57–65
Kline A, Mackley A, Taylor SM, McKenzie SE, Paul DA (2008) Thrombopoietin following transfusion of platelets in preterm neonates. Platelets 19:428–431
Kling PJ, Hutter JJ (2003) Hematologic abnormalities in severe neonatal necrotizing enterocolitis: 25 years later. J Perinatol 23:523–530
Kobayashi SD, Malachowa N, DeLeo FR (2018) Neutrophils and bacterial immune evasion. J Innate Immun 10:432–441
Kocherlakota P, La Gamma EF (1998) Preliminary report: rhG-CSF may reduce the incidence of neonatal sepsis in prolonged preeclampsia-associated neutropenia. Pediatrics 102:1107–1111
Koenig JM, Christensen RD (1989a) Incidence, neutrophil kinetics, and natural history of neonatal neutropenia associated with maternal hypertension. N Engl J Med 321:557–562
Koenig JM, Christensen RD (1989b) Neutropenia and thrombocytopenia in infants with Rh hemolytic disease. J Pediatr 114:625–631

Koenig JM, Christensen RD (1991) The mechanism responsible for diminished neutrophil production in neonates delivered of women with pregnancy-induced hypertension. Am J Obstet Gynecol 165:467–473

Koenig JM, Hunter DD, Christensen RD (1991) Neutropenia in donor (anemic) twins involved in the twin-twin transfusion syndrome. J Perinatol 11:355–358

Kostmann R (1956) Infantile genetic agranulocytosis; agranulocytosis infantilis hereditaria. Acta Paediatr 45(Suppl 105):1–78

Kuhn P, Messer J, Paupe A, Espagne S, Kacet N, Mouchnino G, Klosowski S, Krim G, Lescure S, Le Bouedec S, Meyer P, Astruc D (2009) A multicenter, randomized, placebo-controlled trial of prophylactic recombinant granulocyte-colony stimulating factor in preterm neonates with neutropenia. J Pediatr 155:324–30.e1

Lambert RM, Baer VL, Wiedmeier SE, Henry E, Burnett J, Christensen RD (2009) Isolated elevated blood neutrophil concentration at altitude does not require NICU admission if appropriate reference ranges are used. J Perinatol 29:822–825

Lewin S, Bussel JB (2015) Review of fetal and neonatal immune cytopenias. Clin Adv Hematol Oncol 13(1):35–43

Maheshwari A, Christensen RD, Calhoun DA (2002) Immune-mediated neutropenia in the neonate. Acta Paediatr Suppl 91:98–103

Makeshwari A, Christensen RD, Calhoun DA (2002) Immune neutropenia in the neonate. Adv Pediatr 49:317–339

Manroe BL, Weinberg AG, Rosenfeld CR, Browne R (1979) The neonatal blood count in health and disease. I. Reference values for neutrophilic cells. J Pediatr 95:89–98

Marlow N, Morris T, Brocklehurst P, Carr R, Cowan F, Patel N, Petrou S, Redshaw M, Modi N, Doré CJ (2015) A randomised trial of granulocyte-macrophage colony stimulating factor for neonatal sepsis: childhood outcomes at 5 years. Arch Dis Child Fetal Neonatal Ed 100(4):F320–F326

McPherson RJ, Juul SE (2010) Erythropoietin for infants with hypoxic-ischemic encephalopathy. Curr Opin Pediatr 22:139–145

Metcalf D (1994) Blood. Thrombopoietin--at last. Nature 369(6481):519–520

Miura E, Procianoy RS, Bittar C, Miura CS, Miura MS, Mello C, Christensen RD (2001) A randomized double-masked, placebo controlled trial of recombinant granulocyte colony-stimulating factor administration to preterm infants with the clinical diagnosis of early-onset sepsis. Pediatrics 107:30–35

Mouzinho A, Rosenfeld CR, Sanchez PJ, Risser R (1992) Effect of maternal hypertension on neonatal neutropenia and risk of nosocomial infection. Pediatrics 90:430–435

Murphy MF, Bussel JB (2007) Advances in the management of alloimmune thrombocytopenia. Br J Haematol 136:366–378

Murray NA, Watts TL, Roberts IA (2000) Thrombopoietin in the fetus and neonate. Early Hum Dev 59:1–12

Natalucci G, Latal B, Koller B, Rüegger C, Sick B, Held L, Bucher HU, Fauchère JC, Swiss EPO Neuroprotection Trial Group (2016) Effect of early prophylactic high-dose recombinant human erythropoietin in very preterm infants on neurodevelopmental outcome at 2 years: a randomized clinical trial. JAMA 315:2079–2085

Ohls RK, Christensen RD, Kamath-Rayne BD, Rosenberg A, Wiedmeier SE, Roohi M, Backstrom Lacy C, Lambert DK, Burnett JJ, Pruckler B, Schrader R, Lowe JR (2013) A randomized, masked, placebo controlled study of darbepoetin administered to preterm infants. Pediatrics 132:e119–e127

Ohls RK, Kamath-Rayne BD, Christensen RD, Wiedmeier SE, Rosenberg A, Fuller JA, Backstrom Lacy C, Roohi M, Lambert DK, Burnett JJ, Pruckler B, Peceny H, Cannon DC, Lowe JR (2014) Cognitive outcomes of preterm infants randomized to darbepoetin, erythropoietin or placebo. Pediatrics 133:1023–1030

Ohls RK, Cannon DC, Phillips J, Caprihan A, Patel S, Winter S, Steffen M, Yeo RA, Campbell R, Wiedmeier S, Baker S, Gonzales G, Lowe JR (2016a) Preschool assessment of preterm infants treated with darbepoetin and erythropoietin. Pediatrics 137:1–9

Ohls RK, Cannon DC, Phillips J, Caprihan A, Patel S, Winter S, Steffen M, Yeo RA, Campbell R, Wiedmeier S, Baker S, Gonzales S, Lowe J (2016b) Preschool assessment of preterm infants treated with darbepoetin and erythropoietin. Pediatrics 137(3):e20153859

Ohlsson A, Aher SM (2017) Early erythropoiesis-stimulating agents in preterm or low birth weight infants. Cochrane Database Syst Rev 11:CD004863

Patel S, Ohls RK (2015) Darbepoetin administration in term and preterm neonates. Clin Perinatol 42 (3):557–566

Pierre G, Chakupurakal G, McKiernan P, Hendriksz C, Lawson S, Chakrapani A (2008) Bone marrow transplantation in glycogen storage disease type 1b. J Pediatr 152:286–288

Procianoy RS, Silveira RC, Mussi-Pinhata MM, Souza Rugolo LM, Leone CR, de Andrade Lopes JM, de Almeida MF, Brazilian Network on Neonatal Research (2010) Sepsis and neutropenia in very low birth weight infants delivered of mothers with preeclampsia. J Pediatr 157:434–438

Roberts I, Stanworth S, Murray NA (2008) Thrombocytopenia in the neonate. Blood Rev 22:173–186

Roberts JK, Stockmann C, Ward RM, Beachy J, Baserga MC, Spigarelli MG, Sherwin CM (2015) Population pharmacokinetics of darbepoetin alfa in conjunction with hypothermia for the treatment of neonatal hypoxic-ischemic encephalopathy. Clin Pharmacokinet 54:1237–1244

Saleh MI, Nalbant D, Widness JA, Veng-Pedersen P (2013) Population pharmacodynamic analysis of erythropoiesis in preterm infants for determining the anemia treatment potential of erythropoietin. Am J Physiol Regul Integr Comp Physiol 304:R772–R781

Schibler KR, Osborne KA, Leung LY, Le TV, Baker SI, Thompson DD (1998) A randomized placebo-controlled trial of granulocyte colony-stimulating factor administration to newborn infants with neutropenia and clinical signs of early-onset sepsis. Pediatrics 102:6–13

Schmutz N, Henry E, Jopling J, Christensen RD (2008) Expected ranges for blood neutrophil concentrations of neonates: the Monroe and Mouzinho charts revisited. J Perinatol 28:275–281

Shiou SR, Yu Y, Chen S, Ciancio MJ, Petrof EO, Sun J, Claud EC (2011) Erythropoietin protects intestinal epithelial barrier function and lowers the incidence of experimental neonatal necrotizing enterocolitis. J Biol Chem 286:12123–12132

Sola MC, Calhoun DA, Hutson AD, Christensen RD (1999) Plasma thrombopoietin concentrations in thrombocytopenic and non-thrombocytopenic patients in a neonatal intensive care unit. Br J Haematol 104:90–92

Sparger KA, Ramsey H, Lorenz V, Liu ZJ, Feldman HA, Li N, Laforest T, Sola-Visner MC (2018) Developmental differences between newborn and adult mice in response to romiplostim. Platelets 29:365–372

Stanworth SJ, Clarke P, Watts T, Ballard S, Choo L, Morris T, Murphy MF, Roberts I, Platelets and Neonatal Transfusion Study Group (2009) Prospective, observational study of outcomes in neonates with severe thrombocytopenia. Pediatrics 124:e826–e834

Steward CG, Groves SJ, Taylor CT, Maisenbacher MK, Versluys B, Newbury-Ecob RA, Ozsahin H, Damin MK, Bowen VM, McCurdy KR, Mackey MC, Bolyard AA, Dale DC (2019) Neutropenia in Barth syndrome: characteristics, risks, and management. Curr Opin Hematol 26(1):6–15. https://doi.org/10.1097/MOH.0000000000000472

Sullivan SE, Calhoun DA, Maheshwari A, Ashmeade TL, Auerbach DA, Hudak ML, Beltz SE, Christensen RD (2002) Tolerance of simulated amniotic fluid in premature neonates. Ann Pharmacother 36:1518–1524

Teng RJ, Wu TJ, Garrison RD, Sharma R, Hudak ML (2009) Early neutropenia is not associated with an increased rate of nosocomial infection in very low-birth-weight infants. J Perinatol 29:219–224

Thiel CT, Rauch A (2011) The molecular basis of the cartilage-hair hypoplasia-anauxetic dysplasia spectrum. Best Pract Res Clin Endocrinol Metab 25:131–142

Tsao PN, Teng RJ, Tang JR, Yau KI (1999) Granulocyte colony-stimulating factor in the cord blood of premature neonates born to mothers with pregnancy-induced hypertension. J Pediatr 135:56–59

Vlachodimitropoulou E, Chen YL, Garbowski M, Koonyosying P, Psaila B, Sola-Visner M, Cooper N, Hider R, Porter J (2017) Eltrombopag: a powerful chelator of cellular or extracellular iron(III) alone or combined with a second chelator. Blood 130:1923–1933

Welte K, Zeidler C (2009) Severe congenital neutropenia. Hematol Oncol Clin North Am 223:307–320

Wiedmeier SE, Henry E, Sola-Visner MC, Christensen RD (2009) Platelet reference ranges for neonates, defined using data from over 47,000 patients in a multihospital healthcare system. J Perinatol 29:130–136

Wu YW, Bauer LA, Ballard RA, Ferriero DM, Glidden DV, Mayock DE, Chang T, Durand DJ, Song D, Bonifacio SL, Gonzalez FF, Glass HC, Juul SE (2012) Erythropoietin for neuroprotection in neonatal encephalopathy: safety and pharmacokinetics. Pediatrics 130:683–691

Zeidler C, Boxer L, Dale DC, Freedman MH, Kinsey S, Welte K (2000) Management of Kostmann syndrome in the G-CSF era. Br J Haematol 109:490–495

Zetterstrom R (2002) Kostmann disease--infantile genetic agranulocytosis: historical views and new aspects. Acta Paediatr 91:1279–1281

Pediatric Antiretroviral Therapy

Sahera Dirajlal-Fargo, Wei Li A. Koay, and Natella Rakhmanina

Contents

S. Dirajlal-Fargo (✉)
Pediatric Infectious Diseases, Rainbow Babies and Children's Hospital, Case Western Reserve University School of Medicine, Cleveland, OH, USA
e-mail: sahera.dirajlal-fargo@uhhospitals.org

W. L. A. Koay
Department of Pediatrics, School of Medicine and Health Sciences, The George Washington University, Washington, DC, USA

Division of Infectious Diseases, Children's National Medical Center, Washington, DC, USA

N. Rakhmanina
Department of Pediatrics, School of Medicine and Health Sciences, The George Washington University, Washington, DC, USA

Division of Infectious Diseases, Children's National Medical Center, Washington, DC, USA

Elizabeth Glaser Pediatric AIDS Foundation, Washington, DC, USA

W. Kiess et al. (eds.), *Pediatric Pharmacotherapy*,
Handbook of Experimental Pharmacology 261, https://doi.org/10.1007/164_2019_246

Abstract

Human immunodeficiency virus (HIV) is one of the most serious pediatric infectious diseases, affecting around 3 million children and adolescents worldwide. Lifelong antiretroviral treatment (ART) provides multiple benefits including sustained virologic suppression, restoration and preservation of immune function, decreased morbidity and mortality, and improved quality of life. However, access to ART, particularly among neonates and young infants, continues to be challenging due to limited number of suitable formulations and limited access to pediatric ARV drug. Moreover, children and adolescents living with HIV may experience long-term HIV- and ART-associated comorbidities including cardiovascular, renal, neurological, and metabolic complications. We provide an overview of currently available formulations, dosing, and safety considerations for pediatric antiretroviral drugs by drug classes and according to the three age groups including neonates, children, and adolescents.

Keywords

Adolescents · Antiretroviral drugs · Children · HIV treatment · Infants

1 Introduction

According to the Joint United Nations Programme on HIV/AIDS (UNAIDS), an estimated 36.9 million people were living with HIV worldwide in 2017, including approximately three million children and adolescents under the age of 20 years old (UNAIDS 2018). Of the 940,000 people who died of AIDS-related illnesses in 2017, 130,000 of them were children and adolescents under the age of 20 years old (UNICEF 2018).

Among children under the age of 15 years, there has been a steady decline of new HIV infections due to a significant decrease in mother-to-child transmission (MTCT) of HIV (UNAIDS 2018). The reduction of MTCT of HIV is largely due to the effectiveness of antiretroviral therapy (ART) during pregnancy, labor, and postpartum in infants and breastfeeding mothers (Sperling et al. 1996). Prevention of MTCT (PMTCT), which started with the use of a short course of monotherapy with zidovudine (AZT) in pregnant women, during labor, and postpartum in neonates in the mid-1990s, has evolved to the use of lifelong combination ART for all women living with HIV and combination ART for high-risk infant exposures from 2013 (Sperling et al. 1996; World Health Organization 2013, 2018a; Department of Health and Human Services 2018a; Connor et al. 1994). Improved access to ART among women living with HIV has also contributed to the decline in new perinatal HIV infections, with 80% of pregnant women living with HIV in 2017 having access to combination ART, demonstrating an increase from 51% in 2010 (UNAIDS 2018). These advances in PMTCT could not have been achieved without studies of the pharmacokinetics (PK), efficacy, and safety of antiretroviral (ARV) drugs in pregnant and breastfeeding women and in newborns and infants.

Despite the success of PMTCT globally, there were still 180,000 new cases of perinatal HIV infection in 2017, and as a result of ongoing MTCT, significant number of young children and adolescents are living with HIV and require lifelong combination ART (UNAIDS 2018). Very early initiation of treatment is beneficial in improving the outcomes of children with perinatally acquired HIV infection; however, access to ART, particularly among neonates and young infants, continues to be challenging due to limited number of suitable pediatric formulations and limited access to pediatric ARV drugs (Persaud et al. 2013, 2014; Clarke et al. 2018a). In fact, less than 25% of ARV drugs approved in adults are currently approved for use in children under 2 years of age in the USA and Europe (Penazzato et al. 2017). Compared to the 59% of individuals aged 15 years and older living with HIV having access to ART, an estimated 52% of children (aged 0–14 years) had access to ART in 2017 (UNAIDS 2018). In conjunction with early identification of HIV, new ARV formulations for infants and children along with facilitated procurement of ARV drugs and increased healthcare system capacity are urgently needed to bridge the gap in access to ART and in reducing HIV-related morbidity and mortality in children.

The number of new HIV infections among adolescents (aged 15–19 years) has declined at a significantly slower rate compared to children (UNAIDS 2018). Moreover, the number of AIDS-related deaths among those aged 10–19 years has not decreased and in fact has doubled since 2000 (UNAIDS 2018). Adolescents continue to be underserved by current services across the HIV testing and care continuum, with studies reporting higher rates of loss to follow-up (Kariminia et al. 2018), worse adherence (Ross et al. 2019; Adejumo et al. 2015), and increased needs for psychosocial and sexual reproductive health support (Adejumo et al. 2015) compared to children and adults living with HIV. Sexual acquisition of HIV infection in adolescents and young adults is increasingly prevalent with advanced age, highlighting the importance of HIV testing, safe sex education, and the use of pre- and postexposure prophylaxis with ARV drugs (UNICEF 2016). Pre-exposure prophylaxis (PrEP) was recently approved by the Food and Drug Administration (FDA) for use in pediatric patients weighing ≥35 kg (Food and Drug Administration 2016), thus expanding this option for younger adolescents at high risk for acquiring HIV. Postexposure prophylaxis (nPEP) with ARV drugs is also important for children and adolescents following high-risk exposures, such as sexual abuse and sexual violence.

Lifelong combination ART provides multiple benefits including sustained virologic suppression, restoration and/or preservation of immune function, decreased morbidity and mortality, and improved quality of life (Barlow-Mosha et al. 2017; Lifson et al. 2017; Laurent et al. 2005; Arici et al. 2001). Despite these advantages, children and adolescents living with HIV may experience long-term HIV- and ART-associated comorbidities including cardiovascular (CVD), renal, neurological, and metabolic complications (Vreeman et al. 2015). As HIV-infected children and adolescents continue to get older, more data are being obtained to better understand the long-term complications of HIV and ART in people infected at a young age. With a growing number of HIV-exposed but uninfected children who are exposed to ARV drugs in utero and during infancy, the issue of ARV-associated complications is also a developing area of interest (Van Dyke et al. 2016; Spaulding et al. 2016).

In this manuscript, we provide an overview of formulations, dosing, PK, and safety considerations for currently available pediatric ARV according to the three age groups including neonates and infants, children, and adolescents.

2 ART for Neonates and Infants

Perinatal guidelines recommend postpartum ART prophylaxis with single or dual ARVs for all infants exposed to HIV to reduce the risk of MTCT. The duration and composition of neonatal and infant ART prophylaxis depend on the level of the risk for HIV acquisition and breastfeeding duration for the infants who are breastfed by mothers living with HIV. The current recommendation for uncomplicated neonatal ART prophylaxis without breastfeeding is 4–6 weeks of single or combination ART (Department of Health and Human Services 2018a; Bamford et al. 2018; World Health Organization 2016). For infants at high risk for MTCT and who are breastfed, ARV prophylaxis for 12 weeks is recommended by the World Health Organization (WHO) (World Health Organization 2016). The use of combination triple drug ART during postpartum is recommended for newborns at highest risk of HIV transmission as well as for newborns with confirmed HIV infection. Combination ART initiated in the neonatal period reduces early infant mortality and HIV progression (Violari et al. 2008). Specific interest for early initiation of a triple ART regimen was generated by a case of a "functional cure" of a newborn initiated on a regimen of nucleoside reverse transcriptase inhibitors (NRTIs) AZT plus lamivudine (3TC) and non-nucleoside-reverse transcriptase inhibitor (NNRTI) NVP (Persaud et al. 2013). In this case, the levels of plasma ribonucleic acid (RNA), proviral DNA, and HIV antibodies remained undetectable for over 2 years without ART (Persaud et al. 2013), raising prospective of decreased viral reservoir in those with very early initiation of ART after birth.

There are little data to guide the optimal combination regimen in a newborn with high risk of MTCT. In the HPTN 040 trial, 3TC used for 2 weeks with protease inhibitor (PI) nelfinavir (NFV) and AZT for infant prophylaxis was superior to AZT alone for the prevention of intrapartum HIV transmission (Nielsen-Saines et al. 2012). Higher rates of neutropenia and anemia were associated with this combination therapy compared to AZT alone. High variability in PK parameters have been reported for NFV in neonates (Mirochnick et al. 2011), leading to the US Department of Health and Human Services (DHHS) recommendation to use alternative neonatal prophylaxis for newborns at higher risk for MTCT using AZT plus 3 doses of NVP (birth to 48 h, 48 h after the first dose, 96 h after the second dose). Alternatively, AZT plus 3TC plus NVP and most recently AZT plus 3TC plus integrase strand transfer inhibitor (INSTI) raltegravir (RAL) (Department of Health and Human Services 2018a) can be used.

Early weaning from breastfeeding and substitution with exclusive formula feeding has not been associated with an improved HIV-free survival in neonates (Kuhn et al. 2008). Since 2010, WHO has recommended continued breastfeeding through the first 2 years of life while supporting ART and care for breastfeeding mothers living with HIV (World Health Organization 2010). Breastfed infants remain at risk for MTCT throughout the duration of breastfeeding as the breast milk of HIV-infected mothers on ART may contain reservoirs of HIV, even in light of suppressed maternal plasma viral load (Van de Perre et al. 2012). In fact, breast milk remains responsible for >50% of MTCT in the majority of the priority countries in sub-Saharan Africa (UNAIDS 2016). Data from the IMPAACT PROMISE trial, a randomized controlled trial comparing prolonged infant ARV prophylaxis with NVP vs. maternal ART for the prevention of MTCT through the breastfeeding period, demonstrated, however, very low and comparable breastfeeding transmission in both arms and high infant HIV-free survival at 24 months (Flynn et al. 2018).

There are several challenges for ART prophylaxis to prevent MTCT and to treat an HIV-infected infants and neonates. Those include rapid developmental changes and lack of PK data and limited number of pediatric ARV formulations available. Few ARV drugs are available in formulations suitable for neonates, and limited safety and PK data exist for HIV therapy and prophylaxis in these vulnerable populations (Clarke et al. 2018a).

Dosing of ARV drugs in neonates require special considerations compared with older children. Neonates have differences in drug absorption, distribution, metabolism, and elimination which are affected by the maturation of organ systems within the first weeks of life (Ku and Smith 2015). Challenges associated with oral drug delivery in neonates include changes in stomach pH over the first weeks of life, decreased gastric emptying and intestinal motility, as well as decreased cytochrome metabolism (Linakis et al. 2016). The rapidly changing physiology in this population requires frequent dose titration. The PK data available for the approved ARV drugs in neonates are limited (Rakhmanina and Phelps 2012) and currently only available for AZT, NVP, and PI lopinavir boosted with ritonavir (RTV) (LPV/r) in premature infants, plus RAL in term newborns (Capparelli et al. 2003a; Capretti et al. 2016; Holgate et al. 2012). Accordingly, the formulary of available ARVs in this age group is narrow and includes NRTIs (AZT and 3TC), a NNRTI (NVP), PI (LPV/r), and (INSTI (RAL). Furthermore, safety and efficacy data on neonatal ART are currently very limited. There is even less experience with treating premature and low birth weight neonates. Timing of the transition from prophylactic ART for prevention of transmission to ART regimen aimed at long-term treatment require further investigation (Nuttall 2015).

In addition to limited available formulary of neonatal ARV drugs and limited safety outcome data, the administration of these drugs to neonates poses an additional challenge. Studies in resource-limited settings reveal that mothers place very high value on protecting children from acquiring HIV (Ngarina et al. 2014). However, difficulties of actually administering the medications to infants for caregivers who are also facing their own disease challenges, including widespread stigma, as well as poor palatability especially for liquid pediatric ARV formulations represent significant barriers. Furthermore, liquids formulations may require cold chain storage, as is the case for LPV/r syrup which is prohibitively expensive for resource-limited settings. Granules for oral suspension are available for RAL and require suspending and mixing in a measured amount of water which raises concerns regarding feasibility of administration in resource-limited settings, where access to clean water is limited. Dispersible tablets (tablets for oral solution) for pediatric dosing are available in resource-limited settings and are the preferred solid oral dosage forms over oral liquid solutions for neonates and infants.

Here we review each ARV drug class in relationship to the neonatal and infant use for treatment and/or prophylaxis of HIV.

2.1 Nucleoside and Nucleotide Analogue Reverse Transcriptase Inhibitors (NRTIs)

Emtricitabine (FTC) and AZT are the only NRTIs approved by the FDA since birth. 3TC is approved for use in infants >3 months; however, due to availability of safety and efficacy data (Connor et al. 1994; Mirochnick et al. 2005; Mulenga et al. 2016), both AZT and 3TC are recommended by the DHHS, WHO, and the Paediatric European Network for Treatment of AIDS (PENTA) for infants starting at birth. Abacavir (ABC) is neither approved nor recommended by DHHS for infants <3 months of age; however, it is recommended for use by the WHO for infants starting at 4 weeks of life and with a minimal weight of 3 kg (Department of Health and Human Services 2018a; World Health Organization 2016).

FTC, AZT, and 3TC are available in oral solutions at 10 mg/mL, and ABC is available as 20 mg/mL oral solution. These solutions do not need to be refrigerated and can be given without regard to food. Dispersible pediatric tablets for AZT and ABC are available in resource-limited settings.

Dosing NRTI guidelines for infants <4 weeks of age are limited. Other than for AZT, little PK data exist to fully inform accurate dosing in this population at a time when physiological maturation of the kidneys and liver are occurring rapidly (Capparelli et al. 2003b). Pediatric experience both for treatment with AZT and for prevention of MTCT is extensive. The initial perinatal trial PACTG 076 established the guidelines that AZT given to the mother during pregnancy, labor, and given to the newborn reduced perinatal transmission of HIV by 70% (Connor et al. 1994). For infants who are HIV-exposed but uninfected, AZT is prescribed in prophylactically for the duration of 4–6 weeks. Although the landmark PACTG 076 study used dosing of 2 mg/kg/dose every 6 h, more recent data support more practical twice-daily dosing of AZT at 4 mg/kg (Moodley et al. 2001).

For infants with an HIV infection, AZT and 3TC doses should be increased at 4 weeks of age as the enzymes responsible for glucuronidation reach their maturation over the first 4–6 weeks in full-term neonates (Mirochnick et al. 1999). AZT, 3TC, and ABC are dosed twice daily in infancy, and only FTC in patients older than 3 months of age is dosed once daily (Department of Health and Human Services 2018a).

PK data for preterm infants are available for AZT and 3TC (Capparelli et al. 2003a, b). The renal clearance of AZT and 3TC is further decreased in premature infants requiring a significant decreased in dosing (Capparelli et al. 2003a; Tremoulet et al. 2007). For premature infants diagnosed with HIV, the time to increase the dose from the initial dose is based on post-gestational age and their clinical status, and required careful assessment of hepatic and renal function should be performed prior to dose increase.

For infants unable to tolerate oral agents, the intravenous dose of AZT is available and should be 75% of the oral dose with a similar dosing interval. In fact, AZT is the only ARV drug available for intravenous administration which makes it useful in significantly preterm neonates unable to tolerate oral intake.

2.2 Non-nucleoside Analogue Reverse Transcriptase Inhibitors (NNRTIs)

NVP is the only NNRTI approved for use in neonates (aged $\geq$15 days, Food and Drug Administration 2011a). Efavirenz (EFV) has been approved by the FDA for infants as young as 3 months of age (Food and Drug Administration 2011b); however, it has not been recommended for children aged $<$3 years due to high variation in PK and exposure-related toxicity and functional under dosing concerns (Salem et al. 2014). NVP has, therefore, become a mainstay of ARV prophylaxis for the prevention of MTCT globally despite concerns for low virologic resistance threshold.

NVP is available in a 10 mg/mL suspension which can be stored at room temperature and given without regard to food and is also available in a dispersible pediatric dosing tablet. NVP has a long elimination half-life and is a substrate and inducer of hepatic metabolism by cytochrome P450 family (Food and Drug Administration 2011a). Based on the results of the NICHD-HPTN 040 trial (Nielsen-Saines et al. 2012), 6 weeks of AZT plus 3 doses of NVP is the combination ARV prophylaxis regimen recommended by DHHS for the prophylaxis of the high-risk MTCT exposure (Department of Health and Human Services 2018a). NVP prophylaxis with or without AZT is also recommended for all HIV-exposed infants by WHO regardless of feeding practices (World Health Organization 2010). NVP prophylactic and treatment dosing guidelines by DHHS and WHO for infants starting at 32 weeks of gestational age are based on weight bands and mg/kg dosing. Until 2018, WHO recommended infant prophylaxis with AZT plus NVP for a total of 12 weeks for breastfed infants at high MTCT risk (World Health Organization 2016). Providing multiple drugs to a newborn remained a challenge, specifically the use of both AZT and NVP as AZT is administered twice daily and NVP once daily, making it challenging for caregivers and from an operational programmatic perspective as well.

Furthermore, due to high rates of the NNRTIs resistance observed in young infants in sub-Saharan Africa (Jordan et al. 2017), WHO has recently recommended moving away from using NVP in neonatal period and replacing its use with RAL starting at birth and PI-based regimens with LPV/r starting at 4–6 weeks of life for HIV-infected infants (World Health Organization 2018a).

For premature infants and neonates, data are limited for NVP treatment dosage and are primarily based on PK modeling. In children requiring NVP for treatment and not prophylaxis, traditional dosing of NVP is initiated with a once-daily dose during the first 2 weeks to allow for the induction of the liver enzymes CYP3A and CYP2B6 which are involved in NVP metabolism, so-called lead-in dosing (Food and Drug Administration 2005). Lead-in dosing can reduce the occurrence of rash but can also lead to subtherapeutic plasma NVP levels (Department of Health and Human Services 2018b). Data from the CHAPAS-1 trial suggest that a lead-in dose may not be necessary in young patients and that the risk of rash is more prevalent in older children (Fillekes et al. 2013). Therefore, experts recommend that for children $\leq$2 years of age, NVP may be initiated without a lead-in dose (Department of Health and Human Services 2018b).

2.3 Protease Inhibitors (PI)

LPV/r is approved for treatment of HIV infection in term infants 14 days and older and cannot be administered to neonates before a gestational age of 42 weeks due to toxicity primarily associated with syrup excipients (e.g., propylene glycol and alcohol) (Food and Drug Administration 2011c).

The poor palatability of currently available LPV/r oral solution (20 mg LPV/20 mg RTV) has remained a significant challenge to medication adherence for children and their families. In addition, the syrup requires cold chain storage up to the point of dispersing and once dispensed is stable at 25°C for 6 weeks which is prohibitive for many countries. While evidence demonstrates LPV/r superiority in clinical efficacy over NVP for treatment of HIV regardless of prior exposure to NVP (Violari et al. 2012), this boosted PI is not widely used due to the challenges associated with the liquid formulation. Pediatric LPV/r tablets are available for children; however, they cannot be crushed as crushing tablets result in significant decrease in the plasma drug concentrations (Best et al. 2011). Alternative generic pediatric formulations include mini melt tablets or pellets (in a capsule) which received preliminary approval by the FDA in 2015 (Food and Drug Administration 2015a). This formulation has significant advantages including easy storage and transport and can be administered to infants and young children who cannot swallow tablets. Oral pellets, however, cannot be stirred, dissolved, or crushed in liquid in advance to the administration. For infants not yet taking solid food, the capsule should be open, and pellets can be added to small amount of breast milk or formula or directly placed on the infant's tongue prior to breastfeeding. For those taking solid food, the pellets can be mixed with a small amount of soft food. There are currently limited clinical data on effectiveness and safety of LPV/r pellets in routine care. Data from the CHAPAS-2 trial suggest equivalent bioavailability between LPV/r pellets and syrup in a small number of infants 3–12 months (Musiime et al. 2014). In this study, the proportion of infants and younger children reporting unpleasant taste with pellet was similar to syrup (Kekitiinwa et al. 2016).

LPV/r pellets do not contain propylene glycol and alcohol and could be potentially considered for use starting at birth either as part of infant prophylaxis or combination ART treatment regimen; however, there are currently no data to support its use in infants <3 months of age. The LIVING study, a phase III study led by the Drug for Neglected Diseases *initiative* (DNDi), is an ongoing implementation study of LPV/r pellets in infants and children >3 kg (no age inclusion) who are unable to swallow tablets (US National Library of Medicine 2018). Preliminary data suggest that treatment with LPV/r pellets appears effective and well tolerated with minimal safety concerns (Salami Olawale et al. 2017). Data suggest better acceptability of the new pellet formula, visible positive outcomes of the child's health, and easy administration, all of which support the initiation and maintenance of adherence (Ouma et al. 2018). If the pellets were administered quickly, the development of a bitter taste was avoided (Ouma et al. 2018). Access and cost to LPV/r pellets currently remain barriers to wide implementation in resource-limited settings. LPV/r granules (40 mg/10 mg) are now available from Mylan Laboratories Limited. The granules are recommended for children >3 kg and are expected to be used in the same settings and similar patient populations as the LPV/r pellets. An application is under review to include the granules on WHO Essential Medicines List for Children (World Health Organization 2019).

2.4 Integrase Strand Transfer Inhibitors (INSTI)

RAL is the only INSTI that is FDA-approved for use in newborns and infants weighing ≥ 3 kg (Food and Drug Administration 2013a). RAL for neonates is available in granules for oral suspension: a single-use packet contains 100 mg to be suspended in 10 mL of water (it is not dissolvable in breast milk) for a final concentration of 10 mg/mL (Merck 2017). This formulation requires access to clean drinkable water and, therefore, might pose a challenge in resource-limited settings.

RAL is metabolized by uridine diphosphate glucuronosyltransferase (UGT), the enzyme also responsible for metabolizing bilirubin. UGT activity is low at birth, making it possible for bilirubin and RAL to compete for the enzyme's binding sites (Clarke et al. 2013). RAL may displace bilirubin from albumin and increases the risk of kernicterus in neonates (Clarke et al. 2013). Data suggest that the effect of RAL on neonatal bilirubin binding is unlikely to be clinically significant unless concentrations 50–100-fold higher than typical plasma peak concentrations are reached (Clarke et al. 2013).

RAL crosses the placenta, and if the mother has taken RAL 2–24 h prior delivery, DHHS recommends that the neonate's first dose be delayed until 24–48 h after birth to allow for elimination of transplacentally transferred RAL and to avoid the risk of toxicity in neonate (Clarke et al. 2014). High concentrations of RAL may increase the risk of bilirubinemia and associated neurotoxicity; however, subtherapeutic concentration for the treatment of HIV must be avoided and could increase the risk of acquiring resistance (Clarke et al. 2014). Data from IMPAACT P1110 study suggest that daily use of RAL is safe and well tolerated during the first 6 weeks of life (Clarke et al. 2018b). RAL elimination is highly variable and is prolonged in the first weeks of life. Based on the postpartum maturation of UGT metabolism, RAL dosing is doubled after the first week of life in neonates. Data outside the neonatal period, in infants at least 4 weeks of age, suggest that the granules for oral suspension are well tolerated with good efficacy (Nachman et al. 2015). The 2018 interim HIV treatment guidelines from WHO recommend RAL-based regimen as a preferred first-line regimen for treating HIV-infected neonates (World Health Organization 2018a). The 2018 DHHS guidelines also recommends RAL as a preferred option for empiric HIV therapy for infants at high risk of transmission or those with confirmed HIV infection (Department of Health and Human Services 2018a). To date the data on RAL dosing is limited to infants 37 weeks of gestation, and no data are available for other preterm and low birth weight infants (Department of Health and Human Services 2018a).

RAL has a low genetic barrier to resistance; however, it is yet unclear as to whether early exposure to RAL will result in altered choices of other INSTIs in HIV-infected children. HIV drug resistance testing in resource-limited settings, where treatment options are limited, has been difficult to implement due to high capital and test costs. While there is wide cross-resistance with other INSTIs such as elvitegravir (EVG), there is limited cross-resistance between RAL and dolutegravir (DTG) (Kobayashi et al. 2011). DTG is not approved for use in neonates/infants, and current studies are under way for children weighing $\leq$30 kg in the USA (IMPAACT 2023) and in children $<$25 kg by WHO (Updated Recommendations on first-line and second-line antiretroviral regimens 2018). Children who do not achieve viral suppression on RAL-based regimen will require twice-daily administration of DTG in the future (World Health Organization 2018a).

2.5 Safety Considerations

Several important safety issues in the neonatal population need to be considered when initiating ART either for treatment or prophylaxis. Ideally, all patients initiating ABC should be tested for the HLA-B$*$5701 allele to predict the risk of hypersensitivity reactions. Hypersensitivity reactions with ABC usually occur during the first few weeks of starting therapy and include fever, rash, nausea, vomiting, and respiratory symptoms which should lead to immediate and permanent discontinuation of the drug. This hypersensitivity reaction can affect 3–4% of Caucasian and Asian children but is very rare in African children (Puthanakit et al. 2013).

AZT causes mitochondrial toxicity, and despite extensive experience in pediatrics, experts favor the use of ABC when patient ages do not restrict use because it has less effect on mitochondrial function. The hematologic side effects of AZT appear to be concentration dependent. Granulocytopenia and or anemia are known side effects that may require discontinuation of AZT therapy. In the ARROW trial, severe anemia was found independently of AZT-based regimen; however, AZT was associated with severe neutropenia seen in a small number of children (ARROW Trial Team 2013). Neonatal ARV regimen containing AZT may also represent a higher risk of cardiomyopathy (Patel et al. 2012).

3TC has generally been considered safe in older children and adults; however, hematological toxicity (anemia, thrombocytopenia, and neutropenia) increase when combined with AZT for neonatal prophylaxis with children requiring either discontinuation or blood transfusions (Nielsen-Saines et al. 2012; Mandelbrot et al. 2001).

NVP toxicity includes rash, hypersensitivity reactions, and hepatotoxicity. Close monitoring for rash and liver function test abnormalities is required, and NVP should not be administered to patients with moderate to severe hepatic impairment (Department of Health and Human Services 2018b). Drug-drug interactions are common with NNRTIs and should be addressed prior to initiating and during NVP therapy. The possibility of pre-existing viral resistance because of prior exposure to NVP for PMTCT remains a significant issue in sub-Saharan Africa (Kuhn et al. 2014).

In 2011, the FDA released a statement on LPV/r solution toxicity in neonates which include adrenal insufficiency (Simon et al. 2011), arrhythmias, lactic acidosis, respiratory, and central nervous system depression (Food and Drug Administration 2011c).

2.6 Future Considerations

As a result of lifelong ART in pregnant and breastfeeding mothers, new HIV infections among infants have significantly decreased, while the number of HIV-exposed uninfected infants (HEU) has steadily increased. Numerous studies have reported adverse health outcomes in HEU children including higher mortality (Brennan et al. 2016), mitochondrial toxicity (Jao et al. 2017), infectious disease complications (Slogrove et al. 2016), growth (Powis et al. 2016; Rosala-Hallas et al. 2017), neurodevelopmental outcomes (McHenry et al. 2018), and altered immunity (Reikie et al. 2014). The causes of increased adverse outcomes are likely multifactorial including socioeconomic factors, infant feeding practices, prolonged exposure to ART, postpartum ART regimen, coinfections, and immune activation (Evans et al. 2016). The benefits of ART in reducing vertical transmission and improving maternal health outweigh the risks of ART exposure to children; however, as the number of infants exposed to HIV and ART increase, it remains critical to closely monitor for outcomes and potential adverse effects.

Selected Important Ongoing Neonatal and Infant Studies

1. Ongoing clinical trials including IMPAACT P1115 (ClinicalTrials.gov Identifier: NCT02140255), BHP-074 (ClinicalTrials.gov Identifier: NCT02369406), and the Leopard Study in South Africa (ClinicalTrials.gov Identifier: NCT02431975) will explore early intensive ART regimen in neonates and should provide additional safety and pharmacokinetic data for 3TC, NVP, LPV/r, and RAL.
2. The complete results from the multicountry LIVING study (ClinicalTrials.gov Identifier: NCT02346487) will provide information on efficacy, safety, and acceptability of the LPV/r pellets in infants and children.
3. IMPAACT P1093 (ClinicalTrials.gov Identifier: NCT03016533) is an ongoing phase 1/2 open-label pharmacokinetic and dose finding study of DTG in an oral pediatric granule and dispersible tablet formulation in children aged 4 weeks to <18 years of age.

3 ART for Children

Development changes remain an important consideration in HIV management past infancy for children as they grow and develop. Faster clearance of ARV drugs by younger children often require higher body surface area or weight-based dosing compared to older children and adults. In resource-limited settings, additional challenges in these vulnerable populations include delay in growth, concomitant infectious diseases, and malnutrition, all of which can influence ARV drug clearance and metabolism (Rakhmanina and Phelps 2012). The risk of tuberculosis (TB) and universal isoniazid (INH) prevention therapy in high tuberculosis burden settings further complicate ART options for these children due to multiple drug-drug interactions of INH and other TB drugs such as rifampin with ARV drugs.

Although an increasing number of FDA-approved ARV drugs are available in children, the number of HIV drugs approved for pediatric use still lack behind the number of formulations available for adults. Most pediatric ARV drug and doses approvals are based on the efficacy data from clinical trials in adults with supporting PK and safety data from Phase 1/2 trials in children (Penazzato et al. 2017).

For simplification and ease, doses for most ARV drugs approved in children are broken down by the specific weight bands rather than being calculated by kilogram of weight or body surface area. The dosing recommendations are supported by clinical PK studies, PK modeling, and experts reviews. Based on weight bands, children should not receive more than 25% above the maximum target dose or more than 5% below the minimum target dose (World Health Organization 2016). In addition, several pediatric 2-in-1 and 3-in-1 fixed-dose combinations (FDC) are available and have received quality certification by the WHO and FDA for use in children. Despite progress in scaling up access and introducing WHO guidelines supporting rapid initiation of ART for all children, only 52% of all children living with HIV in 2017 were accessing ARV treatment (UNAIDS 2018).

All current pediatric ART guidelines recommend first line in HIV-infected children to include a dual-NRTI backbone combination plus an agent from a different class including INSTI, NNRTI, or a boosted PI. ART regimen recommendations are often based on age and/or weight limitations. Pediatric studies have compared NNRTI-based regimens to PI-based regimens. The P1060 study demonstrated superiority of LPV/r-based regimens compared to NVP in children aged 2–35 months, regardless of prior maternal or infant exposure prophylaxis (Violari et al. 2012). In the PENPACT-1 study, children either on an NNRTI-based regimen versus a PI-based regimen had similar virologic outcomes after a 4-year follow-up (Babiker et al. 2011). In the PROMOTE trial, children randomized to either an NNRTI- or a LPV/r-based regimen had similar virologic efficacy at 48 weeks (Ruel et al. 2014). Data for INSTI-based regimens in children are currently limited to non-randomized trial studies assessing safety, tolerability, and PK and are largely based on adult efficacy data (Raffi et al. 2013).

Several challenges remain in HIV treatment for children including (a) lack of safety, efficacy, and pharmacokinetics for optimal dosing of some existing and new ARV drugs, particularly with novel drug delivery systems; (b) limited interventions and appropriate drug formulations to improve adherence; (c) variable bioavailability of the FDCs; and (d) short- and long-term ART outcomes particularly as it relates to the risk of remote noncommunicable diseases (Penazzato et al. 2018).

Compared to adults, children living with HIV face a prolonged lifetime journey to remain adherent to ARV drugs. Effective interventions and strategies to support children and their caregivers to ensure improved adherence, disclosure of HIV status, and clinical outcomes are critical. The increased survival of children with HIV into adulthood also poses new challenges in selecting ART regimen with minimal short- and long-term toxicities, preventing the development of resistance and maintaining normal physical growth and neurocognitive development.

Here we review each ARV drug class in relationship to the pediatric use for treatment of HIV.

3.1 Nucleoside and Nucleotide Analogue Reverse Transcriptase Inhibitors (NRTI)

Dual-NRTI form the backbone of combination ART regimens throughout the spectrum of pediatric ages and weight bands. Several NRTIs are approved and available for children <13 years of age and include ABC, FTC, 3TC, AZT, tenofovir disoproxil fumarate (TDF), and tenofovir alafenamide (TAF), as well as didanosine (ddI) and stavudine (D4T) which are both no longer recommended due to drug-related toxicities. In resource-limited settings, AZT, ABC, 3TC, and TDF are available either as single drugs in form of oral solutions, oral powder, scored tablets, or FDCs (including dispersible tablets) for pediatric use (Table 2).

ABC and 3TC comprise the preferred dual-NRTI backbone recommended for children by WHO. Both drugs are dosed twice daily at initiation; however, based on PK studies, data suggest that once-daily dosing of ABC and 3TC is comparable to twice-daily dosing (LePrevost et al. 2006; Bergshoeff et al. 2005; Szubert et al. 2017). DHHS recommends switching to once-daily regimen for 3TC for children $\geq$3 years of age, and for ABC once children are using the pill formulation and are clinical stable with undetectable viral loads (Department of Health and Human Services 2018b). FTC, TAF, and TDF are all dosed once daily. 3TC and FTC are interchangeable and both are well tolerated. Both also select for the M184V resistance mutation, which is associated with high-level resistance to both drugs, a decrease in susceptibility to ABC and improved susceptibility to ZDV and TDF (Borroto-Esoda et al. 2006; Ross et al. 2004).

TAF is an oral prodrug of TDF and is approved by the FDA as a component of FDCs, and based on decreased risk for TDF-associated renal and bone adverse events compared to TDF, it is recommended by DHHS as a preferred dual-NRTI combination with FTC (Table 1). TDF/FTC is available as reduced-strength tablets and oral powder for use in children (Table 2). However, the granules that make up the TDF oral power give the vehicle a gritty consistency, and once mixed TDF should be administered promptly as its taste can become bitter. Finally, FTC, 3TC, TDF, and TAF all have antiviral activity and efficacy against hepatitis B and need to be considered for children with coinfection.

3.2 Non-nucleoside Analogue Reverse Transcriptase Inhibitors (NNRTIs)

Three NNRTIs, specifically EFV (for children aged $\geq$3 months), etravirine (ETR, for children aged $\geq$2 years (Food and Drug Administration 2012)), and NVP (for children starting at birth), are approved for pediatric treatment of HIV (Department of Health and Human Services 2018b). Rilpivirine (RPV) is only approved for children $\geq$12 years (Food and Drug Administration 2011). EFV and NVP are both available in resource-limited settings either as single drug tablet or FDCs. The benefits of NNRTIs as initial therapy include a long half-life requiring less frequent dosing, a lower risk of dyslipidemia, and fat maldistribution compared to PIs and generally a lower pill burden. The major disadvantages of using NNRTI include the low barrier to high-level drug resistance (except for doravirine (DOR)) and cross-resistance within the drug class as well as the potential for multiple drug interactions due to metabolism with hepatic enzymes.

EFV has been approved by the FDA starting at 3 months of age; however, it is not recommended for use in children <3 years by DHHS due to variable PK and associated variability in drug exposure and toxicity (Department of Health and Human Services 2018b). EFV concentrations can also be suboptimal in children $\geq$3 years (Salem et al. 2014). The bioavailability of EFV is affected by food, and it is best administered on an empty stomach. EFV can be swallowed as a whole capsule or can be opened and used as sprinkles with soft foods or formula/breast milk (Food and Drug Administration 2011b). Scored tablets of EFV are available in resource-limited settings. ETR is approved for children >2 years of age and should be administered following a meal (Food and Drug Administration 2012). Available pediatric ETR tablets may be dispersed in liquid. Finally, NVP is available as

Table 1 Summary of current pediatric ART guidelines for the treatment of HIV in children and adolescents from World Health Organization (WHO), US Department of Health and Human Services (DHHS), and Paediatric European Network for Treatment of AIDS (PENTA)

	WHO 2016 and interim guidance 2018 (World Health Organization 2016, 2018a)	DHHS 2018 (Department of Health and Human Services 2018a, b, c)	PENTA 2015 (Paediatric European Network for the Treatment of AIDS 2007)
Preferred regimens (first-line)			
Neonates and infants <12 months	2 NRTIs + RAL	2 NRTIs + NVP 2 NRTIs + RAL	2 NRTIs + NVP 2 NRTIs + LPV/r
Children *<3 years*	2 NRTIs + LPV/r	2 NRTIs + LPV/r 2 NRTIs + RAL	2 NRTIs + NPV 2 NRTIs + LPV/r
3–6 years	2 NRTIs + NNRTI	2 NRTIs + ATV/r 2 NRTIs + DRV/r 2 NRTIs + RAL	2 NRTIs + EFV 2 NRTIs + LPV/r
>6 years	2 NRTIs + DTG	*>6 years to <12 years*: 2 NRTIs + ATV/r 2 NRTIs + DTG	2 NRTIs + ATV/r 2 NRTIs + EFV
Adolescents	2 NRTIs + DTG 2 NRTIs + EFV	*>12 years old and SMR 1–3*: 2 NRTIs + ATV/r 2 NRTIS + DTG 2 NRTIs + DRV 2 NRTIs + EVG/COBI *>12 years old and SMR 4 or 5*: TAF/FTC/BIC (in adults guidelines) 2 NRTIs + DTG 2 NRTIs + RAL	2 NRTIs + ATV/r 2 NRTIs + DRV/r 2 NRTIs + EFV
Alternative regimens (second line)			
Neonates and infants less than 12 months	2 NRTIs + NVP	*>14 days*: 2 NRTIs + NVP *>3 months*: 2 NRTIs + ATV/r	
Children	2 NRTIs + ATV/r or LPV/r 2 NRTIs + DTG DRV/r + DTG + 1–2 NRTIs	*<3 years*: 2 NRTIs + ATV/r *>3–6 years*: 2 NRTIs + EFV 2 NRTIs + LPV/r *6–12 years*: 2 NRTIs + DRV/r 2 NRTIs+ EFV 2 NRTIs + EVB/COBI 2 NRTIs + LPV/r 2 NRTIs + RAL	2 NRTIs + DRV/r 2 NRTIs + NVP

(continued)

Table 1 (continued)

	WHO 2016 and interim guidance 2018 (World Health Organization 2016, 2018a)	DHHS 2018 (Department of Health and Human Services 2018a, b, c)	PENTA 2015 (Paediatric European Network for the Treatment of AIDS 2007)
Adolescents	2 NRTIs + ATV/r or LPV/r 2 NRTIs + DTG	*>12 years old and SMR 1–3:* 2NRTIs + EFV 2 NRTIs + RAL 2 NRTIs + RPV *>12 years old and SMR 4–5:* 2 NRTIs + DRV/r 2 NRTIs + ATV/r 2 NRTIs + EFV 2 NRTIs + RPV	2 NRTIs + NVP 2 NRTIs + LPV/r 2 NRTIs + RAL 2 NRTIs + DTG
Preferred 2-NRTI backbone options			
Neonates and infants less than 12 months	AZT + 3TC	ZDV + (3TC or FTC) *>3 months*: ABC + (3TC or FTC)	ABC (AZT) + 3TC
Children	ABC (AZT) + 3TC	*<6 years*: ABC + (3TC or FTC) ZDV + (3TC or FTC) *>6 years*: ABC + (3TC or FTC) FTC/TAF	ABC+ 3TC
Adolescents	TDF + 3TC (or FTC)	ABC + (3TC or FTC) TAF/FTC	TDF/FTC ABC + 3TC

3TC lamivudine, *ABC* abacavir, *ATV/r* atazanavir/ritonavir, *ART* antiretroviral therapy, *COBI* cobicistat, *DHHS* Department of Health and Human Services, *DRV* darunavir, *DRV/r* darunavir/ritonavir, *DTG* dolutegravir, *EFV* efavirenz, *EVG* elvitegravir, *FTC* emtricitabine, *LPV/r* lopinavir/ritonavir, *NRTI* nucleoside reverse transcriptase inhibitor, *NVP* nevirapine, *PENTA* Pediatric European Network for Treatment of AIDS, *PI* protease inhibitor, *RAL* raltegravir, *RPV* rilpivirine, *SMR* sexual maturity rating, *TAF* tenofovir alafenamide, *TDF* tenofovir disoproxil fumarate, *ZDV* zidovudine, *WHO* World Health Organization

liquid and pediatric single drug tablet formulations and as an extended release formulation. Children ≥6 years of age who are already taking immediate-release NVP twice daily can be switched to NVP extended release once daily without lead-in dosing (Department of Health and Human Services 2018b).

Table 2 ARVs by class and formulation and in comparison between DHHS and WHO guidelines for weight- and age-based dosing limits

Drug	Available formulations (World Health Organization 2016, 2018a; Department of Health and Human Services 2018a, b, c)	Dosing limits DHHS guidelines (Department of Health and Human Services 2018a, b, c)	Dosing limits WHO guidelines (World Health Organization 2016, 2018a)
Nucleoside (nucleotide) reverse transcriptase inhibitors			
ABC	20 mg/mL solution	Age limit (>3 months)	Weight limit (>3 kg)
	60 mg dispersible	N/A	Weight limit (>3 kg)
	300 mg scored tablet	Weight limit (>14 kg)	Higher weight limit (>25 kg)
	ABC 60 mg/3TC 30mg[a]	N/A	Age (>4 weeks) and weight limit (>3 kg)
	ABC 120 mg/3TC 60 mg dispersible[a]	N/A	Age (>4 weeks) and weight limit (>3 kg)
	ABC 600 mg/3TC 300 mg[a]	Weight limit (>25 kg)	Weight limit (>25 kg)
	ABC 300 mg/3TC 150 mg/ AZT 300 mg[a]	Weight limit (>30 kg)	N/A
	ABC 600 mg/DTG 50 mg/ 3TC 300 mg[a]	Weight limit (>25 kg)	N/A
FTC	10 mg/mL solution	Weight-based dosing from birth	N/A
	200 mg capsule	Weight limit (>33 kg)	Age limit (>18 years)
	FTC 100 mg/TDF 150 mg[a]	Weight limit (17–22 kg)	N/A
	FTC 133 mg/TDF 200 mg[a]	Weight limit (22–28 kg)	N/A
	FTC 167 mg/TDF 250mg[a]	Weight limit (28–35 kg)	N/A
	FTC 200 mg/TDF 300 mg[a]	Weight limit (>35 kg)	N/A
	FTC 200 mg/TAF 25 mg[a]	Weight limit (>25 kg)	N/A
	FTC 200 mg/RPV 25 mg/ TDF 300 mg[a]	Age (>12 kg) and weight (>35 kg) limit	N/A
	FTC 200 mg/RPV 25 mg/ TAF 25 mg[a]	Age (>12 kg) and weight (>35 kg) limit	N/A
3TC	Solution: 5 mg/mL and 10 mg/mL	Gestational age (≥32 weeks) limit	Only 10 mg/mL solution available Weight (>2 kg) and gestational age (term) limits
	150 mg scored tablet	Weight limit (>14 kg)	N/A
	Tablets: 100 mg and 300 mg	Weight limit (>25 kg)	Age limit (adolescent[b])
	3TC 300 mg/TDF 300 mg[a]	Weight limit (>35 kg)	N/A
	3TC 150 mg/AZT 300mg[a]	Weight limit (>30 kg)	Lower weight limit (>25 kg)
TAF	25 mg tablet	Weight limit (>25 kg)[c]	N/A

(continued)

Table 2 (continued)

Drug	Available formulations (World Health Organization 2016, 2018a; Department of Health and Human Services 2018a, b, c)	Dosing limits DHHS guidelines (Department of Health and Human Services 2018a, b, c)	Dosing limits WHO guidelines (World Health Organization 2016, 2018a)
TDF	40 mg/1 g oral powder	Age (>2 years) and weight (>10 kg) limit	N/A
	Tablets: 150 mg, 200 mg, 250 mg, and 300 mg	Age (>2 years) and weight (>17 kg) limit	250 mg tabs N/A Lower weight (>14 kg) limit
	TDF 300 mg/3TC 300 mg/ DTG 50mg[a, d]	N/A	Age (adolescent[b]) and weight (>30 kg) limit
AZT	10 mg/mL syrup	Takes gestational age into consideration	Does not consider gestational age
	60 mg dispersible	N/A	Age (>4 weeks) and weight (>3 kg) limit
	100 mg capsule and 300 mg tablet	Age limit (>18 years)	Weight limit (>25 kg)
	AZT 60 mg/3TC 30 mg dispersible[a]	N/A	Age (>4 weeks) and weight (>3 kg) limit
	AZT 60 mg/3TC 30 mg/NVP 50 mg dispersible[a]	N/A	Age (>4 weeks) and weight (>3 kg) limit
	AZT 300 mg/3TC 150 mg/ NVP 200 mg[a]	N/A	Weight limit (>25 kg)
Non-nucleoside reverse transcriptase inhibitors			
DOR	100 mg tablet	Adult dosing available	N/A
	DOR 100 mg/TDF 300 mg/ 3TC 300 mg[a]	Adult dosing available	N/A
EFV	50 mg and 200 mg capsules, 600 mg tablet	Age (>3 years) and weight (>10 kg) limit; higher maximum dose (600 mg)	Age (>3 years) and weight (>10 kg) limit; lower maximum dose (400 mg)
	EFV 600 mg/FTC 200 mg/ TDF 300 mg[a]	Weight limit (>40 kg)	N/A
	EFV 400 mg/3TC 300 mg/ TDF 300 mg[a, e]	Weight limit (>35 kg)	N/A
	EFV 600 mg/3TC 300 mg/ TDF 300 mg[a, e]	Weight limit (>40 kg)	N/A
ETR	Tablets: 25 mg, 100 mg, 200 mg	Age (>2 years) and weight (>10 kg) limit	N/A
NVP	10 mg/mL suspension	Takes gestational age into consideration	Does not consider gestational age
	50 mg dispersible	N/A	Age (>4 weeks) and weight (>3 kg) limit
	Tablets: immediate release 200 mg, extended release 100 mg and 400 mg	Investigational dosing preterm infants (>34 weeks gestation) from birth Regular dosing with age (>1 month) limit	Only immediate release tablet available Weight limit (>25 kg)

(continued)

Table 2 (continued)

Drug	Available formulations (World Health Organization 2016, 2018a; Department of Health and Human Services 2018a, b, c)	Dosing limits DHHS guidelines (Department of Health and Human Services 2018a, b, c)	Dosing limits WHO guidelines (World Health Organization 2016, 2018a)
RPV	25 mg tablet	Age (>12 years) and weight (>35 kg) limit	N/A
Protease inhibitors			
ATV	50 mg power packets	Age (>3 months) and weight (>5 kg) limit	Age (>3 months) and weight (>5 kg) limit
	Capsules: 150 mg, 200, and 300 mg	Age (>6 years) and weight (>15 kg) limit	Weight limit (>10 kg)
	ATV 300 mg/RTV 100 mg[a]	N/A	N/A)
	ATV 300 mg/COBI 150 mg	Adult dosing available	N/A
DRV	100 mg/mL suspension	Age (>3 years) and weight (>10 kg) limit	Age (>3 years) and weight (>10–20 kg) limit
	Tablets: 75 mg, 150, 600, and 800 mg	Age (>3 years) and weight (>15 kg) limit	Lower weight limit (>14 kg)
	DRV 800 mg/COBI 150 mg[a]	Adult dosing available	N/A
	DRV 800 mg/COBI 150 mg/ FTC 200 mg/TAF 10mg[a]	Adult dosing available	N/A
FPV	50 mg/mL suspension	Age (>6 months) limit	N/A
	700 mg tablet	Age limit (adolescent)	N/A
IDV	Capsules: 100 mg, 200 mg and 400 mg	Age limit (adolescent)	N/A
LPV/r	LPV 80 mg/RTV 20 mg/mL solution[a]	Age limit (>14 days)	Weight limit (>2 kg)
	LPV 40 mg/RTV 10 mg pellets[a, d]	N/A	Age (>4 weeks) and weight (>3 kg) limit
	Tablets: LPV 100 mg/RTV 25 mg[a, d] LPV 200 mg/RTV 50 mg[a]	Weight limit (>15 kg)	Only 100/25 mg tablet available Age (>4 weeks) and weight (>10 kg) limit
	LPV 400 mg/RTV 100 mg[a]	N/A	Age limit (adolescent[b])
	LPV 40/RTV 10 mg/ABC 30 mg/3TC 15 mg granules or powder[a, d]	N/A	N/A
NFV	Tablets: 250 mg and 625 mg	Age limit (>2 years)	N/A
RTV	80 mg/mL solution	Dosing recommendations specific to drug combination	Age (>4 weeks) and weight (>3 kg) limit
	Tablets: 25 mg, 50 mg, and 100 mg	N/A	Age (>4 weeks) and weight (>3 kg) limit
	100 mg/packet powder	Dosing recommendation specific to drug combination	Age (>4 weeks) weight (>6 kg) limit

(continued)

Table 2 (continued)

Drug	Available formulations (World Health Organization 2016, 2018a; Department of Health and Human Services 2018a, b, c)	Dosing limits DHHS guidelines (Department of Health and Human Services 2018a, b, c)	Dosing limits WHO guidelines (World Health Organization 2016, 2018a)
SQV	200 mg capsules or 500 mg tabs	Age limit (>16 years)	N/A
TPV	100 mg/mL solution	Age limit (>2 years)	N/A
	250 mg capsule	Age limit (adolescents)	N/A
Integrase inhibitors			
BIC	BIC 50 mg/FTC 200 mg/TAF 25mg[a]	Investigational dosing with age (>6 years) and weight (>25 kg) limit Regular dosing with age limit (>18 years)	N/A
DTG	Tablets: 10 mg, 25 mg, and 50 mg[d]	Weight limit (>25 kg)	Only 50 mg tab available Weight limit (>25 kg)
	DTG 50 mg/RPV 25 mg[a]	Adult dosing available	N/A
EVG	EVG 150 mg/COBI 150 mg/ FTC 200 mg/TAF 10 mg[a]	Weight limit (>25 kg)	N/A
	EVG 150 mg/COBI 150 mg/ FTC 200 mg/TDF 300 mg[a]	Weight (>35 kg) and SMR (4 or 5) limit	N/A
RAL	Single use packet of 100 mg granules for oral suspension, suspended in 10 mL of water for final concentration of 10 mg/mL	Weight (2 kg) and gestational age (>37 weeks) limit	Weight limit (>2 kg)
	400 and 600 mg tablets; 100 mg and 25 mg[d] chewable tablets	Weight limit (>11 kg); higher maximum dose (1,200 mg)	Age (>4 weeks) and weight (>3 kg) limit; lower maximum dose (400 mg)
Fusion and entry inhibitors			
T-20	108 mg of T-20 per vial reconstituted with 1.1 mL of sterile water for a final concentration of 90 mg/1 mL	Age limit (>6 years)	N/A
MVC	20 mg/mL solution	Age (>2 years) and weight (>10 kg) limit	N/A
	Tablets: 25 mg, 75 mg, 150 mg, and 300 mg	Age (>2 years) and weight (>10 kg) limit	N/A
IBA	Single-dose 2 mL vial containing 200 mg/1.33 mL (150 mg/mL)	Age limit (adolescents)	N/A

3TC lamivudine, *ABC* abacavir, *ATV* atazanavir, *ART* antiretroviral therapy, *AZT* zidovudine, *BIC* bictegravir, *COBI* cobicistat, *DHHS* Department of Health and Human Services, *DOR* doravirine, *DRV* darunavir, *DRV/r* darunavir/ritonavir, *DTG* dolutegravir, *EFV* efavirenz, *ETR* etravirine, *EVG* elvitegravir, *FTC* emtricitabine, *FPV* fosamprenavir, *IBA* ibalizumab, *IDV* indinavir, *LPV/r* lopinavir/ritonavir, *MVC* maraviroc, *N/A* formulation and/or dosing guidelines not available, *NFV* nelfinavir, *NRTI* nucleoside reverse transcriptase inhibitor, *NVP* nevirapine, *PEPFAR* President Emergency Plan for AIDS Relief, *PI* protease inhibitor, *RAL* raltegravir, *RPV* rilpivirine,

RTV ritonavir, *SMR* sexual maturity rating, *SQV* saquinavir, *T-20* enfuvirtide, *TAF* tenofovir alafenamide, *TDF* tenofovir disoproxil fumarate, *TPV* tipranavir, *WHO* World Health Organization
[a]Fixed-dose combinations (FDCs) of drug listed under first encountered drug component
[b]WHO defines adolescents as age 10–19 years
[c]Approved only for hepatitis B coinfection treatment
[d]President Emergency Plan for AIDS Relief ARV Formulation Primary Priority
[e]President Emergency Plan for AIDS Relief ARV Formulation Secondary Priority

3.3 Protease Inhibitors (PI)

The boosted PIs, atazanavir/ritonavir (ATV/r), darunavir/ritonavir (DRV/r), fosamprenavir/ritonavir (FPV/r), and LPV/r are FDA-approved in children. PI-based regimens have high clinical, virologic, and immunologic efficacy (Squires et al. 2004; Gatell et al. 2007; Malan et al. 2008; Strehlau et al. 2015; Ortiz et al. 2008; Blanche et al. 2009), and, most importantly, a high barrier to drug resistance. However, their use frequently poses palatability challenges. PIs may increase the pill burden when not taken in FDCs and in solid formulations.

Oral suspensions are available for LPV/r, ritonavir, FPV, and DRV. ATV/r is approved for infants and children ≥3 months (Food and Drug Administration 2003a, b). None of the PIs are approved currently for pediatric use in combination with another pharmacokinetic booster/enhancer without antiviral activity cobicistat (COBI), frequently used in adults. DRV/r is approved for children >3 years and LPV/r is approved for infants >14 days (Food and Drug Administration 2000).

WHO recommends LPV/r as the preferred first-line regimen for children >14 days and <3 years; DHHS recommends LPV/r as the preferred PI-based regimens for infants and ATV/r as the preferred PI-based regimen for children >3 years of age (>6 years of age for PENTA guidelines) (World Health Organization 2018a; Bamford et al. 2018; Department of Health and Human Services 2018b).

3.4 Integrase Strand Transfer Inhibitors (INSTIs)

RAL and DTG are both approved for use in children. RAL is licensed for treatment of infants and children from birth (Food and Drug Administration 2017), and DTG is approved for use in children weighing >30 kg (Food and Drug Administration 2013b) and by the European Medicines Agency (EMA) for children weighing more than 15 kg (European Medical Agency 2011). Recent data from the PENTA ODYSSEY trial, however, suggest that the EMA-approved dose might be suboptimal in children (Bollen et al. 2018), leading to WHO recommending adult 50 mg dose starting at weight of 25 kg and potentially at weight of 20 kg, based on PK modeling (World Health Organization 2018a). EVG is approved only within FDCs in combination with COBI/FTC with TAF for children weighing >25 kg and with TDF for adolescents >35 kg (Department of Health and Human Services 2018b). INSTIs have become the drug within the preferred regimen for children

>6 years worldwide because of their virologic efficacy, high resistance threshold, minimal toxicity, as well as once-daily administration. There are, however, limited data on pediatric dosing and safety.

RAL is available in granules for oral suspension and chewable tablets suitable for younger children. It is generally well-tolerated in children; however, the development of mutations associated with RAL resistance has been a growing concern (Nachman et al. 2018).

DTG is available as once-daily single small size tablet and as an FDC. DTG has a higher threshold for the development of resistance and maintains antiviral activity in the presence of mutations conferring RAL or EVG resistance. DTG is recommended as first-line therapy for children aged ≥6 years by the WHO interim 2018 guidance (World Health Organization 2018a). DTG has advantages over EFV which was previously recommended as first line by the 2016 WHO guidelines. DTG has fewer drug-drug interactions, produces faster viral suppression, is associated with a higher CD4 cell count recovery rates, causes less treatment discontinuations, and has high genetic barrier to developing resistance. In addition, unlike EFV, it is also effective against more rare HIV type 2 (Descamps et al. 2015). The fairly recent availability of this drug as a generic FDC (TDF/3TC/DTG or TLD) at a price comparable to current regimens in low- and middle-income countries further support the use of DTG. WHO recommends that countries with pre-treatment resistance rate to EFV or NVP at 10% or above consider using an alternative regimen that does not contain NNRTI. WHO also recommends DTG as a second-line ART for people who have failed NNRTI or PI-based first-line therapy (World Health Organization 2018a).

3.5 Entry and Fusion Inhibitors

Maraviroc (MVC) is a CCR5 antagonist approved for use in treatment-experience children >2 years of age and weight >10 kg (Food and Drug Administration 2007). Tropism assay needs to be performed prior to use to test for CCR5 tropism of the virus. Clinical failure may still occur and may represent outgrowth of the CXCR4-using HIV variants. MVC requires twice-daily dosing and is available in tablets as well as oral solution for pediatric use. MVC is a substrate of the cytochrome P450 enzyme and has, therefore, a high potential for drug interactions (Department of Health and Human Services 2018b).

Enfuvirtide (T-20) is an injectable fusion inhibitor and is approved for children >6 years of age (Food and Drug Administration 2003a, b). T-20 requires twice-daily subcutaneous injections and is recommended for use in deep salvage regimens only. T-20 is not commonly used because of its high cost, requirement for subcutaneous injections, and high rate of injection site reactions. Its use has declined with the availability of INSTIs.

3.6 Safety Considerations

The use of TDF is associated with decreased bone mineral density in young children, and older children with lower sexual maturity ratings (SMR) may be at higher risk (Department of Health and Human Services 2018c). Some experts recommend screening with a dual-energy absorptiometry (DEXA) before initiation of TDF and at 6–12-month intervals especially in prepubertal children (Department of Health and Human Services 2018c). TDF is also associated with new onset or worsening renal toxicity in children. Urine dipstick and serum creatinine screenings are recommended prior to TDF initiation. Experts also recommend screening serum creatinine every 3–4 months and performing urinalysis every 6–12 months in pediatric patients. TAF achieves high intracellular concentration, but serum concentrations are lower than TDF, therefore reducing bone and renal toxicity. Data in adults and adolescents suggest that there is an increase in cholesterol as early as 24 weeks after initiation of a regimen containing TAF (Food and Drug Administration 2015b). Therefore, monitoring serum lipids in patients on TAF is warranted, given these findings.

Rash with EFV and ETR have been reported in pediatric patients within the first week of treatment at higher rates compared to adults. EFV use has also been associated with significant central nervous system (CNS) neuropsychiatric side effects and can be partially modulated by the bedtime administration of the whole capsule on an empty stomach (Department of Health and Human Services 2018b). Adverse CNS events are generally harder to detect in children and may present as impaired concentration, sleep disturbances, or behavior disorder. An association between suicidal ideation and EFV has been found in adult trials, but has not been reported in children (Mollan et al. 2014). Patients with cytochrome P450 2B6 variants associated with low EFV clearance frequently have increased CNS toxicity, as well as other EFV-associated adverse events such as hepatic injury and QTc prolongation on electrocardiogram (Abdelhady et al. 2016).

DRV cannot be used in children <3 years of age because of toxicity concerns regarding seizures and death observed in animal studies in infant rats with immaturity of the blood-brain barrier (Department of Health and Human Services 2018b). Although many ARVs have variable dyslipidemic properties, use of PIs has been most associated with hypertriglyceridemia and hypercholesterolemia. ATV and DRV have less effect on dyslipidemia compared to LPV/r and FPV/r. PIs may be also associated with cardiometabolic complications including dyslipidemia, fat maldistribution, and insulin resistance (Nolan 2003). RTV which is used in low doses as a booster when co-administered with PIs can increase the risk of hyperlipidemia and drug interactions. ATV causes asymptomatic hyperbilirubinemia.

MVC may cause hepatotoxicity that may be preceded by a systemic allergic reaction such as pruritus, eosinophilia, or elevated immunoglobulin.

Although morbidity and mortality secondary to HIV have significantly decreased for all ages due to ART (GBD 2015 HIV Collaborators 2016), as adults, children living with HIV are at risk of acquiring additional chronic diseases and complications, specifically CVD and metabolic diseases (Feinstein et al. 2016;

Pelchen-Matthews et al. 2018). Metabolic complications of ART that have been described in perinatally HIV-infected children include insulin resistance (Dirajlal-Fargo et al. 2017a; Geffner et al. 2018), fat redistribution (Arrive et al. 2018), and dyslipidemia (Ramteke et al. 2018). CVD complications have also been reported including endothelial dysfunction (Dirajlal-Fargo et al. 2017b), sub-clinical atherosclerosis as measured by carotid ultrasound (Ross et al. 2010), and increased arterial stiffness (Charakida et al. 2009), all of which strongly correlate with CVD events in the general adult population. In these aforementioned studies, complications were described in children on both NNRTI- and PI-based regimen, and data are lacking on the impact of specific ARV drug exposure on the development of cardiometabolic complications. These complications are likely the result of multiple interacting factors including HIV infection, ART, exposure to HIV in utero, race/ethnicity, socioeconomics, and lifestyle factors. HIV in younger populations may play a larger role on CVD risk compared to traditional risk factors (Hanna et al. 2016). Sustained immune activation also seems to persist in HIV-infected children despite ART (Persaud et al. 2014), and few studies in HIV-infected children have already shown that inflammation markers correlate with carotid ultrasound changes (Ross et al. 2010), insulin resistance (Dirajlal-Fargo et al. 2017a), and hyperlipidemia (Miller et al. 2012); however, no sufficiently powered longitudinal studies have been performed to assess the clinical significance of inflammation and immune activation in this population.

Metabolic complications in children raise significant concerns about the cumulative risk of CVD over time in perinatally infected children who face a lifetime of ART exposure. Longitudinal studies of metabolic complications in perinatally infected children in the era of newer-line ARV drugs are warranted.

3.7 Pediatric Adherence Challenges

Pediatric adherence to ART is paramount especially in settings with limited drug choices for further ARV drug substitutions. However, it remains one of the greatest obstacles in pediatric HIV care. Optimal viral suppression requires adherence rates of 95% and above (Bain-Brickley et al. 2011); however, suboptimal adherence to ART in children is common (Reddington et al. 2000; Murphy et al. 2001). Children, unlike adults, face additional adherence challenges. Children depend on caregivers, who may themselves have HIV/AIDS; their adherence is influenced by developmental stages; they may not understand or know the meaning of HIV, their own status, or importance of taking ART; lastly the lack of appropriate and palatable drug formations create an additional and likely most challenging adherence barrier. The WHO promotes peer support strategies and family-centered counseling to support ART (World Health Organization 2016); however, few evidence-based interventions have been developed to date to promote adherence in children.

3.8 Future Considerations

A number of pediatric FDC formulations are currently in the different stages of development including ABC/3TC/LPV/r (four in one) granules, and DTG 10 mg scored dispersible tablets are close to being introduced to the market, while others such as pediatric FDCs of ABC/3TC/DTG, TAF-based FDCs with 3TC and FTC, and DRV/r are in earlier stages of development.

4 ART for Adolescents

Adolescents represent the largest growing population living with HIV worldwide. In 2017 alone, 590,000 between the ages of 15–24 were newly infected with HIV, half of those were adolescents between the ages of 15 and 19 (UNICEF 2018). Among HIV-infected adolescents, the vast majority acquired infection through sexual activity, and a smaller proportion were infected perinatally. There are several factors that place adolescents at high risk for acquiring HIV including inadequate sex and risk behavior education, socioeconomic challenges (e.g., poverty, housing and food insecurity, incarceration, and lack of medical insurance), stigma, and misperceptions about HIV (Services DoHaH 2019).

In the USA, the majority of individuals who acquired HIV through perinatal transmission are now adolescents or young adults (Centers for Disease Control and Prevention 2017). Many of them were initiated on mono or dual combinations of ARV drugs prior to the availability of currently used combination ART regimens. These adolescents frequently face extensive drug resistance, need for more complex regimens, and long-term consequences of living with HIV and using ART.

Compared to children, adolescents have more ART options such as adult FDCs and other ARVs with improved side effects; however, drug dosing during puberty as well as potential drug interactions with hormonal contraceptives or illicit drugs arise as a challenge. Furthermore, dosing for selected ARV drugs in adolescents depends not only on their age and weight but also on the sexual maturation rating (SMR 1 through 5, also known as the Tanner stages I through V). DHHS and WHO generally recommend pediatric dosing for adolescents who are sexually immature (SMR 3 or less) or those with perinatally acquired HIV and stunted sexual maturation (World Health Organization 2016; Department of Health and Human Services 2018b, c). Postpubertal adolescents (SMR 4 or 5) generally follow adult dosing schedules. SMR and age may not predict drug PK, and continued use of pediatric doses in adolescents can result in medication doses that are increased and potentially toxic; however, early introduction of lower adult doses can lead to suboptimal drug concentration and the development of drug resistance. Many drugs including ABC, FTC, 3TC, TDF, and some PIs are administered at significantly higher doses to children compared to adult dosing. In recent years, more and more frequently, DHHS and WHO ARV drugs dosing guidelines are provided without age restrictions merely by definition of adolescence and weight limits (World Health Organization 2016; Department of Health and Human Services 2018c). While this transition simplifies the implementation and providers' tasks, adolescents should be closely monitored during growth spurt periods for drug efficacy and toxicity. Several parameters should be considered when transitioning from pediatric to adult doses including drug formulation, pill burden, adherence, and virologic and immunologic status. Moreover, youth with horizontally acquired HIV are at risk of acquiring resistant virus from partners who are older and ART-experienced and therefore might have baseline resistance negatively affecting treatment outcome (Agwu et al. 2012).

More than 30 ARVs in seven different classes are FDA-approved for treatment of HIV in adolescents. As described below in more detail, several pre-ART and ART-specific characteristics as well as comorbidities or other conditions and other medications should be considered prior to selecting the appropriate regimen in adolescent patient.

Although a three-drug ART regimen is currently recommended as a first line in adolescents, data in adults support two-drug first-line ART regimens such as DTG plus 3TC when ABC, TDF, or TAF cannot be used. DHHS recommend DTF plus 3TC when other backbone drugs cannot be used on the bases of data from phase 3 randomized trials showing that this combination was non-inferior to DTG plus TDF/FTC for virologic efficacy and no drug resistance was seen in either treatment group (Cahn et al. 2019). To date, dual ART regimens including DTG plus 3TC or DTG plus RPV have not been evaluated in adolescents and are not currently recommended for these populations.

4.1 Nucleoside and Nucleotide Analogue Reverse Transcriptase Inhibitors (NRTI)

ABC, FTC, 3TC, TAF, TDF, and AZT are approved and available in FDCs for adolescents. The preferred NRTI backbone for adolescents is TDF or TAF with FTC or 3TC (Department of Health and Human Services 2018c). HLA-B∗507 testing should be performed prior to initiating ABC, and therefore ABC should not be the drug of choice when ART needs to be initiated rapidly. ABC has also been associated with an increased risk of myocardial infarction in adults with pre-existing cardiac risk factors (Worm et al. 2010).

Other factors to consider include renal insufficiency and bone mineral density with TDF and TAF especially when with used with a pharmacologic booster, as well as history of hepatitis B infection (Department of Health and Human Services 2018c). TAF is associated with significantly less renal and bone toxicities than TDF but may have higher risk of dyslipidemia. Currently, most TAF-based FDCs are approved for use adolescents.

4.2 Non-nucleoside Analogue Reverse Transcriptase Inhibitors (NNRTIs)

EFV, ETR, NVP, and RPV are approved for use in adolescents. DOR was approved in August 2018 in HIV-infected adults as an FDC with TDF and 3TC, and the data in the adolescent population are being gathered.

High-level resistance to NVP, EFV, and RPV may occur with a single viral mutation.

Lower dose of EFV (400 mg vs. 600 mg standard dose) has been shown to cause less CNS side effects and fewer treatment discontinuations while preserving the efficacy in adult populations (Cohen et al. 2013). This dose has not been studied in pregnant women or patients co-infected with TB. Recently approved EFV 400 mg-based FDC is now available for use in adolescent populations in the USA and resource-limited settings; however, data efficacy date in adolescents are still lacking.

The use of RPV is limited by the virologic parameters and requires baseline viral load <100,000 copies/mL (Department of Health and Human Services 2018c). ECHO and THRIVE trials have demonstrated that in patients with high viral loads, more participants treated with RPV experienced virologic failure compared to those who were treated with EFV-based ART (Cohen et al. 2013; Domingo and Ribera 2013). EFV can interact with oral hormonal contraceptives, and alternative or additional contraceptive methods may be warranted (Department of Health and Human Services 2018c).

4.3 Protease Inhibitors (PIs)

ATV, DRV, FPV, and LPV/r and TPV/r are Food and Drug Administration (FDA)-approved for use in adolescents. Transmitted PI resistance is usually uncommon, and PI-based regimens may also be useful in adolescents at risk of intermittent therapy due to poor adherence. COBI boosted DRV and ATV are available as single-tablet regimens and are the PI-based regimen recommended by DHHS for ART-naïve patients (Department of Health and Human Services 2018c). Use of COBI boosted PI is limited during pregnancy due to the PK considerations for low plasma concentrations in the second and third trimesters compared to the RTV boosted PIs (Department of Health and Human Services 2018a). Due to several metabolic complications associated with PI use and PK boosting necessary with either RTV or COBI, PI-based regimen is not recommended as first-line regimen; however, due to the high-resistance threshold, they represent viable option for the second- and third-line ART in adolescent treatment-experienced patients.

4.4 Integrase Strand Transfer Inhibitors (INSTI)

DTG, EVG, and RAL are approved in adolescents. Bictegravir (BIC) has not been FDA-approved for patients <18 years of age; however, data from 24 participants in adolescents aged 12–18 years of age show that it was safe and well tolerated

(Aditya Gaur et al. 2018). BIC and COBI boosted EVG are only available in FDC with FTC and TAF or TDF for EVG/COBI. BIC and DTG have the potential of several drug interactions including with polyvalent cations (aluminum, magnesium, antacids, or iron supplements) and should not be co-administered under fasting conditions, with or 2 h after these drugs (Department of Health and Human Services 2018c). BIC is contraindicated with rifampin, which limits considerations for its use in resource-limited setting with high rates of TB coinfection. BIC, DTG, and EVG are all available as components of once-daily single-tablet regimen (STR). RAL has the longest clinical experience but is associated with a higher pill burden and lower barrier to resistance compared to BIC or DTG (Anstett et al. 2017).

DTG is not recommended for pregnant women during the first trimester or for women of childbearing potential (see safety issue section below). DTG is generally well tolerated; however, neuropsychiatric adverse events (such as sleep disturbances, depression, anxiety, and suicidal ideation) have been reported with the use of RAL and DTG (Kheloufi et al. 2015; Harris et al. 2008).

EVG is available as STR; however, it requires boosting with PK enhancer COBI which increases the likelihood of drug-drug interactions. EVG/COBI use is also limited during pregnancy due to the low EVG concentrations in the late pregnancy negatively affecting virologic outcomes (Department of Health and Human Services 2018a).

4.4.1 Entry and Fusion Inhibitors

The CCR5 antagonist MVC has potential for drug-drug interactions, requires twice-daily dosing, and does not offer virologic benefit when compared to other regimen, and is therefore not recommended for initial therapy in adolescents.

T-20 has only been studied in adolescents with virologic failure and is not commonly used. Ibalizumab (IBA) is a recently FDA-approved CD4-directed post-attachment HIV-1 inhibitor, administered intravenously as a single loading dose followed by a maintenance dose infusion every 2 weeks (Food and Drug Administration 2018). It has only been studied in treatment-experienced adults with multidrug-resistant strains, and studies in adolescents are being planned.

4.5 Safety Issues

In 2018, the preliminary data from a cohort study in Botswana suggested an increased rate of neural tube defects among infants born to women who initiated DTG prior to pregnancy and were on DTG at the time of conception (Zash et al. 2018). Four cases of neural tube defects were reported in infants born to women who started DTG prior to conception (0.67% rate). In comparison 0.1% rate were identified among women taking other ART regimens at the time of conception. Currently, it is still unclear if this finding indicates a true increased risk of neural tube defect, and a further analysis with a larger number of exposures is needed to determine risk level. Additional data are being gathered and are expected for release in summer 2019 from Botswana and other cohorts following pregnant women who used DTG-based regimens during conception and throughout the pregnancy. Until further information is available, DTG is not recommended for use in women of childbearing potential who are sexually active and not using effective contraception throughout the first 8 weeks of pregnancy (Department of Health and Human Services 2018a; Updated Recommendations on first-line and second-line antiretroviral regimens 2018). It is also currently unclear whether the risk of neural tube defects is shared by other INSTIs. BIC is similar structurally to DTG, but there are no currently safety data on BIC use near conception or during pregnancy.

For countries that are introducing TLD before new DTG safety data become available, several approaches are considered. The first option is recommending TLD only if use of consistent contraception can be assured, which can be a challenge in settings where women may not have access to consistent contraception or be empowered to make decisions about their own reproductive health. Another option is to recommend TLD not be used in women of childbearing potential, including young adolescent females. This raises concern about equitable access to a regimen that is more effective and better tolerated. Lastly, some countries continue to recommend TLD to women and adolescents using a women-centered approach as recommended by WHO (World Health Organization 2018a). This includes providing counseling and ensuring access to consistent contraception is available. This may be a challenge in settings where simplified guidance is needed and healthcare workers have a high clinical burden (PEPFAR and ICAP 2018).

4.6 Sexual Reproductive Health Considerations

Discussion of family planning and counseling, as well as a discussion of the risks for perinatal transmission, should be provided to all youth. Information about methods to prevent MTCT, as well as choice of ART should be discussed with all women including adolescents.

Important for adolescent and young women, some ARV drugs may interact with hormonal contraceptives. These include drugs that are metabolized by the cytochrome P450 enzyme system (NNRTIs, PIs, MVC, and EVG) and may reduce concentrations and efficacy of oral contraceptive agents or increase the risk of estrogen- or progestin-related side effects (Department of Health and Human Services 2018c). There is also a concern regarding bone mineral density loss following long-term use of depot medroxyprogesterone acetate with or without TDF, prompting recommendations for monitoring bone mineral density via DEXA scans (Department of Health and Human Services 2018c).

Sexual reproductive health including contraception and gynecologic care for female adolescents with HIV as well as screening for sexually transmitted infections should be offered to all adolescents infected with HIV. All adolescents living with HIV should be immunized with the human papilloma virus vaccination where available. Adolescent girls and young women living with HIV should undergo regular screenings for cervical cancer.

4.7 Adherence and Disclosure

Adolescents infected with HIV face additional barriers to adherence including growing independence, misinformation, and lack of disclosure of HIV status, increased peer pressure, risk-taking behavior, lack of support system, and lifestyles with less predictable schedules. Compared to adults, adolescents have lower rates of viral suppression and higher rates of loss to follow-up (Ryscavage et al. 2011; Nachega et al. 2009; Zanoni and Mayer 2014).

Careful assessment of physical and psychosocial maturity, discussions about lifestyle, and existing support systems must take place prior to prescribing combination ART regimen. A once-daily FDC is the preferred choice among adolescents and should be prescribed when feasible (Parienti et al. 2009; Nachega et al. 2014). Current methods that used to support adherence include reminder systems (calendar, text messaging (Belzer et al. 2015), phone calls (Abdulrahman et al. 2017), alarm), direct observed therapy (Purdy et al. 2008), and provision of pill boxes. It is important to make adherence interventions and support inconspicuous, stylish, modern, as well as user-friendly to make it match youth choices. Digital gaming may be a promising intervention strategy for this population in some settings (Hightow-Weidman et al. 2017; Castel et al. 2018). A short-term deference of ART initiation may be necessary until adherence issues can be addressed. Timely viral load testing is important once treatment is initiated and can be used as a proxy for adherence evaluation and support. Prescription or pill count-based methods to estimate adherence are objective estimates of adherence obtained from pharmacy databases and can also be used to guide adherence counseling.

4.8 Mental Health Considerations

Mental health conditions, alcohol, and substance abuse are prevalent in HIV-infected adolescents (West et al. 2019; Earnshaw et al. 2018). Mental health, however, is often a neglected priority for this population. Despite increased access to ART and even in the presence of viral suppression, HIV-infected youth continue to experience neurocognitive complications secondary to HIV-related causes (Crowell et al. 2014) and have socioeconomic factors that increase the risk of mental health problems. Data are lacking in this population, in addition most studies have been done in higher income countries. Lack of screening for mental health disorders can be detrimental to adolescents facing stigma, long-term challenges of retention into care, medication adherence, and transition of care. Youth-focused health services and individual-level interventions improving mental healthcare delivery in adolescents are eventually beneficial to their ART outcomes (Judd et al. 2016).

Healthcare providers should also be aware of clinically important drug-drug interactions of ARVs with antidepressants, anxiolytics, and antipsychotics particularly with PIs and NNRTIs.

5 Conclusion

Significant progress has been made to address the pediatric global HIV epidemic to date. Although HIV remains a major cause of mortality among children and mostly adolescents worldwide, the scale-up of ART has greatly contributed to the prevention and treatment of HIV from infancy to the adulthood. The development of pediatric ARV drugs and formulations has lagged behind the adults and has been prioritized by WHO, which recently published a pediatric drug development toolkit summarizing the challenges and solutions for promoting and accelerating timely quality research and development of ARV formulations suitable for infants, children, and adolescents along with pregnant and breastfeeding women (World Health Organization 2018b).

Better drugs and formulations, including long-term acting and injectable/implant ARVs, need to be developed for use in pediatric and adolescent populations to reduce the complexity of multidrug regimens, increase adherence, and improve treatment outcome and quality of life for infants, children, and adolescents living with HIV. Moreover, studies evaluating simplified drug regimens and novel therapeutic modalities such as neutralizing antibodies for the pediatric population are ongoing and need to be expanded across all ages and developmental stages. Finally, long-term outcomes of perinatal and lifelong ARV drugs exposure need to be consistently evaluated, and preventive interventions to leverage success of ART with the metabolic and CVD complications need to be developed.

Conflict of Interest The authors declare no conflict of interest.

References

Abdelhady AM, Shugg T, Thong N et al (2016) Efavirenz inhibits the human Ether-A-Go-Go related current (hERG) and induces QT interval prolongation in CYP2B6∗6∗6 allele carriers. J Cardiovasc Electrophysiol 27:1206–1213

Abdulrahman SA, Rampal L, Ibrahim F, Radhakrishnan AP, Kadir Shahar H, Othman N (2017) Mobile phone reminders and peer counseling improve adherence and treatment outcomes of patients on ART in Malaysia: a randomized clinical trial. PLoS One 12:e0177698

Adejumo OA, Malee KM, Ryscavage P, Hunter SJ, Taiwo BO (2015) Contemporary issues on the epidemiology and antiretroviral adherence of HIV-infected adolescents in sub-Saharan Africa: a narrative review. J Int AIDS Soc 18:20049

Aditya Gaur CR, McGrath EJ, Hellstrom E, Liberty A, Natukunda E, Kosalaraksa P, Chokephaibulkit K, Coluci A, Majeed SR, Porter D, Wong P, Quirk E, Graham H, Pikora C (2018) Bictegravir/FTC/TAF single-tablet regimen in adolescents: week 24 results. In: Conference on retroviruses and opportunistic infections, Boston

Agwu AL, Bethel J, Hightow-Weidman LB et al (2012) Substantial multiclass transmitted drug resistance and drug-relevant polymorphisms among treatment-naive behaviorally HIV-infected youth. AIDS Patient Care STDs 26:193–196

Anstett K, Brenner B, Mesplede T, Wainberg MA (2017) HIV drug resistance against strand transfer integrase inhibitors. Retrovirology 14:36

Arici C, Ripamonti D, Ravasio V et al (2001) Long-term clinical benefit after highly active antiretroviral therapy in advanced HIV-1 infection, even in patients without immune reconstitution. Int J STD AIDS 12:573–581

Arrive E, Viard JP, Salanave B et al (2018) Metabolic risk factors in young adults infected with HIV since childhood compared with the general population. PLoS One 13:e0206745

ARROW Trial Team (2013) Routine versus clinically driven laboratory monitoring and first-line antiretroviral therapy strategies in African children with HIV (ARROW): a 5-year open-label randomised factorial trial. Lancet 381:1391–1403

Babiker A, Castro nee Green H, Compagnucci A et al (2011) First-line antiretroviral therapy with a protease inhibitor versus non-nucleoside reverse transcriptase inhibitor and switch at higher versus low viral load in HIV-infected children: an open-label, randomised phase 2/3 trial. Lancet Infect Dis 11:273–283

Bain-Brickley D, Butler LM, Kennedy GE, Rutherford GW (2011) Interventions to improve adherence to antiretroviral therapy in children with HIV infection. Cochrane Database Syst Rev 12:CD009513

Bamford A, Turkova A, Lyall H et al (2018) Paediatric European Network for Treatment of AIDS (PENTA) guidelines for treatment of paediatric HIV-1 infection 2015: optimizing health in preparation for adult life. HIV Med 19:e1–e42

Barlow-Mosha L, Musiime V, Davies MA et al (2017) Universal antiretroviral therapy for HIV-infected children: a review of the benefits and risks to consider during implementation. J Int AIDS Soc 20:21552

Belzer ME, Kolmodin MacDonell K, Clark LF et al (2015) Acceptability and feasibility of a cell phone support intervention for youth living with HIV with nonadherence to antiretroviral therapy. AIDS Patient Care STDs 29:338–345

Bergshoeff A, Burger D, Verweij C et al (2005) Plasma pharmacokinetics of once- versus twice-daily lamivudine and abacavir: simplification of combination treatment in HIV-1-infected children (PENTA-13). Antivir Ther 10:239–246

Best BM, Capparelli EV, Diep H et al (2011) Pharmacokinetics of lopinavir/ritonavir crushed versus whole tablets in children. J Acquir Immune Defic Syndr 58:385–391

Blanche S, Bologna R, Cahn P et al (2009) Pharmacokinetics, safety and efficacy of darunavir/ritonavir in treatment-experienced children and adolescents. AIDS 23:2005–2013

Bollen PTA, Mujuru H, Musiime V, Amuge P, Lugenwa A, Colbers A, Spyer M, Lensen S, Moore C, Hakin J, Kityo C, Bbuye D, Atwine L, Giaquinto C, Ford D, Gibb D, Burger D (2018) Steady-state pharmacokinetics and early safety data in HIV-infected African children weighing 14 to<25kg on film-coated dolutegravir 25 mg tablets in the ODYSSEY trial. In: 10th international workshop on HIV pediatrics, Amsterdam

Borroto-Esoda K, Vela JE, Myrick F, Ray AS, Miller MD (2006) In vitro evaluation of the anti-HIV activity and metabolic interactions of tenofovir and emtricitabine. Antivir Ther 11:377–384

Brennan AT, Bonawitz R, Gill CJ et al (2016) A meta-analysis assessing all-cause mortality in HIV-exposed uninfected compared with HIV-unexposed uninfected infants and children. AIDS 30:2351–2360

Cahn P, Madero JS, Arribas JR et al (2019) Dolutegravir plus lamivudine versus dolutegravir plus tenofovir disoproxil fumarate and emtricitabine in antiretroviral-naive adults with HIV-1 infection (GEMINI-1 and GEMINI-2): week 48 results from two multicentre, double-blind, randomised, non-inferiority, phase 3 trials. Lancet 393(10167):143–155

Capparelli EV, Mirochnick M, Dankner WM et al (2003a) Pharmacokinetics and tolerance of zidovudine in preterm infants. J Pediatr 142:47–52

Capparelli EV, Englund JA, Connor JD et al (2003b) Population pharmacokinetics and pharmacodynamics of zidovudine in HIV-infected infants and children. J Clin Pharmacol 43:133–140

Capretti MG, Marsico C, Conti M et al (2016) Nevirapine prophylaxis to prevent HIV-1 mother-to-child transmission: pharmacokinetic considerations in preterm infants. New Microbiol 39:314–316

Castel AD, Qasmieh S, Greenberg D et al (2018) Digital gaming to improve adherence among adolescents and young adults living with HIV: mixed-methods study to test feasibility and acceptability. JMIR Serious Games 6:e10213

Centers for Disease Control and Prevention (2017) HIV surveillance report

Charakida M, Loukogeorgakis SP, Okorie MI et al (2009) Increased arterial stiffness in HIV-infected children: risk factors and antiretroviral therapy. Antivir Ther 14:1075–1079

Clarke DF, Wong RJ, Wenning L, Stevenson DK, Mirochnick M (2013) Raltegravir in vitro effect on bilirubin binding. Pediatr Infect Dis J 32:978–980

Clarke DF, Acosta EP, Rizk ML et al (2014) Raltegravir pharmacokinetics in neonates following maternal dosing. J Acquir Immune Defic Syndr 67:310–315

Clarke DF, Penazzato M, Capparelli E et al (2018a) Prevention and treatment of HIV infection in neonates: evidence base for existing WHO dosing recommendations and implementation considerations. Expert Rev Clin Pharmacol 11:83–93

Clarke DAE, Chain A, Cababasay M, Wang J, Teppler H, Smith B, Hazra H, Popson S, Graham B, Calabrese K, Bryson Y, Spector S, Mirochnik M (2018b) IMPACT P1110: raltegravir pharmacokinetics and safety in HIV-1 exposed neonates: dose-finding study in infants born to mothers receiving raltegravir-containing ART. In: 10th international workshop on HIV pediatrics, Amsterdam

Cohen CJ, Molina JM, Cassetti I et al (2013) Week 96 efficacy and safety of rilpivirine in treatment-naive, HIV-1 patients in two phase III randomized trials. AIDS 27:939–950

Connor EM, Sperling RS, Gelber R et al (1994) Reduction of maternal-infant transmission of human immunodeficiency virus type 1 with zidovudine treatment. Pediatric AIDS Clinical Trials Group Protocol 076 Study Group. N Engl J Med 331:1173–1180

Crowell CS, Malee KM, Yogev R, Muller WJ (2014) Neurologic disease in HIV-infected children and the impact of combination antiretroviral therapy. Rev Med Virol 24:316–331

Department of Health and Human Services (Panel on Treatment of Pregnant Women with HIV Infection and Prevention of Perinatal Transmission) (2018a) Recommendations for the use of antiretroviral drugs in pregnant women with HIV infection and interventions to reduce perinatal HIV transmission in the United States

Department of Health and Human Services (The Panel on Antiretroviral Therapy and Medical Management of Children Living with HIV) (2018b) Guidelines for the use of antiretroviral agents in pediatric HIV infection

Department of Health and Human Services (The Panel on Antiretroviral Guidelines for Adults and Adolescents) (2018c) Guidelines for the use of antiretroviral agents in adults and adolescents living with HIV

Descamps D, Peytavin G, Visseaux B et al (2015) Dolutegravir in HIV-2-infected patients with resistant virus to first-line integrase inhibitors from the French named patient program. Clin Infect Dis 60:1521–1527

Dirajlal-Fargo S, Musiime V, Cook A et al (2017a) Insulin resistance and markers of inflammation in HIV-infected Ugandan children in the CHAPAS-3 trial. Pediatr Infect Dis J 36:761–767

Dirajlal-Fargo S, Sattar A, Kulkarni M, Bowman E, Funderburg N, McComsey GA (2017b) HIV-positive youth who are perinatally infected have impaired endothelial function. AIDS 31:1917–1924

Domingo P, Ribera E (2013) Data on rilpivirine in treatment-naive patients. Lessons from ECHO, THRIVE and STaR. Enferm Infecc Microbiol Clin 31(Suppl 2):20–29

Earnshaw VA, Kidman RC, Violari A (2018) Stigma, depression, and substance use problems among perinatally HIV-infected youth in South Africa. AIDS Behav 22:3892–3896

European Medical Agency (2011) Lopinavir and Ritonavir oral solution drug label

Evans C, Jones CE, Prendergast AJ (2016) HIV-exposed, uninfected infants: new global challenges in the era of paediatric HIV elimination. Lancet Infect Dis 16:e92–e107

Feinstein MJ, Bahiru E, Achenbach C et al (2016) Patterns of cardiovascular mortality for HIV-infected adults in the United States: 1999 to 2013. Am J Cardiol 117:214–220

Fillekes Q, Mulenga V, Kabamba D et al (2013) Is nevirapine dose-escalation appropriate in young, African, HIV-infected children? AIDS 27:2111–2115
Flynn PM, Taha TE, Cababasay M et al (2018) Prevention of HIV-1 transmission through breastfeeding: efficacy and safety of maternal antiretroviral therapy versus infant nevirapine prophylaxis for duration of breastfeeding in HIV-1-infected women with high CD4 cell count (IMPAACT PROMISE): a randomized, open-label, clinical trial. J Acquir Immune Defic Syndr 77:383–392
Food and Drug Administration (2000) Lopinavir and ritonavir oral solution drug label
Food and Drug Administration (2003a) Atazanavir drug label
Food and Drug Administration (2003b) Enfuvirtide drug label
Food and Drug Administration (2005) Nevirapine drug label
Food and Drug Administration (2007) Maraviroc drug label
Food and Drug Administration (2011) Rilpivirine drug label
Food and Drug Administration (2011a) Viramune label
Food and Drug Administration (2011b) Efavirenz prescribing information label
Food and Drug Administration (2011c) Serious health problems seen in premature babies given Kaletra (lopinavir/ritonavir) oral solution
Food and Drug Administration (2012) Etravirine drug label
Food and Drug Administration (2013a) Isentress drug label
Food and Drug Administration (2013b) Dolutegravir drug label
Food and Drug Administration (2015a) Tentative approval for lopinavir and ritonavir oral pellets
Food and Drug Administration (2015b) Clinical review for elvitegravir/cobicistat/emtricitabine/tenofovir alafenamide (Genvoya)
Food and Drug Administration (2016) Truvda (emtricitabine and tenofovir disoproxil fumarate) tablets, for oral use
Food and Drug Administration (2017) Raltegravir supplement approval for infant
Food and Drug Administration (2018) Ibalizumab drug label
Gatell J, Salmon-Ceron D, Lazzarin A et al (2007) Efficacy and safety of atazanavir-based highly active antiretroviral therapy in patients with virologic suppression switched from a stable, boosted or unboosted protease inhibitor treatment regimen: the SWAN Study (AI424-097) 48-week results. Clin Infect Dis 44:1484–1492
GBD 2015 HIV Collaborators (2016) Estimates of global, regional, and national incidence, prevalence, and mortality of HIV, 1980–2015: the Global Burden of Disease Study 2015. Lancet HIV 3:e361–ee87
Geffner ME, Patel K, Jacobson DL et al (2018) Changes in insulin sensitivity over time and associated factors in HIV-infected adolescents. AIDS 32:613–622
Hanna DB, Guo M, Buzkova P et al (2016) HIV infection and carotid artery intima-media thickness: pooled analyses across 5 cohorts of the NHLBI HIV-CVD collaborative. Clin Infect Dis 63:249–256
Harris M, Larsen G, Montaner JS (2008) Exacerbation of depression associated with starting raltegravir: a report of four cases. AIDS 22:1890–1892
Hightow-Weidman LB, Muessig KE, Bauermeister JA, LeGrand S, Fiellin LE (2017) The future of digital games for HIV prevention and care. Curr Opin HIV AIDS 12:501–507
Holgate SL, Rabie H, Smith P, Cotton MF (2012) Trough lopinavir concentrations in preterm HIV-infected infants. Pediatr Infect Dis J 31:602–604
IMPAACT 2023: a phase I trial to evaluate the safety and pharmacokinetics of dolutegravir in HIV-1 exposed neonates at risk of acquiring HIV-1 infection. https://impaactnetwork.org/studies/IMPAACT2023.asp
Jao J, Powis KM, Kirmse B et al (2017) Lower mitochondrial DNA and altered mitochondrial fuel metabolism in HIV-exposed uninfected infants in Cameroon. AIDS 31:2475–2481
Jordan MR, Penazzato M, Cournil A et al (2017) Human immunodeficiency virus (HIV) drug resistance in African infants and young children newly diagnosed with HIV: a multicountry analysis. Clin Infect Dis 65:2018–2025

Judd A, Sohn AH, Collins IJ (2016) Interventions to improve treatment, retention and survival outcomes for adolescents with perinatal HIV-1 transitioning to adult care: moving on up. Curr Opin HIV AIDS 11:477–486
Kariminia A, Law M, Davies MA et al (2018) Mortality and losses to follow-up among adolescents living with HIV in the IeDEA global cohort collaboration. J Int AIDS Soc 21:e25215
Kekitiinwa A, Musiime V, Thomason MJ et al (2016) Acceptability of lopinavir/r pellets (minitabs), tablets and syrups in HIV-infected children. Antivir Ther 21:579–585
Kheloufi F, Allemand J, Mokhtari S, Default A (2015) Psychiatric disorders after starting dolutegravir: report of four cases. AIDS 29:1723–1725
Kobayashi M, Yoshinaga T, Seki T et al (2011) In vitro antiretroviral properties of S/GSK1349572, a next-generation HIV integrase inhibitor. Antimicrob Agents Chemother 55:813–821
Ku LC, Smith PB (2015) Dosing in neonates: special considerations in physiology and trial design. Pediatr Res 77:2–9
Kuhn L, Aldrovandi GM, Sinkala M et al (2008) Effects of early, abrupt weaning on HIV-free survival of children in Zambia. N Engl J Med 359:130–141
Kuhn L, Hunt G, Technau KG et al (2014) Drug resistance among newly diagnosed HIV-infected children in the era of more efficacious antiretroviral prophylaxis. AIDS 28:1673–1678
Laurent C, Ngom Gueye NF, Ndour CT et al (2005) Long-term benefits of highly active antiretroviral therapy in Senegalese HIV-1-infected adults. J Acquir Immune Defic Syndr 38:14–17
LePrevost M, Green H, Flynn J et al (2006) Adherence and acceptability of once daily lamivudine and abacavir in human immunodeficiency virus type-1 infected children. Pediatr Infect Dis J 25:533–537
Lifson AR, Grund B, Gardner EM et al (2017) Improved quality of life with immediate versus deferred initiation of antiretroviral therapy in early asymptomatic HIV infection. AIDS 31:953–963
Linakis MW, Roberts JK, Lala AC et al (2016) Challenges associated with route of administration in neonatal drug delivery. Clin Pharmacokinet 55:185–196
Malan DR, Krantz E, David N, Wirtz V, Hammond J, McGrath D (2008) Efficacy and safety of atazanavir, with or without ritonavir, as part of once-daily highly active antiretroviral therapy regimens in antiretroviral-naive patients. J Acquir Immune Defic Syndr 47:161–167
Mandelbrot L, Landreau-Mascaro A, Rekacewicz C et al (2001) Lamivudine-zidovudine combination for prevention of maternal-infant transmission of HIV-1. JAMA 285:2083–2093
McHenry MS, McAteer CI, Oyungu E et al (2018) Neurodevelopment in young children born to HIV-infected mothers: a meta-analysis. Pediatrics 141:e20172888
Merck (2017) Merck receives FDA approval for isentress [Raltegravir]. In: Combination with other antiretroviral agents, for the treatment of HIV-1 infection in newborns weighing at least 2 kg. Merck, Kenilworth
Miller TI, Borkowsky W, DiMeglio LA et al (2012) Metabolic abnormalities and viral replication are associated with biomarkers of vascular dysfunction in HIV-infected children. HIV Med 13:264–275
Mirochnick M, Capparelli E, Connor J (1999) Pharmacokinetics of zidovudine in infants: a population analysis across studies. Clin Pharmacol Ther 66:16–24
Mirochnick M, Stek A, Acevedo M et al (2005) Safety and pharmacokinetics of nelfinavir coadministered with zidovudine and lamivudine in infants during the first 6 weeks of life. J Acquir Immune Defic Syndr 39:189–194
Mirochnick M, Nielsen-Saines K, Pilotto JH et al (2011) Nelfinavir and lamivudine pharmacokinetics during the first two weeks of life. Pediatr Infect Dis J 30:769–772
Mollan KR, Smurzynski M, Eron JJ et al (2014) Association between efavirenz as initial therapy for HIV-1 infection and increased risk for suicidal ideation or attempted or completed suicide: an analysis of trial data. Ann Intern Med 161:1–10
Moodley D, Pillay K, Naidoo K et al (2001) Pharmacokinetics of zidovudine and lamivudine in neonates following coadministration of oral doses every 12 hours. J Clin Pharmacol 41:732–741

Mulenga V, Musiime V, Kekitiinwa A et al (2016) Abacavir, zidovudine, or stavudine as paediatric tablets for African HIV-infected children (CHAPAS-3): an open-label, parallel-group, randomised controlled trial. Lancet Infect Dis 16:169–179

Murphy DA, Wilson CM, Durako SJ, Muenz LR, Belzer M (2001) Antiretroviral medication adherence among the REACH HIV-infected adolescent cohort in the USA. AIDS Care 13:27–40

Musiime V, Fillekes Q, Kekitiinwa A et al (2014) The pharmacokinetics and acceptability of lopinavir/ritonavir minitab sprinkles, tablets, and syrups in African HIV-infected children. J Acquir Immune Defic Syndr 66:148–154

Nachega JB, Hislop M, Nguyen H et al (2009) Antiretroviral therapy adherence, virologic and immunologic outcomes in adolescents compared with adults in southern Africa. J Acquir Immune Defic Syndr 51:65–71

Nachega JB, Parienti JJ, Uthman OA et al (2014) Lower pill burden and once-daily antiretroviral treatment regimens for HIV infection: a meta-analysis of randomized controlled trials. Clin Infect Dis 58:1297–1307

Nachman S, Alvero C, Acosta EP et al (2015) Pharmacokinetics and 48-week safety and efficacy of raltegravir for oral suspension in human immunodeficiency virus type-1-infected children 4 weeks to 2 years of age. J Pediatric Infect Dis Soc 4:e76–e83

Nachman S, Alvero C, Teppler H et al (2018) Safety and efficacy at 240 weeks of different raltegravir formulations in children with HIV-1: a phase 1/2 open label, non-randomised, multicentre trial. Lancet HIV 5:e715–ee22

Ngarina M, Tarimo EA, Naburi H et al (2014) Women's preferences regarding infant or maternal antiretroviral prophylaxis for prevention of mother-to-child transmission of HIV during breastfeeding and their views on Option B+ in Dar es Salaam, Tanzania. PLoS One 9:e85310

Nielsen-Saines K, Watts DH, Veloso VG et al (2012) Three postpartum antiretroviral regimens to prevent intrapartum HIV infection. N Engl J Med 366:2368–2379

Nolan D (2003) Metabolic complications associated with HIV protease inhibitor therapy. Drugs 63:2555–2574

Nuttall JJC (2015) Antiretroviral therapy during the neonatal period. South Afr J HIV Med 16:361

Ortiz R, Dejesus E, Khanlou H et al (2008) Efficacy and safety of once-daily darunavir/ritonavir versus lopinavir/ritonavir in treatment-naive HIV-1-infected patients at week 48. AIDS 22:1389–1397

Noestlinger C, Nebot Giralt A, Ouma O, Nyamongo I, Salami O, Lallemant M, Lee J, Marchal B (2018) Whether and why caregivers adhere to oral lopinavir/ritonavir pellets: lessons for scaling up an innovative pediatric HIV treatment in Kenya. In: 22nd international AIDS conference, Amsterdam

Paediatric European Network for the Treatment of AIDS (2007) Lamivudine/abacavir maintains virological superiority over zidovudine/lamivudine and zidovudine/abacavir beyond 5 years in children. AIDS 21:947–955

Parienti JJ, Bangsberg DR, Verdon R, Gardner EM (2009) Better adherence with once-daily antiretroviral regimens: a meta-analysis. Clin Infect Dis 48:484–488

Patel K, Van Dyke RB, Mittleman MA, Colan SD, Oleske JM, Seage GR 3rd. (2012) The impact of HAART on cardiomyopathy among children and adolescents perinatally infected with HIV-1. AIDS 26:2027–2037

Pelchen-Matthews A, Ryom L, Borges AH et al (2018) Aging and the evolution of comorbidities among HIV-positive individuals in a European cohort. AIDS 32:2405–2416

Penazzato M, Gnanashanmugam D, Rojo P et al (2017) Optimizing research to speed up availability of pediatric antiretroviral drugs and formulations. Clin Infect Dis 64:1597–1603

Penazzato M, Irvine C, Vicari M et al (2018) A global research agenda for pediatric HIV. J Acquir Immune Defic Syndr 78(Suppl 1):S10–Ss5

PEPFAR U, ICAP (2018) Considerations for the introduction of TLD in national programs

Persaud D, Gay H, Ziemniak C et al (2013) Absence of detectable HIV-1 viremia after treatment cessation in an infant. N Engl J Med 369:1828–1835

Persaud D, Patel K, Karalius B et al (2014) Influence of age at virologic control on peripheral blood human immunodeficiency virus reservoir size and serostatus in perinatally infected adolescents. JAMA Pediatr 168:1138–1146

Powis KM, Smeaton L, Hughes MD et al (2016) In-utero triple antiretroviral exposure associated with decreased growth among HIV-exposed uninfected infants in Botswana. AIDS 30:211–220

Purdy JB, Freeman AF, Martin SC et al (2008) Virologic response using directly observed therapy in adolescents with HIV: an adherence tool. J Assoc Nurses AIDS Care 19:158–165

Puthanakit T, Bunupuradah T, Kosalaraksa P et al (2013) Prevalence of human leukocyte antigen-B*5701 among HIV-infected children in Thailand and Cambodia: implications for abacavir use. Pediatr Infect Dis J 32:252–253

Raffi F, Jaeger H, Quiros-Roldan E et al (2013) Once-daily dolutegravir versus twice-daily raltegravir in antiretroviral-naive adults with HIV-1 infection (SPRING-2 study): 96 week results from a randomised, double-blind, non-inferiority trial. Lancet Infect Dis 13:927–935

Rakhmanina N, Phelps BR (2012) Pharmacotherapy of pediatric HIV infection. Pediatr Clin N Am 59:1093–1115

Ramteke SM, Shiau S, Foca M et al (2018) Patterns of growth, body composition, and lipid profiles in a South African cohort of human immunodeficiency virus-infected and uninfected children: a cross-sectional study. J Pediatric Infect Dis Soc 7:143–150

Reddington C, Cohen J, Baldillo A et al (2000) Adherence to medication regimens among children with human immunodeficiency virus infection. Pediatr Infect Dis J 19:1148–1153

Reikie BA, Adams RCM, Leligdowicz A et al (2014) Altered innate immune development in HIV-exposed uninfected infants. J Acquir Immune Defic Syndr 66:245–255

Rosala-Hallas A, Bartlett JW, Filteau S (2017) Growth of HIV-exposed uninfected, compared with HIV-unexposed, Zambian children: a longitudinal analysis from infancy to school age. BMC Pediatr 17:80

Ross L, Parkin N, Chappey C et al (2004) Phenotypic impact of HIV reverse transcriptase M184I/V mutations in combination with single thymidine analog mutations on nucleoside reverse transcriptase inhibitor resistance. AIDS 18:1691–1696

Ross AC, O'Riordan MA, Storer N, Dogra V, McComsey GA (2010) Heightened inflammation is linked to carotid intima-media thickness and endothelial activation in HIV-infected children. Atherosclerosis 211:492–498

Ross JL, Teeraananchai S, Lumbiganon P et al (2019) A longitudinal study of behavioral risk, adherence and virologic control in adolescents living with HIV in Asia. J Acquir Immune Defic Syndr 81:e28–e38

Ruel TD, Kakuru A, Ikilezi G et al (2014) Virologic and immunologic outcomes of HIV-infected Ugandan children randomized to lopinavir/ritonavir or nonnucleoside reverse transcriptase inhibitor therapy. J Acquir Immune Defic Syndr 65:535–541

Ryscavage P, Anderson EJ, Sutton SH, Reddy S, Taiwo B (2011) Clinical outcomes of adolescents and young adults in adult HIV care. J Acquir Immune Defic Syndr 58:193–197

Salami Olawale KA, Wamalwa D, Obimbo E, Musiime V, Nyandiko W, Ayaya S, Jospeh M, Waweru M, Ouattara G, Odhiambo S, Kyomuhendo F, Simon F, Lee J, Omollo R, Egondi T, Stallaert JF, Oyaro P, Bukusi E, Mwanga J, Wasumma M, Andrieux-Meyer I, Lallemant Marc on behalf of the LIVING Study Team (2017) Prospective study of Lopinavir based ART for HIV infected ChildreN Globally (LIVING study): interim 48-week effectiveness and safety results. In: International conference on AIDS and STIs in Africa, Abidjan, Cote d'Ivoire

Salem AH, Fletcher CV, Brundage RC (2014) Pharmacometric characterization of efavirenz developmental pharmacokinetics and pharmacogenetics in HIV-infected children. Antimicrob Agents Chemother 58:136–143

Services DoHaH (2019) Fact sheets HIV and specific populations

Simon A, Warszawski J, Kariyawasam D et al (2011) Association of prenatal and postnatal exposure to lopinavir-ritonavir and adrenal dysfunction among uninfected infants of HIV-infected mothers. JAMA 306:70–78

Slogrove AL, Goetghebuer T, Cotton MF, Singer J, Bettinger JA (2016) Pattern of infectious morbidity in HIV-exposed uninfected infants and children. Front Immunol 7:164

Spaulding AB, Yu Q, Civitello L et al (2016) Neurologic outcomes in HIV-exposed/uninfected infants exposed to antiretroviral drugs during pregnancy in Latin America and the Caribbean. AIDS Res Hum Retrovir 32:349–356

Sperling RS, Shapiro DE, Coombs RW et al (1996) Maternal viral load, zidovudine treatment, and the risk of transmission of human immunodeficiency virus type 1 from mother to infant. Pediatric AIDS Clinical Trials Group Protocol 076 Study Group. N Engl J Med 335:1621–1629

Squires K, Lazzarin A, Gatell JM et al (2004) Comparison of once-daily atazanavir with efavirenz, each in combination with fixed-dose zidovudine and lamivudine, as initial therapy for patients infected with HIV. J Acquir Immune Defic Syndr 36:1011–1019

Strehlau R, Donati AP, Arce PM et al (2015) PRINCE-1: safety and efficacy of atazanavir powder and ritonavir liquid in HIV-1-infected antiretroviral-naive and -experienced infants and children aged >/=3 months to <6 years. J Int AIDS Soc 18:19467

Szubert AJ, Prendergast AJ, Spyer MJ et al (2017) Virological response and resistance among HIV-infected children receiving long-term antiretroviral therapy without virological monitoring in Uganda and Zimbabwe: observational analyses within the randomised ARROW trial. PLoS Med 14:e1002432

Tremoulet AH, Capparelli EV, Patel P et al (2007) Population pharmacokinetics of lamivudine in human immunodeficiency virus-exposed and -infected infants. Antimicrob Agents Chemother 51:4297–4302

UNAIDS (2016) UNAIDS: on the fast track to an AIDS free generation

UNAIDS (2018) Global HIV and AIDS statistics – 2018 fact sheet

UNICEF (2016) A progress report: ALL IN to end the adolescent aids epidemic. UNICEF, New York

UNICEF (2018) UNICEF HIV report 2018

Updated Recommendations on first-line and second-line antiretroviral regimens and post-exposure prophylaxis and recommendations on early infant diagnosis of HIV (2018). http://apps.who.int/iris/bitstream/handle/10665/273632/WHO-CDS-HIV-18.18-eng.pdf?ua=1. Accessed 12 Oct 2018

US National Library of Medicine (2018) Prospective study of lopinavir based ART for HIV infected children globally (LIVING Study) (LIVING)

Van de Perre P, Rubbo PA, Viljoen J et al (2012) HIV-1 reservoirs in breast milk and challenges to elimination of breast-feeding transmission of HIV-1. Sci Transl Med 4:143sr3

Van Dyke RB, Chadwick EG, Hazra R, Williams PL, Seage GR 3rd (2016) The PHACS SMARTT study: assessment of the safety of in utero exposure to antiretroviral drugs. Front Immunol 7:199

Violari A, Cotton MF, Gibb DM et al (2008) Early antiretroviral therapy and mortality among HIV-infected infants. N Engl J Med 359:2233–2244

Violari A, Lindsey JC, Hughes MD et al (2012) Nevirapine versus ritonavir-boosted lopinavir for HIV-infected children. N Engl J Med 366:2380–2389

Vreeman RC, Scanlon ML, McHenry MS, Nyandiko WM (2015) The physical and psychological effects of HIV infection and its treatment on perinatally HIV-infected children. J Int AIDS Soc 18:20258

West N, Schwartz S, Mudavanhu M et al (2019) Mental health in South African adolescents living with HIV. AIDS Care 31:117–124

World Health Organization (2010) Principles and recommendations for infant feeding in the context of HIV and a summary of evidence. WHO, Geneva

World Health Organization (2013) Consolidated guidelines on the use of antiretroviral drugs for treating and preventing HIV infection. WHO, Geneva

World Health Organization (2016) Consolidated guidelines on the use of antiretroviral drugs for treatment and preventing HIV infection: recommendations for a public health approach. WHO, Geneva

World Health Organization (2018a) Updated recommendations on first-line and second-line antiretroviral regimens and post-exposure prophylaxis and recommendations on early infant diagnosis of HIV

World Health Organization (2018b) Toolkit for research and development of paediatric antiretroviral drugs and formulations
World Health Organization (2019) Application for inclusion of lopinavir/ritonavir oral granules (LPV/r) formulation on WHO model list of essential medicines for children
Worm SW, Sabin C, Weber R et al (2010) Risk of myocardial infarction in patients with HIV infection exposed to specific individual antiretroviral drugs from the 3 major drug classes: the data collection on adverse events of anti-HIV drugs (D:A:D) study. J Infect Dis 201:318–330
Zanoni BC, Mayer KH (2014) The adolescent and young adult HIV cascade of care in the United States: exaggerated health disparities. AIDS Patient Care STDs 28:128–135
Zash R, Makhema J, Shapiro RL (2018) Neural-tube defects with dolutegravir treatment from the time of conception. N Engl J Med 379:979–981

Clinical Pharmacology and Pharmacometrics to Better Understand Physiological Changes During Pregnancy and Neonatal Life

Tamara van Donge, Katrina Evers, Gilbert Koch, John van den Anker, and Marc Pfister

Contents

Abstract

Pregnant women, fetuses, and newborns are particularly vulnerable patient populations. During pregnancy, the body is subject to physiological changes that

T. van Donge (✉) · K. Evers · G. Koch
Pediatric Pharmacology and Pharmacometrics, University of Basel Children's Hospital, Basel, Switzerland
e-mail: tamara.vandonge@ukbb.ch

J. van den Anker
Pediatric Pharmacology and Pharmacometrics, University of Basel Children's Hospital, Basel, Switzerland

Intensive Care and Department of Pediatric Surgery, Erasmus MC-Sophia Children's Hospital, Rotterdam, The Netherlands

Division of Clinical Pharmacology, Children's National Health System, Washington, DC, USA

M. Pfister
Pediatric Pharmacology and Pharmacometrics, University of Basel Children's Hospital, Basel, Switzerland

Certara LP, Princeton, NJ, USA

W. Kiess et al. (eds.), *Pediatric Pharmacotherapy*,
Handbook of Experimental Pharmacology 261, https://doi.org/10.1007/164_2019_210

influence the pharmacokinetics and pharmacodynamics of drugs. Inappropriate dosing in pregnant women can result in sub-therapeutic or toxic effects, putting not only the pregnant woman but also her fetus at risk. During neonatal life, maturation processes also affect pharmacokinetics and pharmacodynamics of drugs. Inappropriate dosing in newborns leads not only to short-term complications but can also have a negative impact on the long-term development of infants and children. For these reasons, it is crucial to characterize physiological changes in pregnant women, describe placental transfer kinetics of drugs, and describe physiological changes related to the transition from intrauterine to extra-uterine life and maturation processes in preterm and term neonates. Quantitative pharmacological approaches such as pharmacometric and physiologically-based modeling and model-based simulations can be useful to better understand and predict such physiological changes and their effects on drug exposure and response. This review article (1) gives an overview of physiological changes in pregnant women, their fetuses, and (pre)term neonates, (2) presents case studies to illustrate applications of new modeling and simulation approaches, and (3) discusses challenges and opportunities in optimizing and personalizing treatments during pregnancy and neonatal life.

Keywords

Drug exposure · Fetus · Newborn · Pediatric pharmacology · Pharmacometrics · Pregnancy

1 Introduction

The core goal of pediatric clinical pharmacology is to improve care through effective and safe use of drugs in fetuses, neonates, infants, children, and adolescents. Studying the effectiveness and safety of drugs in pregnant women and children by conducting clinical trials is less straightforward as compared to performing these in adults due to practical and ethical concerns. This review will present an overview of the physiological changes in pregnant women, their fetuses, and (pre)term neonates with the integration of pharmacometrics in pediatric clinical pharmacology resulting in the development of evidence-based pharmacotherapy during pregnancy and neonatal life.

Physiological changes during pregnancy can influence the disposition of various drugs. Inappropriate dosing in pregnant women can result in sub-therapeutic or even toxic effects, putting not only the pregnant woman but also her fetus at risk (Moore et al. 2002). After birth, the newborn is as well subject to rapid physiological changes related to the transition from intrauterine to extrauterine life and maturational processes affecting the pharmacokinetics and pharmacodynamics of administered drugs (Kearns et al. 2003). Incorrect dosing in neonates results not only in short-term complications but can also have a negative impact on the long-term development of infants and children (Allegaert and Anker 2015). As a consequence, it is very important to characterize these physiological changes in pregnant women, investigate the placental transfer of drugs, and describe the physiological changes and corresponding consequences related to maturation in preterm and term newborns.

Currently, there are various approaches to assess these challenges, such as pharmacometric and physiologically-based modeling together with model-based simulations, which can help us characterize relevant physiological changes and their effects on drug exposure and response during pregnancy and neonatal life. Although there are still challenges to overcome, such as the implementation of these approaches in daily clinical practice, a lot of progress has been made.

2 Understanding the Impact of Physiological Changes on Pharmacotherapy During Pregnancy and Neonatal Life

In the next paragraphs, we will highlight the influence of physiological changes on the pharmacotherapy for the pregnant woman and her unborn fetus and for the newborn during the neonatal period (first 28 days of life).

2.1 Pregnancy and Pharmacotherapy: Something to Worry About?

During pregnancy, women take a variety of medications (either prescribed or over the counter) which can have negative impacts on the pregnant woman and her unborn child. Antenatal medication use during pregnancy has increased over the last three decades (Mitchell et al. 2011). On the other hand, recent study showed that women of child-bearing age in Switzerland have high general health awareness, and when they become pregnant, most of them refrain from using pain killers (Bornhauser et al. 2017). Surveys about their medication use have illustrated that the percentage of pregnant women who took pain killers once a week to several times a week was about half of that in nonpregnant women (25% vs 50%). Of note, in 67% of pregnant women using pain killers, these were prescribed by a physician, as compared to 35% in nonpregnant women (Bornhauser et al. 2017).

Pregnancy affects various physiological processes and alters the body composition of the pregnant woman. These changes can affect the pharmacokinetics of drugs and should therefore be taken into account when prescribing drugs and may even require dosing adjustments to ensure appropriate treatment (Dallmann et al. 2018a). A recent review investigated the alterations in pharmacokinetics during pregnancy studying 121 different medications based on 198 studies in pregnant women (Pariente et al. 2016). Enhanced elimination, resulting in decreased drug exposure at a given dose, was one of the main conclusions. Alterations in drug absorption (k_a)

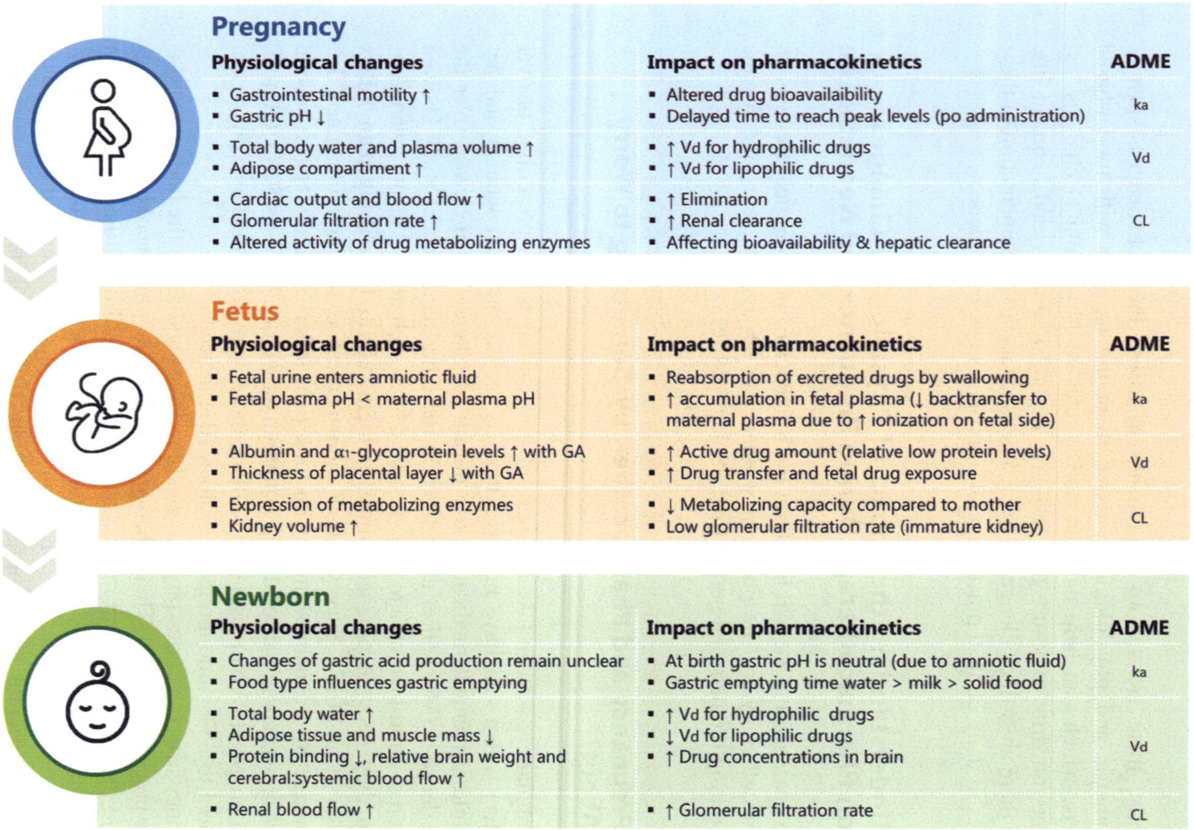

Fig. 1 Schematic overview representing physiological changes and their corresponding impact on pharmacokinetics in pregnant women, their fetus, and newborns. Data retrieved from literature (Anderson 2005; Bonner et al. 2015; Hines 2008; Kearns et al. 2003; Koren 1997; Morton and Brodsky 2016; Pariente et al. 2016; van den Anker et al. 2018; Zhang et al. 2017; Zhang and Unadkat 2017). *ADME* absorption, distribution, metabolism, and excretion, k_a absorption rate, V_d volume of distribution, *CL* clearance, *GA* gestational age

are caused by altered bioavailability and delayed time to reach peak levels after oral administration, which are due to decreased gastrointestinal motility and increased gastric pH (Fig. 1) (Loebstein et al. 1997). For hydrophilic drugs, the volume of distribution (V_d) is increased because of increased total body water and plasma volume, whereas V_d for hydrophobic drugs is increased because of a larger fat compartment. Clearance (CL) of drugs is influenced by many processes such as altered glomerular filtration rate and an adjusted cardiac output (Pariente et al. 2016). Furthermore, diminished plasma albumin concentrations during pregnancy may increase free, and therefore active, drug concentrations associated with a potential increase in drug activity, depending on the physiochemical characteristics of a given drug (Pariente et al. 2016). Unfortunately, for a majority of drugs used during pregnancy, information regarding pharmacokinetic (PK) changes and related effects on safety and efficacy is still lacking.

Physiology-based pharmacokinetics (PBPK) models are increasingly utilized to characterize changes in pharmacokinetics during pregnancy (Dallmann et al. 2018a). In such mechanistic models, physiological parameters (e.g. organ volumes, glomerular filtration rate) are combined with drug-specific parameters (e.g. lipophilicity, molecular mass), and this ensures the assessment of valuable insights into the PK profiles of drugs in this specific population (Hartmanshenn et al. 2016). The prediction of drug exposure could contribute to the adjustment of dosing regimen for drugs prescribed in pregnant women. PBPK modeling can also be deployed to understand effects of concomitantly interacting drugs, which is often the case for HIV-infected women because of their combination antiretroviral therapy. The following example elegantly shows the practical utility of PBPK modeling in the pregnant population to ensure an optimal and practical dose. A recently developed PBPK model predicted a decrease in darunavir/ritonavir exposure and therefore efficacy during pregnancy when taking 800/100 mg once daily. When the dosing regimen was adjusted to 600/100 mg twice daily, the lack in exposure was compensated (Colbers et al. 2016; Ke et al. 2018).

In addition to acquire valuable insights in the pharmacokinetics and pharmacodynamics of drugs during pregnancy, it is of equal importance to understand the physiology of pregnancy-related diseases, for example, with the aid of biomarkers. New biomarkers can help to understand the cause, diagnosis, progression, and treatment of a disease (Mayeux 2004). Hypertensive disorders such as preeclampsia are a major contributor to maternal mortality worldwide (Steegers et al. 2010; Widmer et al. 2015). A lot of research has been done in the field of translational biomarkers which consequently has improved our understanding of preeclampsia and helped us better define the diagnosis of this pregnancy-related disease (Karumanchi 2016). Preeclampsia is diagnosed when there is a combination of increased proteinuria ($\geq$300 mg in 24 h) and pregnancy-induced hypertension (diastolic blood pressure $\geq$90 mmHg) (Evers et al. 2018; Steegers et al. 2010). Various placental anti-angiogenic markers have been investigated, such as soluble endoglin (sEng) and soluble fms-like tyrosine kinase 1 (sFlt-1) that both can cause endothelial dysfunction (Maynard and Karumanchi 2011; Venkatesha et al. 2006). Levels of sEng are correlated with disease severity in preeclamptic pregnant women, together with an increase in sFlt-1 levels (Venkatesha et al. 2006). Furthermore, women suffering from preeclampsia showed decreased levels of free (unbound) serum placental growth factor (PIGF) and free vascular endothelial growth factor (VEGF) before developing clinical signs (Levine et al. 2004). Maternal serum neutrophil gelatinase-associated lipocalin (NGAL) levels are significantly increased in preeclamptic women, and the renal marker cystatin C measured at the end of the third trimester is a predictor of preeclampsia (Artunc-Ulkumen et al. 2015; Risch et al. 2017). In a longitudinal prospective study, it was found that neurofilament light (NfL) concentrations were higher in women with preeclampsia as compared to women who do not develop preeclampsia. Elevated levels of NfL are increasingly recognized as a measure of acute or chronic neuroaxonal damage, and NfL can be used as a predictive value for preeclampsia, especially in women older than 36 years (Evers et al. 2018). New attempts aim at combining biochemical with biophysical markers for a more precise diagnosis of preeclampsia (Kumer et al. 2018). Despite the numerous results, it is important to note that the biomarkers that are listed are not specific for preeclampsia and are also used outside of pregnancy. It is therefore still necessary to search for specific markers and interventions (Huppertz 2018).

2.2 Drug Exposure in the Fetus: Does the Placenta Act as a Barrier?

Contrary to what was assumed decades ago, the placenta does unfortunately not serve as a barrier that prevents drugs from reaching the fetus (Etwel et al. 2014). Drug exposure of the pregnant woman can have an impact on the unborn child. Therapeutic drugs are prescribed to prevent or treat conditions that develop during pregnancy and to guarantee the health of the woman, although in some cases, the target of the treatment is the fetus, as is the case with the prevention of HIV transmission (Kesho Bora Study Group 2011). Regardless whether the fetus is the actual target of pharmacological therapy, the fetus is exposed to almost every drug taken by the pregnant woman. It needs no clarification that the ability to evaluate the fetal exposure to drugs, either their efficacy but most importantly, their risk of toxicity, is imperative.

As it is currently impossible to study drug exposure prior to birth and even at the time of birth, the assessment of fetal exposure to drugs is limited to a single measurement of umbilical cord plasma concentration, which unfortunately does not reflect fetal drug exposure (Zhang et al. 2017). A recent review showed that fetal serum albumin concentrations, in contrast to serum albumin concentrations of pregnant woman, increase with advancing gestational age (GA), although they remain relatively low compared to adult values (Zhang et al. 2017). Fetal serum albumin levels reach 22.1 g/L at week 20 of gestation and 38.3 g/L at week 40 of gestation, a 1.73-fold increase (Zhang et al. 2017). Alpha$_1$-glycoprotein, one of the major drug-binding proteins, was increased from 0.068 g/L at 20 weeks of gestation to 0.23 g/L at 40 weeks of gestation. In addition, the placental transfer layer is the thinnest just before birth, reducing the expression of certain efflux transporters such as P-glycoprotein. Therefore, the transfer of drugs and the fetal exposure may be maximal at term, as compared to earlier gestational ages (Fig. 1) (Etwel et al. 2014). A 29.4-fold increase in the large intestinal volume between 20 and 40 weeks of gestation has been demonstrated (Zhang et al. 2017). Additionally, it has been shown that hepatic organogenesis begins from the fetal mesoderm and endoderm during the fourth week of gestation and transcription of hepatic enzymes involved in drug metabolism has been detected at 8–10 weeks of gestation (Hines 2008). Focusing on the volume of the kidney in a period between 20 and 40 weeks of gestation, the volume increased from 3.39 to 31.21 mL (Zhang et al. 2017). During pregnancy, the homeostasis is assigned to the placenta, and the main task of the fetal kidney is the excretion of urine (hypotonic) as a major component of the amniotic fluid. This might explain why the glomerular filtration rate in the fetus is low, even at the end of gestation (Fig. 1) (Saint-Faust et al. 2014).

Because of ethical and practical constraints of performing clinical trials in this subpopulation, PBPK modeling could provide mechanistic understanding of the fetal drug exposure and might be able to predict the drug exposure during the entire pregnancy until birth. Several research groups have tried to quantify the placental drug transfer to the fetus. Although many of the approaches are substance-specific and therefore cannot be used for other compounds, these are valuable contributions (Abduljalil et al. 2018; Schalkwijk et al. 2018; Zhang et al. 2017; Zhang and Unadkat 2017). We expect that in the near future, more knowledge will be gained in fetal pharmacotherapy and that PBPK modeling will contribute to this.

A recent publication provided understanding on the exposure of ceftazidime in both the pregnant woman and the fetus by the development of a population PK model (Dallmann et al. 2018b). Ceftazidime has been frequently used in pregnant women to treat intrauterine or urinary tract infections. This antibiotic is hydrophilic causing it to mainly distribute into tissues with high water content (e.g. kidneys), and it is purely eliminated by glomerular filtration. Since ceftazidime crosses the placenta, concentrations in the plasma of the pregnant woman and in amniotic fluid are similar. This PK model has provided insights on the pharmacokinetics of ceftazidime in pregnant women and newborns, low drug clearance during the first days of life of newborns is most likely due to the reduced number of perfused glomeruli and reduced renal blood flow (Dallmann et al. 2018b).

Performing clinical trials in newborns is especially cumbersome, not only because of ethical considerations but also due to practical challenges such as limited amount of blood and the corresponding inability to collect multiple samples. Currently, biomarkers to assess fetal drug exposure gain attention; examples are neonatal hair tests or placental corticotrophin-releasing hormone (CRH) levels (Koren et al. 2008; Manokhina et al. 2017; Stout et al. 2015). The ability to diagnose the exposure during pregnancy after birth by neonatal hair has evolved. In neonates, hair grows during the last trimester of pregnancy. A positive neonatal hair test (for cocaine, opioids, cannabinoids, etc.) can reflect fetal exposure, even long after the pregnant woman became aware of her pregnancy, making hair an easily available carrier for biomarkers of maternal drug dependence (Etwel et al. 2014; Koren et al. 2008). Assessing the CRH levels during the third trimester of pregnancy can provide insights on the risk of obesity later in life. Elevated placental CRF has been shown to be associated with catch-up growth, which has been shown to be a prognostic factor for increased metabolic activity and, therefore, obesity (Stout et al. 2015).

2.3 Neonatal Life and Pharmacotherapy: Do We Need New Dosing Strategies?

From a pharmacological point of view, neonates are considered as a separate subpopulation, different from small children and adults (Kearns et al. 2003). In order to provide evidence-based and tailored dosing recommendations, it is clear that we first need to have a clear understanding of the physiological changes that occur during the neonatal period.

Levels of gastric pH after birth are unclear because of contradicting information (Kearns et al. 2003; Koren 1997; van den Anker et al. 2018). An acidic gastric pH has been observed in preterm neonates, but oral ingestion of acid-buffering milk might result in an increase in gastric pH values. Gastric emptying is an important factor for intestinal drug absorption and appears not to be driven by age, but by type of food intake (Bonner et al. 2015). The extracellular and total body water compartments differ vastly between newborns, infants, children, adolescents, and adults (Kearns et al. 2003; Ku and Smith 2014). This causes water-soluble drugs (e.g. aminoglycosides) to distribute into a larger physiological (extracellular) space in neonates; in order to reach effective drug exposure, they require higher dosages (Fig. 1). The distribution of drugs in the central nervous system is different in newborns versus children and adults. Due to decreased protein binding, a higher ratio of cerebral to systemic blood flow, and a higher relative brain weight, the concentrations in brain are likely to be higher in newborns (Ku and Smith 2014; Seyberth and Kauffman 2011). Drug-metabolizing enzymes play an important role in the transformation of xenobiotics. Overall, three different developmental trajectories can be observed according to the ontogeny of drug-metabolizing enzymes (Hines 2008). During gestation, group 1 of these drug-metabolizing enzymes become highly active but are only expressed at low levels after birth (e.g. CYP3A7). The second group consists of enzymes which are expressed at constant levels during gestation and after birth. In the last group, the enzymes are present which expression is observed within the first 2 years of life (Hines 2008). The renal clearance increases with advancing gestational age, postnatal age, and body weight (Kearns et al. 2003). The creatinine clearance remains the best measurement of the assessment of GFR in this population, although it is widely known that assessment of serum creatinine levels during the first days after birth is rather a reflection of the mother's renal function than that of the newborn, since creatinine is easily transferred across the placenta (Kastl 2017). At birth, which is known to be an accelerator for postnatal maturation of renal function, the vascular resistance decreases, and an increase in cardiac output and renal blood flow is observed, which will alter the GFR (Saint-Faust et al. 2014; Sulemanji and Vakili 2013). The renal tubules are not yet structurally or functionally mature at birth and lead to an activity that is approximately 20% of the adult value. By 7–8 months the adult tubular secretion values will be attained (Hines 2008). Although creatinine clearance is currently the best way to determine the renal function, it is probably not the most accurate method to use in newborns. A new renal biomarker such as cystatin C, a protein which is freely filtered by the glomerulus, may reflect the GFR more closely in preterm infants (Saint-Faust et al. 2014). Beta-trace protein is another possible renal marker which does not cross the placental barrier and is subject to increased attention as new indicator of GFR and renal function (Kastl 2017; Saint-Faust et al. 2014).

Integrating pharmacological expertise combined with clinical knowledge on physiological changes provides a strong foundation for innovative and new evidence-based dosing recommendations which are highly necessary for neonates as they are being considered the last therapeutic orphans.

If born prematurely, apnea is often observed due to immaturity of the central nervous system and is primarily treated with caffeine. Although this drug is commonly used across many neonatal intensive care units by a standard dosing regimen consisting of a loading dose (20 mg/kg) followed by a maintenance dose (5 mg/kg/day), not much is known about the effect of the increasing caffeine clearance after birth. Recent research has shown that a higher maintenance dose is required in preterm neonates with apnea to maintain caffeine concentrations above 15 mg/L after the first week of life (Koch et al. 2017). Gentamicin, a widely used antibiotic where the pharmacokinetic understanding has increased over the past years, can be used as another illustration. Despite the increased knowledge, this has resulted in considerable variability in dosing regimen recommendations with respect to dose, dosing interval, and patient characteristics. Model-based simulations for this antibiotic treatment in neonates illustrated that in order to attain an effective peak concentration of 10 mg/L, a dose of 7.5 mg/kg should be administered using an extended dosing interval based on gestational and postnatal age to reduce the risk of renal toxicity (van Donge et al. 2018).

During the first days after birth, newborns will lose body fluids and fat resulting in an initial weight loss. When this weight loss becomes excessive (>10% of birth weight), the risk for serious clinical complications increases (Wilbaux et al. 2016). The use of weight monographs belongs to the current practice, and if a newborn loses 5% of its body weight during the first day of life, this is seen as a critical sign. In 2016, a semi-mechanistic model characterized the weight changes in healthy neonates and quantified key factors (maternal and neonatal) influencing individual weight profiles during the first 7 days of life. It was illustrated that birth weight increases more with advancing gestational age and that boys weigh more than girls at birth. In addition, it was showed that weight gain is influenced by gestational age and that birth weight increases with the maternal age (Wilbaux et al. 2016).

3 Optimize and Personalize Pharmacotherapy During Pregnancy and Neonatal Life

In this new era which is highlighted by technology and innovative approaches, it should not be the case that pregnant women and their newborns are still dependent on off-label drug use. By incorporating knowledge on the physiological changes that happen during these life-changing periods, we can assess the influence on pharmacokinetic profiles and adjust dosing recommendations, ensuring a safe and effective treatment.

Only in the rare circumstance that there is similarity between adults and infants in disease, the mechanism of action of the drug, and the PK/PD relationships, it is justified and allowed to extrapolate the pediatric dose from adult dosages (Manolis and Pons 2009). Otherwise it is required to address all these components before extrapolating pediatric dose from adult standard of care.

Modeling and simulation can not only be applied in order to gain insights in the PK of drugs in this special population; it can also support and optimize the design of pediatric studies. When designing a new pediatric pharmacokinetic/pharmacodynamic study, it is important to know how many samples per patient are required, what the best sampling times are, and how many patients are needed to obtain a statistically powered estimation of the PK/PD parameters. After obtaining clinical data, the first step for PK/PD model-based guidance is to select the appropriate target in the population of interest, such as a desired plasma concentration, target exposure (area under the curve, AUC), time above target exposure, or other measure matrices. Thereafter, one can define the dosage regimen to best achieve this target while taking into account various factors which influence the disposition of the drug (demographic characteristics such as gestational age, weight, or postnatal age).

Development of pregnancy PBPK models makes it possible to assess drug exposure in all trimesters and investigate multiple dosing strategies. Although over the recent years a lot of progress is made with pregnancy PBPK models, knowledge gaps still remain. An integrated fetomaternal PBPK model would be able to examine fetal drug therapy during pregnancy. In order to develop such a complex model, quantitative information on system-specific parameters need to be incorporated into the pregnancy PBPK model, and the characterization of the fetal system in terms of enzyme and transporter tissue abundance remains challenging (Dallmann et al. 2018a). In addition, obtaining data on fetal drug exposure for the evaluation of the fetal PBPK model continues to be cumbersome.

One of the greatest opportunities of using these novel technologies to optimize and personalize pharmacotherapy is at the same time one of the greatest challenges, that is to say, the integration of these research-based models in easily accessible software tools which can become part of daily clinical practice.

Neoweight is an example of such a user-friendly online prediction tool which can forecasts the individual weight changes during the first week of life, based on three weight measurements and standard characteristics of the newborn, and can be found at http://neoweight.mashframe.com (Wilbaux et al. 2016). We hope that in the near future, more validated, user-friendly tools will be developed and integrated in clinical practice. It is rather worrisome that these innovative and novel approaches are being developed in order to ensure safe and effective treatment for the patient but will never fulfill this goal because of problems with translation, implementation, and lack of easy accessibility.

Initiatives to build national and international collaborative networks to facilitate clinical trials and collection and sharing of data are necessary. The Swiss Research Network of Clinical Pediatric Centers (SwissPedNet) and the Swiss Research Center for Pediatric Pharmacology and Pharmacometrics (SwissPedPha) are examples of such national initiatives. In 2012, this research network of pediatric hospitals has been created and has the common goal to facilitate, coordinate, and conduct clinical trials in all pediatric disciplines. Another initiative is the Dutch Center for Pharmacotherapy for Children (NKFK) which aims to improve the quality and safety of pharmacotherapy in children and focuses on improving the provision of information about the use of drugs in children.

4 Conclusion

The characterization of physiological changes in pregnant women, the description of placental transfer kinetics of drugs, the identification of physiological changes related to the transition from intrauterine to extrauterine life, and the characterization of maturation processes in preterm and term neonates are essential in order to ensure safe and effective treatment in both the pregnant women and her fetus or newborn.

Once dosing recommendations based on new biomarkers, pharmacometric approaches, and/or PBPK predictions have been validated in clinical trials, results can be incorporated in clinical practice. Bedside decision support tools should be developed to facilitate optimizing and individualizing treatment strategies in vulnerable patient populations such as pregnant women and their fetuses and newborns. Quantitative pharmacology and pharmacometric approaches have the potential to further personalize and enhance patient care allowing safe and efficacious use of drugs during pregnancy and neonatal life.

Acknowledgment TvD, KE, GK, JvdA, and MP would like to thank the Eckenstein-Geigy Foundation in Basel, Switzerland, for their financial support.

References

Abduljalil K, Johnson TN, Rostami-Hodjegan A (2018) Fetal physiologically-based pharmacokinetic models: systems information on fetal biometry and gross composition. Clin Pharmacokinet 57:1149–1171

Allegaert K, Anker JN (2015) Adverse drug reactions in neonates and infants: a population-tailored approach is needed. Br J Clin Pharmacol 80:788–795

Anderson GD (2005) Pregnancy-induced changes in pharmacokinetics. Clin Pharmacokinet 44:989–1008

Artunc-Ulkumen B, Guvenc Y, Goker A, Gozukara C (2015) Relationship of neutrophil gelatinase-associated lipocalin (NGAL) and procalcitonin levels with the presence and severity of the preeclampsia. J Matern Fetal Neonatal Med 28:1895–1900. https://doi.org/10.3109/14767058.2014.972926

Bonner JJ, Vajjah P, Abduljalil K, Jamei M, Rostami-Hodjegan A, Tucker GT, Johnson TN (2015) Does age affect gastric emptying time? A model-based meta-analysis of data from premature neonates through to adults. Biopharm Drug Dispos 36:245–257

Bornhauser C, Quack KL, Seifert B, Simões-Wüst AP (2017) Diet, medication use and drug intake during pregnancy: data from the consecutive Swiss Health Surveys of 2007 and 2012. Swiss Med Wkly 147:w14572

Colbers A, Greupink R, Litjens C, Burger D, Russel FG (2016) Physiologically based modelling of darunavir/ritonavir pharmacokinetics during pregnancy. Clin Pharmacokinet 55:381–396

Dallmann A, Pfister M, van den Anker J, Eissing T (2018a) Physiologically based pharmacokinetic modeling in pregnancy: a systematic review of published models. Clin Pharmacol Ther 104:1110–1124

Dallmann A, van den Anker J, Pfister M, Koch G (2018b) Characterization of maternal and neonatal pharmacokinetic behavior of ceftazidime. J Clin Pharmacol 59:74–82

Etwel F, Hutson JR, Madadi P, Gareri J, Koren G (2014) Fetal and perinatal exposure to drugs and chemicals: novel biomarkers of risk. Annu Rev Pharmacol Toxicol 54:295–315

Evers KS et al (2018) Neurofilament as neuronal injury blood marker in preeclampsia. Hypertension 117:10314

Hartmanshenn C, Scherholz M, Androulakis IP (2016) Physiologically-based pharmacokinetic models: approaches for enabling personalized medicine. J Pharmacokinet Pharmacodyn 43:481–504. https://doi.org/10.1007/s10928-016-9492-y

Hines RN (2008) The ontogeny of drug metabolism enzymes and implications for adverse drug events. Pharmacol Ther 118:250–267

Huppertz B (2018) An updated view on the origin and use of angiogenic biomarkers for preeclampsia. Expert Rev Mol Diagn:1–9. https://doi.org/10.1080/14737159.2018.1546579

Karumanchi SA (2016) Angiogenic factors in preeclampsia: from diagnosis to therapy. Hypertension 67:1072–1079. https://doi.org/10.1161/HYPERTENSIONAHA.116.06421

Kastl JT (2017) Renal function in the fetus and neonate–the creatinine enigma. In: Seminars in fetal and neonatal medicine, vol 2. Elsevier, Amsterdam, pp 83–89

Ke AB, Greupink R, Abduljalil K (2018) Drug dosing in pregnant women: challenges and opportunities in using physiologically based pharmacokinetic modeling and simulations. CPT Pharmacometrics Syst Pharmacol 7:103–110

Kearns GL, Abdel-Rahman SM, Alander SW, Blowey DL, Leeder JS, Kauffman RE (2003) Developmental pharmacology—drug disposition, action, and therapy in infants and children. N Engl J Med 349:1157–1167

Kesho Bora Study Group (2011) Triple antiretroviral compared with zidovudine and single-dose nevirapine prophylaxis during pregnancy and breastfeeding for prevention of mother-to-child transmission of HIV-1 (Kesho Bora study): a randomised controlled trial. Lancet Infect Dis 11:171–180

Koch G, Datta AN, Jost K, Schulzke SM, van den Anker J, Pfister M (2017) Caffeine citrate dosing adjustments to assure stable caffeine concentrations in preterm neonates. J Pediatr 191:50–56.e51

Koren G (1997) Therapeutic drug monitoring principles in the neonate. Clin Chem 43:222–227

Koren G, Hutson J, Gareri J (2008) Novel methods for the detection of drug and alcohol exposure during pregnancy: implications for maternal and child health. Clin Pharmacol Ther 83:631–634

Ku LC, Smith PB (2014) Dosing in neonates: special considerations in physiology and trial design. Pediatr Res 77:2

Kumer K, Premru-Srsen T, Fabjan-Vodusek V, Tul N, Fabjan T, Osredkar J (2018) Peripheral arterial tonometry and angiogenic biomarkers in preeclampsia. Hypertens Pregnancy 37:197–203. https://doi.org/10.1080/10641955.2018.1524478

Levine RJ et al (2004) Circulating angiogenic factors and the risk of preeclampsia. N Engl J Med 350:672–683. https://doi.org/10.1056/NEJMoa031884
Loebstein R, Lalkin A, Koren G (1997) Pharmacokinetic changes during pregnancy and their clinical relevance. Clin Pharmacokinet 33:328–343
Manokhina I, Del Gobbo GF, Konwar C, Wilson SL, Robinson WP (2017) Review: placental biomarkers for assessing fetal health. Hum Mol Genet 26:R237–R245
Manolis E, Pons G (2009) Proposals for model-based paediatric medicinal development within the current European Union regulatory framework. Br J Clin Pharmacol 68:493–501
Mayeux R (2004) Biomarkers: potential uses and limitations. NeuroRx 1:182–188
Maynard SE, Karumanchi SA (2011) Angiogenic factors and preeclampsia. Semin Nephrol 31:33–46. https://doi.org/10.1016/j.semnephrol.2010.10.004
Mitchell AA, Gilboa SM, Werler MM, Kelley KE, Louik C, Hernández-Díaz S, Study NBDP (2011) Medication use during pregnancy, with particular focus on prescription drugs: 1976-2008. Am J Obstet Gynecol 205:51. e51–51. e58
Moore TJ, Weiss SR, Kaplan S, Blaisdell CJ (2002) Reported adverse drug events in infants and children under 2 years of age. Pediatrics 110:e53–e53
Morton SU, Brodsky D (2016) Fetal physiology and the transition to extrauterine life. Clin Perinatol 43:395–407
Pariente G, Leibson T, Carls A, Adams-Webber T, Ito S, Koren G (2016) Pregnancy-associated changes in pharmacokinetics: a systematic review. PLoS Med 13:e1002160
Risch M et al (2017) High first-trimester maternal blood cystatin C levels despite normal serum creatinine predict pre-eclampsia in singleton pregnancies. Scand J Clin Lab Invest 77:634–643. https://doi.org/10.1080/00365513.2017.1393692
Saint-Faust M, Boubred F, Simeoni U (2014) Renal development and neonatal adaptation. Am J Perinatol 31:773–780
Schalkwijk S, Buaben AO, Freriksen JJ, Colbers AP, Burger DM, Greupink R, Russel FG (2018) Prediction of fetal darunavir exposure by integrating human ex-vivo placental transfer and physiologically based pharmacokinetic modeling. Clin Pharmacokinet 57:705–716
Seyberth HW, Kauffman RE (2011) Basics and dynamics of neonatal and pediatric pharmacology. In: Pediatric clinical pharmacology. Springer, Berlin, pp 3–49
Steegers EA, Von Dadelszen P, Duvekot JJ, Pijnenborg R (2010) Pre-eclampsia. Lancet 376:631–644
Stout SA, Espel EV, Sandman CA, Glynn LM, Davis EP (2015) Fetal programming of children's obesity risk. Psychoneuroendocrinology 53:29–39
Sulemanji M, Vakili K (2013) Neonatal renal physiology. In: Seminars in pediatric surgery, vol 4. Elsevier, Amsterdam, pp 195–198
van den Anker J, Reed MD, Allegaert K, Kearns GL (2018) Developmental changes in pharmacokinetics and pharmacodynamics. J Clin Pharmacol 58:S10–S25
van Donge T, Pfister M, Bielicki J, Csajka C, Rodieux F, van den Anker J, Fuchs A (2018) Quantitative analysis of gentamicin exposure in neonates and infants calls into question its current dosing recommendations. Antimicrob Agents Chemother 62:02004–02017
Venkatesha S et al (2006) Soluble endoglin contributes to the pathogenesis of preeclampsia. Nat Med 12:642–649. https://doi.org/10.1038/nm1429
Widmer M et al (2015) Accuracy of angiogenic biomarkers at $\leq$20 weeks' gestation in predicting the risk of pre-eclampsia: a WHO multicentre study. Pregnancy Hypertens 5:330–338
Wilbaux M, Kasser S, Wellmann S, Lapaire O, Van Den Anker JN, Pfister M (2016) Characterizing and forecasting individual weight changes in term neonates. J Pediatr 173:101–107. e110
Zhang Z, Unadkat JD (2017) Development of a novel maternal-fetal physiologically based pharmacokinetic model II: verification of the model for passive placental permeability drugs. Drug Metab Dispos 45:939–946
Zhang Z, Imperial MZ, Patilea-Vrana GI, Wedagedera J, Gaohua L, Unadkat JD (2017) Development of a novel maternal-fetal physiologically based pharmacokinetic model I: insights into factors that determine fetal drug exposure through simulations and sensitivity analyses. Drug Metab Dispos 45:920–938

Pediatric Pharmacotherapy: Anthelminthic Treatment

Jill E. Weatherhead

Contents

Abstract

Helminths, including nematodes, trematodes, and cestodes, are parasitic worms that infect approximately two billion people worldwide and cause significant morbidity particularly in children. Helminth-induced morbidity is associated with disease burden which typically is greatest in preschool and school-aged children. Preventive chemotherapy through mass drug administration programs has been instituted globally to reduce worm burden and morbidity in children through administration of anthelminthic therapy at regular intervals in helminth endemic areas. Despite these interventions, elimination of these infections remains elusive due to high rates of reinfection and concern for emerging anthelminthic resistance. Although children harbor the greatest burden of disease, minimal pharmacokinetic, safety, and tolerability data is available for young children, limiting their use. Novel anthelminthic therapies are critically needed

J. E. Weatherhead (✉)
Department of Pediatrics, Section of Tropical Medicine, Baylor College of Medicine, Houston, TX, USA

National School of Tropical Medicine, Baylor College of Medicine, Houston, TX, USA

Department of Medicine, Section of Infectious Diseases, Baylor College of Medicine, Houston, TX, USA
e-mail: weatherh@bcm.edu

W. Kiess et al. (eds.), *Pediatric Pharmacotherapy*,
Handbook of Experimental Pharmacology 261, https://doi.org/10.1007/164_2019_254

to combat helminth disease with particular attention paid toward medications that can be used in young children to reduce global helminth-induced morbidity.

Keywords
Anthelminthic vaccine · Anthelminthics · Cestodes · Global health · Helminths · Mass drug administration · Nematodes · Trematodes

1 Introduction

Helminths are multicellular parasitic worms found in subtropical and tropical regions globally and infect approximately two billion people worldwide, nearly 20% of the world's population (Pullan et al. 2014; Li et al. 2018). While these worm infections commonly occur in low-income and middle-income countries, there is significant burden of disease among vulnerable populations living in high-income countries as well, suggesting these worms are infections of poverty (Hotez 2016; Jourdan et al. 2018). Helminths include nematodes, cestodes, and trematodes, with the most prevalent organisms being hookworm (*Necator americanus*, *Ancylostoma duodenale*), roundworm (*Ascaris lumbricoides*), and whipworm (*Trichuris trichiura*), collectively referred to as soil-transmitted helminths (STH), along with schistosomiasis (*S. haematobium*, *S. mansoni*, *S. japonicum*, and *S. mekongi*). Children living in extreme poverty without access to clean water, sanitation, and hygiene (WASH) are at greatest risk of infection and carry the highest burden of disease (Weatherhead et al. 2017; Li et al. 2018). Due to the extensive geographic overlap of helminthic infections, children are commonly infected with more than one worm at a given time (Weatherhead and Hotez 2015).

Helminthic infections are associated with significant morbidity, measured in disability-adjusted life years (DALYS), particularly in young children harboring high burden of disease (Hotez et al. 2006; Weatherhead and Hotez 2015). In these children, morbidity can be severe leading to cognitive and growth development restriction as well as species-specific impairment based on the life cycle of the organism (Hotez et al. 2006; Weatherhead and Hotez 2015). Collectively, helminths cause over ten million DALYs annually, driven largely by the impact of STH, schistosomiasis, lymphatic filariasis, and onchocerciasis (GBD 2017; Li et al. 2018). Transmission of helminth infections in areas of extreme poverty is maintained by the lack of quality hygienic and sanitary conditions within the community perpetuating the life cycle (Weatherhead et al. 2017). Current public health strategies aim to reduce worm burden within the endemic community in order to reduce morbidity in children and ultimately interrupt transmission of infection. These strategies include extensive community public health campaigns and periodic, universal drug administration through mass drug administration (MDA) programs (Urbani and Albonico 2003).

2 Mass Drug Administration

Preventive chemotherapy is a public health strategy to control helminths by providing low-cost, single-dose anthelminthic therapies at regular intervals in order to reduce the burden of disease and helminth-induced morbidity within the community (Urbani and Albonico 2003; World Health Organization 2006). Preventive chemotherapy is administered to selected high-risk populations, irrespective of their infection status, through MDA programs targeting soil-transmitted helminths, schistosomiasis, filarial disease and onchocerciasis in areas of the world with the highest prevalence (Table 1).

Soil-transmitted helminths cause disease in nearly 900 million people worldwide and are associated with a total of 1.9 million DALYS largely secondary to the development of anemia, malnutrition, and cognitive and growth restrictions (Bethony et al. 2006; Weatherhead and Hotez 2015; GBD 2017; Li et al. 2018). Preventive chemotherapy with benzimidazoles (albendazole 400 mg as a single tablet or mebendazole 500 mg as single tablet, orally) is recommended by the World Health Organization for all young children (12–23 months old), preschool children (24–59 months old), school-aged children, and nonpregnant adolescent girls and nonpregnant women of reproductive age (15–59 years old) on an annual basis if baseline prevalence of STH is greater than 20% or biannual if baseline prevalence is greater than 50% within the community (World Health Organization 2017a). Of note children less than 24 months should receive a half-dose of albendazole, 200 mg as a single tablet, orally (World Health Organization 2017a).

Schistosomiasis remains a major public health threat, infecting nearly 120 million people globally and causing 1.4 million DALYs (GBD 2017; Li et al. 2018). Schistosomiasis eggs in the venous plexuses around either the gastrointestinal track or urogenital track causes inflammation that can lead to urogenital tract disease and bladder cancer (*S. haematobium*) or liver failure and portal hypertension (*S. mansoni*, *S. japonicum*) (Hotez et al. 2006). Administration of praziquantel, 40 mg/kg single dose, orally is recommended in all high-risk populations based on current World Health Organization guidelines. In communities with prevalence of schistosomiasis greater than 50%, praziquantel should be administered to all school-age children and high-risk adults annually. High-risk adults include pregnant and lactating women, groups with occupations involving contact with infested water but may also involve treatment of the entire community (World Health Organization 2013). In communities with disease prevalence more than 10% but less than 50%, school-aged children and adults should be treated once every 2 years (World Health Organization 2013). While in low-risk communities, prevalence of less than 10%, school aged children should be treated twice during their primary school (World Health Organization 2013).

Lymphatic filariasis, which includes *Wuchereria bancrofti*, *Brugia malayi*, and *Burgia timori*, infects over 65 million people globally and causes 1.4 million DALYs annually (GBD 2017; Li et al. 2018). The World Health Organization recommendation for lymphatic filariasis MDA programs remains complicated due to vast geographic overlap between lymphatic filariasis and other filarial disease

Table 1 Current mass drug administration recommendations based on disease prevalence and coinfection

Helminth	Mass drug administration recommendations	Additional information
Soil-transmitted helminths (World Health Organization 2017a)	– If prevalence of disease is greater than 50%, benzimidazole should be administered (either albendazole or mebendazole) biannually to high-risk populations – If prevalence of disease is between 20 and 50%, benzimidazole (either albendazole or mebendazole) should be administered annually to high-risk populations	– High-risk populations include children (12–23 months old), preschool children (24–59 months old), school-aged children and nonpregnant adolescent girls and nonpregnant women of reproductive age (15–59 years old) – Children less than 24 months should receive a half-dose of albendazole
Schistosomiasis (World Health Organization 2013)	– If prevalence of disease is greater than 50%, praziquantel should be administered to all school-aged children and high-risk adults annually – If prevalence of disease is more than 10% but less than 50%, school-aged children and adults should be treated once every 2 years – If prevalence of disease is less than 10%, school-aged children should be treated twice during their primary school	– High-risk adults include pregnant and lactating women, groups with occupations involving contact with infested water but may also involve treatment of the entire community
Lymphatic filariasis (World Health Organization 2017b)	– In countries without loiasis or onchocerciasis, diethylcarbamazine with albendazole and ivermectin should be administered annually for eligible populations – In countries co-endemic with onchocerciasis, annual administration of ivermectin plus albendazole – In areas co-endemic with loiasis, biannual administration of albendazole	– Eligible populations include the entire population in area where transmission occurs except pregnant women, children less than 2 years and severely ill – DEC is contraindicated in areas co-endemic for onchocerciasis
Onchocerciasis (World Health Organization 2016)	– Ivermectin administered to over 80% of the community at risk	

such *Loa loa* and *Onchocerca volvulus* restricting anthelminthic use. Despite these restrictions, MDA programs for lymphatic filariasis have transitioned from disease control to a disease elimination focus. To achieve this goal, in countries that are not co-endemic with loiasis or onchocerciasis and have not met the epidemiological thresholds of disease control, the World Health Organization suggests triple combination therapy, known as IDA, with diethylcarbamazine (6 mg/kg, single dose, orally), albendazole (400 mg, single dose, orally), and ivermectin (150–200 μg/kg, single dose, orally) in all eligible population living in at-risk communities. In-eligible community members for lymphatic filariasis MDA include pregnant women, children less than 2 years old and persons who are severely ill (World Health Organization 2017b). Alternative regimens are recommended in areas that are co-endemic with loiasis and onchocerciasis (Table 1).

Onchocerciasis, known as river blindness, is a skin and eye disease caused by the nematode *Onchocerca volvulus* affecting approximately 21 million people around the world and causing 1.3 million DALYS annually (GBD 2017; Li et al. 2018). MDA practices have been organized in collaboration with the World Health Organization by the African Programme for Onchocerciasis Control (APOC) and the Programa para la Eliminacion de la Onchocercosis en las Americas (OEPA) with the use of regular administration of ivermectin to cover over 80% of members living in at-risk communities (World Health Organization 2016). The use of regular, community-wide preventive chemotherapy with ivermectin has led to the interruption of transmission of onchocerciasis in several regions around the world, particularly in the Americas, and cessation of many *Onchocerca* MDA programs globally (Centers for Disease Control and Prevention 2013; World Health Organization 2016).

While MDA provide a mechanism for helminth control and reduction of morbidity, there is no evidence that current strategies will lead to long-term health benefits within the community or global elimination of disease due to the high rate of reinfection and lack of health infrastructure (Groups et al. 2016). An integrative approach that involves community wide coverage, more frequent treatment administration and sustained programming of more than 5 years in combination with appropriate WASH measures, community education, program coordination may be the only way currently to interrupt disease transmission of helminths and allow elimination (Bendavid et al. 2016). However, community-wide programs are difficult to sustain and expansion of preventive chemotherapy may lead to accelerated development of drug resistance as has been documented in numerous nematodes that have significant veterinary importance (Humphries et al. 2017). High-frequency preventive chemotherapy may eliminate drug-sensitive organisms from heterogenous populations and select organisms with resistance genes (Köhler 2001). Thus, stringent monitoring of disease prevalence and drug efficacy is critical to maintain successful MDA programs. Additional barriers to MDA programs include sustainability of high-quality, low-cost anthelminthic medications that are produced under good manufacturing practice standards and the availability of appropriate drug dosing and formulations for infants and young children (Albonico 2003).

3 Anthelminthic Therapies

Various classes of anthelminthic drugs (Table 2) have been well established for preventive chemotherapy programs, treatment of disease and reduction in disease transmission in endemic communities. The efficacy of anthelminthic drugs in children is influenced by many factors, including intensity of infection, age of infection, history of previous anthelminthic treatment, and parasite species and life cycle stage (Moser et al. 2017; Zwang and Olliaro 2018). Anthelminthic drugs are generally well tolerated in children. The rare reports of adverse events are commonly mild and transient. However, the majority of studies evaluating pharmacokinetics, efficacy, and safety of different anthelminthic therapy (Table 3) are lacking for young children and require further investigation.

Benzimidazoles Benzimidazoles, including albendazole, mebendazole, and triclabendazole, are broad-spectrum anthelminthics that selectively and irreversibly bind helminth tubulin. Binding of tubulin by benzimidazoles inhibits tubulin dimer polymerization, disrupting microtubule structure and function (Lacey 1990; Köhler 2001). As benzimidazoles are insoluble in water, the drugs are generally poorly absorbed in the gastrointestinal track; bioavailability is approximately 30–40% of albendazole and <20% of mebendazole after oral administration. Oral absorption can be increased with concurrent intake of fatty foods leading to up to fivefold increase in plasma drug concentration (US Food and Drug Administration; Urbani and Albonico 2003; Moon and Oberhelman 2005; Humphries et al. 2017). Albendazole and mebendazole are available in chewable tablets and liquid suspension allowing for ease of administration to young children (Urbani and Albonico 2003; Moon and Oberhelman 2005). Albendazole is generally preferred for treatment of helminths over mebendazole due to the poor tissue penetration of mebendazole (World Health Organization 1995; Moon and Oberhelman 2005).

Benzimidazoles are first-line therapy for STH as well as other tissue nematodes such as *Toxocara cati* and *T. cani*. For treatment of STH, albendazole 400 mg as a single dose or mebendazole 100 mg twice daily for 3 days is given orally to children older than 24 months of age and albendazole 200 mg as a single dose in children 12–24 months of age (Moon and Oberhelman 2005; The Medical Letter 2013; American Academy of Pediatrics 2015). A single dose of albendazole is most effective to treat ascariasis followed by hookworm, but is relatively ineffective for trichuriasis. Given this low efficacy, treatment of trichuriasis requires 3-day dose schedule to achieve an adequate cure rate (400 mg daily for 3 days, orally) (Kang et al. 2011). Treatment of toxocariasis also requires extended duration of therapy with 400 mg twice daily for 5 days (Moon and Oberhelman 2005). Albendazole is also recommended as first-line therapy for neurocysticercosis (NCC), caused by the larval stage of the trematode *Taenia solium*, a leading cause of seizures and neurologic disease in endemic populations (White et al. 2018). Duration of therapy is dependent on the cysticerci stage and location within the central nervous system. In the setting of 1–2 viable intraparenchymal cysticerci, albendazole 15 mg/kg/day

Table 2 Anthelminthic drugs for the treatment of helminth infections

Anthelminthic	Mechanism of action	Formulation	Adverse events	Additional comments	References
Benzimidazoles (albendazole, mebendazole)	Bind helminth tubulin and inhibit tubulin dimer polymerization	Chewable tablet, suspension	– Gastrointestinal symptoms: anorexia, diarrhea, nausea – Dizziness, headache – Rare: transaminitis, leukopenia	– Avoid in children less than 12 months old – Avoid in first trimester of pregnancy – Take with high fat meal	US Food and Drug Administration, Lacey (1990), World Health Organization (1995, 2017a), Köhler (2001), Montresor et al. (2003), Urbani and Albonico (2003), Moon and Oberhelman (2005), American Academy of Pediatrics (2015), Humphries et al. (2017), and Jourdan et al. (2018)
Praziquantel	Unknown	Tablet, suspension	– Gastrointestinal symptoms: anorexia, diarrhea, nausea – Dizziness, headaches		World Health Organization (1995), Köhler (2001), Moon and Oberhelman (2005), Mutapi (2015), and Babes et al. (2017)
Ivermectin	High affinity to invertebrate glutamate-gated chloride ion channels in helminth motor neurons	Tablet	– Gastrointestinal symptoms: abdominal pain – Fatigue, dizziness – Rash – Rarely: transaminitis, leukopenia – Encephalopathy and immune activation associated with loiasis	– Avoid in children less than 15 kg – Avoid use in pregnancy	Köhler (2001), Moon and Oberhelman (2005), Fox (2006), American Academy of Pediatrics (2015), and Laing et al. (2017)
DEC	Unknown	Tablet	– Mazzotti reaction – Pruritus, maculopapular rash – Fever	– Contraindicated in areas co-endemic with onchocerciasis – Contraindicated in high microfilarial	World Health Organization (1995, 2017b), The Medical Letter (2013), Peixoto and Silva (2014), American Academy of Pediatrics (2015), and Centers

(continued)

Table 2 (continued)

Anthelminthic	Mechanism of action	Formulation	Adverse events	Additional comments	References
			– Edema – Headache	burden of loiasis – Avoid use in pregnancy – Avoid use in children less than 2 years old – Avoid use in severely ill	for Disease Control and Prevention (2017)
Pyrantel and oxantel pamoate	Nicotinic acetylcholine (nACh) surface receptor agonist	Chewable tablet, suspension	– Gastrointestinal symptoms: diarrhea, abdominal pain, nausea, vomiting – Rare: transaminitis	– No data in use of children less than 2 years old – Avoid in first trimester of pregnancy	World Health Organization (1995), Köhler (2001), Urbani and Albonico (2003), and Moser et al. (2018)
Levamisole	Nicotinic acetylcholine (nACh) surface receptors agonist	Tablet	– Gastrointestinal symptoms – Dizziness, headache, and weakness – Encephalitis syndrome	– Avoid in first trimester of pregnancy	Köhler (2001) and Urbani and Albonico (2003)
Niclosamide	Blocks glucose uptake	Tablet	– Gastrointestinal symptoms		World Health Organization (1995)

Table 3 Treatment regimens for helminthic infections in children

	Pediatric dosing of first-line therapies	Alternative therapies	Comments	References
Ascaris lumbricoides	Albendazole 400 mg once	– Mebendazole 100 mg twice daily for 3 days OR 500 once – Ivermectin 150–200 μg/kg once	– If less than 24 months of age, albendazole 200 mg – Benzimidazoles should be taken with fatty meal	Moon and Oberhelman (2005), The Medical Letter (2013), American Academy of Pediatrics (2015), and Jourdan et al. (2018)
Trichuris trichiura	Albendazole 400 mg daily for 3 days	– Mebendazole 100 mg twice daily for 3 days – Pyrantel pamoate (11 mg/kg, maximum of 1 g) daily for 3 days – Ivermectin 200 μg/kg/day for 3 days	– If less than 24 months of age, albendazole 200 mg – Benzimidazoles should be taken with fatty meal	Moon and Oberhelman (2005), American Academy of Pediatrics ((2015), and Jourdan et al. (2018)
Hookworm (*Necator americanus*, *Ancylostoma duodenale*)	Albendazole 400 mg once	– Mebendazole 100 mg twice daily for 3 days OR 500 mg once – Pyrantel pamoate 11 mg/kg (maximum 1 g) daily for 3 days	– If less than 24 months of age, albendazole 200 mg – Benzimidazoles should be taken with fatty meal	Moon and Oberhelman (2005), American Academy of Pediatrics (2015), and Jourdan et al. (2018)
Strongyloides stercoralis	Ivermectin 200 μg/kg daily for 1–2 days	– Albendazole 400 mg oral divided two times daily for 7 days		Moon and Oberhelman (2005), American Academy of Pediatrics (2015), and Jourdan et al. 2018)
Enterobius vermicularis	Pyrantel pamoate 11 mg/kg base once (max 1 g) repeat dose in 2 weeks	– Albendazole 400 mg once, repeat dose in 2 weeks – Mebendazole 100 mg once, repeat dose in 2 weeks	– If less than 24 months of age, albendazole 200 mg recommended	Moon and Oberhelman (2005), The Medical Letter (2013), American Academy of Pediatrics (2015)

(continued)

Table 3 (continued)

	Pediatric dosing of first-line therapies	Alternative therapies	Comments	References
			– Benzimidazoles should be taken with fatty meal	
Toxocara cati, *Toxocara canis*	Albendazole 400 mg twice daily for 5 days	Mebendazole 100–200 mg twice daily for 5 days	– In severe disease, particularly ocular and central nervous system disease, administer anthelminthic in combination with corticosteroids	Moon and Oberhelman (2005), The Medical Letter (2013), American Academy of Pediatrics (2015)
Onchocerca volvulus	Ivermectin 150 μg/kg single dose every 6 months until asymptomatic		– Adjuctive therapy with doxycycline 200 mg orally daily for 6 weeks in non-pregnant children, adolescents and adults over the age of 8 years old can be considered	Moon and Oberhelman (2005), The Medical Letter (2013), and American Academy of Pediatrics (2015)
Lymphatic filariasis (*Wuchereria bancrofti*, *Brugia malayi*, *Brugia timori*)	In areas without co-endemic onchocerciasis or loiasis: DEC 6 mg/kg/day in three divided doses for 12 days OR DEC 6 mg/kg/day as a single oral dose In areas co-endemic with onchocerciasis: ivermectin (150–200 μg/kg) plus albendazole 400 mg In areas co-endemic with loiasis: albendazole 400 mg for 21 days followed by treatment with DEC For tropical pulmonary eosinophilia a longer course of 14–21 days is required		– Ineligible persons include children <2 years old, pregnant women and severely ill persons – DEC is contraindicated in areas with co-endemicity with onchocerciasis – DEC should be used with caution in areas with co-endemicity with *Loa loa*	Moon and Oberhelman (2005), The Medical Letter (2013), and American Academy of Pediatrics (2015)

Loa loa	– Low-burden microfilaria (less than 8,000 MF/mL) DEC 8–10 mg/kg/day in three divided doses daily for 21 days orally – High-burden microfilaria (more than 8,000 MF/mL) albendazole 200 mg twice daily for 21 days prior to treatment with DEC		– DEC is contraindicated in areas with co-endemicity with onchocerciasis	The Medical Letter (2013), American Academy of Pediatrics (2015), and Centers for Disease Control and Prevention (2017)
Taeniasis (*T. saginata* or *T. solium*)	Praziquantel 5–10 mg/kg once	Niclosamide 50 mg/kg (maximum dose 2 g) once (not currently available in United States)		World Health Organization (1995), Moon and Oberhelman (2005), The Medical Letter (2013), and American Academy of Pediatrics (2015)
Cysticercosis (*T. solium*)	– In the setting of 1–2 viable intraparenchymal cysticerci, albendazole 15 mg/kg/day (maximum dose of 1,200 mg/day), divided twice daily, for 14 days – If more than two viable parenchymal cysticerci are present, albendazole should be used in combination with praziquantel for 14 days	Praziquantel 50 mg/kg/day in three divided doses 14–30 days	– In NCC administer anthelminthic in combination with corticosteroids	Moon and Oberhelman (2005), American Academy of Pediatrics (2015), and White et al. (2018)
Diphyllobothrium latum	Praziquantel 5–10 mg/kg once	Niclosamide 50 mg/kg (max 2 g) once		Moon and Oberhelman (2005), The Medical Letter (2013), and American Academy of Pediatrics (2015)

(continued)

Table 3 (continued)

	Pediatric dosing of first-line therapies	Alternative therapies	Comments	References
Echinococcus granulosus and *Echinococcus multilocularis*	Albendazole 15 mg/kg/day divided twice daily (max 800 mg) for minimum of 1–6 months for cystic echinococcosis or 2 years for alveolar echinococcosis		– Monotherapy or combination therapy with PAIR or surgery depends on WHO ultrasound classification	Moon and Oberhelman (2005), The Medical Letter (2013), American Academy of Pediatrics (2015), and Nabarro et al. (2015)
Schistosomiasis	– *S. mansoni* and *S. haematobium*, praziquantel 40 mg/kg/day divided twice daily for 1 day – *S. japonicum*, praziquantel 60 mg/kg/day divided three times per day for 1 day			Moon and Oberhelman (2005), The Medical Letter (2013), World Health Organization (2013), and American Academy of Pediatrics (2015)
Paragonimus westermani, *Paragonimus kellicotti*	Praziquantel 75 mg/kg/day, divided three times daily for 2 days	Triclabendazole 10 mg/kg/day for 1–2 days		Moon and Oberhelman (2005), The Medical Letter (2013), and American Academy of Pediatrics (2015)
Fascioliasis	Triclabendazole 10 mg/kg orally for 1–2 days			Moon and Oberhelman (2005), The Medical Letter (2013), American Academy of Pediatrics (2015), and Kelley et al. (2016)

(maximum dose of 1,200 mg/day), twice daily, orally for 14 days, is the recommended regimen (White et al. 2018). If more than two viable parenchymal cysticerci are present, albendazole should be used in combination with praziquantel for 14–30 days (White et al. 2018). In addition to albendazole, combination with steroids for treatment of viable NCC is recommended (Moon and Oberhelman 2005; White et al. 2018). Treatment of hydatid disease due to the cestode *Echinococcus granulosus* or *E. multilocularis* is dependent on ultrasound classification of the disease stage in either the liver or the lungs (Nabarro et al. 2015). Albendazole is used as monotherapy to treat small (less than 5 cm) simple cysts or small transitional cysts with detached laminated membrane, used in combination with puncture, aspiration, injection, and re-aspiration (PAIR) in large (greater than 5 cm) simple cysts or large transitional cysts with detached laminated membrane or used in combination with surgery in an active multivesicular, multi-septated cyst or complex mass (Nabarro et al. 2015). Albendazole 15 mg/kg/day (maximum of 800 mg) orally should be continued for minimum of 1–6 months for cystic echinococcosis and for more than 2 years for alveolar echinococcosis (The Medical Letter 2013; American Academy of Pediatrics 2015).

Triclabendazole is a chlorinated-thio-benzimidazole compound (Köhler 2001). Unlike albendazole and mebendazole, triclabendazole has a narrow spectrum of activity against helminths but is highly efficacious against the liver fluke *Fasciola hepatica* (Köhler 2001; Kelley et al. 2016). Triclabendazole (10 mg/kg, single tablet daily for 1–2 days, orally) is capable of killing both early immature and adult *Fasciola* (The Medical Letter 2013; Kelley et al. 2016).

There is limited safety data of benzimidazole in children less than 12 months of age, and use is generally not advised in this age group (Montresor et al. 2003; American Academy of Pediatrics 2015; Jourdan et al. 2018). For children between 12 months and 24 months old, a half-dose of albendazole (200 mg, orally) is recommended (Montresor et al. 2003; American Academy of Pediatrics 2015). Benzimidazole use during pregnancy in rabbits and rats was shown to be teratogenic; however, major congenital defects in humans have yet to be demonstrated. Based on the risk of potential teratogenicity, benzimidazoles should be avoided during the first trimester of pregnancy (World Health Organization 1995, 2017a; Urbani and Albonico 2003). Albendazole can be detected in breast milk at low concentrations. However, adverse outcomes with the concurrent use of benzimidazoles and breastfeeding have not been reported (Urbani and Albonico 2003; Abdel-Tawab et al. 2009). Adverse events associated with benzimidazoles are typically mild and may include gastrointestinal upset, anorexia, diarrhea, nausea, headache, and dizziness (Urbani and Albonico 2003; Moon and Oberhelman 2005). Transaminitis and leukopenia have been reported but rarely and most commonly are observed with prolonged use (Urbani and Albonico 2003).

Resistance has not been documented to date in human disease but is well documented in veterinary medicine due to extensive use and improper dosing of benzimidazoles including triclabendazole (Köhler 2001; Kelley et al. 2016). Resistance has been linked to single nucleotide polymorphisms (SNPs) in the β-tubulin gene causing a conformational change in β-tubulin leading to loss of the high-affinity binding site (Köhler 2001; Kang et al. 2011; Furtado et al. 2016). Beyond the concern for the development of drug resistance, benzimidazole drug efficacy varies significantly within populations secondary to treatment history, geographic differences between helminthic species, as well as community diet (Kang et al. 2011).

Ivermectin Ivermectin is a semisynthetic, macrocyclic lactone derived from avermectin B1 which binds selectively and with high affinity to invertebrate glutamate-gated chloride ion channels in helminth motor neurons (Köhler 2001; Fox 2006; Laing et al. 2017). Activation of the chloride ion channels causes an irreversible chloride ion current, hyperpolarization of the cell membrane, and muscle paralysis. The development of flaccid paralysis of the worm limits motility, inhibits pharyngeal coordination causing worm starvation, as well as represses reproduction mechanisms and fecundity (Köhler 2001; Laing et al. 2017). Ivermectin is administered orally as a tablet, has 50–60% bioavailability, and is metabolized in the liver (Fox 2006). Ivermectin is active against a broad range of helminths including *Dirofilaria immitis*, *Strongyloides stercoralis*, *Onchocerca volvulus*, *Loa*, lymphatic filariasis, and several intestinal nematodes (Fox 2006).

Ivermectin is the first-line therapy for *Strongyloides stercoralis*. High cure rates for chronic strongyloidiasis can be achieved in a daily dose (200 μg/kg) of oral ivermectin for 2 consecutive days or two doses administered 2 weeks apart in children (Zaha et al. 2002; Moon and Oberhelman 2005; The Medical Letter 2013). However, severe *Strongyloides* disease in the form of hyperinfection and disseminated infection requires longer treatment regimens. Hyperinfection, a phase of accelerated autoinfection, and disseminated infection, larval migration to organs beyond the lung and gastrointestinal track, are associated with high mortality. This critical form of strongyloidiasis occurs after suppression of the host immune system, commonly due to acute use of corticosteroids (Ramanathan and Nutman 2008; Mejia and Nutman 2012). For *Strongyloides* hyperinfection and disseminated disease, ivermectin 200 μg/kg/day orally should be continued until the stool exam is negative for 2 weeks (Ramanathan and Nutman 2008; Mejia and Nutman 2012). Ivermectin is also the preferential therapy for filarial diseases such as onchocerciasis and alternative therapy for lymphatic filariasis (Fox 2006). Ivermectin is not cidal against adult stage *Onchocerca volvulus* but is microfilaricidal. As a result, ivermectin should be administered every 6–12 months as a single dose of 150 μg/kg for as long as there is evidence of ongoing infection to reduce filarial migration and end-stage organ disease as well as to reduce community transmission (Moon and Oberhelman 2005; Laing et al. 2017). A single dose of ivermectin can decrease circulating *Onchocerca* microfilaria in the skin by 96–99% (Fox 2006). Ivermectin is additionally recommended for treatment of lymphatic filariasis in areas with co-endemicity with onchocerciasis (Fox 2006; World Health Organization 2017b). Similar to onchocerciasis, ivermectin is only microfilaricidal for lymphatic filariasis and is likewise not curative (Moon and Oberhelman 2005; Laing et al. 2017).

Despite the broad use of ivermectin in children, the safety profile for children less than 15 kg has not been established limiting the general use in young children (Moon and Oberhelman 2005; American Academy of Pediatrics 2015). Additionally, use of ivermectin in pregnancy is also not recommended (Fox 2006). Despite these limitations, adverse effects associated with ivermectin are minimal. Minor effects including mild gastrointestinal upset, abdominal pain, fatigue, dizziness, rash, and rarely transaminitis and leukopenia have been reported (Fox 2006). However, attention must be provided when treating filarial infections with ivermectin due to the risk of inflammatory activation as a result of dying microfilariae and posttreatment encephalopathy (Moon and Oberhelman 2005; Fox 2006). These encephalopathy and immune activation phenomena are described specifically in areas with co-endemicity with *Loa loa* and in individuals with high microfilariae burden (Fox 2006). In these select areas, the reduction in microfilaria burden with the use of albendazole is recommended prior to administration of ivermectin (Fox 2006).

Resistance to ivermectin has not been reported to date in humans but remains a global concern for various helminthic infections of veterinary importance with documentation of resistance for intestinal nematodes in ruminants (Fox 2006; Laing et al. 2017). Drug resistance for intestinal nematodes may be secondary to altered binding targets, such as mutations of P-glycoprotein, encoding genes of the glutamate-gated chloride ion channels, or due to increased drug efflux (Köhler 2001). Additionally, ivermectin insensitivity may already exist to onchocerciasis, though the mechanism has not been determined (Fox 2006; Osei-Atweneboana et al. 2011).

Praziquantel Praziquantel is an anthelminthic therapy used for treatment of cestodes including taeniasis (*Taenia solium* and *Taenia saginata*), *Hymenolepis nana*, *Dipylidium caninum*, and *Diphyllobothrium latum* and as adjunct therapy for severe cysticercosis (*Taenia solium*) as well as trematodes such as schistosomiasis, paragonimiasis, and liver flukes (*Clonorchis*, *Opisthorchis*) (Moon and Oberhelman 2005). Despite the broad range of use for both cestodes and trematodes, the mechanism of anthelminthic activity remains unknown (World Health Organization 1995; Köhler 2001). Proposed mechanism of action includes muscular paralysis due to dysregulation of calcium homeostasis leading to rapid calcium influx and disruption of worm tegument causing alteration of cell membrane and antigen exposure to primed schistosome-specific antibodies (Mutapi 2015; Babes et al. 2017). While immune priming and antibody-mediated mechanism have been proposed as a potential mechanism, reduced efficacy of praziquantel has not been demonstrated in immunocompromised hosts (Mutapi 2015). Praziquantel is rapidly absorbed, with approximately 80% bioavailability when administered orally as tablet (which can be crushed) or oral suspension (Stothard et al. 2013; Chai 2013).

Praziquantel is a first-line therapy for adult gastrointestinal-stage cestodes however has minimal efficacy in the treatment of larval tissue-stage cestodes (The Medical Letter 2013). Single-dose administration of 5–10 mg/kg orally leads to high rates of cure for all adult intestinal-stage cestode infection except *Hymenolepis nana*, the dwarf tapeworm, which requires higher doses of 25 mg/kg as a single dose, orally (Moon and Oberhelman 2005; The Medical Letter 2013; American Academy of Pediatrics 2015). Larval tissue-stage cestode infections including echinococcosis and cysticercosis are typically treated with albendazole due to the lack of sufficient efficacy with praziquantel (The Medical Letter 2013). Praziquantel is also a first-line therapy for trematodes such as schistosomiasis. Praziquantel is used as treatment and preventive chemotherapy for all *Schistosoma* spp. with greatest efficacy against *S. japonicum* and *S. haematobium* and least efficacious for mixed infections (Zwang and Olliaro 2018). Praziquantel kills mature schistosomes but not immature worms and thus should not be administered until 6–8 weeks after exposure to contaminated freshwater (Kabuyaya et al. 2018). Treatment dosing for schistosomiasis includes 40 mg/kg/day orally for *S. mansoni* and *S. haematobium* and 60 mg/kg/day orally for *S. japonicum* divided into two doses (Moon and Oberhelman 2005; The Medical Letter 2013). Treatment of schistosomiasis with praziquantel in children reduces chronic morbidity and transmission of schistosomiasis within the community (Kabuyaya et al. 2018).

Safety profiles have not been established in children less than 4 years old, but treatment with praziquantel in children as young as 6 months has been documented without significant adverse events (Moon and Oberhelman 2005; Mutapi 2015; Zwang and Olliaro 2017). Even though young children have high tolerability to praziquantel, use of a standard 40 mg/kg dose of praziquantel in young children was associated with a lower clinical cure rate compared to older children and adults (Sousa-Figueiredo et al. 2012). Clinical trials are underway to determine the optimal dosing of praziquantel in children as young as 3 months (clinicaltrials.gov, NCT02806232). There is minimal data regarding use of praziquantel in pregnant or lactating women; however, no maternal or fetal toxicity has been reported in veterinary studies despite its wide use in treatment of pregnant animals (World Health Organization 2002). As a result, women of childbearing age and pregnant and lactating women with helminth infections such as schistosomiasis should be offered treatment (World Health Organization 2002; Olds 2003). Praziquantel is generally well tolerated with mild adverse effects including abdominal discomfort, headaches, and dizziness dependent on the intensity of the infection (Moon and Oberhelman 2005; Mutapi 2015; Babes et al. 2017). There is ongoing concern of emerging praziquantel resistance of cestodes like schistosomiasis, particularly *S. mansoni*; however, the mechanism of resistance remains unknown (Köhler 2001; Doenhoff et al. 2008; Chai 2013).

Diethylcarbamazine (DEC) DEC is a piperazine derivative anthelmintic drug active against filaria. The mechanism of action of DEC against filaria remains unknown but may be intertwined with activation of the innate immune response through inhibition of arachidonic acid metabolism and inhibition of NF-kB signaling pathway (World Health Organization 1995; Peixoto and Silva 2014). DEC is the first-line therapy for lymphatic filariasis including *Wuchereria bancrofti*, *Brugia malayi*, *Brugia timori*, and *Mansonella* spp. and for *Loa loa* (Moon and Oberhelman 2005) however is contraindicated in onchocerciasis (Moon and Oberhelman 2005). DEC is microfilaricidal for lymphatic filariasis. In children, DEC is administered as 6 mg/kg/day single oral dose or 6 mg/kg/day divided in three doses for 12 days in children more than 2 years in age (World Health Organization 1995; Moon and Oberhelman

2005; The Medical Letter 2013; American Academy of Pediatrics 2015). DEC is cidal against both the adult worms and the microfilaria of *Loa loa* (World Health Organization 1995). However, DEC should not be used to treat loiasis in children with high burden of microfilaria disease due to the risk of severe inflammatory reaction and fatal encephalopathy. Pre-treatment quantitative blood smears are required prior to initiation of DEC therapy for loiasis. DEC (8–10 mg/kg/day orally in three divided doses for 21 days) is the treatment of choice for *Loa loa* in children with low microfilarial burden (<8,000 microfilaria/mL) (The Medical Letter 2013; Centers for Disease Control and Prevention 2017). However, in cases of high microfilarial burden (>8,000 microfilaria/mL), albendazole 200 mg BID daily for 21 days should be administered prior to treatment with DEC to reduce *Loa loa* microfilarial burden and risk of encephalopathy (The Medical Letter 2013; American Academy of Pediatrics 2015; Centers for Disease Control and Prevention 2017).

DEC is currently only available in the United States by investigational new drug protocol through the Centers for Disease Control and Hygiene (CDC) (American Academy of Pediatrics 2015). Prior to treatment of lymphatic filariasis or *Loa loa* with DEC, onchocerciasis should be excluded due to the risk of Mazzotti reaction, a severe reaction manifesting as fever, headache, dizziness, urticarial rash, anorexia, malaise, respiratory failure, and potential death (World Health Organization 1995; American Academy of Pediatrics 2015). If unable to exclude onchocerciasis or if living in co-endemic area, treatment for onchocerciasis with ivermectin prior to use of DEC should be highly considered (American Academy of Pediatrics 2015). Side effects of DEC are otherwise rare but include pruritus, maculopapular rash, fever, edema, and headache (Moon and Oberhelman 2005).

Pyrantel Pamoate and Oxantel Pamoate Pyrantel pamoate and oxantel pamoate are tetrahydropyrimidines that act as agonists on nematode nicotinic acetylcholine (nAch) surface receptors of somatic muscle cells (Moser et al. 2018). Both pyrantel and oxantel pamoates act selectively on the nACh receptor; however, at different targets, pyrantel acts on the L-subtype, while oxantel targets the N-subtype (Moser et al. 2018). Activation of nAch receptor causes depolarization of the muscle cell membrane and subsequent helminth paralysis and elimination (World Health Organization 1995; Köhler 2001; Urbani and Albonico 2003). Nematode nAch receptors have been shown to be pharmacologically distinct from the homologous receptors in mammals permitting increased helminth selectivity (Köhler 2001). Both drugs are administered as single-dose treatments, as solution or chewable tablet, and both drugs have restricted oral bioavailability (Urbani and Albonico 2003; Moon and Oberhelman 2005). Pyrantel pamoate (11 mg/kg dose, maximum of 1 g), administered as two single-dose tablets 2 weeks apart, is a common therapy for treatment of *Enterobius vermicularis*, known as pinworm, in children (World Health Organization 1995; Moon and Oberhelman 2005; The Medical Letter 2013). In comparison to other treatment options for pinworm such as albendazole and mebendazole, pyrantel pamoate is available without prescription in the United States. Pyrantel pamoate is also an alternative treatment for hookworm when administered daily for 3 days orally (11 mg/kg base, maximum 1 g) (The Medical Letter 2013). Oxantel pamoate, a pyrantel analog, has activity against *Trichuris*, and, unlike mebendazole and albendazole, oxantel can be given as a single-dose regimen in the treatment of trichuriasis (Moser et al. 2016). Oxantel pamoate (20 mg/kg, single dose) is more efficacious against trichuriasis than either albendazole or mebendazole monotherapy however has minimal effect against hookworm or ascariasis (Speich et al. 2014). Current validated dosing schemes for oxantel pamoate are lacking in children, particularly in infants. However an optimal dose ranging from 15 to 30 mg/kg has been suggested in school-aged children (Moser et al. 2016). In certain regions globally, oxantel and pyrantel pamoate are marketed in combination, in suspension formulation, for treatment of STH (Moser et al. 2016).

Adverse events are minimal, limited to gastrointestinal symptoms such as diarrhea, abdominal pain, nausea, and vomiting, due to the poor bioavailability of the drugs. In rare occurrences, transaminitis has been reported (Urbani and Albonico 2003). There is no data in use of pyrantel pamoate or oxantel pamoate in children less than 2 years old, but pyrantel pamoate has been widely used in young children, and no reported issues have been documented (Moon and Oberhelman 2005). Additionally, no teratogenic effects have been documented while taking during pregnancy; however, use in pregnancy is not recommended during the first trimester (Urbani and Albonico 2003). Pyrantel pamoate resistance has been reported in hookworm species (*Ancylostoma caninum*, *Ancylostoma duodenale*) (Reynoldson et al. 1997; Kopp et al. 2007). Emerging resistance is likely secondary to structural alterations in the nACh receptor subunits resulting in diminished drug affinity to the binding site (Köhler 2001).

Niclosamide Niclosamide is an oral anthelminthic drug that blocks glucose uptake by intestinal tapeworms. It is administered as a single 2 g dose, orally, in adults and dosed by weight in children (50 mg/kg, maximum of 2 g) as second-line therapy for adult intestinal-stage *Taenia* spp. and *Diphyllobothrium latum* (World Health Organization 1995; The Medical Letter 2013; American Academy of Pediatrics 2015). However, there is no activity against the larvae tissue-stage cysticerci of *Taenia solium* due to the lack of oral bioavailability of niclosamide (World Health Organization 1995; Moon and Oberhelman 2005). Niclosamide is an alternative anthelminthic therapy for *H. nana* but requires prolonged drug administration dosed by weight in children (for weight of 11–34 kg, administer 1 g orally on day 1 and then 500 mg per day for 6 days; if weight is greater than 34 kg, administer 1.5 g orally on day 1 and then 1 g per day for 6 days) (The Medical Letter 2013; American Academy of Pediatrics 2015). Niclosamide has good tolerability owning to the lack of absorption from the intestinal track. Adverse events are mild and transient, most commonly associated with gastrointestinal disturbances (World Health Organization 1995). There is no evidence of teratogenic effects of niclosamide during pregnancy (World Health Organization 1995).

Levamisole Levamisole is an imidazothiazole, (−)-isomer of tetramisole, and nAch receptor agonist on nematode somatic muscle cells and causing paralysis and elimination of STH (Köhler 2001; Urbani and Albonico 2003). The drug is rapidly absorbed with high bioavailability (World Health Organization 1995; Urbani and Albonico 2003). It is an alternative treatment option for ascariasis and mixed *Ascaris* and hookworm infections leading to over 97% cure rate with a single dose (Moser et al. 2017). Levamisole can be easily administered to children with chewable tablet formulation as a single dose (2.5 mg/kg, orally). Adverse events associated with levamisole include gastrointestinal symptoms as well central nervous system symptoms such as dizziness, headache, and weakness (Urbani and Albonico 2003). While these symptoms are commonly mild, cases of levamisole-associated encephalopathy syndrome have been reported. Levamisole-induced encephalopathy syndrome has been attributed to use of generic anthelminthic formulations in the field and lack of adequate quality control, but the syndrome has also been documented in other medical diseases associated with levamisole use (Zheng 1995; Urbani and Albonico 2003; Wu et al. 2006). There are no reported teratogenic effects associated with levamisole; however, use of levamisole is not recommended during the first trimester of pregnancy (Urbani and Albonico 2003). Similar to oxantel pamoate and pyrantel pamoate, drug resistance of intestinal worms to levamisole is possible due to changes in the target site of the nACh subunit permitting less affinity of the drug to the nematode (Köhler 2001).

4 Anthelminthic Drug Discovery

Despite the efforts of MDA, elimination of many helminthic diseases has remained elusive. Efforts toward elimination have been limited by sustainability of community-wide programs and the threat of emerging drug resistance. Not only do current MDA programs and global treatment strategies rely on single drugs without significant alternative options, but the extensive use and improper dosing, typically in children, raise the concern for long-term effectiveness of treatment strategies (Köhler 2001; Walker et al. 2016). Balancing the need of treatment to reduce morbidity in children at high risk of profound morbidity with the cost of maintenance and the potential to lead to resistance due to selective pressure has created a critical need for discovery of new preventative and therapeutic targets and to explore drug combination therapies against helminths (Albonico 2003).

Beyond the concern for emerging resistance of available anthelminthic medications, other anthelminthic needs should be listed as high importance in the drug development pipeline. Novel drugs for the treatment of filarial infections that have fewer associated adverse events particularly in areas of co-endemicity of lymphatic filariasis, loiasis, and onchocerciasis are in significant need. Additionally, novel therapies for the larval tissue stage of cestode infections are in high demand (Köhler 2001). With the availability of complete genomic sequences of many helminthic organisms, drug discovery using the complex, individual life cycles during which organisms undergo changes in morphology and gene expression may be an effective tool to uncover novel targets (Skinner-

Adams et al. 2016). Additionally, encouraging public-private partnership through open-source, resource sharing of the large quantities of known drug compounds will aid in evaluating mechanism of drug targets and pharmacokinetics in order to improve drug discovery efficiency and reduce cost (Weng et al. 2018). However new, novel drug targets will need extensive monitoring and development of formulations that are amenable to treating the most high-risk individuals, children.

Alternative strategies to address urgently needed interventions include repurposing existing drugs to treat helminth infections or use of existing anthelminthic drugs in combinations. The neuromodulatory drugs sertraline, paroxetine, and chlorpromazine have been recently shown to decrease *Trichuris* motility and prevent development of hookworm (Weeks et al. 2018). Other potential repurposed drugs include use of the antimalarial artemisinins for the treatment of trematodes and use of tribendimidine for treatment of both STH (except *Trichuris*) and trematodes (Panic et al. 2014; Robertson et al. 2015). Despite the significant geographic overlap of STH, there is no single drug with high efficacy against all three organisms. As a result, co-administration of current drugs with different modes of action may be a preferable strategy (Huwyler et al. 2017). Combination therapy with albendazole and oxantel pamoate reaches higher cure rates in STH coinfected children, particularly in children with trichuriasis (Speich et al. 2014; Groups et al. 2016). Other combinations including albendazole-ivermectin and tribendimidine-oxantel pamoate have also demonstrated superiority to monotherapy with albendazole for the treatment of trichuriasis (Clarke et al. 2019). Combination therapy of albendazole-ivermectin is currently employed for the treatment of lymphatic filariasis in *Onchocerca* co-endemic regions (Crompton et al. 2003). However, further information on drug-drug interactions and adverse events in children receiving anthelminthic combination therapy are needed.

5 Conclusions

Helminth infection is one of the most common infections of mankind, causing significant morbidity in children living in poverty-stricken, endemic regions globally (Weatherhead and Hotez 2015; Li et al. 2018). Anthelminthic therapy has been used for preventive chemotherapy through mass drug administration and for treatment of infection in order to reduce morbidity in children. However, safety, efficacy, and tolerability of currently available anthelminthic drugs are lacking in young children. Additionally, the threat of evolving drug resistance is ongoing in the setting of escalation of MDA programs aimed at interruption of helminth transmission and elimination. Novel drugs are urgently needed to combat the current limitations of anthelminthics (Weatherhead et al. 2017). In the absence of novel drug targets, alternative approaches such as vaccine development programs could evolve into stand-alone preventative strategies or therapeutic modalities used in combination with MDA programs in the near future (Hotez et al. 2016).

References

Abdel-Tawab AM, Bradley M, Ghazaly EA et al (2009) Albendazole and its metabolites in the breast milk of lactating women following a single oral dose of albendazole. Br J Clin Pharmacol 68:737–742. https://doi.org/10.1111/j.1365-2125.2009.03524.x

Albonico M (2003) Methods to sustain drug efficacy in helminth control programmes. Acta Trop 86:233–242. https://doi.org/10.1016/S0001-706X(03)00043-3

American Academy of Pediatrics (2015) Red book – 2015 report of the Committee on Infectious Diseases, 30th edn. American Academy of Pediatrics, Elk Grove Village

Babes RM, Selescu T, Domocos D, Babes A (2017) The anthelminthic drug praziquantel is a selective agonist of the sensory transient receptor potential melastatin type 8 channel. Toxicol Appl Pharmacol 336:55–65. https://doi.org/10.1016/j.taap.2017.10.012

Bendavid E, Bogoch II, Lai Y-S et al (2016) Assessment of global guidelines for preventive chemotherapy against schistosomiasis and soil-transmitted helminthiasis: a cost-effectiveness modelling study. Lancet Infect Dis 16:1065–1075. https://doi.org/10.1016/s1473-3099(16)30073-1

Bethony J, Brooker S, Albonico M et al (2006) Soil-transmitted helminth infections: ascariasis, trichuriasis, and hookworm. Lancet (London, England) 367:1521–1532. https://doi.org/10.1016/S0140-6736(06)68653-4

Centers for Disease Control and Prevention (2013) Progress toward elimination of onchocerciasis in the Americas – 1993-2012. Morb Mortal Wkly Rep 62:405–408

Centers for Disease Control and Prevention (2017) Parasites – loiasis. https://www.cdc.gov/parasites/loiasis/health_professionals/index.html#tx. Accessed 29 May 2019

Chai J-Y (2013) Praziquantel treatment in trematode and cestode infections: an update. J Infect Chemother 45:32–43. https://doi.org/10.3947/ic.2013.45.1.32

Clarke NE, Doi SAR, Wangdi K et al (2019) Efficacy of anthelminthic drugs and drug combinations against soil-transmitted helminths: a systematic review and network meta-analysis. Clin Infect Dis 68:96–105. https://doi.org/10.1093/cid/ciy423

Crompton DWT, Montresor A, Nesheim MC, Savioli L (2003) Controlling disease due to helminth infections. World Health Organization, Geneva

Doenhoff MJ, Cioli D, Utzinger J (2008) Praziquantel: mechanisms of action, resistance and new derivatives for schistosomiasis. Curr Opin Infect Dis 21:659–667. https://doi.org/10.1097/QCO.0b013e328318978f

Fox LM (2006) Ivermectin: uses and impact 20 years on. Curr Opin Infect Dis 450:588–593

Furtado LFV, de Paiva Bello ACP, Rabelo ÉML (2016) Benzimidazole resistance in helminths: from problem to diagnosis. Acta Trop 162:95–102

GBD (2017) Global, regional, and national disability-adjusted life-years (DALYs) for 333 diseases and injuries and healthy life expectancy (HALE) for 195 countries and territories, 1990–2016: a systematic analysis for the Global Burden of Disease study 201. Lancet 390:1260–1344. https://doi.org/10.1016/S0140-6736(17)32130-X

Groups AP, Hotez PJ, Strych U et al (2016) Efficacy and reinfection with soil-transmitted helminths 18-weeks post-treatment with albendazole-ivermectin, albendazole-mebendazole, albendazole-oxantel pamoate and mebendazole. Parasit Vectors 9:123. https://doi.org/10.1186/s13071-016-1406-8

Hotez P (2016) Blue marble health: an innovative plan to fight diseases of the poor amid wealth. Johns Hopkins University Press, Baltimore

Hotez PJ, Bundy DAP, Beegle K et al (2006) Helminth infections: soil-transmitted helminth infections and schistosomiasis. In: Jamison D, Breman J, Measham A et al (eds) Disease control priorities in developing countries, 2nd edn. The World Bank, Washington

Hotez PJ, Strych U, Lustigman S, Bottazzi ME (2016) Human anthelminthic vaccines: rationale and challenges. Vaccine 34:3549–3555

Humphries D, Nguyen S, Kumar S et al (2017) Effectiveness of albendazole for hookworm varies widely by community and correlates with nutritional factors: a cross-sectional study of school-age children in Ghana. Am J Trop Med Hyg 96:347–354. https://doi.org/10.4269/ajtmh.16-0682
Huwyler J, Moser W, Yapi RB et al (2017) Efficacy and safety of tribendimidine, tribendimidine plus ivermectin, tribendimidine plus oxantel pamoate, and albendazole plus oxantel pamoate against hookworm and concomitant soil-transmitted helminth infections in Tanzania and Côte d'Ivoire: a randomised, controlled, single-blinded, non-inferiority trial. Lancet Infect Dis 17:1162–1171. https://doi.org/10.1016/s1473-3099(17)30487-5
Jourdan PM, Lamberton PHL, Fenwick A, Addiss DG (2018) Soil-transmitted helminth infections. Lancet 391:252–265. https://doi.org/10.1016/S0140-6736(17)31930-X
Kabuyaya M, Chimbari MJ, Mukaratirwa S (2018) Efficacy of praziquantel treatment regimens in pre-school and school aged children infected with schistosomiasis in sub-Saharan Africa: a systematic review. Infect Dis Poverty. 7:73
Kang G, Bethony JM, Behnke JM et al (2011) Assessment of the anthelmintic efficacy of albendazole in school children in seven countries where soil-transmitted helminths are endemic. PLoS Negl Trop Dis 5:e948. https://doi.org/10.1371/journal.pntd.0000948
Kelley J, Elliott T, Beddoe T et al (2016) Current threat of triclabendazole resistance in Fasciola hepatica. Trends Parasitol 32:458–469
Köhler P (2001) The biochemical basis of anthelmintic action and resistance. Int J Parasitol 31:336–345. https://doi.org/10.1016/S0020-7519(01)00131-X
Kopp SR, Kotze AC, McCarthy JS, Coleman GT (2007) High-level pyrantel resistance in the hookworm Ancylostoma caninum. Vet Parasitol 143:299–304. https://doi.org/10.1016/j.vetpar.2006.08.036
Lacey E (1990) Mode of action of benzimidazoles. Parasitol Today 6:112–115. https://doi.org/10.1016/0169-4758(90)90227-U
Laing R, Gillan V, Devaney E (2017) Ivermectin – old drug, new tricks? Trends Parasitol 33:463–472. https://doi.org/10.1016/j.pt.2017.02.004
Li S, Gankpe FG, Wilner LB et al (2018) Global, regional, and national incidence, prevalence, and years lived with disability for 354 diseases and injuries for 195 countries and territories, 1990–2017: a systematic analysis for the Global Burden of Disease study 2017. Lancet 392:1789–1858. https://doi.org/10.1016/s0140-6736(18)32279-7
The Medical Letter (2013) Drugs for parasitic infections. 11:e1–e31
Mejia R, Nutman TB (2012) Screening, prevention, and treatment for hyperinfection syndrome and disseminated infections caused by Strongyloides stercoralis. Curr Opin Infect Dis 25:458–463. https://doi.org/10.1097/QCO.0b013e3283551dbd
Montresor A, Awasthi S, Crompton DWT (2003) Use of benzimidazoles in children younger than 24 months for the treatment of soil-transmitted helminthiasis. Acta Trop 86:223–232. https://doi.org/10.1016/S0001-706X(03)00042-1
Moon TD, Oberhelman RA (2005) Antiparasitic therapy in children. Pediatr Clin N Am 52:917–948. https://doi.org/10.1016/j.pcl.2005.02.012
Moser W, Ali SM, Ame SM et al (2016) Efficacy and safety of oxantel pamoate in school-aged children infected with Trichuris trichiura on Pemba Island, Tanzania: a parallel, randomised, controlled, dose-ranging study. Lancet Infect Dis 16:53–60. https://doi.org/10.1016/S1473-3099(15)00271-6
Moser W, Schindler C, Keiser J (2017) Efficacy of recommended drugs against soil transmitted helminths: systematic review and network meta-analysis. BMJ 358:4307. https://doi.org/10.1136/bmj.j4307
Moser W, Sayasone S, Xayavong S et al (2018) Efficacy and tolerability of triple drug therapy with albendazole, pyrantel pamoate, and oxantel pamoate compared with albendazole plus oxantel pamoate, pyrantel pamoate plus oxantel pamoate, and mebendazole plus pyrantel pamoate and oxantel pamoate against hookworm infections in school-aged children in Laos: a randomised, single-blind trial. Lancet Infect Dis 18:729–737. https://doi.org/10.1016/S1473-3099(18)30220-2

Mutapi F (2015) Changing policy and practice in the control of pediatric schistosomiasis. Pediatrics. 135:536–544. https://doi.org/10.1542/peds.2014-3189

Nabarro LE, Amin Z, Chiodini PL (2015) Current management of cystic echinococcosis: a survey of specialist practice. Clin Infect Dis 60:721–728. https://doi.org/10.1093/cid/ciu931

Olds GR (2003) Administration of praziquantel to pregnant and lactating women. Acta Trop 86:185–195

Osei-Atweneboana MY, Awadzi K, Attah SK et al (2011) Phenotypic evidence of emerging ivermectin resistance in Onchocerca volvulus. PLoS Negl Trop Dis 5:1–11. https://doi.org/10.1371/journal.pntd.0000998

Panic G, Duthaler U, Speich B, Keiser J (2014) Repurposing drugs for the treatment and control of helminth infections. Int J Parasitol Drugs Drug Resist 4:185–200. https://doi.org/10.1016/j.ijpddr.2014.07.002

Peixoto CA, Silva BS (2014) Anti-inflammatory effects of diethylcarbamazine: a review. Eur J Pharmacol 734:35–41

Pullan RL, Smith JL, Jasrasaria R, Brooker SJ (2014) Global numbers of infection and disease burden of soil transmitted helminth infections in 2010. Parasit Vectors 7:37. https://doi.org/10.1186/1756-3305-7-37

Ramanathan R, Nutman T (2008) Strongyloides stercoralis infection in the immunocompromised host. Curr Infect Dis Rep 10:105–110. https://doi.org/10.1007/S11908-008-0019-6

Reynoldson JA, Behnke JM, Pallant LJ et al (1997) Failure of pyrantel in treatment of human Hookworm infections (Ancylostoma duodenale) in the Kimberley region of North West Australia. Acta Trop. https://doi.org/10.1016/S0001-706X(97)00106-X

Robertson AP, Puttachary S, Buxton SK, Martin RJ (2015) Tribendimidine: mode of action and nAChR subtype selectivity in Ascaris and Oesophagostomum. PLoS Negl Trop Dis 9: e0003495. https://doi.org/10.1371/journal.pntd.0003495

Skinner-Adams TS, Sumanadasa SDM, Fisher GM et al (2016) Defining the targets of antiparasitic compounds. Drug Discov Today 21:725–739. https://doi.org/10.1016/j.drudis.2016.01.002

Sousa-Figueiredo JC, Betson M, Atuhaire A et al (2012) Performance and safety of praziquantel for treatment of intestinal schistosomiasis in infants and preschool children. PLoS Negl Trop Dis 6. https://doi.org/10.1371/journal.pntd.0001864

Speich B, Ame SM, Ali SM et al (2014) Oxantel Pamoate–Albendazole for *Trichuris trichiura* infection. N Engl J Med 370:610–620. https://doi.org/10.1056/NEJMoa1301956

Stothard JR, Sousa-Figueiredo JC, Betson M et al (2013) Schistosomiasis in African infants and preschool children: let them now be treated! Trends Parasitol 29:197–205. https://doi.org/10.1016/j.pt.2013.02.001

Urbani C, Albonico M (2003) Anthelminthic drug safety and drug administration in the control of soil-transmitted helminthiasis in community campaigns. Acta Trop 86:215–221. https://doi.org/10.1016/S0001-706X(03)00036-6

US Food and Drug Administration Prescribing Information Albenza. https://www.accessdata.fda.gov/drugsatfda_docs/label/2009/020666s005s006lbl.pdf. Accessed 3 May 2017

Walker M, Mabud TS, Olliaro PL et al (2016) New approaches to measuring anthelminthic drug efficacy: parasitological responses of childhood schistosome infections to treatment with praziquantel. Parasit Vectors 9:41. https://doi.org/10.1186/s13071-016-1312-0

Weatherhead JE, Hotez PJ (2015) Worm infections in children. Pediatr Rev 36:341–352. https://doi.org/10.1542/pir.36-8-341

Weatherhead JE, Hotez PJ, Mejia R (2017) The global state of helminth control and elimination in children. Pediatr Clin N Am 64. https://doi.org/10.1016/j.pcl.2017.03.005

Weeks JC, Roberts WM, Leasure C et al (2018) Sertraline, paroxetine, and chlorpromazine are rapidly acting anthelmintic drugs capable of clinical repurposing. Sci Rep 8:1–17. https://doi.org/10.1038/s41598-017-18457-w

Weng HB, Chen HX, Wang MW (2018) Innovation in neglected tropical disease drug discovery and development. Infect Dis Poverty 7:1–9. https://doi.org/10.1186/s40249-018-0444-1

White AC, Coyle CM, Rajshekhar V et al (2018) Diagnosis and treatment of neurocysticercosis: 2017 clinical practice guidelines by the Infectious Diseases Society of America (IDSA) and the American Society of Tropical Medicine and Hygiene (ASTMH). Am J Trop Med Hyg 98:945–966. https://doi.org/10.4269/ajtmh.18-88751

World Health Organization (1995) WHO model prescribing information: drugs used in parasitic diseases, 2nd edn. World Health Organization

World Health Organization (2002) Report of the WHO informal consultation on the use of praziquantel during pregnancy/lactation and albendazole/mebendazole in children under 24 months

World Health Organization (2006) Preventive chemotherapy in human helminthiasis: coordinated use of anthleminthic drugs in control interventions

World Health Organization (2013) Schistosomiasis: control report 2001–2011 and strategic plan 2012–2020

World Health Organization (2016) Guidelines for stopping mass drug administration and verifying elimination of human onchocerciasis

World Health Organization (2017a) Guideline: preventive chemotherapy to control soil-transmitted helminth infections in at-risk population groups

World Health Organization (2017b) Guideline: alternative mass drug administration regimens to eliminate lymphatic filariasis. World Health Organization

Wu V-C, Huang J-W, Lien H-C et al (2006) Levamisole-induced multifocal inflammatory leukoencephalopathy. Medicine (Baltimore) 85:203–213. https://doi.org/10.1097/01.md.0000230250.95281.60

Zaha O, Hirata T, Kinjo F et al (2002) Efficacy of ivermectin for chronic strongyloidiasis: two single doses given 2 weeks apart. J Infect Chemother 8:94–98. https://doi.org/10.1007/s101560200013

Zheng R (1995) Differential diagnosis of delayed encephalopathy induced by anthelmintic imidazoles. Zhonghua Nei Ke Za Zhi 34:468–471

Zwang J, Olliaro P (2017) Efficacy and safety of praziquantel 40 mg/kg in preschool-aged and school-aged children: a meta-analysis. Parasit Vectors:1–16. https://doi.org/10.1186/s13071-016-1958-7

Zwang J, Olliaro PL (2018) Clinical efficacy and tolerability of praziquantel for intestinal and urinary schistosomiasis – a meta-analysis of comparative and non-comparative clinical trials. PLoS Negl Trop Dis 8:e3286. https://doi.org/10.1371/journal.pntd.0003286

Therapeutics for Inflammatory Bowel Diseases in Children and Adolescents: A Focus on Biologics and an Individualized Treatment Paradigm

Suruchi Batra and Laurie S. Conklin

Contents

Abstract

Pharmacologic treatment of children and adolescents with inflammatory bowel diseases (IBD) [Crohn's disease and ulcerative colitis] requires consideration of disease and medication effects on growth and nutrition, the importance of

S. Batra
Division of Gastroenterology, Hepatology, and Nutrition, Children's National Medical Center, Washington, DC, USA
e-mail: sbatra@childrensnational.org

L. S. Conklin (✉)
George Washington University School of Medicine, Children's National Medical Center, Washington, DC, USA
e-mail: LConklin@childrensnational.org

W. Kiess et al. (eds.), *Pediatric Pharmacotherapy*,
Handbook of Experimental Pharmacology 261, https://doi.org/10.1007/164_2019_255

durability of biologics, and concerns for long-term sequelae of disease and therapies. Achieving early remission in children with Crohn's disease correlates with improved outcomes and therefore allows a window of opportunity for maximizing growth. Thus, there is a great need to treat children and adolescents with the right drug at the right time while achieving adequate exposure. Improved understanding of disease phenotypes, disease natural history, and risk stratification will play a critical role in treatment selection for children, particularly as more therapeutic options become available. Here we summarize data supporting newer concepts of treating the individual child with IBD through targeted early biologic treatment, including utilization of therapeutic drug monitoring to optimize treatment effects and the use of early antitumor necrosis factor (TNF)-α therapies to mitigate long-term sequelae of the disease. Recent inception cohort studies provide important data regarding the risk stratification of children and adolescents with IBD, which support a move toward a personalized therapeutic approach to IBD in children and adolescents.

Keywords
Biologics · Crohn's disease · Inflammatory bowel diseases · Pediatrics · Therapeutics · Ulcerative colitis

1 Introduction

Inflammatory bowel diseases (IBD) are chronic inflammatory diseases of the gastrointestinal tract, which include Crohn's disease (CD) and ulcerative colitis (UC). Clinical manifestations, evolution of the disease, and prognosis are variable. CD may manifest as three different subtypes: inflammatory, penetrating, or stricturing disease. The latter two types may result in life-altering complications including fistulae, abscesses, bowel perforation, bowel obstruction, and intra-abdominal sepsis (Kugathasan et al. 2017). Inflammation in UC is confined to the large intestine; manifestations include hematochezia, anemia, and fatigue. Both are systemic diseases, however, with extraintestinal manifestations affecting approximately one third of patients. IBD is particularly challenging for children and adolescents due to long-term complications, including malnutrition, decreased bone health, and growth failure (Pappa et al. 2011; Gasparetto and Guariso 2014).

Average age of onset follows a bimodal distribution, which peaks in adolescence and middle age. About one quarter of IBD patients are diagnosed prior to 20 years of age (Rosen et al. 2015). The incidence of IBD in children less than 5 years of age has been shown to be rapidly increasing (Benchimol et al. 2017). The approach to treatment of children with IBD has changed in recent years, with increasing knowledge of the disease course, prognosis, and new revelations into optimizing treatment.

2 Treatment Goals in Pediatric IBD

Historically, the treatment target in pediatric IBD was control of symptoms via a step-up approach. Treatment was initiated with a course of glucocorticoids and 5-aminosalicylates. If 5-aminosalicylates failed to maintain symptom-free remission, symptoms were managed with additional glucocorticoids, and maintenance treatment was escalated to immunomodulators, biologics, or a combination. Surgical management was reserved for refractory patients.

It is increasingly appreciated that symptoms and clinical disease indices in children with CD correlate poorly with endoscopic disease activity, while endoscopic healing correlates with improved long-term outcomes for patients, including lower corticosteroid use and decreased hospitalizations (Carman et al. 2019; Kerur et al. 2017; Bossuyt et al. 2019; Colombel et al. 2011; Seow et al. 2010; Maser et al. 2006). Thus, the treatment target in pediatric IBD has evolved from isolated symptom control to an emphasis on endoscopic remission. Mucosal or endoscopic healing has been defined as lack of visible findings on colonoscopy (typically a Mayo score of 0 or 1 in trials), which differs from the absence of histologic findings on biopsies (Lega and Dubinsky 2018). An active area of study, histologic healing and bowel damage are also being considered treatment targets correlated with improved outcomes. Indeed, it has been demonstrated that endoscopically assessed mucosal healing does not eliminate the possibility of progression to bowel damage; in children with CD, residual transmural inflammation often persists despite mucosal healing on endoscopy (Weinstein-Nakar et al. 2018). In addition to endoscopic remission, growth and nutrition optimization, as well as bone health, are important clinical outcome measures, particularly in children and adolescents with CD.

The new treatment paradigm for pediatric IBD focuses on a goal of "deep remission" for ongoing treatment. Disease response is based on clinical response or daily symptoms of disease, serum/fecal biomarkers, and endoscopic evaluation to assess for endoscopic and histologic healing. Patients with IBD are monitored regularly at outpatient clinical visits, at least three to four times per year. These visits allow for assessment of clinical symptoms and biomarkers. There is currently no established guideline regarding the need for surveillance endoscopy and colonoscopy in pediatrics. However, more pediatric gastroenterologists are advocating for surveillance endoscopy and colonoscopy 6–12 months after treatment initiation, following the adult treat-to-target paradigm (Peyrin-Biroulet et al. 2015; Lega and Dubinsky 2018).

Complication-free survival in children with inflammatory CD is increased by early anti-TNFα therapy (Kugathasan et al. 2017). In children with newly diagnosed CD, early monotherapy with biologics, specifically anti-TNFα therapy, was demonstrated to be superior to early treatment with an immunomodulator and corticosteroids and facilitates catch-up growth (Walters et al. 2014; Church et al. 2014). Treatment with concomitant anti-TNFα and immunomodulator therapy has been shown to improve durability and reduce formation of antibodies to infliximab (Cheng et al. 2017; Chi et al. 2018). Proactive infliximab monitoring has also been shown to be a strategy to prevent antibody formation (Lega et al. 2019).

Despite these strategies, early anti-TNFα therapy has not been shown to prevent surgery or complications in stricturing CD and doesn't prevent colectomy in all children with severe, refractory UC (Kugathasan et al. 2017; Kerur et al. 2018; Hyams et al. 2017).

Variation in disease course and response to therapy underscore the growing appreciation for an individualized treatment paradigm for pediatric IBD and need for careful objective assessment of disease following treatment. In addition, it highlights the need for additional therapies for children with refractory inflammatory disease and fibrotic, stricturing disease.

3 Personalized Optimization of Biologics

The utilization of an individualized treatment paradigm is perhaps best illustrated through the use of biologics in pediatric IBD. Biologics used to treat IBD are monoclonal antibodies targeting components in the pathogenesis of IBD, although not all biologics have FDA approval for use in children or adolescents. Biologics used to treat IBD are summarized in Table 1. Anti-TNFα therapies are used as first-line treatment for severe disease or disease that is nonresponsive or poorly controlled by other medications. This class of medications offers various advantages improved efficacy in severe disease, ability to utilize therapeutic drug monitoring (TDM), and potential to mitigate long-term sequelae of poorly controlled IBD in children, such as decreased bone health and growth delay (Thayu et al. 2008; Church et al. 2014; Griffin et al. 2015).

3.1 Therapeutic Drug Concentrations and Achieving Adequate Exposure in Children

The pharmacokinetics of monoclonal antibodies is variable, and doses needed to achieve target serum concentrations are difficult to predict. TDM may be used to assess serum drug concentrations to guide dose adjustments. Several studies have established that consistent anti-TNFα serum drug concentrations are correlated with higher rates of clinical and endoscopic remission in children and adults (Ungar et al. 2016; van Hoeve et al. 2018; van de Casteele et al. 2018). The American Gastroenterology Association has established guidelines for target serum concentrations for adult IBD patients during maintenance anti-TNFα treatment: infliximab serum concentration of $\geq$5 mg/dL and adalimumab serum concentration of $\geq$7.5 mg/dL (Feuerstein et al. 2017). One important challenge in the use of TDM is that target serum drug concentrations may vary with individual patient risk factors and severity of disease. For example, serum concentrations needed to close complex perianal fistulae are likely higher than those needed to maintain remission of luminal inflammatory disease (El-Matary et al. 2019). Patients with a higher inflammatory burden may require higher serum trough concentrations to achieve remission due to increased drug clearance (Fasanmade et al. 2011; Dotan et al. 2014).

Table 1 Summary of biologics used to treat inflammatory bowel disease

Generic name	Trade name	Target	Mechanism of action	Pediatrics FDA-approved?	IBD indication in adults
Infliximab	Remicade®	Chimeric monoclonal antibody against TNFα	Decreases TNFα-related inflammatory cascade	Yes, for CD and UC	CD, UC
Adalimumab	Humira®	Recombinant monoclonal antibody against anti-TNFα	Decreases TNFα-related inflammatory cascade	Yes (for CD only)	CD, UC
Certolizumab pegol	Cimzia®	Humanized antigen-binding fragment (Fab') of a monoclonal antibody that has been conjugated to polyethylene glycol	Decreases TNFα-related inflammatory cascade	No	CD
Golimumab	Simponi®	Binds to both soluble and transmembrane forms of TNFα	Decreases TNFα-related inflammatory cascade	No	UC
Vedolizumab	Entyvio®	Humanized monoclonal antibody to α4β7 integrin	Blocks α4β7 integrin interaction with cell adhesion molecules inhibiting leukocyte migration across endothelium	No	CD, UC
Ustekinumab	Stelara®	Antibody to p40 subunit of IL-12 and IL-23	Decreases IL-12- and IL-23-related pro-inflammatory cascade	No	CD

CD Crohn's disease, *UC* ulcerative colitis

3.2 Utilization of TDM: Reactive vs. Proactive Monitoring

Recent research highlights how TDM may be used to optimize serum concentrations of biologic medication for individual patients. TDM may be used as a "reactive" measure for IBD patients undergoing biologic treatment who may present with concerns for disease flare. In this setting, TDM is used to assess whether the patient has a low drug trough concentration associated with the onset of symptoms. Minar et al. (2016) demonstrated the utility of reactive TDM through assessment of 72 children with CD who presented with signs and symptoms concerning for loss of response to therapy. Twenty-five of 72 (35%) had sub-therapeutic concentrations and required dose escalation. Subsequent to dose escalation, there was significant improvement in remission rates at 6 months. However, relying on reactive TDM may prevent the ability to proactively optimize pharmacokinetics of infliximab. In a pediatric cohort of 50 patients with IBD on infliximab therapy, only a minority had a target trough concentration of 3 μg/mL at week 14. Most patients required more frequent infusions or higher dosing than standard therapy to achieve goal trough concentrations (Lega et al. 2019).

Proactive TDM requires obtaining TDM at set intervals during treatment, even in the absence of active symptoms. If concentrations are found to be suboptimal, they are then proactively optimized to ensure patients maintain a therapeutic drug concentration (Lega et al. 2019). Stronger consideration has been given to the use of proactive TDM as a strategy for personalized optimization of therapy. The Trough Concentration Adapted Infliximab Treatment (TAXIT) trial was a prospective randomized control trial in adults with IBD in which enrolled patients were dose optimized during infliximab induction dosing. Then patients were randomized to dosing based on concentration or dosing based on clinical status. The authors found no benefit to proactive TDM, but there is concern that this 1-year study may not have been long enough in duration to detect a difference in outcomes (van de Casteele et al. 2015). In contrast, other studies of both infliximab and adalimumab have retrospectively found proactive TDM allowed for early identification of patients with low trough concentrations and better probability of patients remaining on drug in remission (Vaughn et al. 2014; Papamichael et al. 2019). A recent meta-analysis found limited existing evidence to support an association between any TDM strategy and superior clinical remission rates but does support a cost-saving benefit for reactive TDM and suggests a potential benefit for anti-TNF durability with proactive TDM. Authors concluded that further longer-term studies are needed, particularly to evaluate proactive TDM and to generate data on other anti-TNF therapies, target drug concentrations during induction, and pediatric populations (Ricciuto et al. 2018).

An important question is whether proactive TDM will be equal or better than use of combination therapy (a biologic with immunomodulator, such as a thiopurine or methotrexate) as a strategy to increase drug concentration and prevent anti-drug antibody formation. In adults with treatment-naïve Crohn's disease, a combination of infliximab with a thiopurine has been demonstrated as superior to either use as monotherapy (Colombel et al. 2010). Combination therapy also optimizes pharmacokinetics and reduces antibodies in adult and pediatric studies (Colombel et al. 2018; Chi et al. 2018). Further studies are needed to compare long-term effectiveness, safety, and cost associated with biologic monotherapy with proactive TDM versus the use of concomitant biologics and immunomodulators.

3.3 PK Modeling and Dashboard Systems

Various clinical factors including anti-drug antibodies, elevated serum C-reactive protein, hypoalbuminemia, and male gender have been identified as risk factors for lower infliximab concentrations (Brandse et al. 2017; Buurman et al. 2015; Dotan et al. 2014). Pharmacokinetic (PK) modeling has emerged as a tool for drug concentration prediction and optimization. Using Bayesian statistics and modeling, dashboard systems may incorporate current clinical information to predict future drug concentrations and target appropriate dosing for an individual patient (Mould and Dubinsky 2015; Dubinsky et al. 2017). Such approaches are likely to provide a new avenue for individualizing biologic treatment optimization for pediatric IBD patients.

3.4 Prevention of Immunogenicity and Anti-drug Antibodies

The prevalence of circulating anti-drug antibodies (ADA) to anti-TNFα treatment is estimated to be between 8 and 60% of IBD patients and is associated with adverse drug reactions and loss of response (Nanda et al. 2013). Development of ADA has been associated with intermittent or inconsistent exposure to treatment and suboptimal serum drug concentrations (Lee et al. 2012). It has been suggestive that proactive TDM may improve the durability of infliximab monotherapy by maintaining higher infliximab concentrations entering into maintenance, ultimately either decreasing antibody formation or modulating the clinical impact of ADA (Lega et al. 2019). Further studies are needed to understand whether maintenance of adequate drug concentrations proactively will prevent clinically relevant complications of anti-drug antibodies.

4 Early Use of Anti-TNF Therapies in Children to Mitigate Long-Term Disease Consequences

4.1 Bone Health

Children with CD are at risk for decreased bone health. Associated risk factors include high levels of inflammation, low serum vitamin D, and albumin concentrations. Bone modeling, remodeling, and turnover are decreased in patients with pediatric IBD. At diagnosis, bone turnover markers are noted to be 30–50% of normal, and biopsies show low bone mineral density (Dubner et al. 2009).

Current guidelines recommend routine bone health screening with dual-energy X-ray absorptiometry as a baseline at diagnosis (Rufo et al. 2012).

Prospective studies have found improvement of trabecular bone mineral density and cortical structure improved by anti-TNFα treatment in children with CD (Dubner et al. 2009). Other studies have shown that bone turnover biomarkers serum insulin-like growth factor-1, bone-specific alkaline phosphatase, and n-terminal propeptide of type-1 collagen were found to increase after initiation of anti-TNF treatment in pediatric IBD (Thayu et al. 2008; DoBoer et al. 2018). These findings highlight the likely advantage of early initiation of anti-TNFα therapy in children with pediatric IBD with impaired bone health.

4.2 Growth

Borrelli et al. (2004) demonstrated improved weight and z-scores in a prospective trial of 18 children with CD after initiation of infliximab therapy. Population-based studies have shown that catch-up growth in pediatric IBD children occurs after initiation of anti-TNFα treatment (Crombé et al. 2011; Church et al. 2014). In a clinical trial of adalimumab in children with CD, this therapy significantly improved and normalized growth rate at weeks 26 and 52 in patients with baseline growth impairment (Walters et al. 2017). Therefore, early anti-TNFα treatment is an example of a personalized treatment intervention for children with CD and linear growth failure.

5 Risk Stratification of Disease Phenotypes and an Individualized Treatment Approach in Pediatric IBD

5.1 Risk Stratification in Crohn's Disease

Increasingly, studies of pediatric CD progression have highlighted the variable course of disease; patients at risk for severe disease or poor response to treatment may need more aggressive or targeted treatment. The RISK trial was a prospective inception cohort study of newly diagnosed children with CD, which aspired to create a risk stratification model. More than 1,800 patients, ages 6–17, were recruited at disease onset and prospectively followed for complications and response to therapies. Certain factors were positively correlated with development of severe CD including African-American race, older age and ASCA, and Cbir1 seropositivity. Notably, patients with a stricturing phenotype were not responsive to early anti-TNFα therapy (started in first 90 days) and had a terminal ileal signature with increased extracellular matrix genes, implying a different biologic process in these patients (Kugathasan et al. 2017). Plasma collagen type III alpha 1 chain has been identified as a biomarker of stricturing disease that may be useful for predicting the need for earlier surgery instead of early anti-TNFα therapy (Ballengee et al. 2018).

Perianal CD is a subset of CD defined as inflammation around or near the anus; manifestations include fissures, fistulae, skin tags, abscesses, and/or stenosis. Complex fistulae may involve the rectum and adjacent structures including the vagina and urinary bladder. The incidence of perianal CD is estimated to be about 13–62%. Anti-TNFα therapies have led to higher rates of clinical remission in perianal CD patients, and the American College of Gastroenterology recommends anti-TNFα treatment as a primary treatment for induction and remission of complex fistulizing perianal disease (Lichtenstein et al. 2018). A prospective, multicenter cohort study of children with newly diagnosed CD assessed clinical response of perianal CD to infliximab therapy; a trough concentration of 12.7 μg/mL predicted fistula healing at week 24 (El-Matary et al. 2019). These data support that higher serum drug concentrations may be required for closure of perianal fistulae and demonstrate an opportunity for tailoring biologic dosing to achieve a specific treatment goal.

5.2 Risk Stratification in UC

The Predicting Response to Standardized Pediatric Colitis Therapy (PROTECT) trial was a natural history study of 428 children with newly diagnosed UC designed to identify characteristics of disease associated with outcomes following standard-of-care therapy for pediatric UC. Clinical presentations ranged from 48% of children with mild-moderate disease treated only with mesalamine, 33% with moderate to severe disease treated initially with oral corticosteroids, and 21% with severe disease treated with intravenous corticosteroids. At 12 weeks, corticosteroid-free remission was achieved in 48% of patients in the mesalamine group, 33% in the oral corticosteroid group, and 21% in the intravenous corticosteroid group. Treatment escalation during the first 12 weeks (to anti-TNFα therapy, immunomodulators, colectomy) was required by 9 (7%) patients in the mesalamine group, 21 (15%) in the oral corticosteroid group, and 52 (36%) in the intravenous corticosteroid group. Eight patients, all of whom were initially treated with intravenous corticosteroids, underwent colectomy. Importantly, the need for biological therapy during the first 12 weeks was confined to those requiring IV steroids as first-line therapy. Moreover, the strongest predictor of corticosteroid-free remission by week 12 without the need for escalation to biologics was clinical response at 4 weeks, regardless of corticosteroid status. Thus, the study highlighted the importance of initial disease severity as a predictor of disease course. Additional risk factors for more severe disease in this population also included lower serum albumin, decreased eosinophils on rectal biopsies, and surface villiform changes on rectal biopsy (Hyams et al. 2017). Higher levels of serum perinuclear anti-neutrophil cytoplasmic antibodies (pANCA) were associated with more extensive disease (Spencer et al. 2018).

6 Conclusion

Recent studies in adults and pediatrics have demonstrated that targeting deep remission improves outcomes for pediatric IBD patients. Individualizing dosing of biologics has translated to improved outcomes for patients, considering clinical risk factors. Additionally, cohort studies in pediatric IBD have highlighted baseline phenotyping of patients to predict the severity of their course. These studies have led to a shift in the treatment paradigm for pediatric IBD, with increasing data demonstrating a need to focus therapeutic choices on individual patients and treatment goals rather than use of a broad, step-up approach for all patients. However, numerous questions remain, including ideal strategies for monitoring patients during induction and in remission. While studies have mainly been focused on anti-TNFα therapies, newer biologics are now approved for use in adults with IBD, with more promising candidates under development. Additional studies are needed to clarify dosing and safety of these drugs in children and adolescents and to understand how various new biologics can be targeted for use in the safest and most efficacious way, alone or in combination with other medications.

References

Ballengee CR, Stidham RW, Liu C et al (2018) Association between plasma level of collagen type III alpha 1 chain and development of strictures in pediatric patients with Crohn's disease. Clin Gastroenterol. pii: S1542-3565(18)30969-8. https://doi.org/10.1016/j.cgh.2018.09.008. [Epub ahead of print]

Benchimol EI, Bernstein CN, Bitton A et al (2017) Trends in epidemiology of pediatric inflammatory bowel disease in Canada: distributed network analysis of multiple population-based provincial health administrative databases. Am J Gastroenterol 112(7):1120–1134

Borrelli O, Bascietto C, Viola F et al (2004) Infliximab heals intestinal inflammatory lesions and restores growth in children with Crohn's disease. Dig Liver Dis 36(5):342–347

Bossuyt P, Baert F, D'Heygere F et al (2019) Early mucosal healing predicts favorable outcomes in patients with moderate to severe ulcerative colitis treated with golimumab: data from the real-life BE-SMART cohort. Inflamm Bowel Dis 25(1):156–162

Brandse JF, Mould D, Smeekes O et al (2017) A real-life population pharmacokinetic study reveals factors associated with clearance and immunogenicity of infliximab in inflammatory bowel disease. Inflamm Bowel Dis 23(4):650–660

Buurman DJ, Maurer JM, Keizer RJ et al (2015) Population pharmacokinetics of infliximab in patients with inflammatory bowel disease: potential implications for dosing in clinical practice. Aliment Pharmacol Ther 42(5):529–539

Carman N, Tomalty D, Church PC et al (2019) Clinical disease activity and endoscopic severity correlate poorly in children newly diagnosed with Crohn's disease. Gastrointest Endosc 89 (2):364–372

Cheng J, Hamilton Z, Smyth M et al (2017) Concomitant therapy with immunomodulator enhances infliximab durability in pediatric inflammatory bowel disease. Inflamm Bowel Dis 23 (10):1762–1773

Chi LY, Zitomersky NL, Liu E et al (2018) The impact of combination therapy on infliximab levels and antibodies in children and young adults with inflammatory bowel disease. Inflamm Bowel Dis 24(6):1344–1351

Church PC, Guan J, Walters TD et al (2014) Infliximab maintains durable response and facilitates catch-up growth in luminal pediatric Crohn's disease. Inflamm Bowel Dis 20(7):1177–1186

Colombel JF, Sandborn WJ, Reinisch W et al (2010) Infliximab, azathioprine, or combination therapy for Crohn's disease. N Engl J Med 362(15):1383–1395

Colombel JF, Rutgeerts P, Reinisch W et al (2011) Early mucosal healing with infliximab is associated with improved long-term clinical outcomes in ulcerative colitis. Gastroenterology 141(4):1194–1201

Colombel JF, Adedokun OJ, Gasink C et al (2018) Combination therapy with infliximab and azathioprine improves infliximab pharmacokinetic features and efficacy: a post hoc analysis. Clin Gastroenterol Hepatol. pii: S1542-3565(18)31024-3. https://doi.org/10.1016/j.cgh.2018.09.033. [Epub ahead of print]

Crombé V, Salleron J, Savoye G et al (2011) Long-term outcome of treatment with infliximab in pediatric-onset Crohn's disease: a population-based study. Inflamm Bowel Dis 17 (10):2144–2152

DoBoer MD, Lee AM, Herbert K et al (2018) Increases in IGF-1 after anti-TNF-α therapy are associated with bone and muscle accrual in pediatric crohn disease. J Clin Endocrinol Metab 103(3):936–945. https://doi.org/10.1210/jc.2017-01916

Dotan I, Ron Y, Yanai H et al (2014) Patient factors that increase infliximab clearance and shorten half-life in inflammatory bowel disease: a population pharmacokinetic study. Inflamm Bowel Dis 20(12):2247–2259

Dubinsky MC, Phan BL, Singh N et al (2017) Pharmacokinetic dashboard-recommended dosing is different than standard of care dosing in infliximab-treated pediatric IBD patients. AAPS J 19 (1):215–222

Dubner SE, Shults J, Baldassano RN et al (2009) Longitudinal assessment of bone density and structure in an incident cohort of children with Crohn's disease. Gastroenterology 136 (1):123–130

El-Matary W, Walters TD, Huynh HQ et al (2019) Higher postinduction infliximab serum trough levels are associated with healing of fistulizing perianal Crohn's disease in children. Inflamm Bowel Dis 25(1):150–155

Fasanmade AA, Adeodokun OJ, Blank M et al (2011) Pharmacokinetic properties of infliximab in children and adults with Crohn's disease: a retrospective analysis of data from 2 phase III clinical trials. Clin Ther 33(7):946–964

Feuerstein JD, Nguyen GC, Kupfer SS et al (2017) American gastroenterological association institute guideline on therapeutic drug monitoring in inflammatory bowel disease. Gastroenterology 153(3):827–834

Gasparetto M, Guariso G (2014) Crohn's disease and growth deficiency in children and adolescents. World J Gastroenterol 20(37):13219–13233

Griffin LM, Thayu M, Baldassano RN et al (2015) Improvements in bone density and structure during anti-TNF-α therapy in pediatric Crohn's disease. J Clin Endocrinol Metab 100 (7):2630–2639

Hyams JS, Davis S, Mack DR et al (2017) Factors associated with early outcomes following standardised therapy in children with ulcerative colitis. Lancet Gastroenterol Hepatol 2 (12):855–868

Kerur B, Litman HJ, Stern JB et al (2017) Correlation of endoscopic disease severity with pediatric ulcerative colitis activity index score in children and young adults with ulcerative colitis. World J Gastroenterol 23(18):3322–3329

Kerur B, Machan JT, Shapiro JM et al (2018) Biologics delay progression of Crohn's disease, but not early surgery, in children. Clin Gastroenterol Hepatol 16(9):1467–1473

Kugathasan S, Denson LA, Walters TD et al (2017) Prediction of complicated disease course for children newly diagnosed with Crohn's disease: a multicentre inception cohort study. Lancet 389(10080):1710–1718. https://doi.org/10.1016/S0140-6736(17)30317-3. Epub 2017 Mar 2

Lee LYW, Sanderson JD, Irving PM (2012) Anti-infliximab antibodies in inflammatory bowel disease: prevalence, infusion reactions, immunosuppression and response, a meta-analysis. Eur J Gastroenterol Hepatol 24(9):1078–1085

Lega S, Dubinsky MC (2018) What are the targets of inflammatory bowel disease management. Inflamm Bowel Dis 24(8):1670–1675

Lega S, Phan BL, Rosenthal CJ et al (2019) Proactively optimized infliximab monotherapy is as effective as combination therapy in IBD. Inflamm Bowel Dis 25(1):134–141

Lichtenstein GR, Loftus EV, Isaacs KL et al (2018) ACG clinical guideline: management of crohn's disease in adults. Am J Gastroenterol 113(4):481–517

Maser EA, Villela R, Silverberg MS et al (2006) Association of trough serum infliximab to clinical outcome after scheduled maintenance treatment for Crohn's disease. Clin Gastroenterol Hepatol 4(10):1248–1254

Minar P, Saeed SA, Afreen M et al (2016) Practical use of infliximab concentration monitoring in pediatric Crohn disease. J Pediatr Gastroenterol Nutr 62(5):715–722

Mould DR, Dubinsky MC (2015) Dashboard systems: pharmacokinetic/pharmacodynamic mediated dose optimization for monoclonal antibodies. J Clin Pharmacol 55(Suppl 3):S51–S59

Nanda KS, Chiefetz AS, Moss AC (2013) Impact of antibodies to infliximab on clinical outcomes and serum infliximab levels in patients with inflammatory bowel disease (IBD): a meta-analysis. Am J Gastroenterol 108(1):40–47

Papamichael K, Juncadella A, Wong D et al (2019) Proactive therapeutic drug monitoring of adalimumab is associated with better long-term outcomes compared to standard of care in patients with inflammatory bowel disease. J Crohns Colitis. https://doi.org/10.1093/ecco-jcc/jjz018. [Epub ahead of print]

Pappa H, Thayu M, Sylvester F et al (2011) Skeletal health of children and adolescents with inflammatory bowel disease. J Pediatr Gastroenterol Nutr 53(1):11–25

Peyrin-Biroulet L, Sandborn W, Sands BE et al (2015) Selecting therapeutic targets in inflammatory bowel disease (STRIDE): determining therapeutic goals for treat-to-target. Am J Gastroenterol 110(9):1324–1338

Ricciuto A, Dhaliwal J, Walters TD et al (2018) Clinical outcomes with therapeutic drug monitoring in inflammatory bowel disease: a systematic review with meta-analysis. J Crohns Colitis 12 (11):1302–1315

Rosen MJ, Dhawan A, Saeed SA (2015) Inflammatory bowel disease in children and adolescents. JAMA Pediatr 169(11):1053–1060

Rufo PA, Denson LA, Sylvester FA et al (2012) Health supervision in the management of children and adolescents with IBD: NASPGHAN recommendations. J Pediatr Gastroenterol Nutr 55 (1):93–108

Seow CH, Newman A, Irwin SP et al (2010) Trough serum infliximab: a predictive factor of clinical outcome for infliximab treatment in acute ulcerative colitis. Gut 59(1):49–54

Spencer EA, Davis SM, Mack DR et al (2018) Serologic reactivity reflects clinical expression of ulcerative colitis in children. Inflamm Bowel Dis 24(6):1334–1343

Thayu M, Leonard MB, Hyams JS et al (2008) Improvement in biomarkers of bone formation during infliximab therapy in pediatric Crohn's disease: results of the REACH study. Clin Gastroenterol Hepatol 6(12):1378–1384

Ungar B, Levy I, Yavne Y et al (2016) Optimizing anti-TNF-α therapy: serum levels of infliximab and adalimumab are associated with mucosal healing in patients with inflammatory bowel diseases. Clin Gastroenterol Hepatol 14(4):550–557

van de Casteele N, Ferrante M, Van Assche G et al (2015) Trough concentrations of infliximab guide dosing for patients with inflammatory bowel disease. Gastroenterology 148 (7):1320–1329

van de Casteele N, Jeyarajah J, Jairath V et al (2018) Infliximab exposure-response relationship and thresholds associated with endoscopic healing in patients with ulcerative colitis. Clin Gastroenterol Hepatol. pii: S1542-3565(18)31200-X. https://doi.org/10.1016/j.cgh.2018.10.036. [Epub ahead of print] van Hoeve K, Dreesen E, Hoffman I et al (2018) Higher infliximab trough levels are associated with better outcome in paediatric patients with inflammatory bowel disease. J Crohns Colitis 12 (11):1316–1325

Vaughn BP, Martinez-Vazquez M, Patwardhan VR et al (2014) Proactive therapeutic concentration monitoring of infliximab may improve outcomes for patients with inflammatory bowel disease: results from a pilot observational study. Inflamm Bowel Dis 20(11):1996–2003

Walters TD, Kim MO, Denson LA et al (2014) Increased effectiveness of early therapy with anti-tumor necrosis factor-α vs an immunomodulator in children with Crohn's disease. Gastroenterology 146(2):383–391

Walters TD, Faubion WA, Griffiths AM et al (2017) Growth impairment with adalimumab treatment in children with moderately to severely active Crohn's disease. Inflamm Bowel Dis 23(6):967–975

Weinstein-Nakar I, Focht G, Church P et al (2018) Associations among mucosal and transmural healing and fecal level of calprotectin in children with Crohn's disease. Clin Gastroenterol Hepatol 16(7):1089–1097

Chronic Functional Constipation in Infants and Children

Gunter Flemming

Contents

Abstract

Functional constipation is a common problem among children. The prevalence worldwide is about 3% and it is accounting for about 3–5% of all visits to pediatricians implicating a significant impact on health care cost. In most children presenting with the symptom constipation no underlying medical disease responsible for the symptom can be found; this is the so-called functional constipation. Functional constipation is characterized by infrequent bowel movements, hard and/or large stools, painful defecation, sometimes in combination with fecal incontinence, and is often accompanied by abdominal pain, without evidence of a structural or biochemical explanation.

The recommendation for the management of FC includes a normal intake of fibers and fluids, normal physical activity, and an additional pharmacologic treatment for fecal disimpaction followed by a pharmacologic maintenance therapy.

In infants constipation is treated somewhat differently as compared with children. When constipation presents early in life, the risk of an underlying organic disease is increased compared to older children.

G. Flemming (✉)
Hospital for Children and Adolescents, Leipzig University, Leipzig, Germany
e-mail: gunter.flemming@medizin.uni-leipzig.de

W. Kiess et al. (eds.), *Pediatric Pharmacotherapy*,
Handbook of Experimental Pharmacology 261, https://doi.org/10.1007/164_2019_223

Keywords
Functional constipation · Osmotic laxatives · Rectal disimpaction · Stimulant laxatives

1 Introduction

Functional constipation is a common problem among children. The prevalence worldwide is about 3% (van den Berg et al. 2006), and it is accounting for about 3–5% of all visits to pediatricians (Thompson et al. 1999) implicating a significant impact on healthcare cost (Liem et al. 2009). In most children presenting with the symptom constipation with no underlying medical disease responsible for the symptom found, this is the so-called functional constipation (Tabbers et al. 2014). Functional constipation is characterized by infrequent bowel movements, hard and/or large stools, and painful defecation, sometimes in combination with fecal incontinence, and is often accompanied by abdominal pain, without evidence of a structural or biochemical explanation (Thompson et al. 1999; Dehghani et al. 2015).

Diagnostic criteria for functional constipation in children and adolescents were updated in 2016 with the Rome IV criteria (Hyams et al. 2016). Diagnostic criteria for functional constipation must include two or more of the following occurring at least once per week for a minimum of 1 month with insufficient criteria for a diagnosis of irritable bowel syndrome:

1. Two or fewer defecations in the toilet per week in a child of a developmental age of at least 4 years
2. At least one episode of fecal incontinence per week
3. History of retentive posturing or excessive volitional stool retention
4. History of painful or hard bowel movements
5. Presence of a large fecal mass in the rectum
6. History of large diameter stools that can obstruct the toilet

AND After appropriate evaluation, the symptoms cannot be fully explained by another medical condition.

According to the Rome IV criteria for functional constipation, the following alarm signs, symptoms, and diagnostic clues should be used to identify an underlying disease responsible for the constipation (Hyams et al. 2016), inevitably resulting in further evaluation (Table 1).

Fecal incontinence (also known as encopresis or soiling) is defined by repetitive passage of stool (voluntary or involuntary) in children 4 years of age and older, at which time a child may be reasonably expected to have completed toilet training and to exercise bowel control. Fecal incontinence is usually associated with chronic constipation and functional fecal retention. However, it may occur in the absence of fecal retention, in which case it is termed nonretentive fecal incontinence.

Table 1 Potential alarm features in constipation (Hyams et al. 2016)

Potential alarm features in constipation
• Passage of meconium >48 h in a term newborn constipation starting in the first month of life
• Family history of Hirschsprung's disease
• Explosive stools
• Ribbon stools
• Blood in the stools in the absence of anal fissures
• Failure to thrive
• Bilious vomiting
• Severe abdominal distension
• Abnormal thyroid gland
• Abnormal position of the anus
• Absent anal or cremasteric reflex
• Decreased lower extremity strength/tone/reflex
• Sacral dimple
• Tuft of hair on spine
• Gluteal cleft deviation
• Anal scars
• Anorectal malformations

Diagnostic Criteria for nonretentive fecal incontinence according to Rome IV (Hyams et al. 2016).

At least a 1-month history of the following symptoms in a child with a developmental age older than 4 years:

1. Defecation into places inappropriate to the sociocultural context.
2. No evidence of fecal retention.
3. After appropriate medical evaluation, the fecal incontinence cannot be explained by another medical condition.

2 General Considerations for the Treatment

The recommendation for the management of FC includes a normal intake of fibers and fluids, normal physical activity, and an additional pharmacologic treatment for fecal disimpaction followed by a pharmacologic maintenance therapy (Tabbers et al. 2014).

In infants constipation is treated somewhat differently as compared with children. When constipation presents early in life, the risk of an underlying organic disease is increased compared to older children (Nurko and Zimmerman 2014). So the clinician should be alert for evidence of organic disease, including cystic fibrosis and Hirschsprung's disease (Tabbers et al. 2014).

3 Specific Pharmaceutical Treatment

The recommendations for pharmaceutical treatment of functional constipation in infants are similar to that in children, but there are some important differences in treatment decisions for infants:

- Osmotic laxatives such as lactulose or sorbitol are frequently used and are usually effective in infants (Nurko and Zimmerman 2014).
- The use of polyethylene glycol without electrolytes (PEG-3350) for infants and toddlers <24 months of age was reported in two small case series (Loening-Baucke et al. 2004; Michail et al. 2004). The treatment was generally effective, and no adverse effects were noted in. But because of the limited data published for infants treated with PEG, safety is less well established than with older age groups.
- Some of the recommended pharmaceuticals for older children with FC are not well investigated in infants, and others are contraindicated in this age group (e.g., mineral oil because of the risk of aspiration) (Tabbers et al. 2014).

3.1 Disimpaction

Most of the children with chronic constipation have fecal impaction and will need disimpaction of the rectum before beginning maintenance therapy (Tabbers et al. 2014; Borowitz et al. 2005).

Oral medications for disimpaction is suggested to be preferred over rectal therapy because this method is noninvasive and may help the child feel in control (Tabbers et al. 2014). However, the parents and child should be involved in the decision regarding the appropriate route (Gleghorn et al. 1991).

Disimpaction is mostly performed in the outpatient setting, but it is very important to assess the response to the regimen as soon as possible after it is completed. In severe cases, patients need a manual disimpaction under general anesthesia before beginning maintenance therapy.

3.1.1 Oral Medication

Polyethylene Glycol (PEG) 3350 and 4000

PEG (also macrogol named) is the basis of a number of laxatives, as well as for whole bowel irrigation and for bowel preparation before surgery or colonoscopy.

The actual guideline from ESPGHAN and NASPGHAN recommends oral PEG as first-line therapy for rectal disimpaction (Tabbers et al. 2014).

Structure

Polyethylene glycol (PEG) is a polyether compound. The structure of PEG is commonly expressed as $H\text{-}(O\text{-}CH_2\text{-}CH_2)_n\text{-}OH$. For initial disimpaction PEG 4000 (molecular weight 4,000 g/mol) and as ingredient in laxative PEG 3350 (molecular weight 3,350 g/mol) is most commonly used.

Mechanism of Action

Due to the high number of polar oxygen atoms of PEG, there is a high affinity to water by forming hydrogen bonds. Hence, PEG is highly hydrophilic. When given orally PEG binds more water in the stool, leading to expansion of the stool volume and a softening of the stool. So the stool is more lubricate and subsequently easier to evacuate.

Pharmacokinetics

PEG is not absorbed and does not undergo biotransformation, and the majority is eliminated with the stool.

Onset of action	Oral – 24–96 h
Absorption	Minimal (<0.28%) (Pelham et al. 2008)
Excretion	Feces (93%); urine (0.2%) (Pelham et al. 2008)

Clinical Trials

No placebo-controlled studies have evaluated the effect of oral laxatives or enemas on disimpaction. One study (90 participants) compared the effect of PEG to enemas but could not detect a difference in effect (Bekkali et al. 2009).

A double-blind uncontrolled study (40 participants) showed that the 3-day administration of polyethylene glycol (PEG) 3350 at a dose of 1 g/kg/day to 1.5 g/kg/day (maximum dose 100 g/day) successfully disimpacted 95% of children and was well tolerated (Youssef et al. 2002).

Dosing Recommendations (for Rectal Disimpaction)

PEG 3350 without electrolytes: Fecal disimpaction 1–1.5 g/kg/day dissolved in approximately 10 mL/kg body weight of water or flavored beverage (for a maximum of six consecutive days) (Tabbers et al. 2014).

PEG 3350 with electrolytes: 25 mL/kg/h to a maximum of 1,000 mL/h by nasogastric tube until stool appears clear or 20 mL/kg/h for 4 h/day (Tabbers et al. 2014).

Adverse Effects

Very common	Nausea, bloating, or feelings of fullness in the stomach/abdomen
Less often	Stomach/abdominal cramps, vomiting, and anal irritation

These adverse reactions are transient and usually subside rapidly. Isolated cases of urticaria, rhinorrhea, dermatitis, and (rarely) anaphylactic reaction have been reported which may represent allergic reactions.

Mineral Oil (Liquid Paraffin)

Oral mineral oil can be used as an alternative for initial disimpaction if PEG is not tolerated or not available (Tolia et al. 1993).

Structure

Mineral oil is any of various colorless, odorless, light mixtures of higher alkanes from a mineral source, particularly a distillate of petroleum.

Molecular formula	C_nH_{2n+2}
Molecular weight	230–700 g/mol

Mechanism of Action

Mineral oil is not absorbed by the intestines, and it functions as a lubricant. Furthermore it may also exert an osmotic effect when it is converted to fatty acids (Plunkett et al. 2007; Sharif et al. 2001).

Pharmacokinetics

Onset of action	Oral, 6–8 h; rectal, 2–15 min
Absorption	Minimal following oral or rectal administration
Distribution	Into intestinal mucosa, liver, spleen, and mesenteric lymph nodes
Excretion	Feces

Clinical Trials

One study (36 participants) compared PEG 3350 to oral-given mineral oil for disimpaction: patients in the lavage group had more frequent bowel movements and showed more effective clearance of abdominal and rectal lumps ($p < 0.01$) (Tolia et al. 1993).

In another study efficacy of mineral oil oral vs. rectal administration was investigated (80 participants). Efficacy of fecal disimpaction was not statistically different, but the patient compliance and family satisfaction were higher in the oral administration group (Farahmand et al. 2010).

Dosing Recommendations (for Rectal Disimpaction)

Oral	15–30 mL/year of age, up to 240 mL
Slow disimpaction	Children and adolescents – 3 mL/kg twice daily for 7 days (Pashankar 2005)

Adverse Effects

Mineral oil should not be used for infants, neurologically impaired children, and others at high risk for gastroesophageal reflux, because of risks of pneumonitis if the oil is aspirated (Zanetti et al. 2007; Bandla et al. 1999).

Gastrointestinal	Abdominal cramps, diarrhea, nausea, and oily rectal leakage (large doses)

3.1.2 Rectal Medication

Enemas are rectally administered fluid containing chemical agents that can influence gut motility, cause an osmotic effect, or both. Common adverse effects of enemas are abdominal pain and anorectal discomfort (Koppen et al. 2015).

In the most current consensus report on childhood functional constipation from ESPGHAN, an NASPGHAN oral disimpaction is preferred, because it is better tolerated by children than enemas (Tabbers et al. 2014; Philichi 2018).

Rectal disimpaction is a choice if oral medication is not tolerated or not available.

Bisacodyl

Bisacodyl is an organic compound that is used as stimulant laxative drugs. It stimulates the enteric nerves to cause colonic contractions (Hoekman and Benninga 2013).

Structure

Bisacodyl belongs to the group of diphenylmethanes.

Molecular formula	$C_{22}H_{19}NO_4$
Molecular weight	361.39 g/mol

Mechanism of Action

Bisacodyl is a prodrug. It has no significant direct physiological effect on the intestine. It is metabolized by gut bacteria into the active compound 4,4′-dihydroxydiphenyl-(2-pyridyl)methane (DPM, BPHM). This compound stimulates peristalsis by directly irritating the smooth muscle of the intestine, possibly the colonic intramural plexus, and so alters water and electrolyte secretion producing net intestinal fluid accumulation and laxation (Hoekman and Benninga 2013).

Pharmacokinetics

Onset of action (rectal)	0.25–1 h (suppository) and 5–20 min (enema) (Koppen et al. 2015)

Metabolism: Bisacodyl is metabolized to an active metabolite (4,4′-dihydroxydiphenyl-(2-pyridyl)methane (DPM, BPHM)). This conversion is mediated by the action of endogenous deacetylase enzymes found on the mucosa of the small intestine and colon (Friedrich et al. 2011).

Absorption	Oral, rectal; systemic, <5% (Wald 2003)
Excretion	BHPM – urine, bile (Friedrich et al. 2011)

Clinical Trials
No randomized clinical trials (RCT) reported for the use of bisacodyl for initial disimpaction.

One study used for the majority of the 37 participants bisacodyl for disimpaction (5-day course), with no reported failure of the initial therapy (Sondheimer and Gervaise 1982).

Dosing Recommendations (Tabbers et al. 2014)

Children 2–10 years	5 mg (1/2 suppository) once daily
Children >10 years and adolescents	5–10 mg (1/2 to 1 enema or suppository) once daily

Adverse Effects

<1%	Abdominal cramps (mild), electrolyte disturbance (metabolic acidosis or alkalosis, hypocalcemia), nausea, rectal irritation (burning), vertigo, vomiting

Sodium Docusate
Docusate sodium is the sodium salt of docusate, a dioctyl salt and an emollient laxative with stool-softening activity.

Structure
Sodium salt of docusate, a dioctyl salt

Molecular formula	$C_{20}H_{37}NaO_7S$
Molecular weight	444.559 g/mol

Mechanism of Action
Sodium docusate belongs to the group of so-called surfactants; they are intended to lower the surface tension of stool, thereby allowing water to more easily enter the stool and so making the stool more soft (Roerig et al. 2010).

Pharmacokinetics

Onset of action	Oral, 12–72 h; rectal, 2–15 min
Excretion	Feces (Gattuso and Kamm 1994)
Metabolism and transport effects	None known

Clinical Trials
No placebo-controlled trials for children

One study (80 participants) found no difference between PEG and rectal sodium docusate in efficacy for treating fecal impaction (Bekkali et al. 2009).

Dosing Recommendations

FDA-approved labeling information

Children 2 to <12 years, 100 mg per 5 mL, 100 mg (1 enema) once daily or 283 mg per 5 mL, 283 mg (1 enema) once daily; children ≥12 years and adolescents, 283 mg per 5 mL up to 3 times daily

Adverse Effects

Rectal administration	None reported

Sodium Phosphate

Sodium phosphate is a saline laxative that works by increasing fluid secretion in the intestine.

Structure

As laxative most often a mixture of monobasic sodium phosphate monohydrate and dibasic sodium phosphate is used.

Molecular formula	Monohydrate, $NaH_2PO_4 \cdot H_2O$; dihydrate, $NaH_2PO_4 \cdot 2H_2O$ or NaH_2PO_4 or H_2NaO_4P
Molecular weight	444.559 g/mol

Mechanism of Action

Sodium phosphate exerts an osmotic effect in the intestine by drawing water into the lumen of the gut, producing distention, and promoting peristalsis and evacuation of the bowel (Hoekman and Benninga 2013).

Pharmacokinetics

Onset of action	Cathartic, 3–6 h; rectal, 2–5 min
Absorption	Oral, ~1–20%; rectal, none
Excretion	Oral forms excreted in feces.

Clinical Trials

No placebo-controlled trials for children

In one pediatric study (96 participants), no statistically significant differences were found between milk and molasses enemas and sodium phosphate enemas (Hansen et al. 2011).

Dosing Recommendations (Tabbers et al. 2014)

1–18 years	2.5 mL/kg, max 133 mL/dose (monobasic sodium phosphate monohydrate 19 g and dibasic sodium phosphate heptahydrate 7 g per 118 mL delivered dose (133 mL))

Adverse Effects
Sodium phosphate enemas are associated with adverse effects including electrolyte abnormalities, metabolic acidosis, and dehydration (Ismail et al. 2000; Harrington and Schuh 1997).

Normal Saline (Sodium Chloride)
Normal saline is widely used as enema for rectal disimpaction, even in neonates.

Structure
NaCl 0.9%

Molecular formula	NaCl
Molecular weight	58.44 g/mol

Mechanism of Action
Fluid distension of the (proximal) colon has been suggested as a mechanism contributing to the generation of propagative motility and stool propulsion (Gomez et al. 2010).

Clinical Trials
No RCT trials for functional childhood constipation reported.

Dosing Recommendations (Tabbers et al. 2014)
Neonate <1 kg, 5 mL; >1 kg, 10 mL
>1 year 6 mL/kg once or twice/day (up to 20 mL/kDa/day)

Adverse Effects
For normal saline enema used in the recommended dosage, no adverse effects are reported.

However, for tap water hyponatremia (Meier et al. 1998) and for twice-normal saline, hypernatremic death has been reported (Schreiber and Stone 1999).

Mineral Oil (Liquid Paraffin)
Rectally administered mineral oil can be used for rectal disimpaction. For further information on mineral oil, see above (Sects. 3.1 and 3.1.1).

Clinical Trials

No RCT for functional childhood constipation reported.

Dosing Recommendations (Tabbers et al. 2014)

2–11 years	30–60 mL once a day
>11 years	60–150 mL once a day

Adverse Effects

Rectal use	Liquid paraffin may leak out of the anus, causing irritation or itching of the skin, and it may stain clothing or furniture (Koppen et al. 2015).

Glycerine/Glycerol

Glycerol can be used as a laxative when introduced into the rectum in suppository or small-volume enema form; it irritates the anal mucosa and induces a hyperosmotic effect (Weisman et al. 1983).

Structure

Glycerol is a simple polyol compound. Glycerol has three hydroxyl groups that are responsible for its solubility in water and its hygroscopic nature.

Molecular formula	$C_3H_8O_3$
Molecular weight	92.09 g/mol

Mechanism of Action

Osmotic dehydrating agent which increases osmotic pressure, draws fluid into colon, and thus stimulates evacuation (Weisman et al. 1983; Constipation Guideline Committee of the North American Society for Pediatric Gastroenterology H, Nutrition 2006)

Pharmacokinetics

Onset of action	Constipation – suppository, 15–30 min
Absorption	Rectal, poorly absorbed

Clinical Trials

No RCT for childhood constipation reported.

Dosing Recommendations

Rectal	Infants and children <2 years, suppository, 1 pediatric suppository once or 2–10 mL enema (Weisman et al. 1983)

Adverse Effects

Rectal	May cause rectal discomfort or a burning sensation (Weisman et al. 1983; Constipation Guideline Committee of the North American Society for Pediatric Gastroenterology H, Nutrition 2006)

3.2 Long-Term Use/Maintenance Therapy

3.2.1 Osmotic Laxatives

Polyethylene Glycol (PEG) 3350

According to the current guideline of NASPGHAN/ESPGHAN, oral PEG is still the first-line medication in maintenance therapy (Tabbers et al. 2014; Philichi 2018).

For further information on the drug, see Sect. 3.1.

Dosing Recommendations (Tabbers et al. 2014)

Maintenance therapy	0.2–0.8 mg/kg/day

Adverse Effects

Side effects include fecal incontinence (especially during disimpaction), flatulence, abdominal pain, nausea, and abdominal bloating.

Isolated cases of urticaria, rhinorrhea, dermatitis, and (rarely) anaphylactic reaction have been reported which may represent allergic reactions (Sari Gokay et al. 2018; Zhang et al. 2015; Wenande and Garvey 2016).

In patients predisposed to water and electrolyte balance disturbances (patients with impaired hepatic or renal function or patients taking diuretics), laboratory electrolyte checks should be considered (Koppen et al. 2015).

Lactulose

Lactulose is recommended in case PEG is not available. It is considered to be safe for all ages (Tabbers et al. 2014).

Mechanism of Action

Lactulose is a hyperosmolar agent that is not hydrolyzed by digestive enzymes in the small intestine and so poorly absorbed by the intestinal mucosa. In the colon, the disaccharide is fermented into hyperosmolar low molecular weight acids by intraluminal bacteria. This results in intraluminal water retention and a decrease in intraluminal pH, which induces an increase in colonic peristalsis. The bacterial fermentation also leads to formation of gas, which induces additional intestinal distension and increases peristalsis (Koppen et al. 2015; Hoekman and Benninga 2013).

Structure

Lactulose is a disaccharide (sugar) synthesized from fructose and galactose.

Molecular formula	$C_{12}H_{22}O_{11}$
Molecular weight	342.297 g/mol

Pharmacokinetics

Onset	Constipation – up to 24–48 h to produce a normal bowel movement
Absorption	Poor
Metabolism	Via colonic flora to lactic acid and acetic acid; requires colonic flora for drug activation
Excretion	Primarily feces; urine ($\leq 3\%$)

Clinical Trials

Cochrane reviews revealed that lactulose is less effective than liquid paraffin or PEG in outcomes of stool frequency per week, consistency, relief of abdominal pain, and need for additional medication (Gordon et al. 2013; Lee-Robichaud et al. 2010). No statistically significant difference in treatment success between lactulose and lactitol, lactulose and senna, or lactulose and dietary fiber has been found (Gordon et al. 2013).

Dosing Recommendations (Tabbers et al. 2014)

1–2 g/kg once or twice/day

Adverse Effects

Side effects of lactulose and lactitol are usually mild and include flatulence, abdominal pain, and abdominal bloating. Chronic use can lead to electrolyte balance disturbances (Koppen et al. 2015).

Magnesium Hydroxide (Also Known as "Milk of Magnesia")

The antacid magnesium hydroxide (also referred to as "milk of magnesia" in its suspension form) has a laxative effect and is used for this indication for many years.

Mechanism of Action

The laxative effect of magnesium hydroxide is considered to derive from the osmotic gradient that is caused by these poorly absorbed hyperosmolar agents (Koppen et al. 2015).

Pharmacokinetics

Onset of action	Laxative – 30 min to 6 h
Absorption	Oral – up to 30%
Excretion	Urine (up to 30% as absorbed magnesium ions); feces (as unabsorbed drug)

Clinical Trials

A randomized controlled (38 participants) open-label trial compared magnesium hydroxide to PEG: the two laxatives showed no difference in effectiveness for the treatment of constipation. However, due to its better acceptance, PEG proved to be a better option for treating chronic functional constipation (Gomes et al. 2011).

Another randomized controlled trial (75 participants) comparing magnesium hydroxide, PEG, and lactulose showed that the number of those who had defecation more than three times a week was significantly more in PEG group than two other groups ($p = 0.040$). Comparing the therapeutic results and satisfaction of the patients, it was concluded that PEG can be used as one of the best alternatives to treat constipation (Saneian and Mostofizadeh 2012).

Dosing Recommendations (Tabbers et al. 2014)

2–5 years	0.4–1.2 g/day, once or divided
6–11 years	1.2–2.4 g/day once or divided
12–18 years	2.4–4.8 g/day, once or divided

Adverse Effects

Side effects include diarrhea, hypotension, weakness, and lethargy. Contraindication for use: severe renal impairment (Koppen et al. 2015).

3.2.2 Stimulant Laxatives

Bisacodyl/Sodium Picosulfate

Both are organic compounds that are used as stimulant laxative drugs. They work directly on the colon to produce a bowel movement. They were recommended as second-line therapy in functional constipation (Tabbers et al. 2014).

Structure

Bisacodyl belongs to the group of diphenylmethanes.

Molecular formula	$C_{22}H_{19}NO_4$
Molecular weight	361.39 g/mol

Sodium Picosulfate

Molecular formula	$C_{18}H_{13}NNa_2O_8S_2$
Molecular weight	481.401 g/mol

Mechanism of Action

Bisacodyl and sodium picosulfate are prodrugs. They have no significant direct physiological effect on the intestine. They are metabolized by gut bacteria into the active compound 4,4′-dihydroxydiphenyl-(2-pyridyl)methane (DPM, BPHM). This compound is a stimulant of intestinal secretion and increases peristalsis in the gut (Hoekman and Benninga 2013; Manabe et al. 2009).

Pharmacokinetics

Onset of action	Oral – 6–12 h
Half-life	BHPM – ~8 h (Friedrich et al. 2011)
Absorption	Oral, rectal; systemic, <5% (Wald 2003)
Excretion	BHPM – urine, bile (Friedrich et al. 2011)

Clinical Trials

No RCT for childhood constipation reported.

Dosing Recommendations (Tabbers et al. 2014)

Bisacodyl

3–10 years	5 mg/day
>10 years	5–10 mg/day

Sodium Picosulfate

1 month–4 years	2.5–10 mg once/day
4–18 years	2.5–20 mg once/day

Adverse Effects

<1%	Abdominal cramps (mild), electrolyte disturbance (metabolic acidosis or alkalosis, hypocalcemia), nausea, vertigo, and vomiting

Senna (Also Known as Sennoside or Senna Glycoside)

Senna contains a variety of anthraquinones and is metabolized into its pharmacologically active metabolite by intestinal bacteria (Koppen et al. 2015; Hoekman and Benninga 2013).

It is recommended as second-line therapy in functional constipation (Tabbers et al. 2014).

Structure

Sennoside is anthraquinone derivatives and dimeric glycosides.

Molecular formula	$C_{42}H_{38}O_{20}$
Molecular weight	862.746 g/mol

Mechanism of Action

The metabolite of senna induces defecation by stimulating peristaltic activity on the intestine by direct action on intestinal mucosa or nerve plexus, while it inhibits absorption of water and electrolytes from the colon (Koppen et al. 2015; Hoekman and Benninga 2013).

Pharmacokinetics

Onset of action (oral)	Within 6–24 h
Metabolism	Hepatic
Excretion	Feces (via bile); urine

Clinical Trials

Only one pediatric study compared senna to PEG in children with anorectal malformations (28 participants). It was conducted as randomized controlled crossover design, including a washout period. This study was terminated early because the interim analysis showed a clear benefit toward senna ($p = 0.026$) (Santos-Jasso et al. 2017).

One crossover study compared senna with lactulose (21 participants) and found no statistically significant difference between the two agents in the number of patients passing stools of any kind each day (Perkin 1977).

Another study (37 participants) reported that liquid paraffin was more effective in comparison to senna for improving defecation frequency and fecal incontinence episodes; however, the evidence was of low quality (Sondheimer and Gervaise 1982).

Dosing Recommendations (Tabbers et al. 2014)

2–6 years	2.5–5 mg once or twice/day
6–12 years	7.5–10 mg/day
>12 years	15–20 mg/day

Adverse Effects

Side effects been reported: abdominal pain, nausea, diarrhea, and flatulence. Melanosis coli is also reported, but this has no medical significance.

In young children, senna may potentially cause severe diaper rash, blisters, and skin sloughing, and it should therefore only be used in children aged >1 year (Koppen et al. 2015; Hoekman and Benninga 2013; Spiller et al. 2003).

3.2.3 Fecal Softeners

Mineral Oil

For further information on mineral oil, see above (Sects. 3.1 and 3.1.1).

Clinical Trials

One study (160 participants) compared liquid paraffin with PEG and revealed no significant difference in treatment response (defined as an increase in bowel movements and a decrease in fecal incontinence frequency) between both groups (Rafati et al. 2011).

Another study (37 participants) reported that liquid paraffin was more effective in comparison to senna for improving defecation frequency and fecal incontinence episodes; however, the evidence was of low quality (Sondheimer and Gervaise 1982).

Dosing Recommendations as Maintenance Therapy (Tabbers et al. 2014)

1–18 years	1–3 mL/kg/day, once or divided, max. 90 mL/day

3.3 Novel Medications Under Investigation

Three medications used successfully for the treatment of adult constipation may have a future role in the management of childhood constipation. These medications are presently not recommended for use in children because of a lack of studies (Tabbers et al. 2014).

Linaclotide is an oligopeptide agonist of guanylate cyclase, acts locally in the intestine to increase fluid secretion and motility (Philichi 2018). So far no clinical trials in children reported.

Lubiprostone is a chloride channel activator, increases intestinal fluid secretion, and facilitates intestinal transit and passage of stool (Philichi 2018). One study (109 subjects completed the study) revealed that the mean spontaneous bowel movements frequency significantly increased compared with baseline at week 1 (3.1 vs. 1.5 SBMs/week, $P < 0.0001$) (Hyman et al. 2014). Lubiprostone was efficacious and well tolerated in children and adolescents with functional constipation.

Prucalopride is a highly selective serotonin 5-HT4 receptor agonist, influences peristalsis, and stimulates secretions (Philichi 2018).

Only one study was conducted in children. Efficacy and safety of prucalopride were assessed in 213 children (106 prucalopride, 107 placebo). It was concluded that prucalopride, although generally well tolerated, was not more effective than placebo in children with functional constipation (Mugie et al. 2014).

References

Bandla HP, Davis SH, Hopkins NE (1999) Lipoid pneumonia: a silent complication of mineral oil aspiration. Pediatrics 103:E19

Bekkali NL, van den Berg MM, Dijkgraaf MG et al (2009) Rectal fecal impaction treatment in childhood constipation: enemas versus high doses oral PEG. Pediatrics 124:e1108–e1115

Borowitz SM, Cox DJ, Kovatchev B et al (2005) Treatment of childhood constipation by primary care physicians: efficacy and predictors of outcome. Pediatrics 115:873–877

Constipation Guideline Committee of the North American Society for Pediatric Gastroenterology H, Nutrition (2006) Evaluation and treatment of constipation in infants and children: recommendations of the North American Society for Pediatric Gastroenterology, Hepatology and Nutrition. J Pediatr Gastroenterol Nutr 43:e1–e13

Dehghani SM, Kulouee N, Honar N et al (2015) Clinical manifestations among children with chronic functional constipation. Middle East J Dig Dis 7:31–35

Farahmand F, Eftekhari K, Modarresi V et al (2010) Comparing oral route paraffin oil versus rectal route for disimpaction in children with chronic constipation; a randomized control trial. Iran J Pediatr 20:291–296

Friedrich C, Richter E, Trommeshauser D et al (2011) Absence of excretion of the active moiety of bisacodyl and sodium picosulfate into human breast milk: an open-label, parallel-group, multiple-dose study in healthy lactating women. Drug Metab Pharmacokinet 26:458–464

Gattuso JM, Kamm MA (1994) Adverse effects of drugs used in the management of constipation and diarrhoea. Drug Saf 10:47–65

Gleghorn EE, Heyman MB, Rudolph CD (1991) No-enema therapy for idiopathic constipation and encopresis. Clin Pediatr (Phila) 30:669–672

Gomes PB, Duarte MA, Melo Mdo C (2011) Comparison of the effectiveness of polyethylene glycol 4000 without electrolytes and magnesium hydroxide in the treatment of chronic functional constipation in children. J Pediatr 87:24–28

Gomez R, Mousa H, Liem O et al (2010) How do antegrade enemas work? Colonic motility in response to administration of normal saline solution into the proximal colon. J Pediatr Gastroenterol Nutr 51:741–746

Gordon M, Naidoo K, Akobeng AK et al (2013) Cochrane review: osmotic and stimulant laxatives for the management of childhood constipation (Review). Evid Based Child Health 8:57–109

Hansen SE, Whitehill JL, Goto CS et al (2011) Safety and efficacy of milk and molasses enemas compared with sodium phosphate enemas for the treatment of constipation in a pediatric emergency department. Pediatr Emerg Care 27:1118–1120

Harrington L, Schuh S (1997) Complications of Fleet enema administration and suggested guidelines for use in the pediatric emergency department. Pediatr Emerg Care 13:225–226

Hoekman DR, Benninga MA (2013) Functional constipation in childhood: current pharmacotherapy and future perspectives. Expert Opin Pharmacother 14:41–51

Hyams JS, Di Lorenzo C, Saps M et al (2016) Functional disorders: children and adolescents. Gastroenterology. https://doi.org/10.1053/j.gastro.2016.02.015

Hyman PE, di Lorenzo C, Prestridge LL et al (2014) Lubiprostone for the treatment of functional constipation in children. J Pediatr Gastroenterol Nutr 58:283–291

Ismail EA, Al-Mutairi G, Al-Anzy H (2000) A fatal small dose of phosphate enema in a young child with no renal or gastrointestinal abnormality. J Pediatr Gastroenterol Nutr 30:220–221

Koppen IJ, Lammers LA, Benninga MA et al (2015) Management of functional constipation in children: therapy in practice. Paediatr Drugs 17:349–360

Lee-Robichaud H, Thomas K, Morgan J et al (2010) Lactulose versus polyethylene glycol for chronic constipation. Cochrane Database Syst Rev 7:CD007570

Liem O, Harman J, Benninga M et al (2009) Health utilization and cost impact of childhood constipation in the United States. J Pediatr 154:258–262

Loening-Baucke V, Krishna R, Pashankar DS (2004) Polyethylene glycol 3,350 without electrolytes for the treatment of functional constipation in infants and toddlers. J Pediatr Gastroenterol Nutr 39:536–539

Manabe N, Cremonini F, Camilleri M et al (2009) Effects of bisacodyl on ascending colon emptying and overall colonic transit in healthy volunteers. Aliment Pharmacol Ther 30:930–936

Meier DE, Foster ME, Guzzetta PC et al (1998) Antegrade continent enema management of chronic fecal incontinence in children. J Pediatr Surg 33:1149–1151; discussion 1151–1142

Michail S, Gendy E, Preud'Homme D et al (2004) Polyethylene glycol for constipation in children younger than eighteen months old. J Pediatr Gastroenterol Nutr 39:197–199

Mugie SM, Korczowski B, Bodi P et al (2014) Prucalopride is no more effective than placebo for children with functional constipation. Gastroenterology 147:1285–1295.e1281
Nurko S, Zimmerman LA (2014) Evaluation and treatment of constipation in children and adolescents. Am Fam Physician 90:82–90
Pashankar DS (2005) Childhood constipation: evaluation and management. Clin Colon Rectal Surg 18:120–127
Pelham RW, Nix LC, Chavira RE et al (2008) Clinical trial: single- and multiple-dose pharmacokinetics of polyethylene glycol (PEG-3350) in healthy young and elderly subjects. Aliment Pharmacol Ther 28:256–265
Perkin JM (1977) Constipation in childhood: a controlled comparison between lactulose and standardized senna. Curr Med Res Opin 4:540–543
Philichi L (2018) Management of childhood functional constipation. J Pediatr Health Care 32:103–111
Plunkett A, Phillips CP, Beattie RM (2007) Management of chronic functional constipation in childhood. Paediatr Drugs 9:33–46
Rafati M, Karami H, Salehifar E et al (2011) Clinical efficacy and safety of polyethylene glycol 3350 versus liquid paraffin in the treatment of pediatric functional constipation. Daru 19:154–158
Roerig JL, Steffen KJ, Mitchell JE et al (2010) Laxative abuse: epidemiology, diagnosis and management. Drugs 70:1487–1503
Saneian H, Mostofizadeh N (2012) Comparing the efficacy of polyethylene glycol (PEG), magnesium hydroxide and lactulose in treatment of functional constipation in children. J Res Med Sci 7:145–149
Santos-Jasso KA, Arredondo-Garcia JL, Maza-Vallejos J et al (2017) Effectiveness of senna vs polyethylene glycol as laxative therapy in children with constipation related to anorectal malformation. J Pediatr Surg 52:84–88
Sari Gokay S, Celik T, Yusuf Sari M et al (2018) Urticaria as a rare side effect of polyethylene glycol-3350 in a child: case report. Acta Clin Croat 57:187–189
Schreiber CK, Stone AR (1999) Fatal hypernatremia associated with the antegrade continence enema procedure. J Urol 162:1433; discussion 1433–1434
Sharif F, Crushell E, O'Driscoll K et al (2001) Liquid paraffin: a reappraisal of its role in the treatment of constipation. Arch Dis Child 85:121–124
Sondheimer JM, Gervaise EP (1982) Lubricant versus laxative in the treatment of chronic functional constipation of children: a comparative study. J Pediatr Gastroenterol Nutr 1:223–226
Spiller HA, Winter ML, Weber JA et al (2003) Skin breakdown and blisters from senna-containing laxatives in young children. Ann Pharmacother 37:636–639
Tabbers MM, DiLorenzo C, Berger MY et al (2014) Evaluation and treatment of functional constipation in infants and children: evidence-based recommendations from ESPGHAN and NASPGHAN. J Pediatr Gastroenterol Nutr 58:258–274
Thompson WG, Longstreth GF, Drossman DA et al (1999) Functional bowel disorders and functional abdominal pain. Gut 45(Suppl 2):II43–II47
Tolia V, Lin CH, Elitsur Y (1993) A prospective randomized study with mineral oil and oral lavage solution for treatment of faecal impaction in children. Aliment Pharmacol Ther 7:523–529
van den Berg MM, Benninga MA, di Lorenzo C (2006) Epidemiology of childhood constipation: a systematic review. Am J Gastroenterol 101:2401–2409
Wald A (2003) Is chronic use of stimulant laxatives harmful to the colon? J Clin Gastroenterol 36:386–389
Weisman LE, Merenstein GB, Digirol M et al (1983) The effect of early meconium evacuation on early-onset hyperbilirubinemia. Am J Dis Child 137:666–668
Wenande E, Garvey LH (2016) Immediate-type hypersensitivity to polyethylene glycols: a review. Clin Exp Allergy 46:907–922
Youssef NN, Peters JM, Henderson W et al (2002) Dose response of PEG 3350 for the treatment of childhood fecal impaction. J Pediatr 141:410–414

Zanetti G, Marchiori E, Gasparetto TD et al (2007) Lipoid pneumonia in children following aspiration of mineral oil used in the treatment of constipation: high-resolution CT findings in 17 patients. Pediatr Radiol 37:1135–1139

Zhang H, Henry WA, Chen LA et al (2015) Urticaria due to polyethylene glycol-3350 and electrolytes for oral solution in a patient with jejunal nodular lymphoid hyperplasia. Ann Gastroenterol 28:148–150

Psychiatric Diseases in Children and Adolescents

Gabrielle Sky Cardwell, Robert L. Findling, and Adelaide S. Robb

Contents

Abstract

Pharmacotherapy of psychiatric illnesses in children and adolescents has grown significantly over the last few decades. However, the body of research examining pharmacological treatments for psychiatric illnesses is much smaller in children and adolescents than it is in adults. As most treatments for psychiatric disorders are more effective if started early in the course of illness, treatment options for youth are especially important in order to ensure better treatment outcomes.

G. S. Cardwell · A. S. Robb (✉)
Department of Psychiatry, Children's National Health System, Washington, DC, USA
e-mail: AROBB@childrensnational.org

R. L. Findling
Department of Psychiatry and Behavioral Sciences, Johns Hopkins University School of Medicine, Baltimore, MD, USA

W. Kiess et al. (eds.), *Pediatric Pharmacotherapy*,
Handbook of Experimental Pharmacology 261, https://doi.org/10.1007/164_2019_262

This chapter discusses currently approved medications to treat psychiatric disorders in children and adolescents. Research on medications that may be effective treatments but are not yet FDA approved is also discussed. The medications are broken down into major categories used in youth with psychiatric disorders including antidepressants, mood stabilizers, ADHD medications, and antipsychotics.

Keywords
Antidepressants · Antipsychotics · Child psychiatry · Mood stabilizers · Pediatric psychopharmacology · Stimulant medications

1 Introduction

Medications to treat psychiatric disorders in children and adolescents are important treatment options and oftentimes should be considered as part of a comprehensive treatment plan. The current body of research on psychopharmacology has led to the FDA approval of a variety of medications used to treat psychiatric illnesses in youth. The aim of this chapter is to discuss the current body of research on psychopharmacology in children and adolescents and to present the pharmacological treatment options available in this population.

2 Antidepressants

Antidepressants are used to treat depression and anxiety disorders in children. The disorders discussed in this section include major depressive disorder (MDD), generalized anxiety disorder (GAD), obsessive-compulsive disorder (OCD), social anxiety disorder (SAD), separation anxiety disorder (SepD), and post-traumatic stress disorder (PTSD). Children diagnosed with MDD must have a 2-week period with at least five of the following symptoms that represent a change from previous functioning: (1) depressed mood by subjective report or as observed by others, (2) decreased interest or pleasure in most activities, (3) significant change in weight or appetite, (4) insomnia or hypersomnia, (5) psychomotor agitation or retardation, (6) fatigue or loss of energy, (7) feelings of worthlessness or guilt, (8) decreased concentration or indecisiveness, and (9) recurrent thoughts of death and dying. Symptoms must not be due to bereavement and must cause impairment in the child's daily function (APA 2013). A diagnosis of GAD requires at least 3 months of excessive anxiety and worry most days about two or more of the following: family, health, finances, or school (APA 2013). SAD is diagnosed in youth who show a marked and persistent fear of one or more social or performance situations in which a person is exposed to strangers or to scrutiny by others and worries about possibly doing something embarrassing (APA 2013). A child with SepD becomes anxious when away from family or their home (APA 2013). A child diagnosed with OCD has obsessions, compulsions, or both. Obsessions are recurrent thoughts, images, or impulses that are experienced as intrusive and inappropriate and cause anxiety or distress. Compulsions are repetitive behaviors (e.g., hand washing) or mental acts (e.g., praying, counting) that are done to neutralize an obsession or as part of following rigid rules. Finally, PTSD is an anxiety disorder that occurs after exposure to a traumatic event. The symptoms of PTSD fall under three categories: re-experiencing the trauma, avoidance and numbing, and increased arousal (APA 2013).

Antidepressant medications used to treat these disorders generally fall under the following major classes: selective serotonin reuptake inhibitors (SSRIs), serotonin and norepinephrine reuptake inhibitors (SNRIs), and tricyclic antidepressants (TCAs). The following sections will describe existing evidence for the use of antidepressants to treat mood and anxiety disorders in children. It is important to note that following the completion of a safety review of the use of nine antidepressants in pediatric populations (fluoxetine, sertraline, paroxetine, fluvoxamine, citalopram, bupropion, venlafaxine, and nefazodone), the FDA issued a boxed warning to indicate an increased risk of suicidal ideation and suicidal attempts in children and adolescents treated with certain antidepressants (Richmond and Rosen 2005). While none of the 4,400 trial participants in the FDA database completed suicide, it is recommended that clinicians closely monitor patients in the immediate weeks after initiating or increasing their dose of an antidepressant (Cheung et al. 2008; Dopheide 2006).

2.1 Selective Serotonin Reuptake Inhibitors (SSRIs)

SSRIs are the most commonly used antidepressants in pediatric populations due to their demonstrated efficacy, low side effect profile, and good tolerability. SSRIs are reported to be helpful in a variety of depressive and anxiety disorders including, but not limited to, MDD, GAD, and OCD. The six main SSRIs are fluoxetine, sertraline, fluvoxamine, citalopram, escitalopram, and paroxetine (Table 1).

Fluoxetine is the most studied SSRI in pediatric populations. Two double-blind, placebo-controlled trials found that children who received fluoxetine showed significantly greater decreases in depression scores than those treated with placebo (Emslie et al. 1997, 2002). These trials led to the FDA labeling of fluoxetine to treat MDD in youth ages 8–17 years. Fluoxetine is also effective in treating pediatric OCD and is FDA approved for OCD treatment in children ages 7–17 years (Geller et al. 2001; Riddle et al. 2001). Fluoxetine was found to be effective in treating anxiety disorders, SAD, GAD, and SepD as well (Birmaher et al. 2003). Long-term use of fluoxetine showed progressive improvement in anxiety symptoms after 6 months, compared to placebo (Clark et al. 2005).

Sertraline has been widely studied in pediatric anxiety and shows consistent benefits in treating children with OCD and OCD with comorbid tic disorder (Alderman et al. 1998; Cook et al. 2001; Garcia et al. 2010; Skarphedinsson et al. 2015; March et al. 2007b; Storch et al. 2013; The Pediatric OCD Treatment Study (POTS) Team 2004; Wagner et al. 2003b). Based on these trials, sertraline was

Table 1 SSRIs and SNRIs FDA indications and positive trials in pediatric population

Medication	FDA indication	Other positive trials	Daily dose (mg)	Schedule
SSRIs				
Fluoxetine	MDD (ages 8–17) OCD (ages 8–17)	SAD, GAD, SepD	10–60	QD
Sertraline	OCD (ages 6–17)	SAD, GAD, SepD	25–200	QD
Citalopram		MDD	10–40	QD
Escitalopram	MDD (ages 12–17)	SAD	5–20	QD
Fluvoxamine	OCD (ages 8–17)	MDD, SAD, GAD, SepD	25–300	QD
SNRIs				
Venlafaxine		MDD, SAD	37.5–300	QD
Desvenlafaxine			25–100	QD
Duloxetine	GAD (ages 7–17)	Chronic pain	30–120	QD
TCAs				
Clomipramine	OCD (ages 10–17)		25–200	QD or BID

FDA approved for the treatment of pediatric OCD in children ages 6–17 years (Alderman et al. 1998; March et al. 1998). Additional RCTs showed significant effects of sertraline in treating GAD, SAD, and SepD and borderline benefit in MDD compared to placebo (Compton et al. 2010; Rynn et al. 2001; Wagner et al. 2003a, b). However, sertraline was not effective in treating PTSD compared to placebo (Robb et al. 2010).

Citalopram was found to be effective in treating MDD and anxiety-induced recurrent abdominal pain in children (Campo et al. 2004; Roohafza et al. 2014; Wagner et al. 2004). Escitalopram (the active enantiomer of citalopram) is FDA approved for treatment of MDD in children between ages 12 and 17 years based on several large trials of children and adolescents (Emslie et al. 2009; Findling et al. 2013c; Von Knorring et al. 2006; Wagner et al. 2006a). An open-label trial of escitalopram for SAD in 20 children (age 10–17) showed significant response (CGI score ≤ 2) in 65% of the population after 12 weeks (Isolan et al. 2007).

Fluvoxamine received FDA approval for treatment of pediatric OCD in children age 8–17 after showing significant efficacy compared to placebo in a 10-week RCT (Riddle et al. 2001). In a large NIH trial of 128 youth with SAD, GAD, or SepD, fluvoxamine showed greater reduction in anxiety symptoms compared with placebo (Walkup et al. 2001). Fluvoxamine showed low evidence of benefit in the treatment of GAD and MDD in a combination trial (Gothelf et al. 2005).

Paroxetine has not shown efficacy over placebo in treating pediatric MDD (Berard et al. 2006; Emslie et al. 2006). Further, in the FDA's safety review of antidepressants, the increase in suicidal ideation was most significant in the paroxetine group, so the FDA added a contraindication warning for use of paroxetine in children (Richmond and Rosen 2005).

2.2 Serotonin and Norepinephrine Reuptake Inhibitors (SNRIs)

SNRIs are the second antidepressant group extensively studied in pediatric MDD and anxiety disorders. The SNRI group includes venlafaxine, desvenlafaxine, duloxetine, and levomilnacipran. None of the SNRIs are FDA approved for the treatment of pediatric MDD, but duloxetine is FDA approved for the treatment of pediatric GAD.

Venlafaxine was found to possibly be effective in treating adolescents with MDD ages 12–17 years, but not in children younger than 12 years based on two large randomized trials (Emslie et al. 2007). The TORDIA (treatment of resistant depression in adolescents) study demonstrated that venlafaxine was equal to other SSRI antidepressants in treating teens with resistant MDD (Brent et al. 2008) but was associated with a higher rate of secondary hypertension compared to SSRIs (Weihs et al. 2018). Venlafaxine has also been found to be effective in treating youth with SAD (March et al. 2007a). Desvenlafaxine was not found to be effective in treating pediatric MDD compared to placebo (Atkinson et al. 2018; Weihs et al. 2018). Duloxetine is FDA approved to treat GAD (Strawn et al. 2015) and was found to be effective in treating chronic pain disorder (Table 1; Kachko et al. 2011; Meighen 2007). However, duloxetine was not effective in treating pediatric MDD (Atkinson et al. 2014). Levomilnacipran pediatric trials are ongoing at the time of this publication.

2.3 Tricyclic Antidepressants (TCAs)

TCAs are known to be effective in treating adults with mood and anxiety disorders; however, they are used as a second-line treatment due to risk of serious side effects (Anderson 2000; Watson and Rees 2008). TCAs commonly used in pediatric populations are clomipramine and imipramine. Clomipramine was the first FDA-approved treatment for pediatric OCD (Anderson 2000). A recent meta-analysis found that clomipramine was more effective than SSRIs including fluoxetine, fluvoxamine, paroxetine, and sertraline in treating pediatric OCD (Varigonda et al. 2016). Imipramine is FDA approved for the treatment of nocturnal enuresis for children older than 6, but RCTs evaluating its effectiveness in treating anxiety related disorders have been mixed (Bernstein et al. 2000; Gittelman-Klein and Klein 1971; Klein et al. 1992).

3 Mood Stabilizers

The main psychiatric use of mood stabilizers in children is to treat pediatric bipolar disorder (BD). BD is a chronic and debilitating mood disorder, characterized by the presence of mixed/manic and/or depressive episodes (APA 2013). Mood stabilizers are a key psychopharmacologic intervention and include lithium, anti-epileptic drugs (AED), and antipsychotic medications (Tables 2 and 5).

Table 2 Lithium and AED FDA psychiatric indications and positive trials in youth

Medication	FDA indication	Other positive trials	Daily dose	Schedule
Lithium	BD (ages 7–17)		Initiate 600–900 mg daily Titrate to trough target level of 1.0 mEq/L Max dose: 40 mg/k/day	BID-TID
Valproic acid		BD	Initiate 125 mg BID and titrate up to max trough level of 125 ug/mL	BID
Lamotrigine		BD (add-on)	Initiate at 25 mg daily Max dose: 152–240 mg daily (initiate with lower doses if on valproic acid or <12 years of age)	BID
Carbamazepine		BD	Initiate 200 mg QPM May titrate up to 1,200 mg/day in divided doses	QPM
Topiramate		BD (showed possible benefit in post hoc analyses)	25–300 mg	QD
Oxcarbazepine		None	150–1,200 mg	BID

Lithium is the oldest and most studied mood stabilizer for the treatment of BD and was recently FDA approved for BD treatment in children ages 7–17 years based on the NICHD Collaborative Lithium Trials (CoLT) that showed the efficacy and safety of using lithium compared to placebo in children (Findling et al. 2015a). Lithium has been used alone or in combination with other medications to treat acute mania (Findling et al. 2005).

Antiepileptic drugs (AEDs) are also used off-label to treat BD. Studies examining the effectiveness of valproic acid (VA) to treat pediatric BD have yielded mixed results (Findling et al. 2005; Geller et al. 2012; Kowatch et al. 2015; Wagner et al. 2009; West et al. 2011). Carbamazepine was found to be effective and safe in treating children with BD in open-label trials (Joshi et al. 2010; Kowatch et al. 2000; Wagner et al. 2006a, b). Oxcarbazepine was not more effective than placebo in treating children with BD manic or mixed episodes (Findling and Ginsberg 2014). A double-blind discontinuation trial found that lamotrigine may be an effective add-on to treat pediatric BD in the 12–17-year-old age group in post hoc analyses (Findling et al. 2015a, b). Moreover, in a small open-label study, lamotrigine was found to be effective in the treatment of bipolar depression (Chang et al. 2006). Results on the effectiveness of topiramate in treating pediatric BD have been mixed (Barzman et al. 2005; DelBello et al. 2002, 2005).

4 ADHD Medications

4.1 Stimulants

For pediatric patients to be diagnosed with attention-deficit hyperactivity disorder (ADHD), the DSM-5 requires six or more persistent (at least 6 months in duration) symptoms of inattention and/or six or more persistent symptoms of hyperactivity-impulsivity that begin before age 12 and impair functioning in two of three settings: home, school (work if adult), and social (APA 2013).

Stimulants are the most frequently used medications for the treatment of ADHD in children and adolescents (National Institute of Mental Health 2016; Table 3). Both methylphenidate- and amphetamine-based products can improve core symptoms of inattention, hyperactivity, and impulsivity within 30 min of administration (Bradley 1937; Conners et al. 1967, 1969; Pelham et al. 1999). The most frequent side effects of stimulant medication include appetite suppression, sleep difficulties, transient headache, and increased heart rate or blood pressure. Less frequent side effects may include nausea, irritability, tics, and rarely, psychosis (Brown et al. 2018).

4.2 Other ADHD Treatments

When children and adolescents fail to respond to stimulant medication, experience significant side effects or if psychostimulant treatment may be either contraindicated or not desired, there are several non-stimulant medications that are effective for treating ADHD (Table 4). The selective norepinephrine reuptake inhibitor (SNRI) atomoxetine has demonstrated efficacy for ADHD with a modestly smaller effect size compared to stimulant treatments (Cheng et al. 2007; Faraone and Glatt 2010; Kratochvil et al. 2008). However, atomoxetine carries an FDA-required boxed warning for suicidality – though at rates lower than those seen in the antidepressants (Lilly USA LLC 2017). Clonidine and guanfacine are alpha-2 adrenergic agents that were initially developed as antihypertensives but have long-acting preparations that are effective in treating pediatric ADHD (Palumbo et al. 2008; Sallee et al. 2009). Both medications are available in short- and long-acting forms and can be used either alone or in conjunction with a stimulant (Kollins et al. 2011; Spencer et al. 2009).

5 Antipsychotics

Antipsychotic medications are generally divided into first-generation or "typical" antipsychotics and second-generation or "atypical" antipsychotics. There is less evidence for the use of first-generation antipsychotics (FGA), such as haloperidol, molindone, and pimozide, in the pediatric population, compared to the second-generation antipsychotics (SGA), including risperidone, quetiapine, olanzapine, and others (Amor 2012). The FDA approved several antipsychotics for the treatment of schizophrenia, BD, and irritability associated with autism spectrum disorder (ASD; Table 5).

Table 3 FDA-approved stimulant medications used in the treatment of ADHD in youth

Medication	Daily dose	Schedule
Dexmethylphenidate (Focalin)	2.5–10 mg	BID
Dexmethylphenidate (Focalin XR)	5–30 mg	QD
Methylphenidate (Methylin chewable tablets)	5–10 mg	BID or TID
Methylphenidate (Methylin solution)	5–10 mg	BID or TID
Methylphenidate (Ritalin)	5–10 mg	BID or TID
Methylphenidate (Ritalin SR)	20–60 mg	QD
Methylphenidate (Metadate ER)	20–60 mg	QD
Methylphenidate (Metadate CD)	20–60 mg	QD
Methylphenidate (Ritalin LA)	20–60 mg	QD
Methylphenidate (Concerta)	Children: 18–54 mg Adolescents: 18–72 mg	QD
Methylphenidate (Quillivant XR)	20–60 mg	QD
Methylphenidate (Quillichew ER)	20–60 mg	QD
Methylphenidate (Contempla XR-ODT)	17.3–51.8 mg	QD
Methylphenidate (Aptensio XR)	10–60 mg	QD
Methylphenidate (Adhansia XR)	25–70 mg	QD
Methylphenidate (Jornay PM)	20–100 mg	QPM
Methylphenidate (Daytrana)	10–30 mg patch	9 h QD
Amphetamine mixed salts (Adderall)	Children 3–5 years old: 2.5 mg QD Children ≥6 years old and adolescents: 5–10 mg	QD or BID
Amphetamine mixed salts (Adderall XR)	5–30 mg	QD
Amphetamine mixed salts (Mydayis)	Not for children under 13 years old Adolescents: 12.5–25 mg	QD
d- and *l*-amphetamine (Adzenys XR-ODT)	Children (6–12 years old): 6.3–18.8 mg Adolescents: 6.3–12.5 mg	QD
d- and *l*-amphetamine (Adzenys ER)	Children (6–12 years old): 6.3–18.8 mg Adolescents: 6.3–12.5 mg	QD
d- and *l*-amphetamine (Dyanavel)	2.5–20 mg	QD
d-amphetamine (Zenzedi)	Children 3–5 years old: 2.5 mg QD Children ≥6 years old and adolescents: 5–15 mg	BID
d-amphetamine (Dexedrine Spansule)	5–15 mg	QD
d-amphetamine (ProCentra)	Children 3–5 years old: 2.5 mg QD Children ≥6 years old and adolescents: 5–15 mg	BID
Lisdexamfetamine (Vyvanse)	30–70 mg	QD

Table 4 FDA-approved non-stimulant medications used in the treatment of ADHD in youth

Medication	Daily dose (mg)	Schedule
SNRI		
Atomoxetine (Strattera)	18–100	QD
Alpha-2 agonists long-acting		
Clonidine (Kapvay)	0.1–0.2	BID
Guanfacine (Intuniv ER)	1–4	QD

Table 5 FDA-approved uses of SGAs in children and adolescents

Medication	FDA-approved indication	Age range, years	Recommended dose range, mg
Risperidone	Schizophrenia	13–17	1–6
	BD (mixed/manic episode)	10–17	1–6
	Irritability, associated with ASD	5–18	0.5–3
Aripiprazole	Schizophrenia	13–17	10–30
	BD (mixed/manic episode)	10–17	10–30
	Irritability, associated with ASD	6–17	5–15
	Tourette's disorder	6–18	<50 kg – 5 to 10 ≥50 kg – 10 to 20
Olanzapine	Schizophrenia	13–17	10
	BD (mixed/manic episode)	13–17	10
Asenapine	BD (mixed/manic episode)	10–17	2.5–10 twice daily
Quetiapine	Schizophrenia	13–17	400–800
	BD (mixed/manic episode)	10–17	400–600
Lurasidone	Schizophrenia	13–17	40–80
	BD (depressive episode)	10–17	20–80
Paliperidone	Schizophrenia	12–17	<51 kg – 3 to 6 ≥51 kg – 3 to 12
Olanzapine/fluoxetine combination	BD (depressive episode)	10–17	3/25–12/50

5.1 Schizophrenia

To be diagnosed with schizophrenia, a child must exhibit two or more of the following symptoms: delusions, hallucinations, disorganized speech, grossly disorganized or catatonic behavior, or negative symptoms. These symptoms must cause severe impairment in the child's daily life and be present for at least 6 months

(American Psychiatric Association 2013). Early-onset schizophrenia (EOS) occurs prior to age 17 and is associated with increased morbidity and functional impairment when compared to the adult-onset form of this disorder (Gillberg 2001). The primary treatment of this disorder focuses on the psychopharmacotherapy (McClellan et al. 2007), but psychosocial interventions are an important adjunct to medication management and should include CBT, social skills training, and family involvement. Several SGAs are currently approved by the FDA for the treatment of EOS, including risperidone, olanzapine, quetiapine, aripiprazole, lurasidone, and paliperidone. Some of the older FGAs are also approved for this indication, but the regulatory approval for these older drugs is not the result of methodologically stringent research.

While most of the trials in adolescents with schizophrenia compared active treatment to placebo, the Treatment of Early-Onset Schizophrenia Spectrum Disorders Study (TEOSS) evaluated the efficacy of olanzapine, risperidone, and molindone in youth with EOS (Sikich et al. 2008). While the side effects did differ across the different medicines, the reduction of psychotic symptoms was similar. However, participants that showed improvement during the first 8 weeks of treatment did not demonstrate additional reduction in psychotic symptoms with longer treatment (Findling et al. 2010). When paliperidone extended release and aripiprazole were compared in adolescents with schizophrenia, both medications were effective in reducing psychotic symptoms (Savitz et al. 2015). Clozapine is considered superior to other antipsychotics for treatment-resistant schizophrenia (Shaw et al. 2006; Siskind et al. 2016). However, due to the requirements for monitoring and side effect profile, it is not used as a first-line agent and is not FDA approved for pediatric patients.

Generally when treating EOS, clinicians should start with one of the FDA-approved SGAs (McClellan 2018). It is recommended that olanzapine should not be the first option due to the increased risk for metabolic AEs. Clozapine may be considered after failure of several other antipsychotic medications.

5.2 Bipolar Disorder

In addition to the mood stabilizers discussed previously, antipsychotics may be used to treat pediatric BD. Based on randomized placebo-controlled trials, the FDA approved several antipsychotic medications for the management of acute mixed and manic episodes of BD, including aripiprazole, asenapine, risperidone, olanzapine, and quetiapine (Stepanova and Findling 2017; Findling et al. 2012, 2013a). Lurasidone and olanzapine/fluoxetine combination are the only two medications that are approved by the FDA for the treatment of bipolar depression (Lee et al. 2018). A trial of ziprasidone showed reduction of manic symptoms in youth but was not FDA approved due to trial design (Findling et al. 2013a, b, c). Quetiapine was not effective for treatment of pediatric bipolar depression (DelBello et al. 2009; Findling et al. 2014).

5.3 Autism Spectrum Disorder

ASD is a pervasive developmental disorder characterized by persistent deficits in social interactions and restricted, repetitive patterns of behavior or interests (APA 2013). In addition to these core symptoms of ASD, many children suffer from irritability, aggression, mood lability, and other emotional and behavioral disturbances (Simonoff et al. 2008). While there is no psychopharmacological intervention for the management of core symptoms of ASD, the FDA has approved two medications (risperidone and aripiprazole) for the management of irritability associated with ASD (Stepanova et al. 2017). In a comparison study, aripiprazole and risperidone similarly reduced irritability scores in children with ASD, but aripiprazole showed effects more quickly (Ghanizadeh et al. 2014). Olanzapine and paliperidone may also be effective in reducing irritability in youth with ASD (Hollander et al. 2006; Kemner et al. 2002; Stigler et al. 2012). Trials of quetiapine showed mixed results (Findling et al. 2004; Golubchik et al. 2011), while lurasidone was not effective in treating irritability associated with ASD (Loebel et al. 2016).

6 Conclusion

The medications discussed in this chapter should be used as part of a comprehensive treatment plan. Before prescribing any medications, clinicians should complete a detailed psychiatric and family history from the patient and their family and identify target symptoms to be treated with medication. Clinicians should initiate all medications at the labeled starting dose and titrate to reach the recommended dose and should clearly explain this process to patients and their families. Side effects should be closely monitored in the first few weeks following initiating or titrating medication, especially in medications with boxed warnings.

Currently, there are far fewer FDA-approved pharmacotherapies available for treating psychiatric illnesses in children and adolescents than for adults. For example, while there are 26 FDA-approved antidepressants to treat MDD in adults, only one medication (fluoxetine) is FDA approved to treat MDD in children and adolescents. For this reason, many medications discussed in this chapter are prescribed off-label. Thus, while the body of research on pharmacotherapy for psychiatric illnesses in children and adolescents has grown substantially over the past few decades, further research is needed to ensure this population receives optimal care.

Disclosure Dr. Findling receives or has received research support, acted as a consultant and/or served on a speaker's bureau for Acadia, Aevi, Akili, Alcobra, Allergan, Amerex, American Academy of Child & Adolescent Psychiatry, American Psychiatric Press, Arbor, Bracket, Daiichi-Sankyo, Epharma Solutions, Forest, Genentech, Insys, Ironshore, KemPharm, Luminopia, Lundbeck, Merck, NIH, Neurim, Noven, Nuvelution, Otsuka, PCORI, Pfizer, Physicians Postgraduate Press, Receptor Life Sciences, Roche, Sage, Shire, Sunovion, Supernus Pharmaceuticals, Syneurx, Teva, TouchPoint, Tris, and Validus.

Dr. Robb receives or has received research support, acted as a consultant and/or served on a DSMB for Allergan, AACAP, American Academy of Pediatrics, Bracket, North American Center for Continuing Medical Education/Psychiatric Congress, Lundbeck, Medgenics Neuroscience

Education Institute, Neuronetics, NCATS, NICHD, NINDS, NIMH, Shire, Supernus, University of Cambridge, I-ACT. Dr. Robb has stock in her IRA in Eli Lilly, Glaxo Smith Kline, Johnson and Johnson, and Pfizer.

References

Alderman J, Wolkow R, Chung M, Johnston HF (1998) Sertraline treatment of children and adolescents with obsessive-compulsive disorder or depression: pharmacokinetics, tolerability, and efficacy. J Am Acad Child Adolesc Psychiatry 37(4):386–394

American Psychiatric Association (2013) Diagnostic and statistical manual of mental disorders (DSM-5®). American Psychiatric Publication, Philadelphia

Amor LB (2012) Antipsychotics in pediatric and adolescent patients: a review of comparative safety data. J Affect Disord 138:S22–S30

Anderson IM (2000) Selective serotonin reuptake inhibitors versus tricyclic antidepressants: a meta-analysis of efficacy and tolerability. J Affect Disord 58(1):19–36

Atkinson SD, Prakash A, Zhang Q, Pangallo BA, Bangs ME, Emslie GJ, March JS (2014) A double-blind efficacy and safety study of duloxetine flexible dosing in children and adolescents with major depressive disorder. J Child Adolesc Psychopharmacol 24(4):180–189

Atkinson S, Lubaczewski S, Ramaker S, England RD, Wajsbrot DB, Abbas R, Findling RL (2018) Desvenlafaxine versus placebo in the treatment of children and adolescents with major depressive disorder. J Child Adolesc Psychopharmacol 28(1):55–65

Barzman DH, DelBello MP, Kowatch RA, Warner J, Rofey D, Stanford K et al (2005) Adjunctive topiramate in hospitalized children and adolescents with bipolar disorders. J Child Adolesc Psychopharmacol 15(6):931–937

Berard R, Fong R, Carpenter DJ, Thomason C, Wilkinson C (2006) An international, multicenter, placebo-controlled trial of paroxetine in adolescents with major depressive disorder. J Child Adolesc Psychopharmacol 16(1–2):59–75

Bernstein GA, Borchardt CM, Perwien AR, Crosby RD, Kushner MG, Thuras PD, Last CG (2000) Imipramine plus cognitive-behavioral therapy in the treatment of school refusal. J Am Acad Child Adolesc Psychiatry 39(3):276–283

Birmaher B, Axelson DA, Monk K, Kalas C, Clark DB, Ehmann M et al (2003) Fluoxetine for the treatment of childhood anxiety disorders. J Am Acad Child Adolesc Psychiatry 42(4):415–423

Bradley C (1937) The behavior of children receiving benzedrine. Am J Psychiatry 94(3):577–585

Brent D, Emslie G, Clarke G, Wagner KD, Asarnow JR, Keller M et al (2008) Switching to another SSRI or to venlafaxine with or without cognitive behavioral therapy for adolescents with SSRI-resistant depression: the TORDIA randomized controlled trial. JAMA 299(8):901–913

Brown KA, Samuel S, Patel DR (2018) Pharmacologic management of attention deficit hyperactivity disorder in children and adolescents: a review for practitioners. Transl Pediatr 7(1):36

Campo JV, Perel J, Lucas A, Bridge J, Ehmann M, Kalas C et al (2004) Citalopram treatment of pediatric recurrent abdominal pain and comorbid internalizing disorders: an exploratory study. J Am Acad Child Adolesc Psychiatry 43(10):1234–1242

Chang K, Saxena K, Howe M (2006) An open-label study of lamotrigine adjunct or monotherapy for the treatment of adolescents with bipolar depression. J Am Acad Child Adolesc Psychiatry 45(3):298–304

Cheng JY, Chen RY, Ko JS, Ng EM (2007) Efficacy and safety of atomoxetine for attention-deficit/hyperactivity disorder in children and adolescents – meta-analysis and meta-regression analysis. Psychopharmacology (Berl) 194(2):197–209

Cheung A, Sacks D, Dewa CS, Pong J, Levitt A (2008) Pediatric prescribing practices and the FDA black-box warning on antidepressants. J Dev Behav Pediatr 29(3):213–215

Clark DB, Birmaher B, Axelson D, Monk K, Kalas C, Ehmann M et al (2005) Fluoxetine for the treatment of childhood anxiety disorders: open-label, long-term extension to a controlled trial. J Am Acad Child Adolesc Psychiatry 44(12):1263–1270

Compton SN, Walkup JT, Albano AM, Piacentini JC, Birmaher B, Sherrill JT et al (2010) Child/adolescent anxiety multimodal study (CAMS): rationale, design, and methods. Child Adolesc Psychiatry Ment Health 4(1):1

Conners CK, Eisenberg L, Barcai A (1967) Effect of dextroamphetamine on children: studies on subjects with learning disabilities and school behavior problems. Arch Gen Psychiatry 17(4):478–485

Conners CK, Rothschild G, Eisenberg L, Schwartz LS, Robinson E (1969) Dextroamphetamine sulfate in children with learning disorders children with learning disorders: effects on perception, learning and achievement. Arch Gen Psychiatry 21(2):182–190

Cook EH, Wagner KD, March JS, Biederman J, Landau P, Wolkow R, Messig M (2001) Long-term sertraline treatment of children and adolescents with obsessive-compulsive disorder. J Am Acad Child Adolesc Psychiatry 40(10):1175–1181

DelBello MP, Kowatch RA, Warner J, Schwiers ML, Rappaport KB, Daniels JP et al (2002) Adjunctive topiramate treatment for pediatric bipolar disorder: a retrospective chart review. J Child Adolesc Psychopharmacol 12(4):323–330

Delbello MP, Findling RL, Kushner S, Wang D, Olson WH, Capece JA et al (2005) A pilot controlled trial of topiramate for mania in children and adolescents with bipolar disorder. J Am Acad Child Adolesc Psychiatry 44(6):539–547

DelBello MP, Chang K, Welge JA, Adler CM, Rana M, Howe M et al (2009) A double-blind, placebo-controlled pilot study of quetiapine for depressed adolescents with bipolar disorder. Bipolar Disord 11(5):483–493

Dopheide JA (2006) Recognizing and treating depression in children and adolescents. Am J Health Syst Pharm 63(3):233–243

Emslie GJ, Rush AJ, Weinberg WA, Kowatch RA, Hughes CW, Carmody T, Rintelmann J (1997) A double-blind, randomized, placebo-controlled trial of fluoxetine in children and adolescents with depression. Arch Gen Psychiatry 54(11):1031–1037

Emslie GJ, Heiligenstein JH, Wagner KD, Hoog SL, Ernest DE, Brown E et al (2002) Fluoxetine for acute treatment of depression in children and adolescents: a placebo-controlled, randomized clinical trial. J Am Acad Child Adolesc Psychiatry 41(10):1205–1215

Emslie GJ, Wagner KD, Kutcher S, Krulewicz S, Fong R, Carpenter DJ et al (2006) Paroxetine treatment in children and adolescents with major depressive disorder: a randomized, multicenter, double-blind, placebo-controlled trial. J Am Acad Child Adolesc Psychiatry 45(6):709–719

Emslie GJ, Findling RL, Yeung PP, Kunz NR, Li Y (2007) Venlafaxine ER for the treatment of pediatric subjects with depression: results of two placebo-controlled trials. J Am Acad Child Adolesc Psychiatry 46(4):479–488

Emslie GJ, Ventura D, Korotzer A, Tourkodimitris S (2009) Escitalopram in the treatment of adolescent depression: a randomized placebo-controlled multisite trial. J Am Acad Child Adolesc Psychiatry 48(7):721–729

Faraone SV, Glatt SJ (2010) A comparison of the efficacy of medications for adult attention-deficit/hyperactivity disorder using meta-analysis of effect sizes. J Clin Psychiatry 71(6):754

Findling RL, Ginsberg LD (2014) The safety and effectiveness of open-label extended-release carbamazepine in the treatment of children and adolescents with bipolar I disorder suffering from a manic or mixed episode. Neuropsychiatr Dis Treat 10:1589

Findling RL, McNamara NK, Gracious BL, ORiordan MA, Reed MD, Demeter C, Blumer JL (2004) Quetiapine in nine youths with autistic disorder. J Child Adolesc Psychopharmacol 14(2):287–294

Findling RL, Mcnamara NK, Youngstrom EA, Stansbrey R, Gracious BL, Reed MD, Calabrese JR (2005) Double-blind 18-month trial of lithium versus divalproex maintenance treatment in pediatric bipolar disorder. J Am Acad Child Adolesc Psychiatry 44(5):409–417

Findling RL, Johnson JL, McClellan J, Frazier JA, Vitiello B, Hamer RM et al (2010) Double-blind maintenance safety and effectiveness findings from the treatment of early-onset schizophrenia spectrum (TEOSS) study. J Am Acad Child Adolesc Psychiatry 49(6):583–594

Findling RL, Youngstrom EA, McNamara NK, Stansbrey RJ, Wynbrandt JL, Adegbite C et al (2012) Double-blind, randomized, placebo-controlled long-term maintenance study of aripiprazole in children with bipolar disorder. J Clin Psychiatry 73(1):57

Findling RL, Çavuş I, Pappadopulos E, Vanderburg DG, Schwartz JH, Gundapaneni BK, DelBello MP (2013a) Efficacy, long-term safety, and tolerability of ziprasidone in children and adolescents with bipolar disorder. J Child Adolesc Psychopharmacol 23(8):545–557

Findling RL, Correll CU, Nyilas M, Forbes RA, McQuade RD, Jin N et al (2013b) Aripiprazole for the treatment of pediatric bipolar I disorder: a 30-week, randomized, placebo-controlled study. Bipolar Disord 15(2):138–149

Findling RL, Robb A, Bose A (2013c) Escitalopram in the treatment of adolescent depression: a randomized, double-blind, placebo-controlled extension trial. J Child Adolesc Psychopharmacol 23(7):468–480

Findling RL, Pathak S, Earley WR, Liu S, DelBello MP (2014) Efficacy and safety of extended-release quetiapine fumarate in youth with bipolar depression: an 8 week, double-blind, placebo-controlled trial. J Child Adolesc Psychopharmacol 24(6):325–335

Findling RL, Chang K, Robb A, Foster VJ, Horrigan J, Krishen A et al (2015a) Adjunctive maintenance lamotrigine for pediatric bipolar I disorder: a placebo-controlled, randomized withdrawal study. J Am Acad Child Adolesc Psychiatry 54(12):1020–1031

Findling RL, Robb A, McNamara NK, Pavuluri MN, Kafantaris V, Scheffer R et al (2015b) Lithium in the acute treatment of bipolar I disorder: a double-blind, placebo-controlled study. Pediatrics 136(5):885

Garcia AM, Sapyta JJ, Moore PS, Freeman JB, Franklin ME, March JS, Foa EB (2010) Predictors and moderators of treatment outcome in the pediatric obsessive compulsive treatment study (POTS I). J Am Acad Child Adolesc Psychiatry 49(10):1024–1033

Geller DA, Hoog SL, Heiligenstein JH, Ricardi RK, Tamura ROY, Kluszynski S et al (2001) Fluoxetine treatment for obsessive-compulsive disorder in children and adolescents: a placebo-controlled clinical trial. J Am Acad Child Adolesc Psychiatry 40(7):773–779

Geller B, Luby JL, Joshi P, Wagner KD, Emslie G, Walkup JT et al (2012) A randomized controlled trial of risperidone, lithium, or divalproex sodium for initial treatment of bipolar I disorder, manic or mixed phase, in children and adolescents. Arch Gen Psychiatry 69(5):515–528

Ghanizadeh A, Sahraeizadeh A, Berk M (2014) A head-to-head comparison of aripiprazole and risperidone for safety and treating autistic disorders, a randomized double blind clinical trial. Child Psychiatry Hum Dev 45(2):185–192

Gillberg C (2001) Epidemiology of early onset schizophrenia. In: Remschmidt H (ed) Schizophrenia in children and adolescents. Cambridge University Press, Cambridge, pp 43–59

Gittelman-Klein R, Klein DF (1971) Controlled imipramine treatment of school phobia. Arch Gen Psychiatry 25(3):204–207

Golubchik P, Sever J, Weizman A (2011) Low-dose quetiapine for adolescents with autistic spectrum disorder and aggressive behavior: open-label trial. Clin Neuropharmacol 34(6):216–219

Gothelf D, Rubinstein M, Shemesh E, Miller O, Farbstein I, Klein A et al (2005) Pilot study: fluvoxamine treatment for depression and anxiety disorders in children and adolescents with cancer. J Am Acad Child Adolesc Psychiatry 44(12):1258–1262

Hollander E, Wasserman S, Swanson EN, Chaplin W, Schapiro ML, Zagursky K, Novotny S (2006) A double-blind placebo-controlled pilot study of olanzapine in childhood/adolescent pervasive developmental disorder. J Child Adolesc Psychopharmacol 16(5):541–548

Isolan L, Pheula G, Salum GA Jr, Oswald S, Rohde LA, Manfro GG (2007) An open-label trial of escitalopram in children and adolescents with social anxiety disorder. J Child Adolesc Psychopharmacol 17(6):751–760

Joshi G, Wozniak J, Mick E, Doyle R, Hammerness P, Georgiopoulos A et al (2010) A prospective open-label trial of extended-release carbamazepine monotherapy in children with bipolar disorder. J Child Adolesc Psychopharmacol 20(1):7–14

Kachko L, Ben Ami S, Liberman A, Birk E, Kronenberg S (2011) Duloxetine contributing to a successful multimodal treatment program for peripheral femoral neuropathy and comorbid 'reactive depression' in an adolescent. Pain Res Manag 16(6):457–459

Kemner C, Willemsen-Swinkels SH, de Jonge M, Tuynman-Qua H, van Engeland H (2002) Open-label study of olanzapine in children with pervasive developmental disorder. J Clin Psychopharmacol 22(5):455–460

Klein RG, Koplewicz HS, Kanner A (1992) Imipramine treatment of children with separation anxiety disorder. J Am Acad Child Adolesc Psychiatry 31(1):21–28

Kollins SH, Jain R, Brams M, Segal S, Findling RL, Wigal SB, Khayrallah M (2011) Clonidine extended-release tablets as add-on therapy to psychostimulants in children and adolescents with ADHD. Pediatrics 127(6):e1406

Kowatch RA, Suppes T, Carmody TJ, Bucci JP, Hume JH, Kromelis M et al (2000) Effect size of lithium, divalproex sodium, and carbamazepine in children and adolescents with bipolar disorder. J Am Acad Child Adolesc Psychiatry 39(6):713–720

Kowatch RA, Scheffer RE, Monroe E, Delgado S, Altaye M, Lagory D (2015) Placebo-controlled trial of valproic acid versus risperidone in children 3–7 years of age with bipolar I disorder. J Child Adolesc Psychopharmacol 25(4):306–313

Kratochvil CJ, Milton DR, Vaughan BS, Greenhill LL (2008) Acute atomoxetine treatment of younger and older children with ADHD: a meta-analysis of tolerability and efficacy. Child Adolesc Psychiatry Ment Health 2(1):25

Lee ES, Vidal C, Findling RL (2018) A focused review on the treatment of pediatric patients with atypical antipsychotics. J Child Adolesc Psychopharmacol 28(9):582–605

Lilly USA LLC (2017) Straterra [Product information]. Lilly, Indianapolis

Loebel A, Brams M, Goldman RS, Silva R, Hernandez D, Deng L et al (2016) Lurasidone for the treatment of irritability associated with autistic disorder. J Autism Dev Disord 46(4):1153–1163

March JS, Biederman J, Wolkow R, Safferman A, Mardekian J, Cook EH et al (1998) Sertraline in children and adolescents with obsessive-compulsive disorder: a multicenter randomized controlled trial. JAMA 280(20):1752–1756

March JS, Entusah AR, Rynn M, Albano AM, Tourian KA (2007a) A randomized controlled trial of venlafaxine ER versus placebo in pediatric social anxiety disorder. Biol Psychiatry 62(10):1149–1154

March JS, Franklin ME, Leonard H, Garcia A, Moore P, Freeman J, Foa E (2007b) Tics moderate treatment outcome with sertraline but not cognitive-behavior therapy in pediatric obsessive-compulsive disorder. Biol Psychiatry 61(3):344–347

McClellan J (2018) Psychosis in children and adolescents. J Am Acad Child Adolesc Psychiatry 57(5):308–312

McClellan J, Kowatch R, Findling RL (2007) Practice parameter for the assessment and treatment of children and adolescents with bipolar disorder. J Am Acad Child Adolesc Psychiatry 46(1):107–125

Meighen KG (2007) Duloxetine treatment of pediatric chronic pain and co-morbid major depressive disorder. J Child Adolesc Psychopharmacol 17(1):121–127

National Institute of Mental Health (2016) Attention-deficit/hyperactivity disorder. https://www.nimh.nih.gov/health/topics/attention-deficit-hyperactivity-disorder-adhd/index.shtml

Palumbo DR, Sallee FR, Pelham WE Jr, Bukstein OG, Daviss WB, McDermott MP, CAT Study Team (2008) Clonidine for attention-deficit/hyperactivity disorder: I. Efficacy and tolerability outcomes. J Am Acad Child Adolesc Psychiatry 47(2):180–188

The Pediatric OCD Treatment Study (POTS) Team (2004) Cognitive-behavior therapy, sertraline, and their combination for children and adolescents with obsessive-compulsive disorder: the Pediatric OCD Treatment Study (POTS) randomized controlled trial. JAMA 292(16):1969

Pelham WE, Aronoff HR, Midlam JK, Shapiro CJ, Gnagy EM, Chronis AM et al (1999) A comparison of Ritalin and Adderall: efficacy and time-course in children with attention-deficit/hyperactivity disorder. Pediatrics 103(4):e43

Richmond TK, Rosen DS (2005) The treatment of adolescent depression in the era of the black box warning. Curr Opin Pediatr 17(4):466–472

Riddle MA, Reeve EA, Yaryura-Tobias JA, Yang HM, Claghorn JL, Gaffney G et al (2001) Fluvoxamine for children and adolescents with obsessive-compulsive disorder: a randomized, controlled, multicenter trial. J Am Acad Child Adolesc Psychiatry 40(2):222–229

Robb AS, Cueva JE, Sporn J, Yang R, Vanderburg DG (2010) Sertraline treatment of children and adolescents with posttraumatic stress disorder: a double-blind, placebo-controlled trial. J Child Adolesc Psychopharmacol 20(6):463–471

Roohafza H, Pourmoghaddas Z, Saneian H, Gholamrezaei A (2014) Citalopram for pediatric functional abdominal pain: a randomized, placebo-controlled trial. Neurogastroenterol Motil 26(11):1642–1650

Rynn MA, Siqueland L, Rickels K (2001) Placebo-controlled trial of sertraline in the treatment of children with generalized anxiety disorder. Am J Psychiatry 158(12):2008–2014

Sallee FR, Lyne A, Wigal T, McGough JJ (2009) Long-term safety and efficacy of guanfacine extended release in children and adolescents with attention-deficit/hyperactivity disorder. J Child Adolesc Psychopharmacol 19(3):215–226

Savitz AJ, Lane R, Nuamah I, Gopal S, Hough D (2015) Efficacy and safety of paliperidone extended release in adolescents with schizophrenia: a randomized, double-blind study. J Am Acad Child Adolesc Psychiatry 54(2):126–137

Shaw P, Sporn A, Gogtay N, Overman GP, Greenstein D, Gochman P et al (2006) Childhood-onset schizophrenia: a double-blind, randomized clozapine-olanzapine comparison. Arch Gen Psychiatry 63(7):721–730

Sikich L, Frazier JA, McClellan J, Findling RL, Vitiello B, Ritz L et al (2008) Double-blind comparison of first-and second-generation antipsychotics in early-onset schizophrenia and schizo-affective disorder: findings from the treatment of early-onset schizophrenia spectrum disorders (TEOSS) study. Am J Psychiatry 165(11):1420–1431

Simonoff E, Pickles A, Charman T, Chandler S, Loucas T, Baird G (2008) Psychiatric disorders in children with autism spectrum disorders: prevalence, comorbidity, and associated factors in a population-derived sample. J Am Acad Child Adolesc Psychiatry 47(8):921–929

Siskind D, McCartney L, Goldschlager R, Kisely S (2016) Clozapine v. first-and second-generation antipsychotics in treatment-refractory schizophrenia: systematic review and meta-analysis. Br J Psychiatry 209(5):385–392

Skarphedinsson G, Compton S, Thomsen PH, Weidle B, Dahl K, Nissen JB et al (2015) Tics moderate sertraline, but not cognitive-behavior therapy response in pediatric obsessive-compulsive disorder patients who do not respond to cognitive-behavior therapy. J Child Adolesc Psychopharmacol 25(5):432–439

Spencer TJ, Greenbaum M, Ginsberg LD, Murphy WR (2009) Safety and effectiveness of coadministration of guanfacine extended release and psychostimulants in children and adolescents with attention-deficit/hyperactivity disorder. J Child Adolesc Psychopharmacol 19(5):501–510

Stepanova E, Findling RL (2017) Psychopharmacology of bipolar disorders in children and adolescents. Pediatr Clin 64(6):1209–1222

Stepanova E, Dowling S, Phelps M, Findling RL (2017) Pharmacotherapy of emotional and behavioral symptoms associated with autism spectrum disorder in children and adolescents. Dialogues Clin Neurosci 19(4):395

Stigler KA, Mullett JE, Erickson CA, Posey DJ, McDougle CJ (2012) Paliperidone for irritability in adolescents and young adults with autistic disorder. Psychopharmacology (Berl) 223(2):237–245

Storch EA, Bussing R, Small BJ, Geffken GR, McNamara JP, Rahman O et al (2013) Randomized, placebo-controlled trial of cognitive-behavioral therapy alone or combined with sertraline in the treatment of pediatric obsessive–compulsive disorder. Behav Res Ther 51(12):823–829

Strawn JR, Prakash A, Zhang Q, Pangallo BA, Stroud CE, Cai N, Findling RL (2015) A randomized, placebo-controlled study of duloxetine for the treatment of children and adolescents with generalized anxiety disorder. J Am Acad Child Adolesc Psychiatry 54(4):283–293

Varigonda AL, Jakubovski E, Bloch MH (2016) Systematic review and meta-analysis: early treatment responses of selective serotonin reuptake inhibitors and clomipramine in pediatric obsessive-compulsive disorder. J Am Acad Child Adolesc Psychiatry 55(10):851–859

Von Knorring AL, Olsson GI, Thomsen PH, Lemming OM, Hultén A (2006) A randomized, double-blind, placebo-controlled study of citalopram in adolescents with major depressive disorder. J Clin Psychopharmacol 26(3):311–315

Wagner KD, Ambrosini P, Rynn M, Wohlberg C, Yang R, Greenbaum MS et al (2003a) Efficacy of sertraline in the treatment of children and adolescents with major depressive disorder: two randomized controlled trials. JAMA 290(8):1033–1041

Wagner KD, Cook EH, Chung H, Messig M (2003b) Remission status after long-term sertraline treatment of pediatric obsessive-compulsive disorder. J Child Adolesc Psychopharmacol 13(2, Supplement 1):53–60

Wagner KD, Robb AS, Findling RL, Jin J, Gutierrez MM, Heydorn WE (2004) A randomized, placebo-controlled trial of citalopram for the treatment of major depression in children and adolescents. Am J Psychiatry 161(6):1079–1083

Wagner KD, Jonas J, Findling RL, Ventura D, Saikali K (2006a) A double-blind, randomized, placebo-controlled trial of escitalopram in the treatment of pediatric depression. J Am Acad Child Adolesc Psychiatry 45(3):280–288

Wagner KD, Kowatch RA, Emslie GJ, Findling RL, Wilens TE, McCague K et al (2006b) A double-blind, randomized, placebo-controlled trial of oxcarbazepine in the treatment of bipolar disorder in children and adolescents. Am J Psychiatry 163(7):1179–1186

Wagner KD, Redden L, Kowatch RA, Wilens TE, Segal S, Chang K et al (2009) A double-blind, randomized, placebo-controlled trial of divalproex extended-release in the treatment of bipolar disorder in children and adolescents. J Am Acad Child Adolesc Psychiatry 48(5):519–532

Walkup JT, Labellarte MJ, Riddle MA, Pine DS, Greenhill L, Klein R et al (2001) Fluvoxamine for the treatment of anxiety disorders in children and adolescents. N Engl J Med 344(17):1279–1285

Watson HJ, Rees CS (2008) Meta-analysis of randomized, controlled treatment trials for pediatric obsessive-compulsive disorder. J Child Psychol Psychiatry 49(5):489–498

Weihs KL, Murphy W, Abbas R, Chiles D, England RD, Ramaker S, Wajsbrot DB (2018) Desvenlafaxine versus placebo in a fluoxetine-referenced study of children and adolescents with major depressive disorder. J Child Adolesc Psychopharmacol 28(1):36–46

West AE, Weinstein SM, Celio CI, Henry D, Pavuluri MN (2011) Co-morbid disruptive behavior disorder and aggression predict functional outcomes and differential response to risperidone versus divalproex in pharmacotherapy for pediatric bipolar disorder. J Child Adolesc Psychopharmacol 21(6):545–553

Pharmacotherapy in Children and Adolescents: Oncology

Georg Hempel

Contents

G. Hempel (✉)
Westfälische Wilhelms-Universität Münster, Institut für Pharmazeutische und Medizinische Chemie, Klinische Pharmazie, Münster, Germany
e-mail: georg.hempel@wwu.de

W. Kiess et al. (eds.), *Pediatric Pharmacotherapy*,
Handbook of Experimental Pharmacology 261, https://doi.org/10.1007/164_2019_306

Abstract
Pharmacotherapy in paediatric oncology is a difficult task. It is challenging to determine the optimal dose in children of different age groups. In addition, anticancer drugs display severe side effects reducing the quality of life. Late effects like secondary tumours and cardiotoxicity can be apparent years after treatment and must be taken into account when planning treatment schedules. Classical cytoreducing agents are still of great importance in treating children with leukaemia and solid tumours. In addition, drugs developed by rational drug design (targeted drugs) are a very important part of many treatment protocols, and newer drugs are emerging in several types of cancer. Unfortunately, there is only limited experience with newer drugs in children, because new drugs are mostly developed for adults. Complicated therapy regimens require a solid knowledge of the pharmacology of the drugs applied. This chapter attempts to introduce some pharmacological knowledge for the most important anticancer drugs in children with a focus on side effects and age-specific considerations.

Keywords
Busulfan · Cancer · Cytarabine · Daunorubicin · Doxorubicin · Leukaemia · Methotrexate

1 Introduction

Cytotoxic drugs generally target all proliferating cells. As cancer cells are rapidly proliferating, this explains in part their selective killing of cancer cells and their side effects: rapidly proliferating cells in the bone marrow and skin are mainly affected. However, this does not explain the high anticancer activity of certain cytotoxic drugs for specific tumour types, such as platinum derivatives in germ cell tumours. Some aspects to be considered to explain are specific tissue distribution but also the distribution of drugs and/or their active metabolites into cells of different types (Peterson 2011).

Several malignancies occurring in children and adolescents are curable with chemotherapy including acute lymphoblastic leukaemia (ALL), lymphoma, germ cell tumours, osteo- and Ewing sarcoma and neuroblastoma, among others (Nygren 2001). In general, haematopoiesis recovers much better after chemotherapy in children in comparison with older patients. Therefore, high-dose therapy is usually much better tolerated than in older patients.

Changes in the pharmacokinetic properties of anticancer drugs in children occur mainly in the first 3 years of life. In children 3 years or older, the pharmacokinetic parameters correlate with size parameters such as weight or body surface area, and dose adjustment can be done using these size parameters. With cytotoxic drugs, however, one needs to consider possible late effects after therapy, which may be less relevant in adults with their reduced life expectancy. In addition, younger children are more prone to certain toxicities than adults.

Toxicities like hearing loss due to platinum chemotherapy has much more serious consequences in small children than in adults, because language development will be impaired by hearing loss early in life. Secondary malignancies after treatment with topoisomerase inhibitors are a severe problem in children with up to 5% of patients concerned. Children are more prone to cardiotoxicity of anthracyclines than adults, and they need their heart to work for many decades.

Dosing based on body surface area (BSA) is used in clinical routine. BSA is calculated according to the formula of Mosteller (1987):

$$\mathrm{BSA} = \sqrt{\frac{W \cdot H}{3600}} \text{ with } W \text{ weight } [\mathrm{kg}] \text{ and } H \text{ height } [\mathrm{cm}]. \tag{1}$$

This formula produces slightly other results than the formula of Du Bois and Du Bois (1916) commonly used in adults. Especially for smaller children and infants with a body weight of less than 10 kg, clearance better correlates with weight according to the 3/4 power law (Anderson et al. 1997). This concept is often termed allometry. However, for dosing of anticancer drugs in practise, the use of BSA is justified, because BSA correlates with the clearance of most anticancer drugs and the deviation to allometry is negligible (Hempel and Boos 2007). For children less than 12 months of age, it is common practise to reduce the dose by 25–33% due to toxicity concerns.

2 Alkylating Agents

Alkylating agents directly interact with DNA and produce DNA strand breaks resulting in cell death. Due to the mentioned better recovery of the bone marrow in children, they tolerate higher dose intensity of alkylating agents than adults. However, this finding is only applicable for drugs without substantial non-haematological toxicity. For example, cisplatin has substantial nephro- and ototoxicity.

2.1 Busulfan

Busulfan (Fig. 1) is part of many conditioning regimens before haematopoietic stem cell transplantation (HCT) for the treatment of leukaemia and other malignancies. Since the 1950s, the drug was used for the treatment of chronic myeloid leukaemia in low doses. Today, it is used in combination with cyclophosphamide or fludarabine in high-dose therapy regimens. The intravenous formulation should be standard of care

Fig. 1 Busulfan

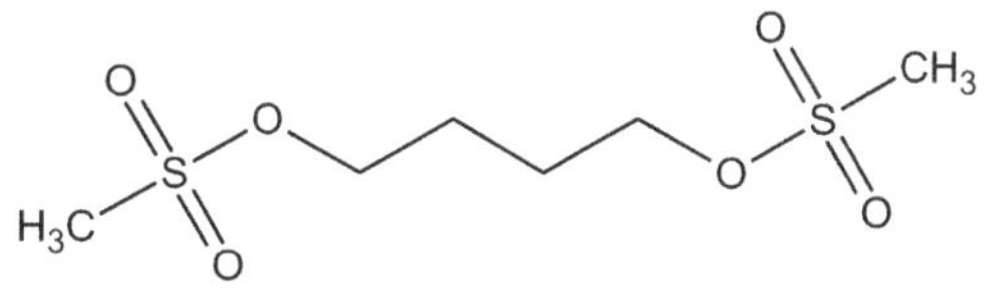

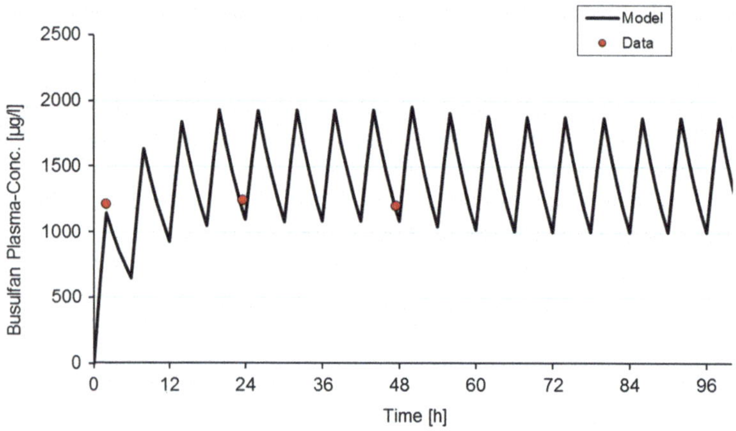

Fig. 2 Plasma concentration time curve in a 6-year-old child receiving 1 h infusions of 0.8 mg/kg busulfan every 6 h for 4 days. The line represents post hoc estimates of a population pharmacokinetic model (Trame et al. 2011)

in children, because oral busulfan results in highly variable AUCs due to fluctuation in the absorption of the drug. In addition, it is much more convenient for the patients, because swallowing of a great number of busulfan tablets is unpleasant and may cause vomiting.

For conditioning before HCT, 16 administrations every 6 h are the standard schedules. Figure 2 shows a typical plasma-concentration time curve. With i.v. busulfan, once-daily dosing offers some practical advantages and appears to be as safe and effective as the standard schedule (Bartelink et al. 2008).

The drug is metabolised in the liver, mainly by the enzyme glutathione S-transferase (GST), by forming a sulphonium ion and subsequent oxidation resulting in inactive products (Myers et al. 2017). Genotyping of patients for polymorphisms in genes encoding for GST was extensively investigated, but there is no recommendation to genotype patients before busulfan administration, because GST polymorphism can only explain a part of the variability in busulfan clearance. Therefore, therapeutic drug monitoring is recommended in order to reduce the variability in individual exposure (Palmer et al. 2016).

Busulfan is hepatotoxic with sinusoidal obstruction syndrome (SOS, formerly termed veno-occlusive disease (VOD)) occurring with an incidence of about 20% (Kerl et al. 2014). VOD is lethal in a substantial number of patients. Other severe side effects are myelosuppression, convulsions and interstitial pneumonia. Anticonvulsive prophylaxis with midazolam or phenytoin is recommended.

2.2 Treosulfan

Although treosulfan (Fig. 3) is an old drug which is on the market for more than 50 years, it has gained interest in the last years as an alternative to busulfan in HCT due to reduced hepatotoxicity (ten Brink et al. 2014). Treosulfan is infused in a dose of 10–14 g/m^2 on three consecutive days, often in combination with fludarabine or cyclophosphamide.

Activation of the drug requires no drug-metabolising enzymes. Therefore, polymorphisms in the genes encoding for the enzymes as a source of pharmacokinetic variability are not relevant. The active metabolite diepoxybutane is formed when the pH is higher than six with a half-live of about 2.2 h (medac Gmbh 2014). Myelosuppression is the dose-limiting toxicity making the drug a suitable option for HCT. Other important toxicities in children are mucositis, skin toxicity, diarrhoea and some liver toxicity with an SOS rate of 5% in older and 12% in younger children, respectively (ten Brink et al. 2014). Seizures were also reported, but a general anticonvulsive prophylaxis is not routinely done (Slatter et al. 2011). Drug monitoring of treosulfan requires immediate stabilisation of blood samples due to the spontaneous degradation of the treosulfan and is therefore difficult to apply in clinical routine (Hilger et al. 1998).

2.3 Melphalan

Melphalan (Fig. 4) belongs to the group of N-Lost derivatives. The chloroethyl side chains bound to the nitrogen form highly reactive metabolites after removal of the chlorine and subsequent cyclisation to an aziridinium ion displaying alkylating properties. Of note, activation requires no drug-metabolising enzymes.

It is used in conditioning regimes for autologous or allogenic HCT in combination with busulfan, fludarabine or cyclophosphamide in patients with high-risk neuroblastoma or other severe malignancies such as relapsed Ewing sarcoma. High-dose melphalan is administered in a dose range of 140–200 mg/m^2 (total dose). It is questionable if dose escalation above 140 mg/m^2 is useful. Busulfan in

Fig. 3 Treosulfan

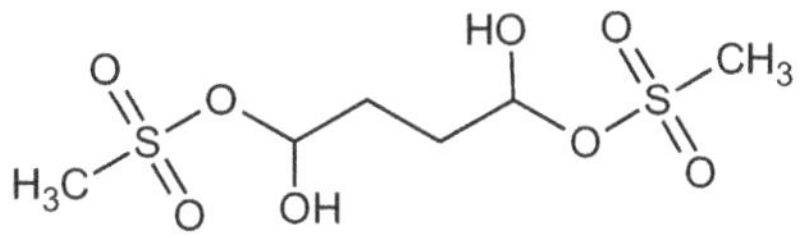

Fig. 4 Melphalan

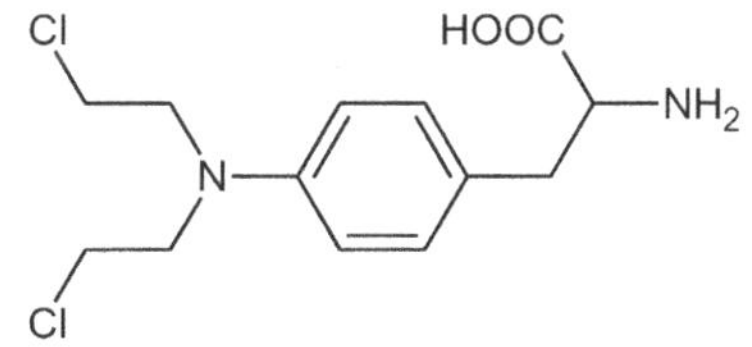

combination with melphalan (BuMel) appears to be better than BuCy in adult AML patients (Gorin et al. 2018). BuMel also appears in many treatment protocols for Ewing sarcoma patients (Abate et al. 2018). However, this scheme is hepatotoxic with a 7% incidence of SOS. Defibrotide appears to offer some protection against hepatotoxicity (Park et al. 2013). Adjustment of melphalan dose in renally impaired patients is required. Typical side effects are alopecia, myelosuppression and musculoskeletal toxicity. In high-dose therapy, gastrointestinal toxicity (diarrhoea, vomiting and stomatitis) is dose-limiting. More seldom, interstitial pneumonia is a serious side effects, which can also occur with many alkylating agents.

A population pharmacokinetic analysis in children revealed that weight, GFR and previous carboplatin therapy influenced the clearance of melphalan (Nath et al. 2007). These factors must be taken into account when selecting the dose of melphalan. The terminal half-live was found to be about 1 hour.

2.4 Cyclophosphamide and Ifosfamide

Cyclophosphamide (Fig. 5) is one of the oldest anticancer drugs. It was discovered as early as 1958 and introduced into cancer therapy in 1959. It remains a mainstay in the therapy of haematological malignancies as well as of various tumours. The drug is applied in many conditioning regimens before HCT for haematological malignancies (AML, MDS) as well as for aplastic anaemia.

Important side effects are leuco- and thrombocytopenia, anaemia and cardio- and bladder toxicity. To avoid haemorrhagic cystitis, MESNA (sodium 2-sulfanylethanesulfonate) must be administered before cyclophosphamide administration to neutralise the toxic metabolite acrolein in the urine. In addition, nephrotoxicity, cardiotoxicity and liver toxicity occur. All these effects are highly dose-dependent. Cardiotoxicity is dose-limiting in high-dose schedules of cyclophosphamide. Ifosfamide appears to be less cardiotoxic; however, neurotoxicity appears more often after ifosfamide administration.

Similar to melphalan, the active metabolite phosphoramide mustard forms a highly reactive cyclic aziridinium cation, which can react with the N(7) of the guanine and with cytidine from the DNA. The active metabolite of ifosfamide, ifosfamide mustard, is formed in a similar same way.

Although cyclophosphamide is in therapeutic use for many decades, new therapies were developed such as metronomic- and high-dose therapy. Currently, low-dose cyclophosphamide is used in many experimental protocols with the aim to overcome immunosuppression in advanced cancer (Ahlmann and Hempel 2016).

Fig. 5 Cyclophosphamide and ifosfamide

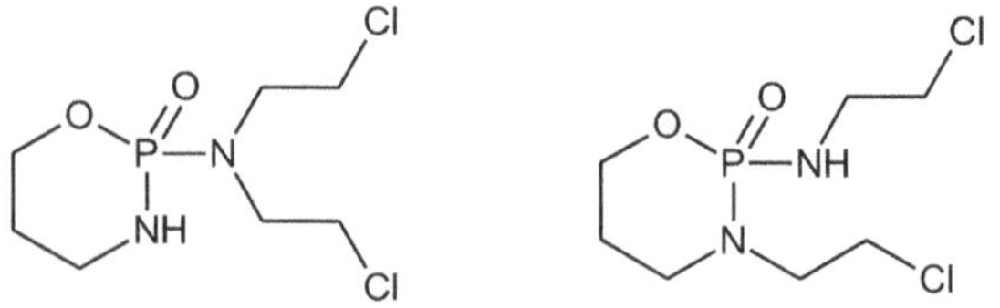

Ifosfamide (Fig. 5) displays similar efficacy and toxicity profiles, although neurotoxicity occurs more often in children with ifosfamide. The drug is usually applied as a daily dose of up to 3 g/m^2 for 5 days in one cycle. Continuous infusions over 24 h were associated with a higher rate of neurotoxicity than 1 h infusions. Urotoxicity was less pronounced with continuous infusions (Carli et al. 2003). As an inactivating pathway, cleavage of one dichloroethyl side chains occurs parallel with the activation, and chloroacetaldehyde is formed. This also occurs with cyclophosphamide, however, to a much lesser extent (Kamen et al. 1995). Both activation and deactivation are catalysed by CYP 2B6 and CYP3A4, and autoinduction of the metabolism can be observed after repeated courses (Boddy et al. 1995). This phenomenon can be observed with both drugs, whereas saturation of the activation pathway was only observed with cyclophosphamide given at doses higher than 4 g/m^2 (Boddy and Yule 2000). The co-administration of inhibitors of P450 enzymes such as voriconazole or aprepitant often used in supportive care may reduce the anticancer effect of the drugs. Fatal encephalopathy was observed in adults receiving aprepitant in combination with ifosfamide (Séjourné et al. 2014). This observation may be explained by a shift in the metabolite pattern in favour of the inactive dichloroethyl metabolites and the neurotoxic chloroacetaldehyde (Durand et al. 2007).

2.5 Cisplatin and Carboplatin

Platinum complexes like cisplatin and carboplatin (Fig. 6) exert their antitumour effects by forming DNA adducts and subsequent inhibition of DNA replication and transcription. The active form is the aquo-complex Pt $(NH_3)_2(H_2O)_2$ which is formed intracellularly due to the low chloride concentration. Formation of this complex from carboplatin is much slower than from cisplatin (Murry 1997). Consequently, the dose administered for cisplatin is 40–80 mg/m^2, whereas carboplatin can be administered in about fivefold higher amounts.

Platinum derivatives have an important role in the treatment of several solid tumours. Besides myelosuppression, nephrotoxicity and ototoxicity are dose-limiting for cisplatin, whereas thrombocytopenia is dose-limiting for carboplatin. Cisplatin significantly reduces fertility in male patients (Chow et al. 2016).

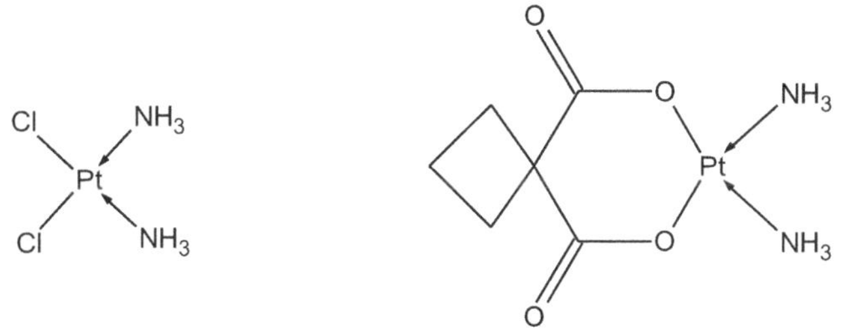

Fig. 6 Cisplatin and carboplatin

Cisplatin is extensively bound to plasma proteins, and clear pharmacokinetic-pharmacodynamic correlations have been identified for the ultrafiltrable, i.e., unbound fraction of the drug in plasma and toxicity as well as therapeutic effect (de Waal et al. 1990).

As carboplatin is preferentially eliminated through the kidney, clearance can be predicted using parameters of the renal function. Calvert et al. proposed and validated a formula to calculate the dose of carboplatin for a desired AUC from the glomerular filtration rate calculated using ^{51}Cr-EDTA clearance (Calvert et al. 1989). For children, modified formulae have been developed (Newell et al. 1993; Chatelut et al. 1996).

Formulae to calculate the carboplatin dose are today widely applied in clinical routine. They can reduce the variability in the AUC to about 25% in comparison with an up to fourfold variability in AUC when the dose is adjusted to BSA (Calvert and Egorin 2002). Dose individualisation based on plasma concentration measurements is recommended for infants. More recent studies suggested a bodyweight-based dose calculation for neuroblastoma patients (Duong et al. 2019). Of note, neuroblastoma patients are very young (median age 3.5 years in the study of Duong), and the findings of this relatively small study cannot be applied for all children. In summary, the optimal method for carboplatin dosing differs between age groups and, possibly, tumour entities.

2.6 Other Alkylating Agents: Dacarbazine, Procarbazine and Temozolomide

The hydrazine derivatives dacarbazine and procarbazine are used for the treatment of melanoma and brain tumours and display substantial toxicity. Procarbazine inhibits spermatogenesis and results in azoospermia in males treated with the drug for Hodgkin disease (Howell and Shalet 2005). Therefore, this drug should be avoided in post-pubertal boys. Girls and boys with poor prognostic features with Hodgkin lymphoma receive procarbazine as part of a polychemotherapy protocol (Dörffel et al. 2013). The typical daily dose is 100 mg/m^2 for up to 14 days.

In an attempt to develop similar anticancer alkylating agents with reduced toxicity, temozolomide (Fig. 7) was developed (Stevens et al. 1987). The drug is mainly used for the treatment of brain tumours such as gliomas, because it shows some activity in this very difficult to treat tumour and can be administered orally.

Fig. 7 Temozolomide

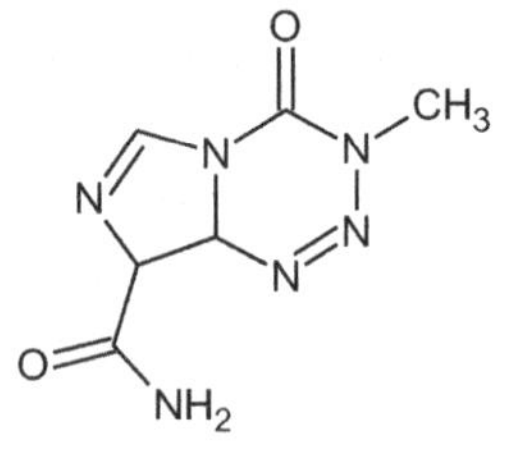

However, the activity in children with brain tumours is limited (Lashford et al. 2002; Cohen et al. 2011). Temozolomide is administered orally in a dose of 150–200 mg/m^2 for 28 days following a 23-day therapy-free interval. The drug is hepatotoxic, and neutropenia is usually dose-limiting.

3 Antimetabolites

The group of antimetabolites show similarity to endogenous compounds necessary for normal cell functions. The drugs or their metabolites bind to their target enzymes resulting in inhibition of essential cell functions. Many of the antimetabolites are also used as immunosuppressant or anti-inflammatory drugs in other diseases such as multiple sclerosis, rheumatoid arthritis, or autoimmune disorders.

3.1 Methotrexate

Methotrexate (Fig. 8) is used in the treatment of childhood ALL, osteosarcoma in children, as well as for non-Hodgkin lymphoma. It belongs to the group of antimetabolite cytostatics as they were developed to replace endogenous substances necessary for cell metabolism resulting in subsequent inhibition of proliferation. The drug is an inhibitor of dihydrofolate reductase, an enzyme responsible for the formation of tetrahydrofolate, which is the carrier for the transfer of carbon units. Inhibition of dihydrofolate reductase results in reduced thymine production necessary for DNA synthesis.

The main metabolites found in plasma are 7-hydroxy-methotrexate and 4-amino-4-deoxy-N10-methylpteroic acid. However, the drug is mainly excreted unchanged through the kidneys. When entering the cell, methotrexate is conjugated with two to seven glutamate moieties to methotrexate polyglutamates and can be stored in this form. The polyglutamates also display pharmacological activity. Similarly, 7-hydroxy-methotrexate can be polyglutamated and stored inside the cell.

Figure 9 shows the serum concentration time curve after administration as a 24 h infusion. Methotrexate is the only cytotoxic drug where a specific antidote, folinic acid, is available. This fact allows dose escalations beyond the usually lethal dose of the drug by administering folinic acid at least 36 h after starting the methotrexate infusion. In fact, for certain tumour entities like osteosarcoma, a positive correlation between dose intensity and therapeutic outcome has been found in retrospective analyses (Graf et al. 1994).

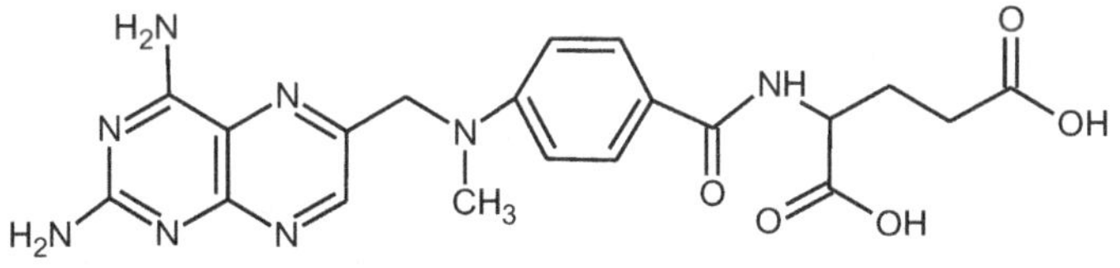

Fig. 8 Methotrexate

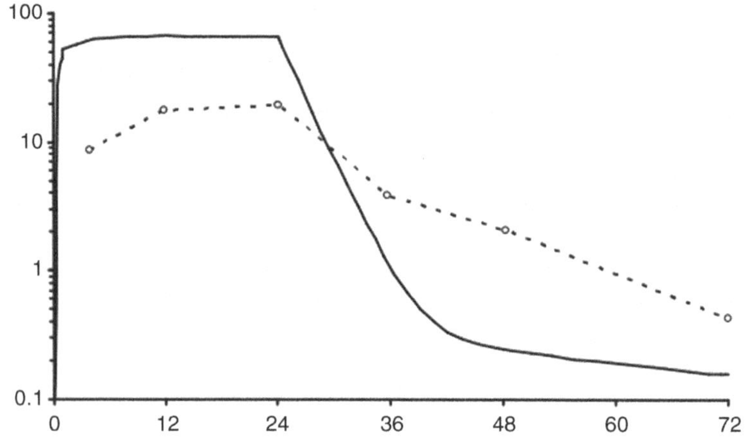

Fig. 9 Serum concentration of methotrexate (solid line) and 7-OH methotrexate (dotted line) in a child receiving 1 g/m^2 as a 24 h infusion

Sufficient hydration, alkalisation of the urine by infusion of hydrogen carbonate and avoiding drugs which may impair Mtx elimination such as benzimidazoles (i.e. omeprazole or pantoprazole), ciprofloxacin or nonsteroidal antirheumatic drugs (NSAIDs) are essential for the safe administration of Mtx. Monitoring of serum concentrations during high-dose therapy is necessary in order to identify delayed elimination which can be lethal without adequate treatment. Methotrexate is both nephro- and hepatotoxic at higher doses.

Low-dose oral methotrexate is part of maintenance therapy in the therapy of ALL. Children receive a weekly dose of 20 mg/m^2. It is very important for patients and other caregivers that methotrexate is administered only once in a week, whereas mercaptopurine is administered daily, because daily administration of methotrexate may result in serious overdosing. Other drugs influencing the folate pathway such as sulfamethoxazole/trimethoprim cannot be administered on the same day due to increased toxicity.

3.2 Thiopurines: 6-Mercaptopurine

Mercaptopurine (Fig. 10) is one of the oldest cytostatic drugs and is used in remission induction and maintenance therapy of ALL in children (Burchenal et al. 1953). Mercaptopurine requires activation by conjugation to the respective nucleotide catalysed by the enzyme hypoxanthine phosphoribosyltransferase. The monophosphate can be converted to the respective triphosphates which can subsequently be incorporated into DNA or RNA (Bostrom and Erdmann 1993). Another route catalysed by xanthine oxidase leads to inactive metabolites. Further, mercaptopurine is methylated at the sulphur leading to products which can also catabolised to the respective nucleotides. The enzyme responsible for the methylation, thiopurine

Fig. 10 Mercaptopurine

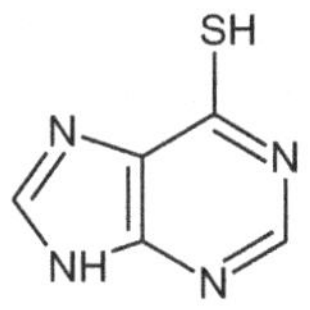

methyltransferase (TPMT), displays a genetic polymorphism with up to 0.6% of patients showing very low activity of this enzyme (Stanulla et al. 2005). Patients receive the drug as a daily oral dose of 50 mg/m^2 for several months. Dose adjustment is usually done according to the leucocyte count. Hepatotoxicity is apparent, and liver enzymes must be controlled during therapy.

3.3 Cytosine-Arabinoside (Cytarabine, Ara-C)

1-β-d-arabinofuranosylcytosine (Fig. 11) is a mainstay in the treatment of acute myeloid leukaemia (AML) and also shows activity in ALL. Combination with anthracyclines is standard in induction therapy for AML. The standard dose is 200 mg/m^2 for 7 days, but high-dose Ara-C with twice-daily dosing of up to 3 g/m^2 is very popular as induction therapy (Boos 1992). It remains an open question if high-dose therapy is superior to standard-dose Ara-C (Magina et al. 2017). In adolescents and adults, a slight advantage for high-dose Ara-C can only be seen for disease-free survival, but not overall survival (Löwenberg 2013).

Ara-C needs to be transformed to the respective nucleotide to be cytotoxic. Deoxycytidine kinase is responsible for the formation of the monophosphate Ara-CMP. After catabolism to the respective triphosphate Ara-CTP, inhibition of the DNA polymerase due to its similarity to deoxycytidine triphosphate (dCTP) is the main mechanism of action.

Fig. 11 Cytarabine

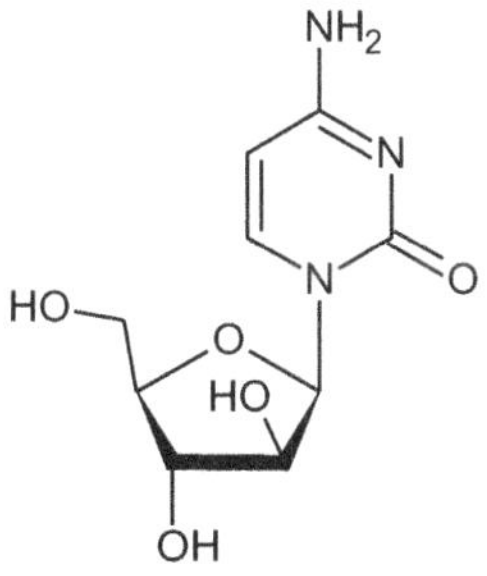

Ara-C is one of the few drugs which can be administered by the intrathecal route, although the drug is potentially neurotoxic. Such a CNS therapy is necessary to protect CNS relapse and avoid CNS irradiation. A liposomal formulation (DepoCyte) has been developed with the aim to achieve extended exposure after intrathecal administration (Peyrl et al. 2014).

CPX-351 is a liposomal formulation containing Ara-C and daunorubicin as a fixed combination in a ratio of 5:1. It shows promising results in the treatment of leukaemia in adults and could be a good option for children in the future (Carol et al. 2015).

3.4 Cladribine (2-CdA)

This drug (Fig. 12) is used in the treatment of AML and ALL in children during induction and maintenance therapy. It can be administered both i.v. and orally. 2-CdA is an inhibitor of ribonucleotide reductase and can augment the bioactivation of Ara-C. By inhibiting ribonucleotide reductase, concentrations of deoxyadenosine (dAdo) decrease. dAdo inhibits deoxycytidine kinase, the key enzyme responsible for the activation of Ara-C. Therefore, combination with cytarabine was tested in several investigations (Freyer et al. 2015). For children with newly diagnosed or relapsed/refractory AML, 2-CdA alone and in combination with Ara-C, topotecan or idarubicin was evaluated. 2-CdA was mostly administered as a continuous infusion over 5 days with a daily dose of up to 9 mg/m^2 (Chaleff et al. 2012). Besides myelosuppression, neurotoxicity occurs when administered in higher doses. Progressive multifocal leukoencephalopathy (PML) is a severe neurological disease which is believed to be the result of proliferation of the polyomavirus JC due to immunosuppression. PML was reported, sometimes years after treatment with cladribine, however, JC virus could not be detected (Berghoff et al. 2013).

Fig. 12 Cladribine

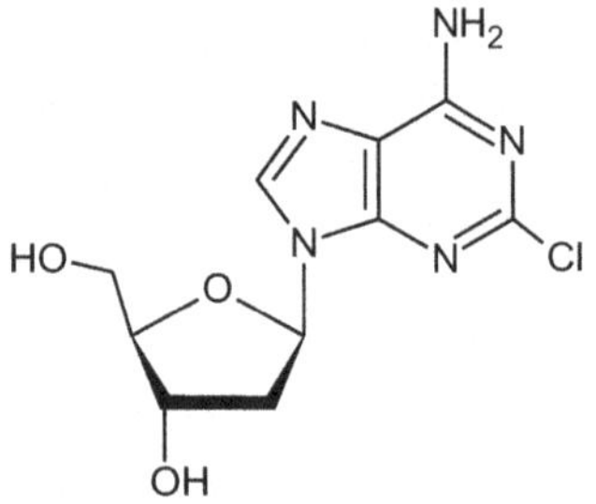

Fig. 13 Clofarabine

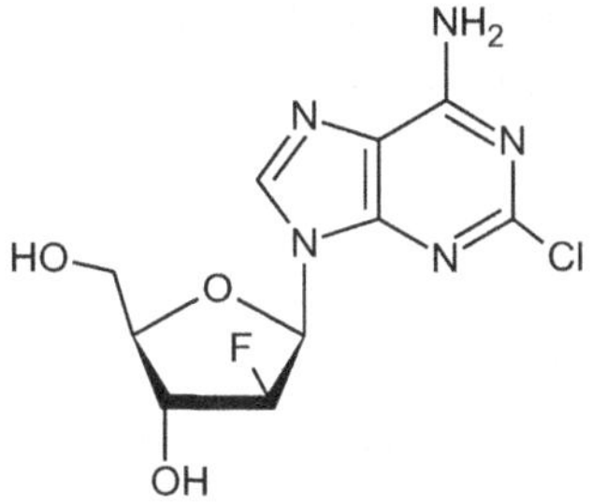

3.5 Clofarabine

This nucleoside analogue is approved for the treatment of leukaemia in children since 2004. As with other drugs of this class, clofarabine (Fig. 13) requires phosphorylation to the respective trinucleotide to exert its anticancer effect. The drug not only acts on proliferating blasts but also on quiescent nondividing lymphocytes (Hijiya et al. 2012). It can be administered in combination with cytarabine. The drug is administered as a 2-h infusion in a dose of 52 mg/m^2 on 5 consecutive days. About 60% of the administered dose is excreted unchanged in the urine within 24 h. A recent study indicates that clofarabine may replace anthracyclines in remission induction for children with AML (Rubnitz et al. 2019). Reducing the cumulative anthracycline dose for children is desirable due to the cumulative cardiotoxicity of this class of cytostatics (see below). As with cladribine, the risk of infections due to neutropenia is very high. Systemic inflammatory response syndrome (SIRS) occurred in 5% of paediatric patients treated with clofarabine for AML.

3.6 Fludarabine

For intravenous administration, the monophosphate ester is used because of the good solubility in water (Fig. 14). It is used during conditioning before bone marrow transplantation. It is also used in combination with Ara-C in AML patients in order to increase the accumulation of Ara-C within malignant cells (FLAG

Fig. 14 Fludarabine phosphate

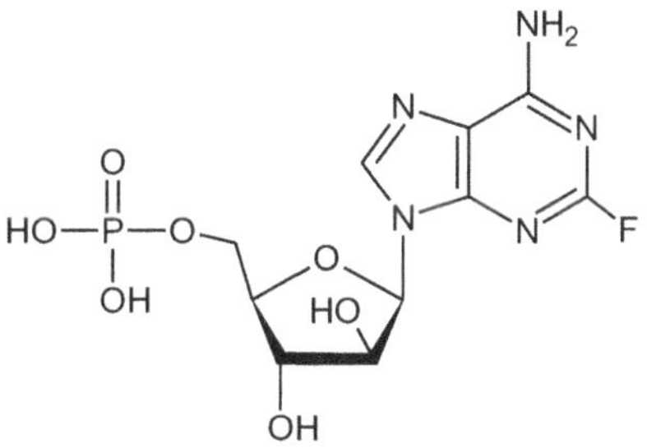

schemes), often in combination with anthracyclines like the Ida-FLAG with idarubicin and G-CSF (Fleischhack et al. 1998). Fludarabine is administered with a daily dose of 30 mg/m^2 for 4 days. Besides myelosuppression, upper respiratory tract infections, herpes virus infections and fever of unknown origin are quite common after therapy with fludarabine (Schmitt et al. 2002).

4 Topoisomerase Inhibitors

Topoisomerase is necessary for DNA unlinking and thus for normal DNA replication. The topoisomerase inhibitors discussed here interact with topoisomerase IIa forming a topoisomerase-drug-DNA complex which is poisonous by inhibition of the elongation reaction. Unfortunately, this mode of action is associated with the development of secondary cancers and cardiotoxicity (Delgado et al. 2018). Topoisomerase I poisons like topotecan and irinotecan are not often used in children and are therefore not discussed here.

4.1 Anthracyclines

The first drug from the group of anthracyclines, daunorubicin (Fig. 15), was isolated from *Streptomyces* strains in 1961 (Cassinelli 2016). They are still the most active anticancer agents available (Peterson 2011) and exert their anticancer effect mainly by inhibiting or poisoning of the eukaryotic topoisomerase II. Other mechanisms like formation of free radicals or DNA intercalation identified in vitro with high concentrations do not appear to play a role in vivo at therapeutic concentrations (Gewirtz 1999).

Daunorubicin and idarubicin are mainly used for the treatment of leukaemia, whereas the less lipophilic doxorubicin is part of many treatment protocols for solid tumours including neuroblastoma, Ewing- and osteosarcoma. Epirubicin, an epimer of doxorubicin, is rarely used in children.

Anthracyclines are metabolised by carbonyl reductase and aldo-keto reductase to their respective 13-hydroxy metabolites. Less than 10% are excreted renally,

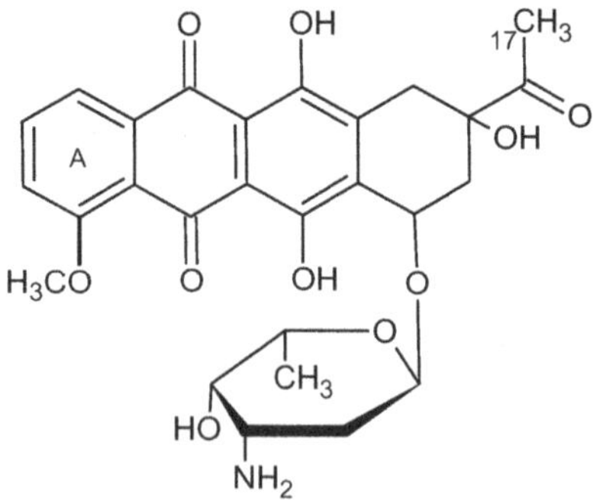

Fig. 15 Daunorubicin; doxorubicin has a hydroxyl function on C-17; idarubicin lacks the methoxy group on the aromatic ring A

while most of the drug and the metabolites undergo biliary excretion. Age-dependent pharmacokinetics was observed in a recent study analysing plasma concentrations from children receiving doxorubicin for leukaemia and solid tumours (Völler et al. 2015) (Fig. 16).

Dauno- and doxorubicin are administered in a dose of 20–60 mg/m^2, whereas idarubicin is administered in fourfold to fivefold lower doses. Only for idarubicin, an oral formulation is available, because the bioavailability of the other anthracyclines is very low. The duration of infusion should not be shorter than 1 h, because preclinical and clinical evidence exists that shorter infusion times resulting in high peak plasma concentrations are more cardiotoxic than longer infusion times (Loeffen et al. 2018). Nevertheless, some paediatric oncologists are in favour of short infusions and the addition of dexrazoxane as a cardioprotectant (Asselin et al. 2016). However, dexrazoxane inhibits topoisomerase II and may increase the risk for secondary malignancies (Tebbi et al. 2007). In a retrospective investigation, no higher incidence of secondary tumours with dexrazoxane was found (Seif et al. 2015). Another approach to reduce cardiotoxicity is the administration as a liposomal formulation (Creutzig et al. 2013). Unfortunately, liposomal daunorubicin is currently not available.

Cardiotoxicity is a very serious side effect especially for children because heart failure due to anthracyclines may appear decades after treatment. Risk factors for

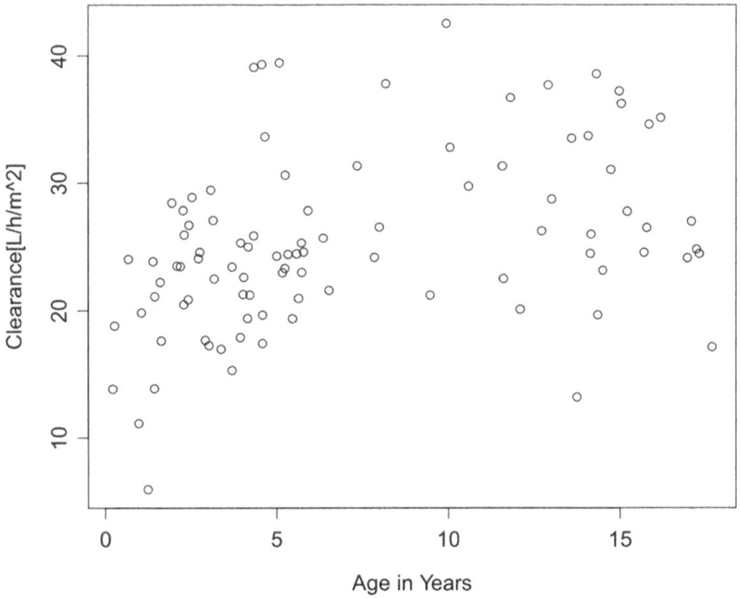

Fig. 16 Clearance of doxorubicin vs. age in a population of 99 children receiving doxorubicin for different tumour entities. Data from Völler et al. (2015)

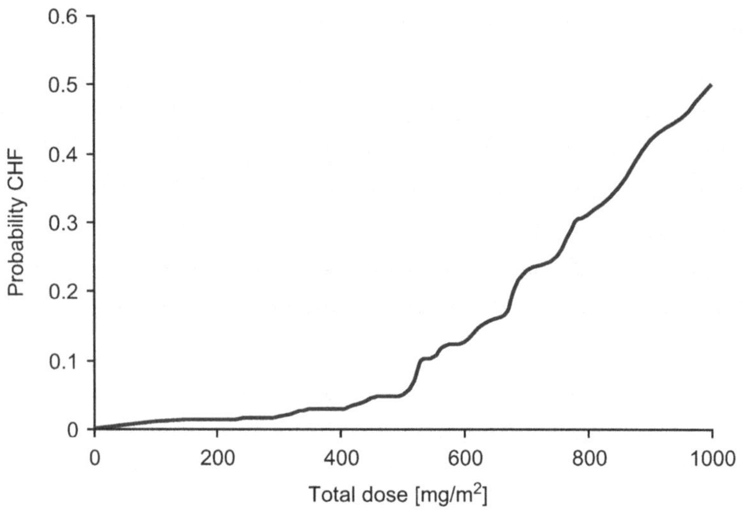

Fig. 17 Probability of developing congestive heart failure (CHF) vs. cumulative anthracycline dose (von Hoff et al. 1979). Data from adult patients. Note that children tend to be more sensitive to cardiotoxicity

anthracycline-induced cardiotoxicity are the cumulative dose, mediastinal radiation, younger age and female sex (Kremer et al. 2002; Fig. 17).

4.2 Etoposide

Etoposide (VP-16), Fig. 18) is a semi-synthetic drug derived from podophyllotoxin, a poison found in *Podophyllum peltatum*, a plant in medical use for more than 1,000 years. It is a topoisomerase II poison that is used extensively in the treatment of leukaemia and germ cell tumours. It is administered in an i.v. formulation containing polyethylene glycol, Tween 80, ethanol and benzylalcohol due to the low water solubility of the compound. Especially the latter two excipients are not suited for the use in children due to their potential neurotoxicity. Therefore, etoposide phosphate as a more hydrophilic prodrug should be preferred in children. Etoposide can also be administered orally, and capsules containing 50 or 100 mg are on the market. The bioavailability is approximately 50% with a high variability (Slevin 1991).

The elimination of etoposide is highly dependent on renal function, because 20–50% of the applied dose are excreted in the urine (Lowis et al. 1993). In addition, the drug is metabolised by P450 3A4 and is a substrate of several ABC transporters (Lagas et al. 2010). Etoposide is highly protein-bound, and interindividual changes in protein binding are apparent (Würthwein et al. 2002).

Fig. 18 Etoposide

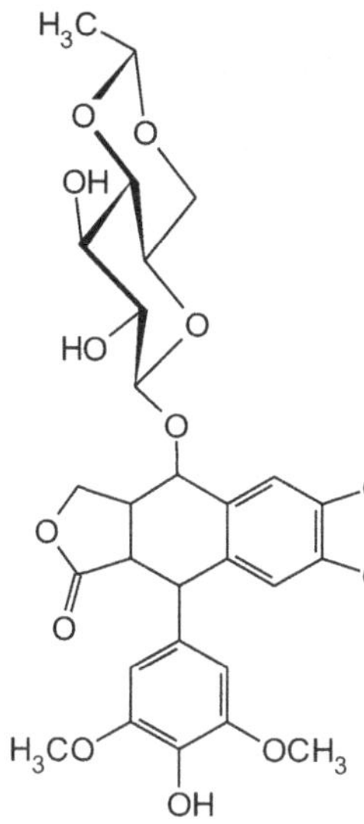

Conventional dosing of etoposide is in the range of 50–150 mg/m^2 administered on 3–5 days. In high-dose schemes before SCT, up to 50 mg/kg are administered. High-dose therapy is possible because neutropenia is the dose-limiting toxicity. Secondary malignancies occur mainly as AML in about 8% of patients receiving etoposide-containing polychemotherapy. Oral etoposide is administered with daily dosing of 25–50 mg/m^2.

4.3 Drugs Interacting with Tubulin

α- and β-tubulin form the microtubule responsible for the separation of the chromosomes during cell division. Drugs inhibiting the formation like *Vinca* alkaloids or drugs stabilising microtubuli like taxanes lead to cell cycle arrest in the metaphase and apoptosis. Of therapeutic interest in children is vincristine, whereas taxanes like paclitaxel do not show a clear benefit in children over other anticancer drugs due to toxicity like neuropathy and pseudo-allergic reactions (Doz et al. 2001). These side effects were mainly due to formulation for i.v. use containing Cremophor EL as a surfactant. However, even when administered in the novel innovative formulation nab-paclitaxel adsorbed to nanoparticular albumin, the response rates with paclitaxel are only modest (Moreno et al. 2018).

4.4 Vinca Alkaloids: Vincristine

Vinca alkaloids are a group of endogenous compounds from *Catharanthus roseus*. They bind to the β-subunit of tubulin and thereby impose the formation of microtubuli. Vincristine is the most important drug from this group of drugs. It is used in the treatment of ALL as part of the multiagent induction therapy in combination with several other drugs in a dose of 1–2 mg/m^2 in weekly intervals. Elimination of vincristine from the body is mainly by biliary excretion and metabolism by cytochrome P450 3A4. Neurotoxicity is dose-limiting starting with neuropathy. Accidentally administered intrathecal vincristine due to confusion in the multiagent therapy results in ascending paralysis and death within days (Hennipman et al. 2009). ABCB1 (also called P-glycoprotein, PGP) is – at least in part – responsible for keeping the drug out of the CNS. Therefore, combining vincristine with inhibitors of ABCB1 such as voriconazole and related drugs increases neurotoxicity and should therefore be avoided (Moriyama et al. 2012).

5 "Targeted" Drugs

Since the beginning of this century, many authors and textbooks distinguish anticancer agents in the newer targeted drugs like imatinib which were invented by rational drug design and the older nontargeted drugs mainly developed by screening for cytotoxicity in cell lines.

However, it must be noted that these categories are not correctly assigned as many of the old drugs like the antimetabolites target specific enzymes within the cell. Moreover, it was found that the so-called targeted drugs address several targets in the body. Tyrosine kinase inhibitors inhibit several enzymes which is usually desirable, because blocking a single pathway can be easily circumvented by the cancer cell. An exemption is the Bcr-Abl protein targeted by imatinib, which is obviously the protein responsible for the proliferation of certain types of leukaemia (see below).

5.1 Asparaginase

This enzyme is already in use for decades but should be categorised as a targeted drug, because it depletes asparagine from the serum. ALL blasts lack the enzyme asparagine synthetase, and treatment with asparaginase results in cell death, whereas other cells are able to synthetize asparagine (Asselin and Rizzari 2015). Currently, a recombinant asparaginase (originally derived from *E.coli*), a product derived from *Erwinia chrysanthemi* called Erwinase, and a PEGylated asparaginase (Oncaspar) are on the market in Europe. The recombinant asparaginase is administered i.m. or i.v. as a 1-h infusion with a dose of 2,500–10,000 U/m^2 every 2–3 days, whereas therapy with Erwinase requires a higher dose of up to 25,000 U/m^2. Oncaspar is the preparation of choice, because it can administered with a dose of 1,000 U/m^2 in dosing intervals of 14 days due to its lower clearance in comparison to the preparation without polyethylene glycol (Würthwein et al. 2017).

Thrombosis, pancreatitis and hepatotoxicity are very relevant toxicities. Patients may develop antibodies binding to the protein and/or to PEG inactivating the enzyme (Tong et al. 2014). In this case, therapy has to be modified by applying asparaginase from another biological source, which does not cross-react with the antibodies to ensure sufficient therapy intensity (Boos 1997). Antibody formation can occur with or without an allergic reaction. In the latter case, the so-called silent inactivation results in worse outcome for the patients (Salzer et al. 2018). Monitoring of asparaginase activity in patients serum is now generally recommended in order to identify patients with inactivating antibodies (van der Sluis et al. 2016).

5.2 Bortezomib

Bortezomib (Fig. 19) was the first proteasome inhibitor introduced to the clinic. Proteasome inhibition means inhibition of protein degradation within the cell resulting in cumulation of proteins in the cytosol. Nuclear factor kappa-light-chain-enhancer of activated B cells (NF-κB) appears to play a key role for the anticancer effect as bortezomib is able to block the tumorigenic and pro-inflammatory NF-κB pathway by inhibition of the degradation of i-κB (Cvek and Dvorak 2011). It was developed for the treatment of multiple myeloma in adults and showed clear benefits over existing therapies with regard to overall survival (Scott et al. 2016). Some efficacy was demonstrated in paediatric patients with relapsed ALL in combination with vincristine, dexamethasone, PEG-asparaginase and doxorubicin (Messinger et al. 2010), whereas the antileukemic effect as a single agent is low (Horton et al. 2007). Additional studies in relapsed ALL with bortezomib in different combinations show some activity, for example, in T-ALL (Kaspers et al. 2018; Horton et al. 2007). The drug is administered i.v. in a dose of 1.3 mg/m^2 in weekly or shorter intervals depending on the combination partners. Febrile neutropenia is dose-limiting in contrast to the situation in adults where neuropathy is the most serious toxicity. Bortezomib clearance increases linearly with body surface area in an age range from 2 to 16 years justifying dosing based on BSA (Hanley et al. 2017).

Fig. 19 Bortezomib

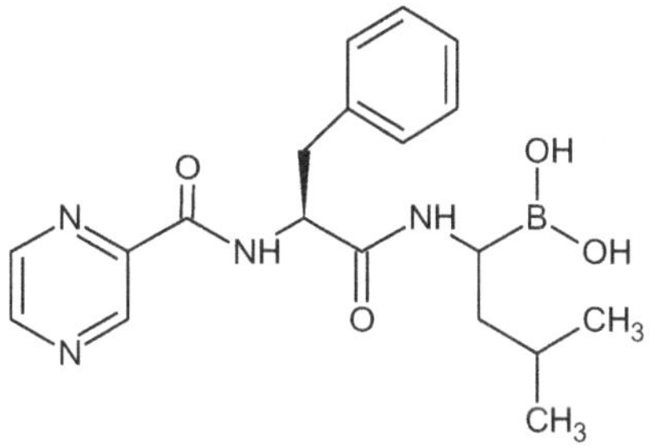

5.3 Tyrosine Kinase Inhibitors (TKIs): Imatinib, Dasatinib, Ponatinib, Sorafenib and Vemurafenib

The breakpoint cluster region – Abelson (Bcr-Abl) tyrosine kinase inhibitor imatinib (Fig. 20) – is probably the most extensively used TKI in children because it was the first drug of this class approved in 2001. Bcr-Abl displays tyrosine kinase activity and is formed as a fusion gene product as a result of a t(9;22) translocation known as Philadelphia chromosome (Barr 2010). Imatinib blocks the dysregulated proliferative signal of Bcr-Abl. This protein is expressed in chronic myeloid leukaemia, which is a rare disease in children. In a subgroup of children with ALL, the t(9;22) translocation is also present, and imatinib shows high activity in this subgroup. Response rates were almost doubled in comparison with other treatment options by introduction of imatinib (Schultz et al. 2009).

TKI's are administered daily over longer time periods in comparison with classical anticancer drugs. Oral administration is much more convenient to the patient but introduces an additional source of variability and the risk of nonadherence. 300 mg/m^2 is a standard daily dose for imatinib. Bioavailability is very high, and the drug can be metabolised by CYP 3A after entering the hepatocyte with the help of the organic cation transporter 1 (OCT1). However, the first-pass effect is low with an oral bioavailability of more than 95%. Elimination via the bile is achieved after glucuronidation (Takahashi and Miura 2011). Enterohepatic recirculation occurs which means that diarrhoea, use of antibiotics or any other disturbance of the normal gastrointestinal function may influence exposure to imatinib. Dasatinib, nilotinib and ponatinib are drugs showing activity if resistance to imatinib occurs. In addition, TKIs targeting other proteins with tyrosine kinase domains such as the epidermal growth factor receptor (EGFR), platelet-derived growth factor receptor (PDGFR) or members of the vascular endothelial growth factor receptor (VEGF) family are increasingly used in solid tumours such as neuroblastoma or sarcomas. However, so far the results of clinical studies with TKI's in children with solid tumours are disappointing (Kim et al. 2015; Okada et al. 2016).

Fig. 20 Imatinib

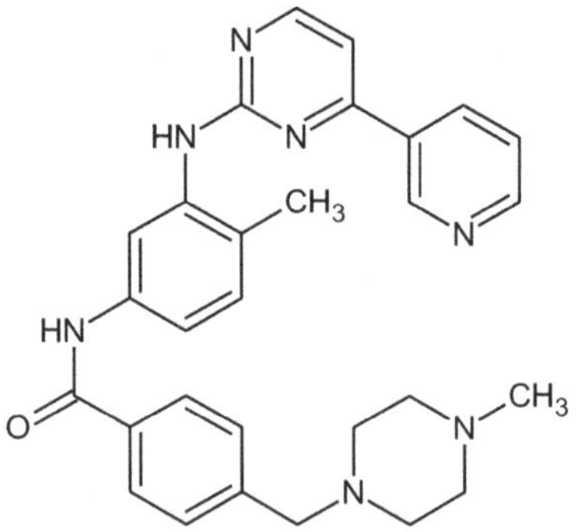

Side effects of TKI's are substantial and include hypertension, obstruction, diarrhoea, hepatotoxicity and many more. Growth retardation during imatinib therapy has been observed but is reversible after drug cessation (Vandyke et al. 2009).

References

Abate ME, Paioli A, Cammelli S, Cesari M, Longhi A, Palmerini E, Ferrari S, Carretta E, Picci P, Piscaglia F (2018) Sinusoidal obstruction syndrome/veno-occlusive disease after high-dose intravenous busulfan/melphalan conditioning therapy in high-risk Ewing Sarcoma. Bone Marrow Transplant 53(5):591–599

Ahlmann M, Hempel G (2016) The effect of cyclophosphamide on the immune system. Implications for clinical cancer therapy. Cancer Chemother Pharmacol 78(4):661–671

Anderson BJ, McKee AD, Holford NH (1997) Size, myths and the clinical pharmacokinetics of analgesia in paediatric patients. Clin Pharmacokinet 33(5):313–327

Asselin B, Rizzari C (2015) Asparaginase pharmacokinetics and implications of therapeutic drug monitoring. Leuk Lymphoma 56(8):2273–2280

Asselin BL, Devidas M, Chen L, Franco VI, Pullen J, Borowitz MJ, Hutchison RE, Ravindranath Y, Armenian SH, Camitta BM, Lipshultz SE (2016) Cardioprotection and Safety of Dexrazoxane in patients treated for newly diagnosed t-cell acute lymphoblastic leukemia or advanced-stage lymphoblastic non-hodgkin lymphoma: a report of the Children's Oncology Group randomized trial Pediatric Oncology Group 9404. J Clin Oncol 34(8):854–862

Barr RD (2010) Imatinib mesylate in children and adolescents with cancer. Pediatr Blood Cancer 55 (1):18–25

Bartelink IH, Bredius RGM, Ververs TT, Raphael MF, van Kesteren C, Bierings M, Rademaker CMA, den Hartigh J, Uiterwaal CSPM, Zwaveling J, Boelens JJ (2008) Once-daily intravenous busulfan with therapeutic drug monitoring compared to conventional oral busulfan improves survival and engraftment in children undergoing allogeneic stem cell transplantation. Biol Blood Marrow Transplant 14(1):88–98

Berghoff M, Schänzer A, Hildebrandt GC, Dassinger B, Klappstein G, Kaps M, Gizewski ER, Acker T, Grams A (2013) Development of progressive multifocal leukoencephalopathy in a patient with non-Hodgkin lymphoma 13 years after treatment with cladribine. Leuk Lymphoma 54(6):1340–1342

Boddy AV, Yule SM (2000) Metabolism and pharmacokinetics of oxazaphosphorines. Clin Pharmacokinet 38(4):291–304

Boddy AV, Cole M, Pearson AD, Idle JR (1995) The kinetics of the auto-induction of ifosfamide metabolism during continuous infusion. Cancer Chemother Pharmacol 36(1):53–60

Boos J (1992) Ist die Pharmakokinetik von Cytarabin klinisch relevant? (Is the pharmacokinetic profile of cytarabine clinically relevant?). Klin Padiatr 204(4):198–203

Boos J (1997) Pharmacokinetics and drug monitoring of L-asparaginase treatment. Int J Clin Pharmacol Ther 35(3):96–98

Bostrom B, Erdmann G (1993) Cellular pharmacology of 6-mercaptopurine in acute lymphoblastic leukemia. Am J Pediatr Hematol Oncol 15(1):80–86

Burchenal JH, Murphy ML, Ellison RR, Sykes MP, Tan TC, Leone LA, Karnofsky DA, Craver LF, Dargeon HW, Rhoads CP (1953) Clinical evaluation of a new antimetabolite, 6-mercaptopurine, in the treatment of leukemia and allied diseases. Blood 8(11):965–999

Calvert AH, Egorin MJ (2002) Carboplatin dosing formulae. Gender bias and the use of creatinine-based methodologies. Eur J Cancer 38(1):11–16

Calvert AH, Newell DR, Gumbrell LA, O'Reilly S, Burnell M, Boxall FE, Siddik ZH, Judson IR, Gore ME, Wiltshaw E (1989) Carboplatin dosage. Prospective evaluation of a simple formula based on renal function. J Clin Oncol 7(11):1748–1756

Carli M, Passone E, Perilongo G, Bisogno G (2003) Ifosfamide in pediatric solid tumors. Oncology 65(Suppl 2):99–104

Carol H, Fan MMY, Harasym TO, Boehm I, Mayer LD, Houghton P, Smith MA, Lock RB (2015) Efficacy of CPX-351, (cytarabine:daunorubicin) liposome injection, against acute lymphoblastic leukemia (ALL) xenograft models of the Pediatric Preclinical Testing Program. Pediatr Blood Cancer 62(1):65–71

Cassinelli G (2016) The roots of modern oncology: from discovery of new antitumor anthracyclines to their clinical use. Tumori 2016(3):226–235

Chaleff S, Hurwitz CA, Chang M, Dahl G, Alonzo TA, Weinstein H (2012) Phase II study of 2-chlorodeoxyadenosine plus idarubicin for children with acute myeloid leukaemia in first relapse: a paediatric oncology group study. Br J Haematol 156(5):649–655

Chatelut E, Boddy AV, Peng B, Rubie H, Lavit M, Dezeuze A, Pearson AD, Roché H, Robert A, Newell DR, Canal P (1996) Population pharmacokinetics of carboplatin in children. Clin Pharmacol Ther 59(4):436–443

Chow EJ, Stratton KL, Leisenring WM, Oeffinger KC, Sklar CA, Donaldson SS, Ginsberg JP, Kenney LB, Levine JM, Robison LL, Shnorhavorian M, Stovall M, Armstrong GT, Green DM (2016) Pregnancy after chemotherapy in male and female survivors of childhood cancer treated between 1970 and 1999. A report from the Childhood Cancer Survivor Study cohort. Lancet Oncol 17(5):567–576

Cohen KJ, Pollack IF, Zhou T, Buxton A, Holmes EJ, Burger PC, Brat DJ, Rosenblum MK, Hamilton RL, Lavey RS, Heideman RL (2011) Temozolomide in the treatment of high-grade gliomas in children. A report from the Children's Oncology Group. Neuro Oncol 13(3):317–323

Creutzig U, Zimmermann M, Bourquin J-P, Dworzak MN, Fleischhack G, Graf N, Klingebiel T, Kremens B, Lehrnbecher T, von Neuhoff C, Ritter J, Sander A, Schrauder A, von Stackelberg A, Starý J, Reinhardt D (2013) Randomized trial comparing liposomal daunorubicin with idarubicin as induction for pediatric acute myeloid leukemia: results from Study AML-BFM 2004. Blood 122(1):37–43

Cvek B, Dvorak Z (2011) The ubiquitin-proteasome system (UPS) and the mechanism of action of bortezomib. Curr Pharm Des 17(15):1483–1499

de Waal WA, Maessen FJ, Kraak JC (1990) Analytical methodologies for the quantitation of platinum anti-cancer drugs and related compounds in biological media. J Pharm Biomed Anal 8(1):1–30

Delgado JL, Hsieh C-M, Chan N-L, Hiasa H (2018) Topoisomerases as anticancer targets. Biochem J 475(2):373–398

Dörffel W, Rühl U, Lüders H, Claviez A, Albrecht M, Bökkerink J, Holte H, Karlen J, Mann G, Marciniak H, Niggli F, Schmiegelow K, Schwarze E-W, Pötter R, Wickmann L, Schellong G (2013) Treatment of children and adolescents with Hodgkin lymphoma without radiotherapy for patients in complete remission after chemotherapy: final results of the multinational trial GPOH-HD95. J Clin Oncol 31(12):1562–1568

Doz F, Gentet JC, Pein F, Frappaz D, Chastagner P, Moretti S, Vassal G, Arditti J, Tellingen OV, Iliadis A, Catalin J (2001) Phase I trial and pharmacological study of a 3-hour paclitaxel infusion in children with refractory solid tumours: a SFOP study. Br J Cancer 84(5):604–610

Du Bois D, Du Bois EF (1916) A formula to estimate the approximate surface area if height and weight be known. 1916. Nutrition 5(5):303–311; discussion 312–3

Duong JK, Veal GJ, Nath CE, Shaw PJ, Errington J, Ladenstein R, Boddy AV (2019) Population pharmacokinetics of carboplatin, etoposide and melphalan in children. A re-evaluation of paediatric dosing formulas for carboplatin in patients with normal or mild impairment of renal function. Br J Clin Pharmacol 85(1):136–146

Durand J-P, Gourmel B, Mir O, Goldwasser F (2007) Antiemetic neurokinin-1 antagonist aprepitant and ifosfamide-induced encephalopathy. Ann Oncol 18(4):808–809

Fleischhack G, Hasan C, Graf N, Mann G, Bode U (1998) IDA-FLAG (idarubicin, fludarabine, cytarabine, G-CSF), an effective remission-induction therapy for poor-prognosis AML of

childhood prior to allogeneic or autologous bone marrow transplantation: experiences of a phase II trial. Br J Haematol 102(3):647–655
Freyer CW, Gupta N, Wetzler M, Wang ES (2015) Revisiting the role of cladribine in acute myeloid leukemia. An improvement on past accomplishments or more old news? Am J Hematol 90 (1):62–72
Gewirtz DA (1999) A critical evaluation of the mechanisms of action proposed for the antitumor effects of the anthracycline antibiotics adriamycin and daunorubicin. Biochem Pharmacol 57:727–741
Gorin NC, Labopin M, Blaise D, Dumas P-Y, Pabst T, Trisolini SM, Arcese W, Houhou M, Mohty M, Nagler A (2018) Optimizing the pretransplant regimen for autologous stem cell transplantation in acute myelogenous leukemia. Better outcomes with busulfan and melphalan compared with busulfan and cyclophosphamide in high risk patients autografted in first complete remission: A study from the acute leukemia working party of the EBMT. Am J Hematol 93 (7):859–866
Graf N, Winkler K, Betlemovic M, Fuchs N, Bode U (1994) Methotrexate pharmacokinetics and prognosis in osteosarcoma. J Clin Oncol 12(7):1443–1451
Hanley MJ, Mould DR, Taylor TJ, Gupta N, Suryanarayan K, Neuwirth R, Esseltine D-L, Horton TM, Aplenc R, Alonzo TA, Lu X, Milton A, Venkatakrishnan K (2017) Population pharmacokinetic analysis of bortezomib in pediatric leukemia patients: model-based support for body surface area-based dosing over the 2- to 16-year age range. J Clin Pharmacol 57(9):1183–1193
Hempel G, Boos J (2007) Flat-fixed dosing versus body surface area based dosing of anticancer drugs. There is a difference. Oncologist 12(8):924–926
Hennipman B, de Vries E, Bökkerink JPM, Ball LM, Veerman AJP (2009) Intrathecal vincristine: 3 fatal cases and a review of the literature. J Pediatr Hematol Oncol 31(11):816–819
Hijiya N, Barry E, Arceci RJ (2012) Clofarabine in pediatric acute leukemia. Current findings and issues. Pediatr Blood Cancer 59(3):417–422
Hilger RA, Harstrick A, Eberhardt W, Oberhoff C, Skorzec M, Baumgart J, Seeber S, Scheulen ME (1998) Clinical pharmacokinetics of intravenous treosulfan in patients with advanced solid tumors. Cancer Chemother Pharmacol 42(2):99–104
Horton TM, Pati D, Plon SE, Thompson PA, Bomgaars LR, Adamson PC, Ingle AM, Wright J, Brockman AH, Paton M, Blaney SM (2007) A phase 1 study of the proteasome inhibitor bortezomib in pediatric patients with refractory leukemia: a Children's Oncology Group study. Clin Cancer Res 13(5):1516–1522
Howell SJ, Shalet SM (2005) Spermatogenesis after cancer treatment. Damage and recovery. J Natl Cancer Inst Monogr 34:12–17
Kamen BA, Frenke LA, Colvin OM (1995) Ifosfamide: should the honeymoon be over? J Clin Oncol 13(2):307–309
Kaspers GJL, Niewerth D, Wilhelm BAJ, Scholte-van Houtem P, Lopez-Yurda M, Berkhof J, Cloos J, de Haas V, Mathôt RA, Attarbaschi A, Baruchel A, de Bont ES, Fagioli F, Rössig C, Klingebiel T, de Moerloose B, Nelken B, Palumbo G, Reinhardt D, Rohrlich P-S, Simon P, von Stackelberg A, Zwaan CM (2018) An effective modestly intensive re-induction regimen with bortezomib in relapsed or refractory paediatric acute lymphoblastic leukaemia. Br J Haematol 181(4):523–527
Kerl K, Diestelhorst C, Bartelink I, Boelens J, Trame MN, Boos J, Hempel G (2014) Evaluation of effects of busulfan and DMA on SOS in pediatric stem cell recipients. Pediatr Blood Cancer 61 (2):306–311
Kim A, Widemann BC, Krailo M, Jayaprakash N, Fox E, Weigel B, Blaney SM (2015) Phase 2 trial of sorafenib in children and young adults with refractory solid tumors: a report from the Children's Oncology Group. Pediatr Blood Cancer 62(9):1562–1566
Kremer LCM, van der Pal HJH, Offringa M, van Dalen EC, Voûte PA (2002) Frequency and risk factors of subclinical cardiotoxicity after anthracycline therapy in children: a systematic review. Ann Oncol 13(6):819–829

Lagas JS, Fan L, Wagenaar E, Vlaming MLH, van Tellingen O, Beijnen JH, Schinkel AH (2010) P-glycoprotein (P-gp/Abcb1), Abcc2, and Abcc3 determine the pharmacokinetics of etoposide. Clin Cancer Res 16(1):130–140

Lashford LS, Thiesse P, Jouvet A, Jaspan T, Couanet D, Griffiths PD, Doz F, Ironside J, Robson K, Hobson R, Dugan M, Pearson ADJ, Vassal G, Frappaz D (2002) Temozolomide in malignant gliomas of childhood. A United Kingdom Children's Cancer Study Group and French Society for Pediatric Oncology Intergroup Study. J Clin Oncol 20(24):4684–4691

Loeffen EAH, van Dalen EC, Mulder RL, van de Wetering MD, Kremer LCM, Tissing WJE (2018) The duration of anthracycline infusion should be at least one hour in children with cancer: a clinical practice guideline. Pediatr Blood Cancer 65(2):e26867

Löwenberg B (2013) Sense and nonsense of high-dose cytarabine for acute myeloid leukemia. Blood 121(1):26–28

Lowis SP, Pearson AD, Newell DR, Cole M (1993) Etoposide pharmacokinetics in children: the development and prospective validation of a dosing equation. Cancer Res 53(20):4881–4889

Magina KN, Pregartner G, Zebisch A, Wölfler A, Neumeister P, Greinix HT, Berghold A, Sill H (2017) Cytarabine dose in the consolidation treatment of AML. A systematic review and meta-analysis. Blood 130(7):946–948

medac Gmbh (2014) Summary of product characteristics. Ovastat 1000/5000 mg. www.fachinfo.de. Assessed Apr 2019

Messinger Y, Gaynon P, Raetz E, Hutchinson R, Dubois S, Glade-Bender J, Sposto R, van der Giessen J, Eckroth E, Bostrom BC (2010) Phase I study of bortezomib combined with chemotherapy in children with relapsed childhood acute lymphoblastic leukemia (ALL): a report from the therapeutic advances in childhood leukemia (TACL) consortium. Pediatr Blood Cancer 55(2):254–259

Moreno L, Casanova M, Chisholm JC, Berlanga P, Chastagner PB, Baruchel S, Amoroso L, Gallego Melcón S, Gerber NU, Bisogno G, Fagioli F, Geoerger B, Glade Bender JL, Aerts I, Bergeron C, Hingorani P, Elias I, Simcock M, Ferrara S, Le Bruchec Y, Slepetis R, Chen N, Vassal G (2018) Phase I results of a phase I/II study of weekly nab-paclitaxel in paediatric patients with recurrent/refractory solid tumours: A collaboration with innovative therapies for children with cancer. Eur J Cancer 100:27–34

Moriyama B, Henning SA, Leung J, Falade-Nwulia O, Jarosinski P, Penzak SR, Walsh TJ (2012) Adverse interactions between antifungal azoles and vincristine. Review and analysis of cases. Mycoses 55(4):290–297

Mosteller RD (1987) Simplified calculation of body-surface area. N Engl J Med 317(17):1098

Murry DJ (1997) Comparative clinical pharmacology of cisplatin and carboplatin. Pharmacotherapy 17(5 Pt 2):140S–145S

Myers AL, Kawedia JD, Champlin RE, Kramer MA, Nieto Y, Ghose R, Andersson BS (2017) Clarifying busulfan metabolism and drug interactions to support new therapeutic drug monitoring strategies. A comprehensive review. Expert Opin Drug Metab Toxicol 13(9):901–923

Nath CE, Shaw PJ, Montgomery K, Earl JW (2007) Population pharmacokinetics of melphalan in paediatric blood or marrow transplant recipients. Br J Clin Pharmacol 64(2):151–164

Newell DR, Pearson AD, Balmanno K, Price L, Wyllie RA, Keir M, Calvert AH, Lewis IJ, Pinkerton CR, Stevens MC (1993) Carboplatin pharmacokinetics in children. The development of a pediatric dosing formula. The United Kingdom Children's Cancer Study Group. J Clin Oncol 11(12):2314–2323

Nygren P (2001) What is cancer chemotherapy? Acta Oncol 40(2–3):166–174

Okada K, Nakano Y, Yamasaki K, Nitani C, Fujisaki H, Hara J (2016) Sorafenib treatment in children with relapsed and refractory neuroblastoma: an experience of four cases. Cancer Med 5 (8):1947–1949

Palmer J, McCune JS, Perales M-A, Marks D, Bubalo J, Mohty M, Wingard JR, Paci A, Hassan M, Bredeson C, Pidala J, Shah N, Shaughnessy P, Majhail N, Schriber J, Savani BN, Carpenter PA (2016) Personalizing Busulfan-based conditioning. Considerations from the American society for blood and marrow transplantation practice guidelines committee. Biol Blood Marrow Transplant 22(11):1915–1925

Park M, Park HJ, Eom H-S, Kwon YJ, Park JA, Lim YJ, Yoon JH, Kong S-Y, Ghim TT, Lee HW, Yun T, Park B-K (2013) Safety and effects of prophylactic defibrotide for sinusoidal obstruction syndrome in hematopoietic stem cell transplantation. Ann Transplant 18:36–42

Peterson C (2011) Drug therapy of cancer. Eur J Clin Pharmacol 67(5):437–447

Peyrl A, Sauermann R, Chocholous M, Azizi AA, Jäger W, Höferl M, Slavc I (2014) Pharmacokinetics and toxicity of intrathecal liposomal cytarabine in children and adolescents following age-adapted dosing. Clin Pharmacokinet 53(2):165–173

Rubnitz JE, Lacayo NJ, Inaba H, Heym K, Ribeiro RC, Taub J, McNeer J, Degar B, Schiff D, Yeoh AE-J, Coustan-Smith E, Wang L, Triplett B, Raimondi SC, Klco J, Choi J, Pounds S, Pui C-H (2019) Clofarabine can replace anthracyclines and etoposide in remission induction therapy for childhood acute myeloid leukemia. The AML08 multicenter, randomized phase III trial. J Clin Oncol 37(23):2072–2081

Salzer W, Bostrom B, Messinger Y, Perissinotti AJ, Marini B (2018) Asparaginase activity levels and monitoring in patients with acute lymphoblastic leukemia. Leuk Lymphoma 59 (8):1797–1806

Schmitt B, Wendtner CM, Bergmann M, Busch R, Franke A, Pasold R, Schlag R, Hopfinger G, Hiddemann W, Emmerich B, Hallek M (2002) Fludarabine combination therapy for the treatment of chronic lymphocytic leukemia. Clin Lymphoma 3(1):26–35

Schultz KR, Bowman WP, Aledo A, Slayton WB, Sather H, Devidas M, Wang C, Davies SM, Gaynon PS, Trigg M, Rutledge R, Burden L, Jorstad D, Carroll A, Heerema NA, Winick N, Borowitz MJ, Hunger SP, Carroll WL, Camitta B (2009) Improved early event-free survival with imatinib in Philadelphia chromosome-positive acute lymphoblastic leukemia: a children's oncology group study. J Clin Oncol 27(31):5175–5181

Scott K, Hayden PJ, Will A, Wheatley K, Coyne I (2016) Bortezomib for the treatment of multiple myeloma. Cochrane Database Syst Rev 4:CD010816

Seif AE, Walker DM, Li Y, Huang Y-SV, Kavcic M, Torp K, Bagatell R, Fisher BT, Aplenc R (2015) Dexrazoxane exposure and risk of secondary acute myeloid leukemia in pediatric oncology patients. Pediatr Blood Cancer 62(4):704–709

Séjourné A, Noal S, Boone M, Bihan C, Sassier M, Andrejak M, Chauffert B (2014) Two cases of fatal encephalopathy related to Ifosfamide: an adverse role of aprepitant? Case Rep Oncol 7 (3):669–672

Slatter MA, Rao K, Amrolia P, Flood T, Abinun M, Hambleton S, Nademi Z, Goulden N, Davies G, Qasim W, Gaspar HB, Cant A, Gennery AR, Veys P (2011) Treosulfan-based conditioning regimens for hematopoietic stem cell transplantation in children with primary immunodeficiency. United Kingdom experience. Blood 117(16):4367–4375

Slevin ML (1991) The clinical pharmacology of etoposide. Cancer 67:319–329

Stanulla M, Schaeffeler E, Flohr T, Cario G, Schrauder A, Zimmermann M, Welte K, Ludwig W-D, Bartram CR, Zanger UM, Eichelbaum M, Schrappe M, Schwab M (2005) Thiopurine methyltransferase (TPMT) genotype and early treatment response to mercaptopurine in childhood acute lymphoblastic leukemia. JAMA 293(12):1485–1489

Stevens MF, Hickman JA, Langdon SP, Chubb D, Vickers L, Stone R, Baig G, Goddard C, Gibson NW, Slack JA (1987) Antitumor activity and pharmacokinetics in mice of 8-carbamoyl-3-methyl-imidazo5,1-d-1,2,3,5-tetrazin-4(3H)-one (CCRG 81045; M & B 39831), a novel drug with potential as an alternative to dacarbazine. Cancer Res 47(22):5846–5852

Takahashi N, Miura M (2011) Therapeutic drug monitoring of imatinib for chronic myeloid leukemia patients in the chronic phase. Pharmacology 87(5–6):241–248

Tebbi CK, London WB, Friedman D, Villaluna D, de Alarcon PA, Constine LS, Mendenhall NP, Sposto R, Chauvenet A, Schwartz CL (2007) Dexrazoxane-associated risk for acute myeloid leukemia/myelodysplastic syndrome and other secondary malignancies in pediatric Hodgkin's disease. J Clin Oncol 25(5):493–500 ten Brink MH, Zwaveling J, Swen JJ, Bredius RGM, Lankester AC, Guchelaar HJ (2014) Personalized busulfan and treosulfan conditioning for pediatric stem cell transplantation. The role of pharmacogenetics and pharmacokinetics. Drug Discov Today 19(10):1572–1586

Tong WH, Pieters R, Kaspers GJL, te Loo DMWM, Bierings MB, van den Bos C, Kollen WJW, Hop WCJ, Lanvers-Kaminsky C, Relling MV, Tissing WJE, van der Sluis IM (2014) A prospective study on drug monitoring of PEGasparaginase and Erwinia asparaginase and asparaginase antibodies in pediatric acute lymphoblastic leukemia. Blood 123(13):2026–2033

Trame MN, Bergstrand M, Karlsson MO, Boos J, Hempel G (2011) Population pharmacokinetics of busulfan in children. Increased evidence for body surface area and allometric body weight dosing of busulfan in children. Clin Cancer Res 17(21):6867–6877

van der Sluis IM, Vrooman LM, Pieters R, Baruchel A, Escherich G, Goulden N, Mondelaers V, Sanchez de Toledo J, Rizzari C, Silverman LB, Whitlock JA (2016) Consensus expert recommendations for identification and management of asparaginase hypersensitivity and silent inactivation. Haematologica 101(3):279–285

Vandyke K, Dewar AL, Fitter S, Menicanin D, To LB, Hughes TP, Zannettino ACW (2009) Imatinib mesylate causes growth plate closure in vivo. Leukemia 23(11):2155–2159

Völler S, Boos J, Krischke M, Würthwein G, Kontny NE, Boddy AV, Hempel G (2015) Age-dependent pharmacokinetics of doxorubicin in children with cancer. Clin Pharmacokinet 54(11):1139–1149

von Hoff DD, Layard MW, Basa P, Davis HL, von Hoff AL, Rozencweig M, Muggia FM (1979) Risk factors for doxorubicin-induced congestive heart failure. Ann Intern Med 91(5):710–717

Würthwein G, Klingebiel T, Krümpelmann S, Metz M, Schwenker K, Kranz K, Lanvers-Kaminsky C, Boos J (2002) Population pharmacokinetics of high-dose etoposide in children receiving different conditioning regimens. Anticancer Drugs 13:101–110

Würthwein G, Lanvers-Kaminsky C, Hempel G, Gastine S, Möricke A, Schrappe M, Karlsson MO, Boos J (2017) Population pharmacokinetics to model the time-varying clearance of the PEGylated asparaginase Oncaspar® in children with acute lymphoblastic leukemia. Eur J Drug Metab Pharmacokinet 42(6):955–963

Immunosuppressants in Organ Transplantation

Burkhard Tönshoff

Contents

Abstract

The goal of immunosuppressive therapy post-transplantation in pediatric renal transplant recipients is to prevent acute and chronic rejection while minimizing drug side effects. Most therapies alter immune response mechanisms but are not immunologically specific, and a careful balance is required to find the dose that prevents rejection of the graft while minimizing the risks of overimmunosuppression leading to infection and cancer. While this chapter because of space constraints focuses on immunosuppressive therapy in pediatric renal transplant recipients, many aspects can be applied on pediatric recipients of other solid organ transplants such as the liver and heart. The major maintenance immunosuppressive agents currently used in various combination regimens are tacrolimus, cyclosporine, mycophenolate mofetil, azathioprine, everolimus, sirolimus, and glucocorticoids (steroids). Although data from adult renal transplantation trials are used to help guide management decisions in pediatric

B. Tönshoff (✉)
Department of Pediatrics I, University Children's Hospital, Heidelberg, Germany
e-mail: Burkhard.Toenshoff@med.uni-heidelberg.de

W. Kiess et al. (eds.), *Pediatric Pharmacotherapy*,
Handbook of Experimental Pharmacology 261, https://doi.org/10.1007/164_2019_331

patients, immunosuppressive therapy in pediatric renal transplant recipients often must be modified because of the unique dosage requirements and clinical effects of these agents in children, including their impact on growth and development. The optimal immunosuppressive therapy post-transplant is not established. The goal remains to find the best combination of immunosuppressive agents that optimizes allograft survival by preventing acute rejection while limiting drug toxicities.

Keywords
Calcineurin inhibitors · Cyclosporine · Everolimus · Glucocorticoids (steroids) · Immunosuppressive induction therapy · Immunosuppressive maintenance therapy · Mycophenolate mofetil · Pediatric renal transplantation · Tacrolimus

1 Introduction

Ideally, a host would accept a renal transplant by induction of antigen-specific non-responsiveness (immunologic tolerance). Current immunosuppressive agents reduce acute rejection but do not induce tolerance. It is true that a few patients with organ transplants successfully can withdraw their immunosuppression without rejecting their grafts for long periods of time. However, these are rare exceptions, and such patients may eventually reject, even after years. Even though antigen-specific T cells with reactivity to the foreign antigen persist in the host indefinitely, some graft and host adaptation must occur, since the level of immunosuppression required long-term is very low compared to the levels required within the first weeks. This adaptation makes long-term immunosuppression possible; however, the long-term risk of cancer in the immunosuppressed patient remains increased. Thus, the distinction between immunosuppression and tolerance induction is partly artificial: any immunosuppression involves some apparent antigen-specific adaptation, i.e., downregulation of the host response to the graft; and many tolerance protocols involve some nonspecific immunosuppressive therapies.

The common immunosuppressive agents used in pediatric renal transplantation include antibodies to cell surface antigens on lymphocytes (antithymocyte globulin (ATG)), anti-interleukin 2 (IL-2) receptor antibodies, the calcineurin inhibitors tacrolimus and cyclosporine, the lymphocyte proliferation inhibitors mycophenolate mofetil (MMF) and azathioprine, and the mammalian target of rapamycin (mTOR) inhibitors sirolimus and everolimus and glucocorticoids. Although an adequate maintenance level of immunosuppression is required to dampen the immune response to the allograft, the level of chronic immunosuppression is slowly decreased over time to help lower the overall risk of infection and malignancy; these risks directly correlate with the degree of overall immunosuppression. Maintenance regimens consist of a combination of immunosuppressive agents that differ in their mechanism of action. This strategy minimizes morbidity and mortality associated with each class of agent while maximizing overall effectiveness. Allograft survival rates vary among the various immunosuppressive agents due to patient-specific clinical characteristics, such as age, obesity, ethnicity, hyperlipidemia,

Table 1 Immunosuppressive agents categorized according to mechanism of action

Mechanism of action	Drugs
Polyclonal antibodies	Antithymocyte globulin
	Thymoglobulin (rabbit)
	ATGAM (equine)
Monoclonal antibodies	Anti-CD3 antibody: OKT3 (murine)
	Anti-CD52 antibody: Alemtuzumab (human)
	Anti-CD20 antibody: Rituximab
	Anti-CD25 antibody: Daclizumab (human) Basiliximab (chimeric)
	Selective blocker of CD86-CD28 costimulation: Belatacept
Calcineurin inhibitors	Cyclosporine
	Tacrolimus
Target of rapamycin inhibitors	Sirolimus
	Everolimus
Antimetabolites	Azathioprine
Purine synthesis inhibitors	Mycophenolate mofetil
Others	Glucocorticoids
	Intravenous immunoglobulin G

arterial hypertension, and/or delayed allograft function. Immunosuppressive agents should therefore be chosen in part based on patient characteristics. Other issues to be taken into account are related to the immunologic history of the patient, such as the degree of HLA matching, pre-sensitization, re-transplant, history of acute rejection episodes, and the risk of recurrent disease.

The immunosuppressive and immunomodulatory drugs can be pharmacologically categorized on the basis of their mechanism of action (Table 1). Figure 1 depicts a schematic representation of the three-signal model along with the site of action of common immunosuppressive drugs. The three-signal model of T-cell activation and proliferation is helpful in understanding the molecular mechanisms and site of action of various immunosuppressive drugs (Halloran 2004). Signal 1 features antigen-presenting cells (APCs; macrophages and dendritic cells) presenting the foreign antigen to the T lymphocyte, activating the T-cell receptor (TCR), which further relays the signal through the transduction apparatus known as the CD3 complex. Signal 2 is a nonantigen-specific costimulatory signal which occurs as a result of binding of the B7 molecule on the APC to CD28 on the T cell. Both signal 1 and signal 2 activate signal transduction pathways: the calcium–calcineurin pathway, mitogen-activated protein (MAP) pathway, and the nuclear factor-κB (NF-κB) pathway. This in turn leads to increased expression of interleukin-2 (IL-2), which through its receptor (IL-2R) activates the cell cycle (signal 3). Signal 3 activation requires the enzyme target of rapamycin for translation of mRNA and cell proliferation. Thus, various drugs act on different cellular signals and achieve immunosuppression by a number of mechanisms: depleting lymphocytes, diverting lymphocyte traffic, or blocking lymphocyte response pathways.

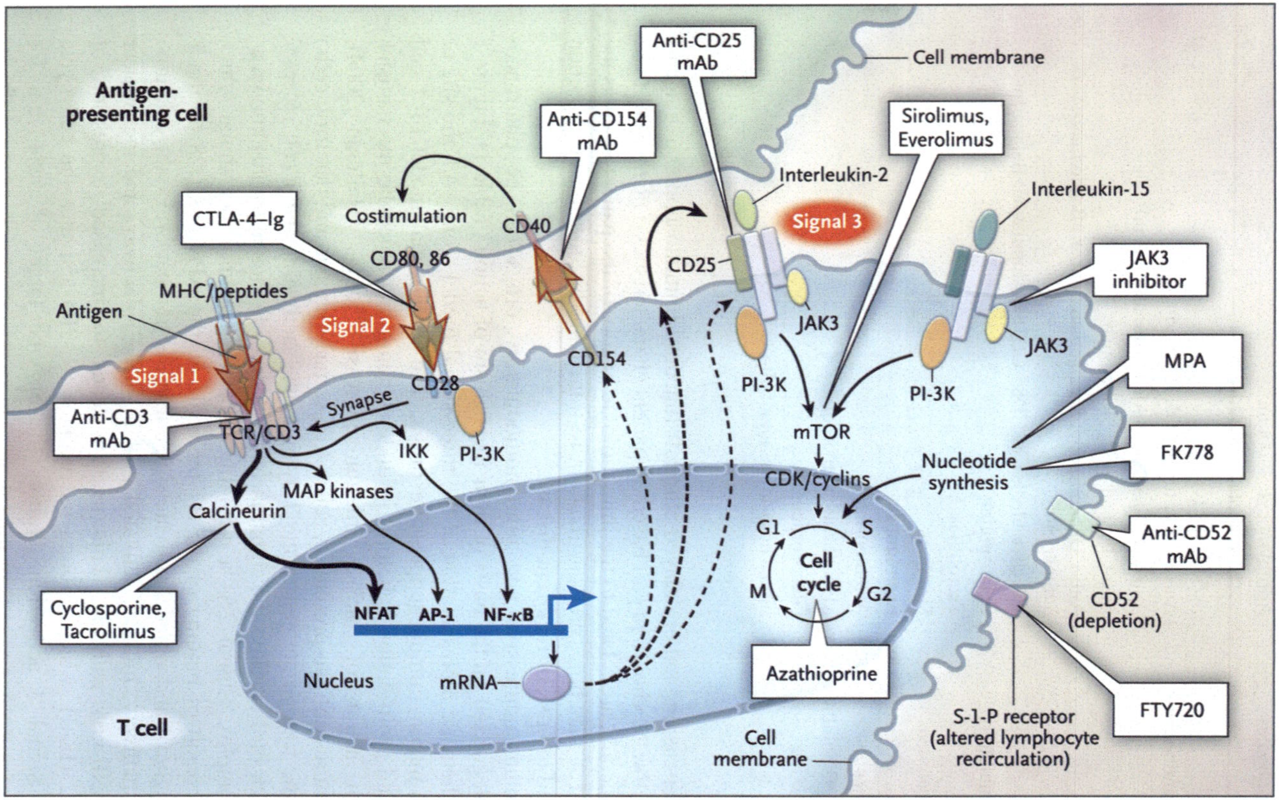

Fig. 1 Individual immunosuppressive drugs and sites of action in the three-signal model. Anti-CD154 antibody has been withdrawn from clinical trials but remains of interest. FTY720 engagement of sphingosine-1-phosphate (S-1-P) receptors triggers and internalizes the receptors and alters lymphocyte recirculation, causing lymphopenia. Antagonists of chemokine receptors (not shown) are also being developed in preclinical models. MPA denotes mycophenolic acid. Modified according to (Halloran 2004)

Table 2 Immunosuppressive agents categorized according to phase of immunosuppression

Phase of immunosuppression	Drugs
Induction phase	Basiliximab
	Thymoglobulin
	Glucocorticoids
Maintenance phase	Tacrolimus
	Cyclosporine
	Mycophenolate mofetil, azathioprine
	Sirolimus, everolimus
	Glucocorticoids
	Belatacept
Treatment of rejection	Glucocorticoids
	Thymoglobulin
	Intravenous immunoglobulin G
	Rituximab

Immunosuppressive agents are also classified on the basis of the phase of transplantation for which they are used (Table 2). Different immunosuppressive drugs are used for induction versus maintenance of immunosuppression, while others may be used for the treatment and reversal of graft rejection. The commonly used agents in immunosuppressive protocols are discussed in greater detail in the following section.

2 Induction Immunosuppressive Therapy

Induction refers to the administration of an intensive immunosuppressive regimen during the perioperative period. The rationale behind this approach is that the risk of acute rejection is greatest in the first weeks or months post-transplant. Induction therapies often involve the use of polyclonal or monoclonal antibodies to achieve rapid and profound early immunosuppression. Polyclonal antibodies used for this purpose include those against thymocytes (antithymocyte globulin (ATG)); monoclonal antibodies include basiliximab (a chimeric human–murine anti-CD25 or anti-interleukin (IL)-2 receptor antibody) and alemtuzumab (an anti-CD52 antibody targeting both B and T cells); the latter is not readily available and will therefore not be discussed here.

Each protocol may have specific advantages and/or disadvantages in a particular patient population, none is yet proven to be superior when all relevant factors are taken into account. The optimal prophylactic induction immunosuppressive therapy to prevent renal transplant rejection therefore remains controversial. Figure 2 presents the induction antibody use from 1996 to 2013, as reported by North American Renal Trials and Collaborative Studies (NAPRTCS) 2014 Annual Report (The NAPRTCS 2014), Fig. 3 reports the respective use in Europe reported by the Cooperative European Paediatric Renal Transplant Initiative (CERTAIN)

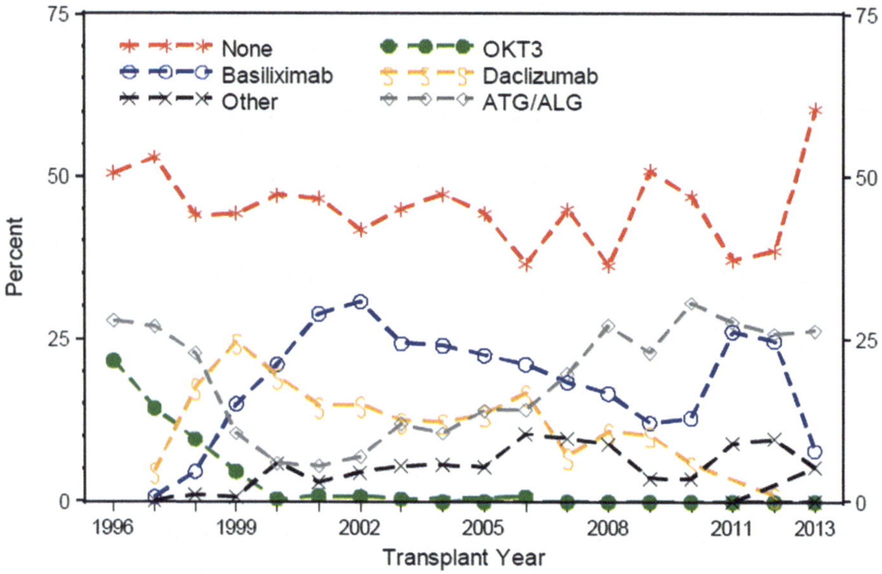

Fig. 2 Induction antibody use in North American pediatric renal transplant recipients, by year of renal transplantation (Data are from The NAPRTCS 2014 Annual Report. https://web.emmes.com/study/ped/index.htm)

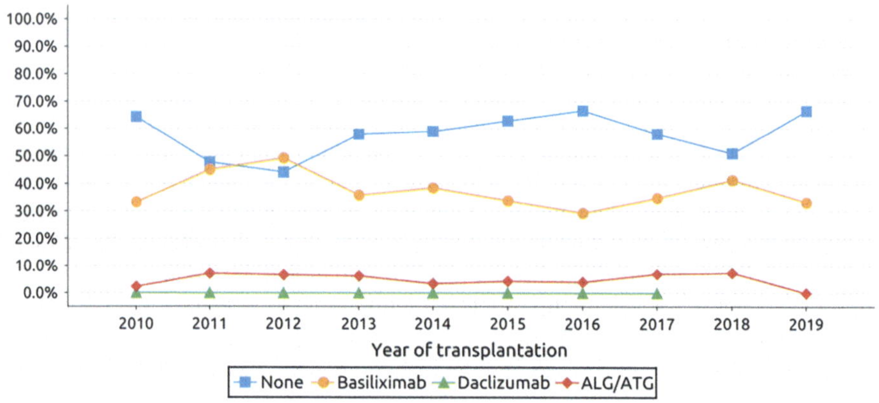

Fig. 3 Induction antibody use in European pediatric renal transplant recipients, by year of renal transplantation (Data are from the Cooperative European Paediatric Renal Transplant Initiative (CERTAIN) registry. www.certain-registry.eu)

(Cooperative European Paediatric Renal Transplant Initiative (CERTAIN) Registry 2019). The frequency of use of the different immunosuppressive antilymphocyte regimens for induction therapy varies markedly between North America and Europe.

Induction therapy produces the greatest benefits in groups at high risk for allograft rejection. These high-risk groups include African-Americans, recipients of kidneys with prolonged (>24 h) cold ischemia time, and those at high immunologic risk, particularly individuals who are presensitized. The sequential induction regimen of thymoglobulin followed by tacrolimus or cyclosporine is recommended in these high-risk groups.

2.1 Polyclonal Lymphocyte-Depleting Antibody Thymoglobulin

Because of the redundancy of the immune system, polyclonal antibodies, which have a broad specificity, should theoretically be more effective in induction therapy than monoclonal antilymphocyte agents. Thymoglobulin is a rabbit-derived polyclonal antibody preparation approved for the treatment of rejection and recently also for induction therapy by the US Federal Drug Administration (FDA). Thymoglobulin contains antibodies to a wide variety of T-cell and major histocompatibility complex (MHC) antigens. Polyclonal antibodies act in three ways: By activating or altering the function of lymphocytes, by lysing lymphoid cells, and by altering the traffic of lymphoid cells and sequestering them. These antibodies are potently immunosuppressive but often produce side effects. By triggering T cells, they generate significant first-dose effects, with the release of tumor necrosis factor alpha (TNFα), interferon γ (IFN-γ), and other cytokines, causing a first-dose reaction (flu-like syndrome, fever, and chills).

Thymoglobulin induction is usually dosed from 1 to 6 mg/kg per dose, and the duration may range from 1 to 10 days, although a more typical regimen is 1.5 mg/kg per dose for 3 to 5 days (Peddi et al. 2002; Stratta et al. 2005; Wong et al. 2006; Gurk-Turner et al. 2008). The optimal induction dose is felt to total 6 mg/kg (Wong et al. 2006; Stevens et al. 2008). Higher doses and prolonged duration of induction agents are thought to be associated with an increased risk of infection and the potential development of lymphoma, whereas cumulative doses of less than 3 mg/kg may not effectively prevent acute rejection (Goggins et al. 2003).

2.2 Monoclonal IL-2 Receptor Antibody Basiliximab

Full T-cell activation leads to the calcineurin-mediated stimulation of the transcription, translation, and secretion of IL-2, a key autocrine growth factor that induces T-cell proliferation. Thus, an attractive therapeutic option is abrogation of IL-2 activity via the administration of anti-IL-2 receptor antibodies. The only anti-IL-2 receptor antibody currently available is basiliximab, a chimeric monoclonal antibody that has been approved by the FDA for use in renal transplantation in adults and pediatric patients. Basiliximab is directed against CD25, the IL-2 receptor 55 kDa α-chain. However, IL-2 receptor functions are partially redundant, because other cytokine receptors have overlapping functions, e.g., IL-15 receptors. Therefore, saturating IL-2 receptors produces stable but relatively mild immunosuppression and is only effective in combination with other immunosuppressants.

The dosing schedule for basiliximab is the following: Intravenous administration of two 10 mg doses to children <35 kg body weight and two 20 mg doses to children ≥35 kg, with the first dose given during transplant surgery and the second on post-transplant day four. In patients on concomitant immunosuppression with cyclosporine and azathioprine, the mean duration of IL-2 receptor saturation is 42 ± 16 days (Sterkers et al. 2000). In patients on cyclosporine in conjunction with MMF, MMF reduces basiliximab clearance and prolongs CD25 saturation from 5 to 10 weeks (Höcker et al. 2008).

In pediatric renal transplant recipients, two large prospective randomized controlled trials showed that induction therapy with basiliximab in patients with low to standard immunological risk on maintenance therapy with tacrolimus in conjunction with azathioprine and steroids or on cyclosporine in conjunction with MMF and steroids did not lead to a statistically significant reduction in the incidence of acute rejection episodes (Grenda et al. 2006; Offner et al. 2008). As a result, there is presently no consensus among pediatric renal transplantation centers regarding the use and regimen for immunosuppressive induction therapy. Considerations in choosing the appropriate agent include the efficacy in the patient population (e.g., recipients with high or low risk of graft loss), the side effect profile, and the concomitant immunosuppressive therapy (steroid avoidance, early steroid withdrawal, or conventional steroid therapy).

3 Maintenance Immunosuppressive Therapy

Maintenance immunosuppressive therapy is administered to renal transplant recipients to help prevent acute rejection. Although an adequate level of immunosuppression is required to dampen the immune response to the allograft, the level of chronic immunosuppression is slowly decreased over time to help lower the overall risk of infection and malignancy; these risks directly correlate with the degree of overall immunosuppression. The type of immunosuppression may also be varied to decrease the risk of developing chronic antibody-mediated rejection, the most common underlying long-term cause of allograft loss. Conventional maintenance regimens consist of a combination of immunosuppressive agents that differ in their mechanism of action. This strategy minimizes morbidity and mortality associated with each class of agent while maximizing overall effectiveness. Such regimens may vary by transplant center and geographic area.

There are a number of important issues to consider when deciding upon the immunosuppressive protocol to administer in a particular patient: The risk for acute rejection and allograft loss is highest in the first 3 months after transplantation. As a result, immunosuppression should be at its highest during this period. The occurrence of the most serious side effects of immunosuppressive therapy, infections and malignancy, correlate with the total amount of immunosuppression. It is therefore essential that immunosuppression is gradually tapered to a maintenance level by 6–12 months post-transplant.

Allograft survival rates vary among the various immunosuppressive agents due to patient-specific clinical characteristics, such as age, obesity, ethnicity, hyperlipidemia, arterial hypertension, and/or delayed allograft function. Immunosuppressive agents should therefore be chosen in part based on patient characteristics. Other issues to be taken into account are related to the "immunologic" history of the patient such as the degree of HLA matching, presensitization, re-transplant, number and severity of previous acute rejection episodes, and the risk of recurrent disease.

The optimal maintenance immunosuppressive therapy in pediatric renal transplantation is not established. The major immunosuppressive agents currently used in various combination regimens are tacrolimus, cyclosporine, MMF, azathioprine, everolimus, sirolimus, and glucocorticoids (primarily oral prednisone or methylprednisolone). Most transplant centers currently utilize a maintenance regimen consisting of triple immunosuppression therapy with a calcineurin inhibitor (tacrolimus or cyclosporine), an anti-metabolite (MMF or azathioprine), and in some patients methylprednisolone. Everolimus or sirolimus are also used by some transplant centers in triple therapy regimens, sometimes in place of the calcineurin inhibitor or the antimetabolite. Within the NAPRTCS registry, marked changes in the type of maintenance immunosuppression and dosing strategies have been observed over time (The NAPRTCS 2014). These are substantially caused by the introduction of newer drugs such as MMF and tacrolimus (Table 3).

3.1 The Calcineurin Inhibitors Cyclosporine and Tacrolimus

Cyclosporine, a lipophilic cyclic peptide of 11 amino acid residues, and tacrolimus, a macrolide antibiotic, are drugs with similar mechanisms of action that have become major maintenance immunosuppressive agents used in transplantation. Cyclosporine and tacrolimus act by inhibiting the calcium-dependent serine phosphatase calcineurin, which normally is rate-limiting in T-cell activation.

3.1.1 Pharmacokinetics and Dosing

Cyclosporine and tacrolimus are both variably absorbed and are metabolized extensively by the liver (via the cytochrome P450 system). Neither cyclosporine nor tacrolimus is affected by alterations in renal function. Both cyclosporine and tacrolimus bind to cells and to plasma components (primarily lipoproteins for cyclosporine and albumin for tacrolimus) in the blood; consequently, they must be assayed in whole blood. Many drugs and agents can affect cyclosporine and tacrolimus levels through effects on their absorption or metabolism (Table 4).

Since the absorption of cyclosporine is decreased and its metabolism increased in children compared to adults, relatively higher dosages are required in pediatric patients. Cyclosporine is usually administered initially as 8–15 mg/kg daily in two divided doses (or intravenously using one third the oral dose over a 24-h period) during the induction phase, with target trough blood levels of 150–300 μg/L for the first 3–6 months post-transplant. Doses are reduced after 3–6 months (typically 4–6 mg/kg daily); long-term target trough blood levels of 75–125 μg/L appear to

Table 3 Observed drug utilization rates in North American pediatric renal transplant recipients among transplanted grafts with ≥30 days function that have occurred since 1996

Percent drug utilization – post transplant (patients with functioning grafts)												
	Transplant Era 1996–2001				Transplant Era 2002–2007				Transplant Era 2008–2013			
	30 days	1 year	3 years	5 years	30 days	1 year	3 years	5 years	30 days	1 year	3 years	5 years
Prednisone/CsA/MMF	35.6	38.2	30.7	22.5	10.0	8.8	8.0	7.9	1.7	2.4	0.9	–
Prednisone/CsA/Aza	23.1	17.7	14.2	8.9	0.8	0.8	0.6	0.7	0.2	0.1	0.4	–
Prednisone/Csa	11.5	5.4	4.8	5.4	3.4	1.6	1.0	1.4	0.8	0.3	0.0	–
Prednisone-/TAC/MMF	14.6	19.7	24.5	30.2	52.0	50.3	44.6	42.7	52.0	46.8	42.3	–
Prednisone-/TAC/Aza	2.3	4.9	6.5	6.9	1.8	2.4	2.6	4.0	2.2	2.1	4.0	–
Prednisone/TAC	6.1	7.7	10.5	11.8	9.6	11.4	11.5	8.4	4.0	10.9	13.2	–
TAC/MMF	0.4	1.1	1.7	2.7	10.7	9.7	11.8	13.5	28.7	22.3	22.5	–
Other combination	6.3	5.3	7.2	11.6	11.6	15.1	20.0	21.5	10.4	15.1	16.7	–

Data are from the NAPRTCS 2014 annual report. https://web.emmes.com/study/ped/index.htm

Table 4 Examples of common drug interactions of immunosuppressants used in solid-organ transplantation: cyclosporine, tacrolimus, sirolimus, and everolimus

Common types of drug interactions	Examples of interacting drugs
Coadministration of drugs that inhibit CYP3A metabolism and/or P-gp efflux can increase immunosuppressant whole blood concentrations, leading to significant toxicities	Amiodarone ART-boosting agents (e.g., ritonavir, cobicistat) Azole antifungals (e.g., fluconazole, posaconazole, voriconazole) HIV protease inhibitors (e.g., atazanavir, nelfinavir, saquinavir) Macrolide antibiotics (except azithromycin) Non-dihydropyridine calcium channel blockers Ombitasvir-paritaprevir-ritonavir with or without dasabuvir (an HCV, direct-acting antiviral regimen) Grapefruit juice
Coadministration of drugs that induce CYP3A metabolism and/or P-gp efflux pumping can decrease immunosuppressant whole blood concentrations, increasing the risk of organ rejection	Antiseizure drugs, enzyme inducing (e.g., carbamazepine, fosphenytoin, oxcarbazepine, phenobarbital, phenytoin, primidone) Enzalutamide Nafcillin Rifamycins (e.g., rifabutin, rifampin, rifapentine) St. John's wort
Coadministration of nephrotoxic drugs with cyclosporine or tacrolimus can cause additive or synergistic kidney injury	Aminoglycosides Amphotericin B Colchicine Nonsteroidal anti-inflammatory drugs (NSAIDs)
Coadministration of drugs that increase serum potassium with cyclosporine or tacrolimus may cause severe hyperkalemia	ACE inhibitors/ARBs Amiloride Spironolactone Triamterene Trimethoprim, trimethoprim-sulfamethoxazole (cotrimoxazole)
Coadministration of statin drugs with cyclosporine can increase statin levels and risk of myotoxicity	Atorvastatin Lovastatin Pitavastatin Rosuvastatin Simvastatin

CYP cytochrome P450 metabolism, *P-gp* P-glycoprotein drug efflux pump, *ART* HIV antiretroviral therapy, *HIV* human immunodeficiency virus, *HCV* hepatitis C virus, *ACE* angiotensin-converting enzyme, *ARB* angiotensin II receptor blocker

provide comparable patient and graft survival as higher blood levels but with less risk of malignancy (Dantal et al. 1998). Generic forms of cyclosporine are available, but they may not be equivalent and readily interchangeable, and knowledge of the characteristics of the oral formulations is necessary before switching between them.

Tacrolimus is 20- to 30-fold more potent than cyclosporine and, therefore, is administered at a 20-fold lower dose. Initial dosing is usually 0.2–0.3 mg/kg daily in two divided doses orally (or 0.05–0.1 mg/kg daily intravenously over 24 h), and target trough levels are 5–15 μg/L. Since tacrolimus is more water-soluble than cyclosporine, it is not as dependent upon bile salts for absorption. However, food intake can reduce the absorption of tacrolimus by up to 40%; thus, it is recommended that this agent be taken on an empty stomach (Venkataramanan et al. 1991). In addition, tacrolimus is best absorbed in the morning. Tacrolimus granules (Modigraf™) are also available, developed for patients who are unable to swallow capsules, in particular infants (Webb et al. 2019). The guidelines for dosing and therapeutic drug monitoring are the same as for tacrolimus capsules. There is also a prolonged-release tacrolimus formulation available for older children and adolescents (Advagraf™ in Europe, Astagraf™ in the United States). Comparative pharmacokinetic studies have shown that stable pediatric transplant recipients can be converted from immediate-release to prolonged-release-tacrolimus at the same total daily dose, using the same therapeutic drug monitoring method (Rubik et al. 2019a, b).

3.1.2 Drug Interactions

Because of the prime importance of the intestinal *P*-glycoprotein and the CYP3A4 and CYP3A5 systems in absorption and metabolism of CNIs, a large number of drugs that affect these systems can cause significant interactions (van Gelder 2002; Campana et al. 1996), as shown in Table 4. Additive toxicity may also occur with other drugs, such as hyperkalemia with ACE inhibitors; nephrotoxicity with aminoglycosides, amphotericin B, and nonsteroidal anti-inflammatory drugs; and myopathy and rhabdomyolysis with lipid-lowering statins.

3.1.3 Efficacy and Adverse Effects

The overall conclusion from data in adult renal transplant recipients is that tacrolimus-based immunosuppression is associated with decreased acute rejection rates, a superior long-term renal function, and more favorable cardiovascular risk profile than cyclosporine microemulsion-based immunosuppression which translates into improved long-term renal allograft survival. In pediatric patients, the efficacy and safety of tacrolimus and cyclosporine were compared in one multicenter trial in 196 patients, who were randomly assigned to receive either tacrolimus or cyclosporine microemulsion administered concomitantly with azathioprine and corticosteroids (Trompeter et al. 2002). Tacrolimus therapy resulted in a significantly lower incidence of acute rejection (36.9%) compared with cyclosporine therapy (59.1%) ($P = 0.003$). The incidence of steroid-resistant rejection was also significantly lower in the tacrolimus group compared with the cyclosporine group (7.8% vs. 25.8%, $P = 0.001$). The difference was also significant for biopsy-confirmed acute rejection (16.5% vs. 39.8%, $P < 0.001$). At 1 year, patient survival was similar (96.1% vs. 96.6%); ten grafts were lost in the tacrolimus group compared with 17 graft losses in the cyclosporine group ($P = 0.06$). At 1 year, the tacrolimus group had a significantly better estimated glomerular filtration rate (GFR). A follow-up study at 4 years showed that patient survival was similar (94% vs. 92%, $P = 0.86$), but graft survival (86% vs. 69%; $P = 0.025$) and mean estimated GFR significantly favored tacrolimus (Filler et al. 2005). Cholesterol remained significantly higher with cyclosporine throughout follow-up. Three patients in each arm developed PTLD. Incidence of insulin-dependent diabetes mellitus was not different. Hence, tacrolimus is significantly more effective than cyclosporine in preventing acute rejection in pediatric renal transplant recipients, and renal function and graft survival are also superior with tacrolimus.

Cyclosporine and tacrolimus have similarities and differences in their toxicity profiles (Table 5). Both can cause nephrotoxicity, hyperkalemia, hyperuricemia with occasional gouty attacks, hypomagnesemia secondary to urinary loss, arterial hypertension, diabetes mellitus, and neurotoxicity, especially tremor. In the European pediatric study, the incidence of hypomagnesemia was significantly higher in the tacrolimus-treated group (34%) compared with the cyclosporine-treated group (12.9%) (Trompeter et al. 2002). Similarly, diarrhea was more frequent in tacrolimus-treated patients (13.6% vs. 3.2%). Hypertrichosis, gum hyperplasia, and flu syndrome were reported only in cyclosporine-treated patients, and tremor was reported only in tacrolimus-treated patients (Trompeter et al. 2002). Those results are similar to adults where tremor is consistently more common with tacrolimus and hirsutism and gum disease more common in cyclosporine (Tanabe 2003). Also arterial hypertension and hyperlipidemia are more commonly observed with cyclosporine. In the European pediatric study, the mean total cholesterol levels were reported to decrease in the tacrolimus group and increase in the cyclosporine group at the end of 6 months (Trompeter et al. 2002). In the multicenter analysis from the European CERTAIN Registry, the prevalence of dyslipidemia was 95% before engraftment and 88% at 1 year post-transplant; the use of tacrolimus and of MMF was associated with significantly lower concentrations of all lipid parameters compared to regimens containing cyclosporine and mTOR inhibitors (Habbig et al. 2017). Regimens consisting of cyclosporine, MPA, and steroids as well as of cyclosporine, mTOR inhibitors, and steroids were associated with a 3- and 25-fold increased risk of having more than one pathologic lipid parameter as compared to the use of tacrolimus, MMF, and steroids (Habbig et al. 2017). Similarly in adults, several studies have shown that lipid levels are much lower in tacrolimus-treated patients than in those receiving cyclosporine (Tanabe 2003). The improved lipid profiles on tacrolimus may contribute to a better long-term outcome with less cardiovascular morbidity.

On the other hand, tremor and glucose intolerance are more common with tacrolimus. In the pediatric multicenter European study, there was, however, no difference in the incidence of new onset insulin-dependent diabetes mellitus between tacrolimus- (3%) and cyclosporine-treated patients (2.2%) (Trompeter et al. 2002; Filler et al. 2005). The incidence of diabetes mellitus with tacrolimus immunosuppression has become less frequent in recent randomized trials comparing these two calcineurin inhibitors. Post-transplant diabetes regresses after dose reduction in some but not all patients. Both reduction of steroid dosage and a low target trough tacrolimus concentrations contribute to the recent marked reduction of the incidence

Table 5 Semiquantitative comparison of safety profiles of current primary immunosuppressive compounds

	Tacrolimus	Cyclosporine	Mycophenolate mofetil	Sirolimus/everolimus	Glucocorticoids
Nephrotoxicity[a]	++(+)	+++	–	+	–
Hyperlipidemia	+(+)	++	–	+++	++
Arterial hypertension	++	+++	–	–	+
Neurotoxicity	+++	+++	–	–	+
Post-transplant diabetes mellitus	+++	++	–	–	++
Bone marrow suppression	–	–	++	++	–
Gastrointestinal adverse effects[b]	+	+	+++	+	–
Hepatotoxicity	+	+	–	+	–
Esthetical changes	+	++	–	–	++
Wound healing problems[c]	–	–	+	++	+
Pulmonary toxicity	–	–	–	+	–
Fetal toxicity	+	+	++	NA	–
Osteoporosis	+	+	–	?	++
Inhibition of longitudinal growth	–	–	–	+	+++

– Indicates the drug has no effect on this adverse effect, + indicates mild, ++ indicates moderate, +++ indicates severe, ? indicates clinical data available, but insufficient to provide conclusions, *NA* no information available

[a]Sirolimus without calcineurin inhibitor

[b]Gastrointestinal disorders: diarrhea, abdominal pain, nausea and vomiting, ileus, rectal disorders, mucosal ulcerations

[c]Wound healing problems including lymphocele formation

of diabetes mellitus under tacrolimus immunosuppression in both adults and children. Cyclosporine may also be associated with coarsening of facial features, especially in young children. Bone pain that is responsive to calcium channel inhibitors may also occur with cyclosporine use and sometimes may require changing to tacrolimus.

The most common serious problem with the calcineurin inhibitors is nephrotoxicity, with both a reversible vasomotor component and an irreversible component (Tönshoff and Höcker 2006; Nankivell et al. 2003). Both cyclosporine and tacrolimus can cause acute elevations in serum creatinine that reverse with reduction of the dose, apparently caused by renal vasoconstriction which itself may be mediated by calcineurin inhibition. Chronically, cyclosporine and tacrolimus can induce tubular atrophy and interstitial fibrosis with characteristic hyalinosis of the afferent arteriole (Nankivell et al. 2003). The importance of this lesion is apparent from studies in cardiac and liver transplant recipients, in whom cyclosporine or tacrolimus use is associated with chronic kidney disease progressing to end-stage renal disease in a significant fraction of patients (Ojo et al. 2003). This problem was more acute at a time, when higher doses of cyclosporine were administered for longer periods. Currently, cyclosporine and tacrolimus toxicity is associated with only mild-to-moderate declines in renal function. However, as the number of patients with long-standing nonrenal transplants increases, there is increasing concern about future end-stage renal disease in this population. It is important to establish the diagnosis of calcineurin inhibitor toxicity by renal biopsy and reduce or stop calcineurin inhibition whenever possible (Tönshoff and Höcker 2006; Höcker and Tönshoff 2009, 2011).

There is no difference in the incidence of PTLD between tacrolimus-treated and cyclosporine-microemulsion-treated recipients when used in combination with azathioprine and steroids [1% (1/103) vs. 2.1% (2/93)] (Filler et al. 2005) or when used in conjunction with MMF/steroids (1.4% vs. 2%) (Neu et al. 2003). This is similar to adults, in whom recent large, randomized studies could not show any difference in the incidence of malignancy between patients treated with tacrolimus or cyclosporine (Tanabe 2003).

3.1.4 Therapeutic Drug Monitoring

Tacrolimus and cyclosporine are drugs with a narrow therapeutic index and a broad intraindividual and interindividual pharmacokinetic variability. Serious clinical consequences may occur because of underdosing or overdosing. Hence, individualization of calcineurin inhibitor dosage by therapeutic drug monitoring is required. When tacrolimus is utilized, a monitoring strategy based on trough levels is in general sufficient, because trough levels are good indicators of systemic exposure. In most transplant centers, doses are adjusted to attain target whole-blood trough concentrations of 8–12 μg/L during the first 3 months after transplantation, between 5 and 10 μg/L during month 4–12, and 4–8 μg/L thereafter. It must be emphasized that these target ranges are dependent on the concomitant immunosuppressive therapy. In the SYMPHONY trial for example, low tacrolimus exposure (trough levels between 3 and 7 μg/L) in the first year post-transplant in conjunction with

MMF, prednisone and daclizumab induction was associated with excellent efficacy and little tacrolimus-associated toxicity (Ekberg et al. 2007). Also for cyclosporine individualization of dosage by therapeutic drug monitoring is required. The traditional monitoring strategy for cyclosporine is based on pre-dose trough level measurements (C_0). Many centers aim for the following trough levels in conjunction with MMF therapy and prednisone: months 0–3 post-transplant, 120–200 μg/L, thereafter 80–160 μg/L.

3.2 Antiproliferative Agents

3.2.1 Mycophenolate Mofetil

Mycophenolate mofetil (MMF) impairs lymphocyte function by blocking purine biosynthesis via inhibition of the enzyme inosine monophosphate dehydrogenase (IMPDH). MMF was developed as a replacement for azathioprine for maintenance immunosuppression. It is not nephrotoxic and has less bone marrow toxicity than azathioprine. However, gastrointestinal toxicity can occur, usually manifested by gastritis and diarrhea. Mycophenolic acid (MPA), the active ingredient of the prodrug MMF, acts by blocking de novo purine synthesis in lymphocytes. Furthermore, MPA impairs the ability of dendritic cells to present antigen, suppresses the recruitment of monocyte lineage cells, suppresses the glycosylation of adhesion molecules, inhibits vascular smooth muscle proliferation, improves endothelial function, and inhibits mononuclear cell recruitment into allografts and nephritic kidneys (Allison and Eugui 2005). MPA also decreases cytokine-induced nitric oxide synthesis and prevents the formation of reactive species such as peroxynitrite. Furthermore, MPA exhibits antioxidant effects in experimental nephropathies. These properties of MPA likely augment its immunosuppressive properties by limiting fibrosis and vascular sclerosis after immunological injury (van Leuven et al. 2006).

Pharmacokinetics and Dosing

MMF, a semisynthetic ethyl ester of MPA, is rapidly and completely absorbed and hydrolyzed by esterases to yield the active drug MPA. The recommended dose in pediatric patients in conjunction with cyclosporine is 1,200 mg/m^2 per day in two divided doses, the recommended MMF dose in conjunction with tacrolimus is 800 mg/m^2 per day in two divided doses. However, data from a large prospective randomized study in both pediatric and adult renal transplant recipients on fixed dose MMF vs. a concentration-controlled regimen, the FDCC study, indicate that a higher initial MMF dose, for example, 1,800 mg MMF/m^2 per day in conjunction with cyclosporine and 1,200 mg MMF/m^2 per day in conjunction with tacrolimus for the first 2–4 weeks post-transplant, is required to achieve adequate MPA exposure in the majority of patients (van Gelder et al. 2008; Höcker et al. 2011). The MMF dose should be reduced with active CMV infection. When MMF is associated with diarrhea (a side effect of MMF, see below), dividing up the daily dosing to three to four doses per day may be effective in controlling the diarrhea.

The difference in MMF dosing depending on the concomitant calcineurin inhibitor is explained by a pharmacokinetic interaction of cyclosporine with the main MPA metabolite 7-O-MPA glucuronide (7-O-MPAG). Cyclosporine inhibits the multidrug resistance protein 2-mediated transport of 7-O-MPAG into the bile. MPAG is subject to enzymatic and nonenzymatic hydrolysis in the bile and more importantly in the intestine, thereby liberating the unconjugated drug MPA, which is then reabsorbed into the systemic circulation. This enterohepatic circulation is responsible for a secondary MPA peak occurring 6–12 h after administration. The impact of the enterohepatic cycle on the MPA plasma concentration varies within and between individuals due to factors such as meal times or co-medication of drugs that interrupt the enterohepatic circulation (e.g., bile acid sequestrants, antibiotics). These factors should be considered when evaluating MPA concentrations (particularly pre-dose concentrations) in clinical practice. Furthermore, genetic abnormalities and disease can affect enterohepatic cycling and thus the bioavailability of MPA (Shipkova et al. 2005). When using MMF in combination with tacrolimus, lower MMF doses can be used to achieve comparable MPA exposure, guided by therapeutic drug monitoring, to that seen with cyclosporine (Shipkova et al. 2005).

The metabolism of MPA due to glucuronidation can also be affected by drug induction. Glucocorticoids are known inducers of UDP-glucuronosyltransferases in vitro. When steroids were completely withdrawn 12 months after transplantation, a 33% increase in the mean dose-normalized MPA pre-dose concentrations and MPA-AUCs was observed compared with concentrations at 6 months, when the patients were still receiving maintenance doses of steroids (Cattaneo et al. 2002). The relevant drug-drug interactions are summarized in Table 6.

Efficacy and Adverse Effects

Following the success of the early MMF studies in adults, MMF was investigated in pediatric renal transplant recipients in open-label studies with historical controls. Data from three large multicenter studies (Bunchman et al. 2001; Höcker et al. 2005; Staskewitz et al. 2001; Jungraithmayr et al. 2003; Cransberg et al. 2005) and one smaller study (Ferraris et al. 2005) provided support for the safety and efficacy of MMF in the pediatric renal transplant population when used with cyclosporine and prednisone. The incidence of acute rejection within the first 6 months to 1 year for patients receiving MMF in these studies ranged from 28% to 37% (Bunchman et al. 2001; Staskewitz et al. 2001; Cransberg et al. 2005). Those studies comparing MMF patient groups to historical controls reported significant reductions in the incidence of acute rejection with MMF versus AZA (Staskewitz et al. 2001; Cransberg et al. 2005). There was also a significant improvement in the incidence of acute rejection between patients receiving MMF and those receiving azathioprine at 3 years in a follow-up report to one study (Jungraithmayr et al. 2003). In one large study (Bunchman et al. 2001; Höcker et al. 2005), there were no differences in the incidence of acute rejection when the results were stratified by age. Long-term (3-year) graft and patient survival were excellent, with a 30% incidence of acute rejection (Höcker et al. 2005). MMF has a role in the prevention and/or treatment of

Table 6 Drug interactions between mycophenolate mofetil and frequently used comedications

Drug	Effect	Site of interaction
Antacids	MPA AUC ↓	Absorption
Cholestyramine	MPA AUC ↓ MPAG AUC ↓	Absorption
Corticosteroids	MPA trough ↓ MPA AUC ↓ MPAG ↑	Glucuronidation
Cyclosporine	MPA trough ↓ MPA AUC ↓	Enterohepatic cycling
Metronidazole	MPA AUC ↓ MPAG AUC ↓	Enterohepatic cycling Suppression of anaerobic bacterial glucuronidase
Norfloxacin	MPA AUC ↓ MPAG AUC ↓	Enterohepatic cycling Suppression of anaerobic bacterial glucuronidase
Phosphate binder	MPA AUC ↓ Cmax ↓	Absorption

MPA-AUC area under the concentration-time curve of mycophenolic acid, *MPAG* mycophenolic acid glucuronide

chronic rejection. Among children with chronic rejection, some evidence suggests that substituting MMF for azathioprine may improve renal function (Ferraris et al. 2000; Henne et al. 2003).

The major toxicity of MMF is gastrointestinal, mainly diarrhea, possibly as a result of the high concentrations of acyl-MPAG in the gut. In the MMF suspension trial in pediatric renal transplant recipients, safety of MMF was evaluated based on the occurrence of adverse events, including the development of opportunistic infections and malignancies. The most frequently noted adverse events were hematological problems such as leukopenia and gastrointestinal disorders such as diarrhea, which occurred in 25% and 16% of all patients, respectively, and were observed more often in the youngest age group. In general, the risk of developing side effects declines with increasing age. MMF is devoid of intrinsic renal, cardiovascular, or metabolic toxicities but can increase the risk for CMV infections, leukopenia, and mild anemia (Table 5). MMF should not be used in pregnant transplant patients.

Therapeutic Drug Monitoring

Patients on standard-dose MMF therapy show considerable between-patient variability in pharmacokinetic parameters. This variability is attributable to factors that influence exposure to MMF, such as patient renal function, serum albumin levels, concomitant medications such as cyclosporine that inhibit enterohepatic recirculation of the active metabolite of MMF, MPA (Table 6) and genetic polymorphisms of MPA-metabolizing enzymes. This variability is clinically relevant, as higher plasma concentrations of MPA are correlated with reduced risk of acute rejection after kidney transplantation (Weber et al. 2002; van Gelder et al. 2006; Tönshoff et al. 2011). These findings have suggested that individualizing the dose regimen of MMF may further improve clinical outcomes compared with a standard-dose regimen.

There has been considerable debate regarding the utility of measuring MPA levels. Advocation for MPA monitoring is based on the premise that monitoring will result in avoiding both underdosing, which prevents rejection, and overdosing, which increases the risk of adverse reactions (van Gelder et al. 2006; Tönshoff et al. 2011). One study in adults, for example, showed significantly fewer treatment failures and acute rejection episodes in the monitoring arm compared with the fixed dose arm with no significant difference in side effects (Le Meur et al. 2007). Within this study, MMF dosing and MPA exposure were higher in the monitoring arm based on three levels measured over the first 3 h post-dose (limited sampling strategy for the calculation of the area under the concentration time curve (MPA-AUC). Therefore, some transplant centers monitor MPA levels and target levels between 1.5 and 4 mg/L. In addition, they use therapeutic drug monitoring as a measure of adherence to the immunosuppression plan. In general, monitoring of MPA exposure by MPA pre-dose plasma levels is more popular in clinical practice than monitoring of the area under the concentration time curve (MPA-AUC), for example, by a limited sampling strategy, but less precise. A MPA-AUC > 40 mg $\times$ L/12 h has been recommended for sufficient MPA exposure in conjunction with a calcineurin inhibitor for the prevention of acute rejection episodes (Tönshoff et al. 2011).

3.2.2 Azathioprine

Azathioprine is a purine analog derived from 6-mercaptopurine (6-MP). It has been widely used in renal transplantation for four decades but is now substituted by the more efficacious MMF in most transplant centers. Azathioprine is metabolized in the liver to 6-MP and further converted to the active metabolite thioinosinic acid (TIMP) by the enzyme hypoxanthine–guanine phosphoribosyltransferase. Some but not all of the immunosuppressive activity of azathioprine is attributable to 6-MP. Azathioprine acts mainly as an antiproliferative agent by interfering with normal purine pathways, by inhibiting DNA synthesis, and by being incorporated itself into DNA, thereby affecting the synthesis of DNA and RNA (Elion 1993). By inhibiting the synthesis of DNA and RNA, azathioprine suppresses the proliferation of activated B and T lymphocytes. In addition, azathioprine has been shown to reduce the number of circulating monocytes by arresting the cell cycle of promyelocytes in the bone marrow.

Azathioprine is administered orally at 1.5 mg/kg per day in conjunction with calcineurin inhibitors and 2.5 mg/kg per day, when used without calcineurin inhibitors. It is metabolized in the liver to 6-MP and further converted to the active metabolite TIMP. Because 6-MP is degraded by xanthine oxidase, allopurinol (a xanthine oxidase inhibitor) will increase the levels of TIMP. Severe leukopenia can occur if allopurinol (used for the treatment of hyperuricemia and gout) is given with azathioprine. Thus, allopurinol should generally be avoided in patients treated with azathioprine. The major side effect of azathioprine is bone marrow suppression. All three hematopoietic cell lines can be affected, leading to leukopenia, thrombocytopenia, and anemia. The hematologic side effects are dose-related and can occur late in the course of therapy. They are usually reversible upon dose reduction or temporary discontinuation of the drug. Azathioprine should be temporarily withheld if the white cell count falls below 3,000/mm^3 or if the count drops by 50% between blood draws. Recovery usually occurs within 1–2 weeks. The drug can then be restarted at a lower dose and increased gradually to the usual maintenance dose while monitoring the white cell count. Another potentially serious side effect of azathioprine, which requires decreasing the dose or even stopping the drug, is hepatotoxicity. Azathioprine has also been linked to the development of skin cancer, the most common malignancy in renal transplant patients. As a result, patients taking azathioprine for a prolonged period should be instructed to avoid direct exposure to sunlight or to use heavy sunscreens when exposed. Other side effects include increased susceptibility to infection and hair loss.

3.3 The Target of Rapamycin (TOR) Inhibitors Everolimus and Sirolimus

Sirolimus (rapamycin) is a macrocyclic triene antibiotic that is produced by the actinomycete *Streptomyces hygroscopicus*. Sirolimus was approved in September 1999 by the United States Food and Drug Administration and in December 2000 by the European Medicines Agency for use in adult renal transplant recipients. Everolimus is an analog of sirolimus that has similar effectiveness and side effect profile as sirolimus, but different pharmacokinetics (shorter half-life). Sirolimus and everolimus display a novel mechanism of immunosuppressive action, which is distinct from that of the other immunosuppressive drugs. They first bind to the cytosolic immunophilin FK-binding protein 12 (FKBP12). This complex binds to and inhibits the activation of the mammalian target of rapamycin (mTOR), a key regulatory kinase. This inhibition suppresses cytokine-mediated T-cell proliferation inhibiting the progression from the G1 to the S-phase of the cell cycle. Thus, sirolimus and everolimus act at a later stage in the cell cycle than do the calcineurin inhibitors cyclosporine and tacrolimus (Fig. 1). Everolimus can, therefore, be used in combination with the calcineurin inhibitors to produce a synergistic effect (Ganschow et al. 2013).

3.3.1 Pharmacokinetics and Dosing

Everolimus and sirolimus are both macrolide derivatives and share many pharmacokinetic features, including a close correlation between total exposure and trough concentration, low absorption that varies between and within patients, and differences in absorption between adults and children (Mahalati and Kahan 2001; Kirchner et al. 2004). Everolimus is the 40-O-(2-hydroxyethyl) derivative of sirolimus, a modification that results in some important pharmacokinetic differences between the two drugs. Everolimus is more hydrophilic than sirolimus and is absorbed more rapidly from the gut with more systemic clearance than sirolimus (Crowe et al. 1999). As a result, the elimination half-life of everolimus is shorter than for sirolimus (mean 28 h vs. 62 h) (Rapamune 2011; Certican 2012). The clinical effect is that no loading dose is required for everolimus and that is administered twice a day both in adults in children. Because more data are available on the use of everolimus than sirolimus in pediatric renal transplantation, only data on everolimus are presented here.

Everolimus is available as tablets and dispersible tablets for administration in water. The current evidence from pediatric kidney transplantation suggests that everolimus be administered at an initial dose of 0.8 mg/m^2 body surface area twice daily when given in combination with cyclosporine therapy, adjusted to target a trough concentration of 3–8 μg/L (Ettenger et al. 2008; Pape et al. 2007). There is a well-documented drug–drug interaction between mTOR inhibitors and cyclosporine (Kirchner et al. 2004), arising from a shared metabolic pathway (via the cytochrome P450 CYP3A4 isoenzyme system) and the fact that both are substrates for the drug transporter *P*-glycoprotein. Everolimus exposure is increased by up to threefold in patients receiving concomitant cyclosporine (Kovarik et al. 2002, 2006), while tacrolimus exerts only a minimal effect (Kovarik et al. 2002; Brandhorst et al. 2008). In patients receiving everolimus with concomitant tacrolimus, a dose of 2 mg/m^2 BSA twice daily is therefore appropriate (Kovarik et al. 2006).

3.3.2 Efficacy and Adverse Events

The most frequent reason to include an mTOR inhibitor in the immunosuppressive regimen is to facilitate a reduction in calcineurin inhibitor exposure or to eliminate calcineurin inhibitor therapy entirely. The current evidence suggests that de novo administration of everolimus with low-exposure calcineurin inhibitor therapy in children undergoing renal transplantation is efficacious and safe. The recently published 12-month, multicenter, open-label randomized study investigated everolimus with reduced-dose tacrolimus and steroid elimination from month 5 post-transplant compared with a standard-dose tacrolimus regimen with MMF and steroids (control) (Tönshoff et al. 2019). The cumulative incidence of a co-primary efficacy end point (biopsy-proven acute rejection, graft loss, or death from randomization to month 12) was 10.3% in the everolimus group and 5.8% in control. Biopsy-proven acute rejections occurred in 9.6% and 5.6% of patients, respectively. Patient and renal allograft survival were 100%. The co-primary end point of mean estimated glomerular filtration rate at month 12 was comparable. Longitudinal growth and sexual maturation were equivalent between groups. The randomized drug regimen was discontinued in 34.6% and 13% of patients in the everolimus group and control group, respectively ($P = 0.024$), and discontinued due to adverse events/infections in 25.0% and 11.1% of patients ($P = 0.062$). These data show that early conversion of pediatric kidney transplant patients from standard-dose tacrolimus, MMF, and steroids to everolimus in conjunction with reduced dose tacrolimus and steroid withdrawal maintains immunosuppressive efficacy and preserves renal function (Tönshoff et al. 2019).

Use of de novo everolimus with complete calcineurin inhibitor avoidance has not been explored in large trials in pediatric transplant recipients but is unlikely to be preferable to concomitant reduced-exposure calcineurin inhibitor. Switching maintenance patients to an mTOR inhibitor to facilitate calcineurin inhibitor minimization can improve renal function or avoid further functional deterioration, particularly when undertaken before irreversible damage has developed. Late switch below an eGFR of 40 mL/min/1.73 m^2, however, may be associated with an increase in preexisting proteinuria due to podocytopenia, favoring early conversion. It remains unresolved whether calcineurin inhibitor therapy should be reduced or, indeed, eliminated in maintenance patients regardless of whether renal dysfunction is believed to be due to calcineurin inhibitor-related nephrotoxicity. Currently, many transplant centers use mTOR inhibitors as part of a maintenance immunosuppressive regimen only in the following patient subsets in which this drug class may have particular utility: (1) in patients who have histologically proven calcineurin inhibitor nephrotoxicity despite low levels and doses of the calcineurin inhibitor; (2) in patients with malignancy (e.g., skin cancers and Kaposi sarcoma), either in remission or being actively treated; (3) during and after treatment of B-cell PTLD; and (4) in patients with recurrent CMV viremia, because everolimus has anti-CMV activity in vitro and is associated with less CMV replication and disease in vivo compared to MMF (Tedesco-Silva et al. 2015; Höcker et al. 2016). Notably, the incidence of Epstein–Barr virus (EBV) or BK polyoma virus infection is not lower in everolimus- compared to MMF-treated patients (Tönshoff et al. 2019).

Clinically relevant adverse effects of everolimus that require a specific therapeutic response or can potentially influence short- and long-term patient morbidity and mortality as well as graft survival include hypercholesterolemia, hypertriglyceridemia, infectious and noninfectious pneumonia, anemia, lymphocele formation, and impaired wound healing (Table 5). These drug-related adverse effects are important determinants in the choice of a tailor-made immunosuppressive drug regimen that complies with the individual patient risk profile. Equally important in the latter decision is the lack of severe intrinsic nephrotoxicity associated with everolimus and its advantageous effects on arterial hypertension, post-transplantation diabetes mellitus, and esthetic changes induced by calcineurin inhibitors. Mild and transient thrombocytopenia, leukopenia, gastrointestinal adverse effects, and mucosal ulcerations are all minor complications of everolimus therapy that have less impact on the decision for choosing this drug as the basis for tailor-made immunosuppressive therapy.

3.4 Glucocorticoids

Glucocorticoids, developed in the early 1950s, represent one of the principal agents used for both maintenance immunosuppression and treatment of acute rejection. Glucocorticoids have both anti-inflammatory and immunosuppressive actions (Franchimont 2004). Lymphopenia and monocytopenia occur with the inhibition of lymphocyte proliferation, survival, activation, homing, and effector functions.

3.4.1 Pharmacokinetics and Dosing

The major glucocorticoids used are prednisone or prednisolone (given orally with comparable efficacy) and methylprednisolone (given orally or intravenously with 25% more potency). These agents are rapidly absorbed and have short plasma half-lives (60–180 min) but long biological half-lives (18–36 h).

In many transplant centers, the initial dose of glucocorticoids is usually administered during surgery as intravenous methylprednisolone, at doses between 2 and 10 mg/kg body weight. The oral dose of glucocorticoids used for maintenance therapy varies between 15 and 60 mg/m^2 per day (0.5–2 mg/kg body weight per day), which is gradually tapered over time to approximately 3–5 mg prednisone per m^2 surface area, usually taken as a single morning dose. Alternate-day dosing is often administered 6–12 months post-transplant to minimize the effect of corticosteroids on growth.

3.4.2 Adverse Effects

Glucocorticoids (steroids) have multiple side effects in children, including growth impairment, susceptibility to infections, cushingoid appearance, body disfigurement, acne, cardiovascular complications, arterial hypertension, hyperglycemia, aseptic bone necrosis, osteopenia, cataracts, poor wound healing, and psychological effects (Table 5). The negative impact that steroids have on appearance may play a role in poor adherence, especially in the body image-conscious adolescent. The risk for infection is excessive if high-dose pulse therapy is prolonged (typically >3 g per 1.73 m^2). Steroid dosage should, therefore, be decreased gradually during rejection treatment even if serum creatinine fails to improve. Interestingly, glucocorticoids are not associated with increased risk for malignancy. One of the most important reasons for stopping corticosteroids or switching to alternate day therapy is statural growth impairment, which is frequently observed in those on continuous treatment.

3.4.3 Steroid Minimization Protocols

Because of the multiple adverse effects of maintenance corticosteroid therapy, attempts have been made to withdraw or minimize corticosteroid therapy in children with a renal allograft (Ingulli and Tejani 1994; Benfield et al. 2010; Sutherland et al. 2009; Barletta et al. 2009; Höcker et al. 2009, 2010; Sarwal et al. 2003). There are two major approaches in steroid minimization in pediatric renal transplantation: (1) late steroid withdrawal (>1 year post-transplantation) and (2) either complete steroid avoidance or early steroid withdrawal (<7 days post-transplantation). In the late steroid withdrawal approach, the patients suitable for minimization are identified by stable post-transplant clinical course and renal function. In late steroid withdrawal, there is no need for an antibody induction in the perioperative period (Höcker et al. 2009, 2010). In early withdrawal or complete avoidance protocols, the criteria of suitability are predefined before transplantation (e.g., criteria of low immunological risk), and antibody induction is used in all enrolled patients (Sarwal et al. 2003, 2012; Shapiro et al. 2006; Chavers et al. 2009; Grenda et al. 2010; Webb et al. 2015). There is also an "intermediate" approach, combining elements from early and late withdrawal protocols, in which antibody induction is used; however, the decision of steroid withdrawal is delayed until 6–9 months post-transplant, when stable renal graft function (sometimes combined with normal picture of protocol biopsy) allows to identify suitable candidates (as in the late withdrawal approach) (Pape et al. 2010). Steroid withdrawal has the advantage over steroid avoidance that immunologically high-risk patients and those with unstable graft function can easily be identified beforehand and be excluded from steroid-free immunosuppression.

Steroid avoidance or early withdrawal protocols have been used successfully both in the United States and in Europe. However, many of these protocols have chosen low-risk individuals and utilized intensive induction therapy with induction therapy with thymoglobulin, tacrolimus, and MMF (Sarwal et al. 2003). Regarding the efficacy and safety of early steroid withdrawal or complete steroid avoidance, in a randomized controlled study of 196 pediatric renal transplant recipients, two doses of daclizumab in patients treated with a regimen of tacrolimus and MMF allowed early steroid withdrawal on day 5 post-transplant (Grenda et al. 2010). There was a comparable rate of biopsy-proven acute rejection rates after 6 months in patients off steroids compared with controls (10.2% vs. 7.1%). In addition, prepubertal patients with early steroid withdrawal showed better growth and lipid and glucose metabolism profiles compared with controls, without increases in graft rejection or loss. These favorable effects were confirmed in a follow-up study over a 2-year observation period (Webb et al. 2015). The results of the North American randomized controlled multicenter study with a follow-up of 3 years post-transplant showed that the steroid-free group showed lower systolic blood pressure and lower cholesterol levels (Sarwal et al. 2012). The authors concluded that complete steroid avoidance is safe and effective in nonsensitized children receiving primary kidney transplants (Sarwal et al. 2012).

Nevertheless, steroid withdrawal or avoidance following renal transplantation remains a controversial issue. Although the benefits of using steroid-free protocols in pediatric patients shows great promise, further study is needed to determine the impact on long-term allograft function and to identify patients (e.g., low immunologic risk) who can be successfully converted to steroid-free immunosuppression without increasing the risk of acute rejection.

4 Conclusions

Transplantation in children carries unique challenges. While issues such as controlling rejection and minimizing side effects are similar between adults and children, maintenance immunosuppressant regimens that affect developmental processes have a disproportionate impact on children. This is particularly true for glucocorticoids (steroids) which have many side effects including some that can be quite devastating in pediatric patients. Steroid avoidance has been successful in the short term, when MMF is combined with tacrolimus and either basiliximab or antithymocyte globulin is added. With the goal of eliminating steroids, the combination of MMF and tacrolimus may strike the correct balance between adequate and overimmunosuppression (Fig. 4). Recently, the use of everolimus has been advocated for minimizing calcineurin inhibitor exposure after renal transplantation, but its use is limited by mTOR-related side effects. There is at present no consensus for immunosuppressive therapy following renal transplantation in children.

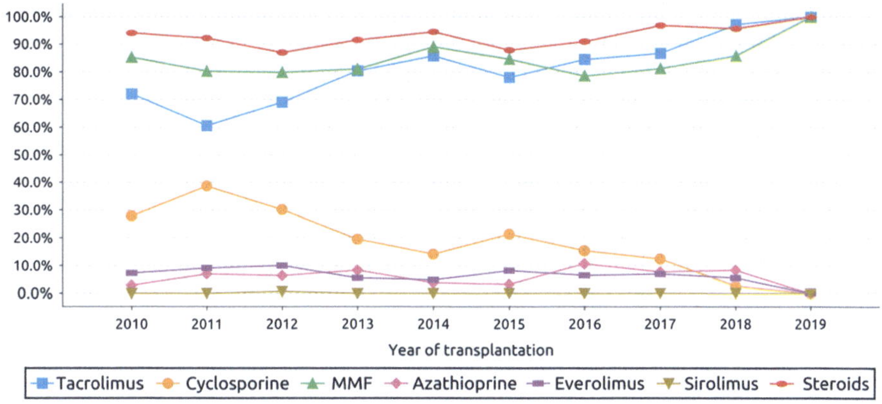

Fig. 4 Observed drug utilization rates in European pediatric renal transplant recipients among transplanted grafts with ≥30 days function, by year of renal transplantation (Data are from the Cooperative European Paediatric Renal Transplant Initiative (CERTAIN) registry. www.certain-registry.eu)

Newer drugs such as belatacept have not been systematically studied in the pediatric transplant patient population. Since the approval of belatacept in 2011 for use in de novo adult kidney transplantation, this CD80/86–CD28 co-stimulation blocker has been shown to be a valuable treatment option for maintenance immunosuppression (Noble et al. 2019). Belatacept in adults has been associated with superior glomerular filtration rate as compared to calcineurin inhibitor-based treatments because of the absence of nephrotoxicity. Additionally, belatacept avoids the cardiovascular side effects (e.g., hypertension and dyslipidemia) caused by a calcineurin inhibitor-based regimen (Noble et al. 2019). Clearly, much additional work is needed to define optimal immunosuppressive regimens in pediatric renal transplant patients, particularly with respect to newer and evolving regimens. The safety and efficacy of these protocols with special emphasis on long-term graft survival and PTLD need to be established.

References

Allison AC, Eugui EM (2005) Mechanisms of action of mycophenolate mofetil in preventing acute and chronic allograft rejection. Transplantation 80:181–190

Barletta GM, Kirk E, Gardner JJ et al (2009) Rapid discontinuation of corticosteroids in pediatric renal transplantation. Pediatr Transplant 13:571–578

Benfield MR, Bartosh S, Ikle D et al (2010) A randomized double-blind, placebo controlled trial of steroid withdrawal after pediatric renal transplantation. Am J Transplant 10:81–88

Brandhorst G, Tenderich G, Zittermann A et al (2008) Everolimus exposure in cardiac transplant recipients is influenced by concomitant calcineurin inhibitor. Ther Drug Monit 30:113–116

Bunchman T, Navarro M, Broyer M et al (2001) The use of mycophenolate mofetil suspension in pediatric renal allograft recipients. Pediatr Nephrol 16:978–984

Campana C, Regazzi MB, Buggia I et al (1996) Clinically significant drug interactions with cyclosporin. An update. Clin Pharmacokinet 30:141–179
Cattaneo D, Perico N, Gaspari F et al (2002) Glucocorticoids interfere with mycophenolate mofetil bioavailability in kidney transplantation. Kidney Int 62:1060–1067
Certican (2012) Basic prescribing information. Novartis Pharma AG, Basel
Chavers BM, Chang C, Gillingham KJ et al (2009) Pediatric kidney transplantation using a novel protocol of rapid (6-day) discontinuation of prednisolone: 2-year results. Transplantation 88:237–241
Cooperative European Paediatric Renal Transplant Initiative (CERTAIN) Registry (2019) www.certain-registry.eu. Accessed 15 Aug 2019
Cransberg K, Marlies Cornelissen EA, Davin JC et al (2005) Improved outcome of pediatric kidney transplantations in the Netherlands–effect of the introduction of mycophenolate mofetil? Pediatr Transplant 9:1004–1011
Crowe A, Bruelisauer A, Duerr L et al (1999) Absorption and intestinal metabolism of SDZ-RAD and rapamycin in rats. Drug Metab Dispos 27:627–632
Dantal J, Hourmant M, Cantarovich D et al (1998) Effect of long-term immunosuppression in kidney-graft recipients on cancer incidence: randomised comparison of two cyclosporin regimens. Lancet 351:623–628
Ekberg H, Tedesco-Silva H, Demirbas A et al ELITE-Symphony Study (2007) Reduced exposure to calcineurin inhibitors in renal transplantation. N Engl J Med 357:2562–2575
Elion GB (1993) The pharmacology of azathioprine. Ann N Y Acad Sci 685:400–407
Ettenger R, Hoyer PF, Grimm P et al (2008) Multicenter trial of everolimus in pediatric renal transplant recipients: results at three year. Pediatr Transplant 12:456–463
Ferraris JR, Tambutti ML, Redal MA et al (2000) Conversion from azathioprine [correction of azathioprina] to mycophenolate mofetil in pediatric renal transplant recipients with chronic rejection. Transplantation 70:297–301
Ferraris JR, Ghezzi LF, Vallejo G et al (2005) Improved long-term allograft function in pediatric renal transplantation with mycophenolate mofetil. Pediatr Transplant 9:178–182
Filler G, Webb NJ, Milford DV et al (2005) Four-year data after pediatric renal transplantation: a randomized trial of tacrolimus vs. cyclosporin microemulsion. Pediatr Transplant 9:498–503
Franchimont D (2004) Overview of the actions of glucocorticoids on the immune response: a good model to characterize new pathways of immunosuppression for new treatment strategies. Ann N Y Acad Sci 1024:124–137
Ganschow R, Pape L, Sturm E et al (2013) Growing experience with mTOR inhibitors in pediatric solid organ transplantation. Pediatr Transplant 17:694–706
Goggins WC, Pascual MA, Powelson JA et al (2003) A prospective, randomized, clinical trial of intraoperative versus postoperative thymoglobulin in adult cadaveric renal transplant recipients. Transplantation 76:798–802
Grenda R, Watson A, Vondrak K et al (2006) A prospective, randomized, multicenter trial of tacrolimus-based therapy with or without basiliximab in pediatric renal transplantation. Am J Transplant 6:1666–1672
Grenda R, Watson A, Trompeter R et al (2010) A randomized trial to assess the impact of early steroid withdrawal on growth in pediatric renal transplantation: the TWIST study. Am J Transplant 10:828–836
Gurk-Turner C, Airee R, Philosophe B et al (2008) Thymoglobulin dose optimization for induction therapy in high risk kidney transplant recipients. Transplantation 85:1425–1430
Habbig S, Volland R, Krupka K et al (2017) Dyslipidemia after pediatric renal transplantation-the impact of immunosuppressive regimens. Pediatr Transplant 21(3):e12914
Halloran PF (2004) Immunosuppressive drugs for kidney transplantation. N Engl J Med 351:2715–2729
Henne T, Latta K, Strehlau J et al (2003) Mycophenolate mofetil-induced reversal of glomerular filtration loss in children with chronic allograft nephropathy. Transplantation 76:1326–1330

Höcker B, Tönshoff B (2009) Treatment strategies to minimize or prevent chronic allograft dysfunction in pediatric renal transplant recipients: an overview. Paediatr Drugs 11:381–396

Höcker B, Tönshoff B (2011) Calcineurin inhibitor-free immunosuppression in pediatric renal transplantation: a viable option? Paediatr Drugs 13:49–69

Höcker B, Weber LT, Bunchman T et al (2005) Mycophenolate mofetil suspension in pediatric renal transplantation: three-year data from the tricontinental trial. Pediatr Transplant 9:504–511

Höcker B, Kovarik JM, Daniel V et al (2008) Pharmacokinetics and immunodynamics of basiliximab in pediatric renal transplant recipients on mycophenolate mofetil comedication. Transplantation 86:1234–1240

Höcker B, Weber LT, Feneberg R et al (2009) Prospective, randomized trial on late steroid withdrawal in pediatric renal transplant recipients under cyclosporine microemulsion and mycophenolate mofetil. Transplantation 87:934–941

Höcker B, Weber L, Feneberg R et al (2010) Improved growth and cardiovascular risk after late steroid withdrawal: 2-year results of a prospective, randomized trial in paediatric renal transplantation. Nephrol Dial Transplant 25:617–624

Höcker B, van Gelder T, Martin-Govantes J et al (2011) Comparison of MMF efficacy and safety in paediatric vs. adult renal transplantation: subgroup analysis of the randomised, multicentre FDCC trial. Nephrol Dial Transplant 26:1073–1079

Höcker B, Zencke S, Pape L et al (2016) Impact of everolimus and low-dose cyclosporin on cytomegalovirus replication and disease in pediatric renal transplantation. Am J Transplant 16:921–929

Ingulli E, Tejani A (1994) Steroid withdrawal after renal transplantation. In: Tejani AH, Fine RM (eds) Pediatric renal transplantation. Wiley-Liss, New York, pp 221–238

Jungraithmayr T, Staskewitz A, Kirste G et al (2003) Pediatric renal transplantation with mycophenolate mofetil-based immunosuppression without induction: results after three years. Transplantation 75:454–461

Kirchner GI, Meier-Wiedenbach I, Manns MP (2004) Clinical pharmacokinetics of everolimus. Clin Pharmacokinet 43:83–95

Kovarik JM, Kalbag J, Figuerredo J et al (2002) Differential influence of two cyclosporine formulations on everolimus pharmacokinetics: a clinically relevant pharmacokinetic interaction. J Clin Pharmacol 42:95–99

Kovarik JM, Curtis JJ, Hricik DE et al (2006) Differential pharmacokinetic interaction of tacrolimus and cyclosporine on everolimus. Transplant Proc 38:3456–3458

Le Meur Y, Büchler M, Thierry A et al (2007) Individualized mycophenolate mofetil dosing based on drug exposure significantly improves patient outcomes after renal transplantation. Am J Transplant 7:2496–2503

Mahalati K, Kahan BD (2001) Clinical pharmacokinetics of sirolimus. Clin Pharmacokinet 40:573–585

Nankivell BJ, Borrows RJ, Fung CL et al (2003) The natural history of chronic allograft nephropathy. N Engl J Med 349:2326–2333

Neu AM, Ho PL, Fine RN et al (2003) Tacrolimus vs. cyclosporine A as primary immunosuppression in pediatric renal transplantation: a NAPRTCS study. Pediatr Transplant 7:217–222

Noble J, Jouve T, Janbon B et al (2019) Belatacept in kidney transplantation and its limitations. Expert Rev Clin Immunol 15:359–367

Offner G, Toenshoff B, Höcker B et al (2008) Efficacy and safety of basiliximab in pediatric renal transplant patients receiving cyclosporine, mycophenolate mofetil, and steroids. Transplantation 86:1241–1248

Ojo AO, Held PJ, Port FK et al (2003) Chronic renal failure after transplantation of a nonrenal organ. N Engl J Med 349:931–940

Pape L, Ahlenstiel T, Ehrich JH et al (2007) Reversal of loss of glomerular filtration rate in children with transplant nephropathy after switch to everolimus and low-dose cyclosporine A. Pediatr Transplant 11:291–295

Pape L, Offner G, Kreuzer M et al (2010) De novo therapy with everolimus, low-dose cyclosporine A, basiliximab and steroid elimination in pediatric kidney transplantation. Am J Transplant 10:2349–2354
Peddi VR, Bryant M, Roy-Chaudhury P et al (2002) Safety, efficacy, and cost analysis of thymoglobulin induction therapy with intermittent dosing based on CD3+ lymphocyte counts in kidney and kidney-pancreas transplant recipients. Transplantation 73:1514–1518
Rapamune (2011) Summary of product characteristics. Pfizer, New York
Rubik J, Debray D, Iserin F et al (2019a) Comparative pharmacokinetics of tacrolimus in stable pediatric allograft recipients converted from immediate-release tacrolimus to prolonged-release tacrolimus formulation. Pediatr Transplant 23:e13391
Rubik J, Debray D, Kelly D et al (2019b) Efficacy and safety of prolonged-release tacrolimus in stable pediatric allograft recipients converted from immediate-release tacrolimus – a Phase 2, open-label, single-arm, one-way crossover study. Transpl Int. https://doi.org/10.1111/tri.13479
Sarwal MM, Vidhun JR, Alexander SR et al (2003) Continued superior outcomes with modification and lengthened follow-up of a steroid-avoidance pilot with extended daclizumab induction in pediatric renal transplantation. Transplantation 76:1331–1339
Sarwal MM, Ettenger RB, Dharnidharka V et al (2012) Complete corticosteroid avoidance is effective and safe in children with renal transplants: a multicentre randomized trial with three year follow-up. Am J Transplant 12:2719–2729
Shapiro R, Ellis D, Tan HP et al (2006) Antilymphoid antibody preconditioning and tacrolimus monotherapy for pediatric kidney transplantation. J Pediatr 148:813–818
Shipkova M, Armstrong VW, Oellerich M et al (2005) Mycophenolate mofetil in organ transplantation: focus on metabolism, safety and tolerability. Expert Opin Drug Metab Toxicol 1:505–526
Staskewitz A, Kirste G, Tönshoff B et al (2001) Mycophenolate mofetil in pediatric renal transplantation without induction therapy: results after 12 months of treatment. Transplantation 71:638–644
Sterkers G, Baudouin V, Ansart-Pirenne H et al (2000) Duration of action of a chimeric interleukin-2 receptor monoclonal antibody, basiliximab, in pediatric kidney transplant recipients. Transplant Proc 32:2757–2759
Stevens RB, Mercer DF, Grant WJ et al (2008) Randomized trial of single-dose versus divided-dose rabbit anti-thymocyte globulin induction in renal transplantation: an interim report. Transplantation 85:1391–1399
Stratta RJ, Sundberg AK, Farney AC et al (2005) Experience with alternate-day thymoglobulin induction in pancreas transplantation with portal-enteric drainage. Transplant Proc 37:3546–3548
Sutherland S, Li L, Concepcion W et al (2009) Steroid-free immunosuppression in pediatric renal transplantation: rationale for and outcomes following conversion to steroid based therapy. Transplantation 87:1744–1748
Tanabe K (2003) Calcineurin inhibitors in renal transplantation: what is the best option? Drugs 3:1535–1548
Tedesco-Silva H, Felipe C, Ferreira A et al (2015) Reduced incidence of cytomegalovirus infection in kidney transplant recipients receiving everolimus and reduced tacrolimus doses. Am J Transplant 15:2655–2664
The NAPRTCS (2014) Annual report. https://web.emmes.com/study/ped/index.htm
Tönshoff B, Höcker B (2006) Treatment strategies in pediatric solid organ transplant recipients with calcineurin inhibitor-induced nephrotoxicity. Pediatr Transplant 10:721–729
Tönshoff B, David-Neto E, Ettenger R et al (2011) Pediatric aspects of therapeutic drug monitoring of mycophenolic acid in renal transplantation. Transplant Rev (Orlando) 25:78–89
Tönshoff B, Ettenger R, Dello Strologo L et al (2019) Early conversion of pediatric kidney transplant patients to everolimus with reduced tacrolimus and steroid elimination: results of a randomized trial. Am J Transplant 19:811–822

Trompeter R, Filler G, Webb NJ et al (2002) Randomized trial of tacrolimus versus cyclosporin microemulsion in renal transplantation. Pediatr Nephrol 7:141–149
van Gelder T (2002) Drug interactions with tacrolimus. Drug Saf 25:707–712
van Gelder T, Le Meur Y, Shaw LM et al (2006) Therapeutic drug monitoring of mycophenolate mofetil in transplantation. Ther Drug Monit 28:145–154
van Gelder T, Silva HT, de Fijter JW et al (2008) Comparing mycophenolate mofetil regimens for de novo renal transplant recipients: the fixed-dose concentration-controlled trial. Transplantation 86:1043–1051
van Leuven SI, Kastelein JJ, Allison AC et al (2006) Mycophenolate mofetil (MMF): firing at the atherosclerotic plaque from different angles? Cardiovasc Res 69:341–347
Venkataramanan R, Jain A, Warty VW et al (1991) Pharmacokinetics of FK 506 following oral administration: a comparison of FK 506 and cyclosporine. Transplant Proc 23:931–933
Webb N, Douglas S, Rajai A et al (2015) Corticosteroid-free kidney transplantation improves growth: two-year follow-up of the TWIST randomised controlled trial. Transplantation 99:1178–1185
Webb NJA, Baumann U, Camino M et al (2019) Pharmacokinetics of tacrolimus granules in pediatric de novo liver, kidney, and heart transplantation: the OPTION study. Pediatr Transplant 23:e13328
Weber LT, Shipkova M, Armstrong VW et al (2002) The pharmacokinetic-pharmacodynamic relationship for total and free mycophenolic acid in pediatric renal transplant recipients: a report of the German study group on mycophenolate mofetil therapy. J Am Soc Nephrol 13:759–768
Wong W, Agrawal N, Pascual M et al (2006) Comparison of two dosages of thymoglobulin used as a short-course for induction in kidney transplantation. Transpl Int 19:629–635

Pharmacotherapy in Pediatric Hematopoietic Cell Transplantation

R. Admiraal and J. J. Boelens

Contents

Abstract

Hematopoietic cell transplantation (HCT) is a curative treatment option for both malignant and nonmalignant diseases. Success of the procedure mainly depends on disease control and treatment-related complications. Pharmacotherapy plays a major role in HCT and significantly impacts the outcomes. Main drug use within HCT includes conditioning, GvHD prophylaxis, and prevention/treatment of infections.

R. Admiraal
Blood and Marrow Transplantation Program, Prinses Maxima Center for Pediatric Oncology, Utrecht, The Netherlands

J. J. Boelens (✉)
Stem Cell Transplantation and Cellular Therapies Pediatrics, New York, NY, USA

Memorial Sloan Kettering Cancer Center, New York, NY, USA
e-mail: J.J.Boelens@prinsesmaximacentrum.nl; boelensj@mskcc.org

W. Kiess et al. (eds.), *Pediatric Pharmacotherapy*,
Handbook of Experimental Pharmacology 261, https://doi.org/10.1007/164_2019_247

Increasing evidence suggests individualized dosing in (pediatric) HCT may improve outcome. Dose individualization may result in a better predictable drug treatment in terms of safety and efficacy, including timely immune reconstitution after HCT and optimal tumor or disease control, which may result in improved survival chances.

Keywords
Cellular therapies · Conditioning · Graft-versus-host disease · Hematopoietic cell transplantation · Individualized dosing · Relapse · Therapeutic drug monitoring

1 Allogeneic Hematopoietic Cell Transplantation

Allogeneic hematopoietic cell transplantation (HCT) is a potentially life-saving procedure by transplanting donor-derived hematopoietic stem cells and lymphocytes into a patient. The technique is also referred to as stem cell transplantation; however this is not fully correct due to co-infusion of lymphocytes and other hematopoietic cells. Indications for HCT include malignant (leukemia, lymphoma) and nonmalignant disorders (primary immune deficiencies, bone marrow failure, inborn errors of metabolism, and hemoglobinopathies) (Tolar et al. 2012; Gratwohl et al. 2000; Passweg et al. 2014). During this procedure, the diseased bone marrow and cellular immune system are replaced by a healthy, donor-derived hematopoietic system.

The donor cells can be harvested from a donor in several ways and can be either from related or unrelated donors. Historically, an identical sibling was the most predominant stem cells source used in HCT. As two siblings only have a 25% chance of being human leukocyte antigen (HLA) identical, expansion of the donor pool was needed to be able to offer HCT to more patients. Bone marrow donor registries for unrelated donors were established; the first registry was introduced in 1973 in the United Kingdom (Apperley et al. 2012). During the late 1980s, better HLA typing expanded the possibilities to use grafts from both related and unrelated donors (Apperley et al. 2012; Heemskerk et al. 2005). Nowadays, transplanted donor cells can be either derived from bone marrow (BM), mobilized peripheral blood stem cells (PBSC), or umbilical cord blood (CB), from either related or unrelated donors. Each source has its advantages and disadvantages. Compared to BM, the main advantage of PBSC includes the harvesting of cells that can be performed without anesthesia and sedation (Molineux et al. 1990). Cord blood on the other hand has less stringent HLA-matching criteria and has the advantage to be promptly available (Heemskerk et al. 2005). However, the number of cells is lower in CB and BM when compared to PBSC, although the latter is associated with a higher incidence of chronic graft-versus-host disease (Holtick et al. 1996).

In 2014, approximately 1 in 40,000 US inhabitants received an allogeneic HCT (Pasquini and Zhu 2018). In the Netherlands a total of 350 first HCTs are performed annually, of which approximately 80–90 in children (Claas et al. 2016).

2 Principles of HCT

This paragraph highlights the most important aspects of HCT and thus serves as an overview of the procedure. A more in-depth focus on pharmacotherapy involved in HCT can be found in the paragraph *Pharmacotherapy in HCT*.

The treatment plan for HCT depends on the disease, age, comorbidities, previous treatments, stem cell source, and local protocols and can therefore vary considerably between patients. Still, the main components for any HCT are the same and are depicted in Fig. 1.

The *donor search* starts when a patient becomes eligible for HCT and is registered to the HCT unit. Based on center preference and donor availability, HLA matching, and donor cell counts, the most optimal donor is selected (Heemskerk et al. 2005).

The *conditioning* phase starts approximately 1 week before infusion of the stem cells; however some centers start conditioning earlier (Lindemans et al. 2014). The main goal of the conditioning is to deplete the bone marrow and suppress the host immune system. Additionally, in case of malignancy, the conditioning regimen depletes any residual leukemic cells. Bone marrow depletion, or myeloablation, is mostly performed using chemotherapy, while some patients receive chemotherapy combined with total body irradiation (TBI) (Uberti et al. 2011; Davies et al. 2000). Chemotherapy-based conditionings mostly consist of an alkylating agent (busulfan, melphalan, treosulfan) combined with a second cytostatic drug (fludarabine, cyclophosphamide) (Rambaldi et al. 2015; Nagler et al. 2015; Hough et al. 2015). The alkylators mainly give myeloablation, while fludarabine and cyclophosphamide are used for immunosuppression and immune ablation. Clofarabine, a purine antinucleotide, can be added to the conditioning regimen for malignant indications (El-Jawahri et al. 2016). In TBI-containing regimens, TBI is used for myeloablation as well as immunosuppression and is combined with one or more cytostatic drug. In recent years, non-myeloablative regimens or reduced intensity conditioning (RIC) has been increasingly used for older patients (>60 years) and those in poor clinical

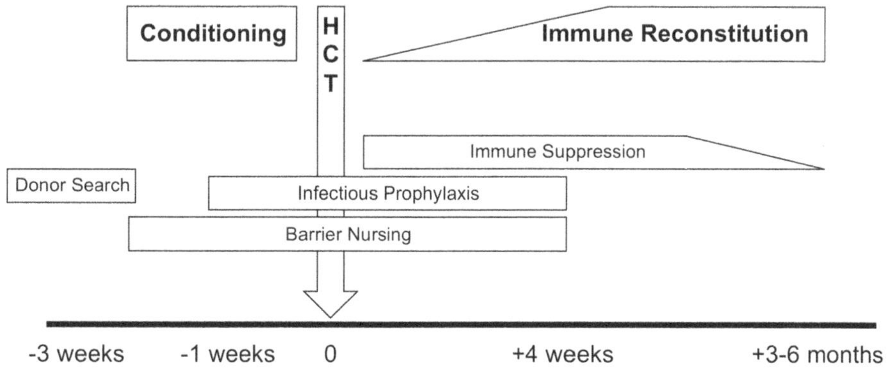

Fig. 1 Overview of treatment plan for HCT

condition (Gyurkocza and Sandmaier 2014; Passweg et al. 2015; Sengsayadeth et al. 2015). In children, RIC conditioning is reserved for patients with DNA instability who are expected to experience significant toxicity from standard protocols. These patients usually receive either low-dose TBI, cyclophosphamide, or low-dose busulfan or thiotepa, all combined with fludarabine. The choice of chemotherapy agents depends on the conditioning intensity (myeloablative versus RIC), underlying disease, stem cell source, and center preferences. This introduces substantial variation in actual treatment between centers, which can be suboptimal for comparing results between centers and getting optimal experience and control over the conditioning used in a single center. Besides differences in the choice of drugs, the actual drug exposure varies due to variability in pharmacokinetics and pharmacodynamics between patients. By using individualized dosing regimens, this variability in PK and PD is accounted for, resulting in more patients reaching optimal drug exposure and thereby drug effects. An individualized dosing regimen is available and being used in clinical care for busulfan (Bartelink et al. 2013a) and is being developed for fludarabine (Langenhorst et al. 2019a, b; McCune et al. 2014a). Additionally, exposure of ATG before and after HCT has shown to have impact on the outcomes. Individualized dosing regimen for ATG seems therefore crucial to influence the outcomes; currently clinical studies for individualized ATG are recruiting. To our best knowledge, these are the only drugs used in the conditioning regimen in allogeneic HCT for which individualized dosing regimens are available. However, efforts have been made to characterize the PK and PD of other drugs used including fludarabine (Long-Boyle et al. 2011; McCune et al. 2014a), treosulfan (Brink et al. 2014), and cyclophosphamide (Laínez et al. 2014), which however did not yet result in practical guidelines or dosing recommendations.

Serotherapy is another important component of the conditioning regimen, introduced to prevent graft-versus-host disease (GvHD) and rejection (Theurich et al. 2013). The main mechanism of action of serotherapy is in vivo lymphodepletion, mainly of T cells, although it is thought to have some immune-modulatory properties as well (Mohty 2007). Anti-thymocyte globulin (ATG) and alemtuzumab (Campath®) are the two drugs used for this indication (Willemsen et al. 2015; Marsh et al. 2014; Soiffer et al. 2011). ATG is the product of vaccinating rabbits or horses with human lymphocytes or whole thymus tissue and is therefore a polyclonal non-humanized IgG antibody with many epitopes directed to various human cell-bound targets (Mohty 2007; Storek et al. 2015). Additionally, the number of IgG molecules targeted against human markers (referred to as active ATG) may differ from animal to animal (Mohty 2007). Therefore, IgG from many immunized animals is pooled aiming for a stable and comparable product. Additionally, the percentage of active ATG differs between the different ATG products. In thymoglobulin, the most commonly used ATG preparation in HCT, approximately 9% of total rabbit IgG is directed to human markers (Jol-van der Zijde et al. 2009; Waller et al. 2003). Alemtuzumab on the other hand is a monoclonal humanized anti-CD52 IgG antibody. At first, Campath was a monoclonal rat antihuman IgM antibody and was later humanized. This served as the basis for the currently used drug alemtuzumab, an anti-CD52 IgG antibody (Riechmann et al. 1988). CD52 is mainly expressed on cells originating from the lymphoid lineage and is not expressed on hematopoietic stem cells. In 1991, alemtuzumab was approved as a treatment for chronic lymphatic leukemia and as serotherapy in HCT. Nowadays it is most frequently used in the United Kingdom and in selected treatment protocols.

Starting with the infusion of the stem cells, *immune suppression* is given to prevent GvHD. GvHD can be prevented by strategies both before (serotherapy or T-cell depletion of the graft) and after (GvHD prophylaxis, posttransplant cyclophosphamide) graft infusion.

The cornerstone of GvHD prophylaxis is cyclosporin A (CsA), a calcineurin inhibitor, which is combined with prednisolone, methotrexate (MTX), mycophenolate mofetil (MMF), and tacrolimus (TAC), depending on the stem cell source (Apperley et al. 2012). For bone marrow and peripheral blood with MAC conditioning, CsA and MTX remains the most often used combination of agents in Europe. Some trials in adults suggest that TAC combined with MTX is equally safe as GvHD prophylaxis and made TAC-MTX the most often used regimen in America (Ratanatharathorn et al. 1998; Nash et al. 2000). For cord blood transplant, most centers resort to CsA in combination with prednisolon (Apperley et al. 2012). CsA or TAC in combination with MMF is the preferred combination in patients receiving reduced intensity conditioning. In case of CsA toxicity, patients are switched to tacrolimus or sirolimus (Wang et al. 2015). Immune suppressive therapy is given up to 3–4 weeks after HCT, after which it is carefully tapered, starting with the second agent, after which CsA is tapered.

Despite numerous strategies to prevent GvHD, still 20–30% of children develop severe GvHD. Two forms of GvHD after HCT are recognized: acute (aGvHD) and chronic (cGvHD) GvHD. Historically, GvHD occurring before or after day +100 was classified as aGvHD and cGvHD, respectively. With recent criteria, there is no time limit on either classification. The diagnosis is currently made based on the clinical features with the addition of an overlap syndrome. Both aGvHD and cGvHD can be staged, where aGvHD is graded 1–4 and cGvHD is graded as mild, moderate, and severe. Acute GvHD manifests in the skin, gut, and liver and is graded based on percentage affected and erythrodermia (skin), quantity of diarrhea, and ileus (gut) and bilirubin levels (liver). Chronic GvHD can affect many organ systems, mainly involving the skin and mucous membranes, eyes, lungs, and the gastrointestinal tract.

Grade 1 aGvHD and mild cGvHD (skin only) are usually treated with topical steroids alone. More advanced grades of GvHD are treated in the first line with steroids, either prednisolone or methylprednisolone for 7–14 days. Patients failing to respond to this therapy are treated with second-line therapy, mainly consisting of steroids combined with monoclonal antibodies (daclizumab, basiliximab, inolimomab; interleukin-2 receptor blockers, abatacept; CD80/86 blocker, ATG, or alemtuzumab; both serotherapy) or mesenchymal stem cells. GvHD remains an important cause for mortality and morbidity. More effective treatment is needed, either as new agents or by optimizing current therapies.

Supportive care consists of infectious prophylaxis as well as treatment in high-efficiency, particle-free, positive-pressure rooms (Apperley et al. 2012; Mank and Davies 2008; O'Grady et al. 2002). All medical and nursing staff perform *barrier nursing* during the admission of any patient to minimize changes of infections. Main threats during neutropenia and intensive immune suppression include bacteria and fungi. Most patients receive infectious prophylaxis to prevent bacterial and/or fungal infections. These can be divided in gut decontamination, aiming to completely or selectively deplete the gut of mainly gram-negative bacterial burden. Main drugs used for gut decontamination include ciprofloxacin and oral nonabsorbable drugs like piperacilline/tazobactam, amphotericin B, gentamicin, and vancomycin. Furthermore, patients are at a high risk for pneumocystis jiroveci pneumonia (PJP) and therefore receive co-trimoxazole as PJP prophylaxis. Fungi and yeasts are another serious cause of morbidity and mortality, mainly by the *Aspergillus* and *Candida* species. Patients receive fungal prophylaxis, mainly consisting of voriconazole or posaconazole. Both drugs have a narrow therapeutic window, and serum concentrations should be monitored.

Immune reconstitution following HCT can be separated in neutrophil recovery and lymphocyte reconstitution. When focusing on neutrophil recovery, patients will experience a phase of neutropenia starting approximately 14 days after the first dose of busulfan or TBI, which reflects the transit time for neutrophils (Friberg et al. 2002; Van Kesteren et al. 2005). From this moment onward, the patient will depend on donor-stem cell-derived neutrophils, which will enter the peripheral blood around day 14–25 after HCT (Bartelink et al. 2013b). Patients are highly susceptible for bacterial and fungal infections during this time of neutropenia. Lymphocytes on the other hand are mainly depleted by serotherapy, which causes a rapid decline in peripheral blood lymphocyte counts and to a lesser extent of tissue lymphocytes (Willemsen et al. 2015; Petersen et al. 2003). Within the lymphocyte compartment, reconstitution of NK cells occurs parallel to neutrophil reconstitution, while B cells start to be detectable on day +40 after HCT (Petersen et al. 2003). Reconstitution of T cells following HCT is markedly different compared to other lymphocytes (Willemsen et al. 2015; Bosch et al. 2012; Veys et al. 2012). Two distinct routes of T-cell reconstitution can be identified: peripheral expansion and thymopoiesis. Under the influence of interleukin (IL)-7, IL-15, and IL-21 and tumor growth factor (TGF) β, graft-infused T cells divide to give rise to a relatively oligoclonal T-cell population (Bosch et al. 2012; Williams et al. 2008). However, although this T-cell population has a skewed T-cell receptor (TCR) repertoire, these cells seem effective in clearing viral infections, which is most pronounced in CB (Williams et al. 2008; Chiesa et al. 2012). Depending on thymic function, output of naïve T cells through thymopoiesis commences 3–6 months after HCT (Krenger et al. 2011; Kanda et al. 2012). Several factors negatively influence thymic function, including steroid use, GvHD, and age (Krenger et al. 2011). In light of the relatively long time window between HCT and thymopoiesis, patients fully depend on peripheral expansion during the most critical time after HCT in terms of mortality (Bartelink et al. 2013b; Williams et al. 2008; Parkman et al. 2006). Hence, the graft-infused T cells are crucial and must be protected against rigorous depletion (Bosch et al. 2012; Szabolcs and Niedzwiecki 2007; Lucchini et al. 2015; Oshrine et al. 2013). Exposure of donor T cells to serotherapy and immuno-ablative cytotoxic agents as fludarabine can potentially result in severe lymphodepletion, thereby abrogating early T-cell immune reconstitution. Serotherapy is more potent and has a significantly longer half-life compared to fludarabine (McCune et al. 2014a; Waller et al. 2003; Call et al. 2009; Kakhniashvili et al. 2005) and therefore has a greater influence on T-cell immune reconstitution following HCT.

3 Limitations of HCT

The major limitations of HCT include (1) transplant-related mortality, (2) relapse of disease, and (3) late effects.

3.1 Transplant-Related Mortality

The main causes of transplant-related mortality include alloreactivity and infections. Alloreactivity in HCT can manifest as either GvHD or graft rejection. GvHD can present acutely, manifesting in the skin, gut, or liver or in a more chronic way, mainly in the skin, mucous membranes, and lungs and as cytopenias (Shulman et al. 1980; Filipovich et al. 2005; Glucksberg et al. 1974). A three-step model is mostly used to describe the pathophysiology of acute GvHD (Ferrara et al. 2009). First, tissue damage, either pre-existing or caused by the conditioning regimen, leads to antigen-presenting cell (APC) activation. Next, host APCs activate donor T cells, which finally give rise to an inflammatory reaction. This process leads to tissue damage, followed by more APC activation, resulting in a self-reinforcing process. The pathophysiology of chronic GvHD on the other hand is poorly understood. The main treatment for acute and chronic GvHD is steroids; steroid refractory GvHD has abominable outcome.

As opposed to GvHD, graft rejection is an immunological reaction of host cells toward the donor. Here, host T cells give rise to a cellular response against the donor stem cells (Locatelli et al. 2014). Outcome following graft rejection is negatively impacted by infections as well as a high chance on developing a second graft failure (Lund et al. 2015).

The main predictor for GvHD and rejection is HLA disparity between donor and recipient; however many other factors including viral reactivations, the gut microbiome, and pharmacotherapy may also play a role (Ferrara et al. 2009; Locatelli et al. 2014; Lindemans et al. 2015; Kanda 2013).

Infections are another important contributor to morbidity and mortality. Following the conditioning regimen, patients will go through a period of 2–3 weeks of neutropenia dependent on rate of engraftment, leaving the patient vulnerable for bacterial and fungal infections for which prophylaxis is given (Akan et al. 2013; Robinson et al. 2016). During and after this neutropenic period, cellular immunity may be hampered up to months after HCT depending on the level of immunosuppression and T-cell depletion (Willemsen et al. 2015; Bartelink et al. 2013b; Bosch et al. 2012). The main effector cells for cellular immunity are lymphocytes, including T cells, B cells, and NK cells. This puts patients at risk for reactivations of previously encountered viral infections, including adenovirus (AdV), cytomegalovirus (CMV), human herpes virus 6 (HHV-6), and Epstein-Barr virus (EBV) (Hiwarkar et al. 2013; Park et al. 2014; Servais et al. 2014; Gotoh et al. 2014; Bruno et al. 2003; Admiraal et al. 2017a) but also relapse. Antiviral drugs are available for most of these viral infections. These include ganciclovir and foscarnet for CMV and HHV-6, with cidofovir as a second-line treatment for CMV. Cidofovir is the first-line treatment for AdV reactivations. EBV can be treated with rituximab, thereby depleting B cells as the reservoir for the viral infection. The use of most antiviral drugs is limited by their toxicity, mainly hepato- and nephrotoxicity. Another possibility to treat viral reactivations is by infusion of virus-specific T cells cultured from the graft donor, which is mainly used for AdV and CMV infections. Moreover, promoting early and adequate T-cell reconstitution seems an attractive solution to prevent viral reactivations post-HCT. As dosage and timing of serotherapy play a major role in the early T-cell reconstitution, optimization of serotherapy may help prevent the incidence of viral reactivations (Admiraal et al. 2015, 2017a; de Koning et al. 2017).

3.2 Relapse of Disease

Relapse of the underlying malignancy is another major limitation of HCT, occurring in 10–30% of patients (Wagner et al. 2014; Ponce et al. 2015; Eapen et al. 2010). Disease status, remission status, and tumor burden before HCT expressed in minimal residual disease (MRD) are predictors for relapse (Krejci et al. 2003; Knechtli et al. 2014; Lankester et al. 2010; Grimwade and Freeman 2014). The main mechanisms for tumor control by HCT include high doses of myeloablative chemotherapy and the so-called graft-versus-leukemia (GvL) effect, a donor T-cell-driven response against residual leukemic blasts (Falkenburg and Warren 2011). This stresses the importance of T-cell reconstitution after HCT for preventing relapse (Parkman et al. 2006).

3.3 Late Effects

With the higher survival rates after HCT, late effects become increasingly important. Late effects may have a significant impact on the quality of life, which particularly in children is pivotal. Chronic GvHD requiring systemic immune suppression is associated with infections, poor quality of life, and premature death. Growth and cognitive capabilities may be impaired in children following HCT, the latter mainly following central nervous system irradiation (Bieri et al. 2011). Fertility may be hampered in patients receiving a HCT as a child due to ovarian dysfunction or decreased spermatogenesis (Sayan et al. 2016; Leader et al. 2011; Green et al. 2009). Secondary malignancies as a result of any chemotherapy treatment and/or radiation are rare but serious late effects.

In recent years, HCT has become a safer procedure through less toxic conditioning regimens, novel therapeutic options for treatment and prevention of relapse and GvHD, improvements in donor selection, promising alternative donor sources, and better supportive care (Gratwohl et al. 2000; Passweg et al. 2014; Pai et al. 2014; Boelens et al. 2013). However, therapy- and relapse-related mortality as well as long-term morbidity remains to be a limitation of HCT. Further enhancement of the safety of the procedure as well as getting better disease control can further improve the outcomes of HCT (Mohty et al. 2014). As pointed out above, the number of characteristics introduced to the treatment is significant, including patient, donor, conditioning, and supportive care. A uniform treatment plan for all patients may therefore lead to under- or overtreatment in certain part of patients. Therefore, a promising approach to improve outcomes is by individualizing the treatment. This includes risk stratification for treatment intensity, individualized dosing of agents used in the conditioning regimen, and adjuvant cellular therapies targeting specific tumor markers (Lankester et al. 2010; McCune et al. 2014b; de Haar et al. 2015). Besides improved outcomes, safer and more effective treatment may extend the indications for HCT toward lower-risk malignancies and milder phenotypes of benign disease.

4 Pharmacological Considerations in HCT

Most commonly used drugs and their indications are described in the paragraphs above. Some special considerations frequently apply to drugs used in HCT, including drug interactions and therapeutic drug monitoring, which are further explored in the following paragraphs.

4.1 Drug Interactions

Most patients receive multiple drugs during the treatment, which may result in pharmacological interactions. These can be either pharmacokinetic or pharmacodynamic interactions, where the former is most important and perhaps best understood. Most pharmacokinetic interactions involve competition for metabolic enzymes (i.e., cytochrome P450 [CYP]) and drug transporters (i.e., P-glycoprotein [PgP]). An important group of interactions is competition on CYP-3A4, which is involved in many pharmacological pathways including drugs frequently used in HCT. Examples on CYP-3A4 inhibitors include azoles, ciprofloxacin, and erythromycin, while phenytoin, carbamazepine, and corticosteroids induce the enzyme. Many immunosuppressants used in HCT including cyclosporin A, tacrolimus, and sirolimus are metabolized by CYP-3A4, and concentrations of these drugs will be influenced by introduction of an inductor or inhibitor. As the number of potential drug interactions of drugs used in HCT is high and cannot be summarized in a book chapter, involvement of a clinical pharmacist in daily clinical care is highly recommended.

4.2 Therapeutic Drug Monitoring

A significant number of drugs used in HCT have a narrow and/or critical therapeutic window and may also be involved in drug-drug interactions. Individualized dosing regimens are available for some drugs to minimize variability in drug exposures (see also Sect. 5). In order to address remaining variability, therapeutic drug monitoring (TDM) is often performed in HCT. Most centers use standard TDM for drugs including busulfan, voriconazole, posaconazole, cyclosporin A, tacrolimus, and sirolimus.

5 Toward Individualized Dosing

Historically, the vast majority of drug development studies were performed in adults. Many drugs are not evaluated in children, contributing to off-label or unlicensed use in as high as 49–87% of drugs used in tertiary care hospitals (Kimland and Odlind 2012; Knibbe et al. 2011). Pediatric dosing regimens are often empirical, linearly extrapolated from adult dosing based on body weight. When using a per kilogram dose, the assumption is made that the PK (e.g., clearance, volume of distribution) also increases linearly with body weight in order to reach comparable concentrations. In addition, the assumption is made that the concentration-effect relationship is comparable between children and adults. However, since developmental changes are mostly nonlinear (Kearns et al. 2003), empirical dosing can lead to underdosing or overdosing. This is especially true in the very young children and adolescents, thereby introducing toxicity or reduced efficacy (Knibbe et al. 2011; Knibbe and Danhof 2011). In order to reach optimal exposure in all patients, the PK and pharmacodynamics (PD) need to be described, including the influence of predictors such as body size on PK and PD. With these models, the optimal dose for any individual patient can be predicted to reach optimal exposure. This approach has been demonstrated in pediatric HCT (Bartelink et al. 2012a). While most cytostatic agents used in HCT are dosed using a fixed mg/kg or mg/m^2 dose for all patients, busulfan dose is fully individualized and controlled using therapeutic drug monitoring (TDM) (Bartelink et al. 2012a). Recent work has shown that actual exposure to busulfan impacts outcome in terms of toxicity, graft failure, and relapse (Bartelink et al. 2009, 2012b; Lalmohamed et al. 2015).

The population approach, using advanced nonlinear mixed effects modeling and high computing power, is the preferred method for PK analyses according to both the FDA and EMEA guidelines (EMEA 2007; FDA 1999). Previously, the so-called two-step approach was the method of choice. In this approach, PK parameters are individually determined for which full sampling is required in all patients. Next, descriptive statistics are applied to the PK parameters in the whole population. In the population approach, data from all patients is pooled to estimate a population mean for all PK parameters (Bauer 2011). Next, based on individual concentrations, interindividual variability and residual error are calculated for each patient. Main advantage of the population approach is the ability to use sparsely sampled and unbalanced (differences in number of samples and sample times between patients, as often the case) data (Sheinerm 1984). This makes the population approach particularly attractive in pediatrics, where few samples are available and the absolute dose varies significantly between children. Additionally, the estimation of PK parameters is more robust as the software is able to differentiate between real interindividual variability and residual error (a combination of incorrect sample times, measurement errors, and model misspecification) (Sheiner and Beal 1980). Altogether, from an ethical, practical, and methodological point of view, the population approach is the preferred method for PK analyses.

After describing the population pharmacokinetics, the relationship between concentrations or exposure and effects or toxicity (PD) needs to be determined. The PD analysis will give further insight into the therapeutic window and will set an optimal target exposure. Next, an individualized dosing regimen can be designed using the population PK model, aiming for optimal exposure. The proposed individualized dosing regimen should be evaluated in a prospective trial, both for external validation of the PK model and the clinical safety and efficacy (Ince et al. 2009).

Individualized drug dosing is increasingly incorporated, especially in pediatrics where differences in PK between children of different age groups are major. While individualized dosing regimens are designed according to the above in many fields, we feel HCT is at the front of incorporating the individualized dosing in clinical practice. As such, most centers use individualized busulfan dosing with therapeutic drug monitoring (Bartelink et al. 2012a, 2016). Individualized dosing for ATG has been designed and is currently evaluated in clinical trials (Admiraal et al. 2015, 2017b). In the coming years, we expect to see more individualized dosing regimens emerging in the field of HCT, especially in pediatric transplantations, where differences in PK are major. In our view, we need fully individualized conditioning regimens including all drugs used. This way, outcome will be predictable and adjustable based on individual patients' needs. Additionally, other drugs used in HCT may need individualization as well, including GvHD prophylaxis and the treatment and prophylaxis for infectious diseases. Finally, the currently available models may be further sophisticated, describing not only PK or PD but rather the complete spectrum of drug treatment, including dose, PK, biomarker response, clinical efficacy, and toxicity in one comprehensive model. We expect development and implementation of individualized dosing to take place in the next 10 years, thereby improving the knowledge and efficacy of clinical drug therapy and improving clinical outcome following HCT. With individualized dosing, unwanted variability in drug exposure will be reduced, leading to predictable, adjustable, and improved outcome of HCT. Such a predictable conditioning regimen can also be used as a transplantation platform in the context of harmonized clinical trial design to study the effects of adjuvant therapies, e.g., concomitant chemotherapy in conditioning or adjuvant immunotherapies.

Currently, cost-effectiveness is playing an increasingly larger role in healthcare decision-making. In this perspective, we hypothesize that dose individualization may be quite cost-effective, especially in the field of HCT where all complications are very costly (e.g., treatment of GvHD, expensive antiviral drugs, VOD, graft failure) (Bartelink et al. 2013a; Corbacioglu et al. 2012). Additionally, the costs of the development of individualized dosing regimens are relatively low.

6 Adjuvant Cellular Therapies

Adjuvant cellular therapies, given posttransplantation, are strategies being used and developed to get better disease control in patients receiving a HCT, including CBT for malignant disease as this remains an unmet need for certain indications.

Historically and still in some protocols, unmanipulated lymphocyte infusions are given, while nowadays also more specific cell therapies are being developed, such as engineered T cells and cellular vaccines.

As relapse remains the main obstacle even after potentially curative HCT, novel combinational immunotherapeutic strategies are being developed aiming at preventing relapse after HCT. Currently the most widely used type of additional immunotherapy combined with allogeneic HCT is donor lymphocyte infusion (DLI), where alloreactive T cells may help to eradicate residual tumor cells. Unfortunately, this "non-specific" strategy suffers from severe toxic side effects, such as GvHD (Deol and Lum 2010). Other approaches aim to increase innate or adaptive antitumor responses by transferring ex vivo-generated cells, such as (chimeric antigen receptor (CAR)-modified) tumor-specific cytotoxic T lymphocytes (CTL) or natural killer (NK) cells (Lee et al. 2015; Grupp et al. 2013; Maude et al. 2014; Brentjens et al. 2013; Porter et al. 2011; Louis et al. 2011; Zhou et al. 2014). Although initial results seem promising, these procedures are often time-consuming (up to months) and may have limitations, such as HLA restriction and uncertain functionality. Additionally, there is a highly variable induction of immunological memory upon transfer in the patient, which may restrict the broad eligibility of these treatments. Although CAR-modified T cells look promising, at least on the short term, several drawbacks, such as (life)-long B-cell lymphopenia in CAR T cells against CD19. Furthermore, the duration of effect, which may reflects the life span of these engineered T cells, remains unclear.

Another intriguing option is development of cell vaccines: increased antigen presentation provided by a dendritic cell (DC) vaccine combined with the intrinsic increased proliferative capacity of the grafted CB cells may result in fast differentiation and proliferation of tumor-specific CTL early after CBT (de Haar et al. 2015; Palucka and Banchereau 2013). This early and mass expansion of tumor-specific CTL may subsequently result in clearance of minimal residual disease and prevention of relapses in cancer patients. Naïve CB T cells display exceptional proliferative capacities, suggesting that efficient priming of these cells using a tumor-specific DC vaccine will provide powerful antitumor activity. This may result in clearance of, and long-term immunological memory against, tumor cells. That CB T cells mediate a stronger antileukemic activity compared to adult cells was recently shown (Hiwarkar et al. 2015).

For all these adjuvant immunotherapies, predictable T-cell immune reconstitution is essential as the effect relies on the absence of circulation ATG but also on presence of adequate number of T cells to mediate the desired antitumor effect.

7 Conclusion

HCT provides a final and potentially curative treatment option for a number of malignant and benign disorders. However, there is a need for improved survival chances after HCT, which may be accomplished by improving disease control and reducing the toxicity of the procedure. Pharmacotherapy plays a major role in both the conditioning phase as in the prevention and treatment of GvHD and infectious complications. There is a stringent need for an evidence-based, individualized dosing regimen agents used in HCT.

References

Admiraal R, van Kesteren C, Jol-van Der Zijde CM et al (2015) Association between anti-thymocyte globulin exposure and CD4+ immune reconstitution in paediatric haematopoietic cell transplantation: a multicentre, retrospective pharmacodynamic cohort analysis. Lancet Haematol 2:e194–e203

Admiraal R, de Koning C, Lindemans CA et al (2017a) Viral reactivations and associated outcomes in context of immune reconstitution after pediatric hematopoietic cell transplantation. J Allergy Clin Immunol 140(6):1643–1650

Admiraal R, Nierkens S, de Witte MA et al (2017b) Association between anti-thymocyte globulin exposure and survival outcomes in adult unrelated haemopoietic cell transplantation: a multicentre, retrospective, pharmacodynamic cohort analysis. Lancet Haematol. https://doi.org/10.1016/S2352-3026(15)00045-9

Akan H, Antia VP, Kouba M et al (2013) Preventing invasive fungal disease in patients with haematological malignancies and the recipients of haematopoietic stem cell transplantation: practical aspects. J Antimicrob Chemother 68(Suppl 3):iii5–ii16

Apperley J, Carreras E, Gluckman E, Masszi T (eds) (2012) ESH-EBMT handbook on haematopoietic stem cell transplantation. Forum Service Editore, Genoa

Bartelink IH, Bredius RGM, Belitser SV et al (2009) Association between busulfan exposure and outcome in children receiving intravenous busulfan before hematologic stem cell transplantation. Biol Blood Marrow Transplant 15:231–241

Bartelink IH, van Kesteren C, Boelens JJ et al (2012a) Predictive performance of a busulfan pharmacokinetic model in children and young adults. Ther Drug Monit 34:574–583

Bartelink IH, Boelens JJ, Bredius RGM et al (2012b) Body weight-dependent pharmacokinetics of busulfan in paediatric haematopoietic stem cell transplantation patients: towards individualized dosing. Clin Pharmacokinet 51:331–345

Bartelink IH, van Reij EML, Gerhardt CE et al (2013a) Fludarabine and exposure-targeted busulfan compares favorably with busulfan/cyclophosphamide-based regimens in pediatric hematopoietic cell transplantation: maintaining efficacy with less toxicity. Biol Blood Marrow Transplant 20:1–9

Bartelink IH, Belitser SV, Knibbe CAJ et al (2013b) Immune reconstitution kinetics as an early predictor for mortality using various hematopoietic stem cell sources in children. Biol Blood Marrow Transplant 19:305–313

Bartelink IH, Lalmohamed A, van Reij EML et al (2016) Association of busulfan exposure with survival and toxicity after haemopoietic cell transplantation in children and young adults: a multicentre, retrospective cohort analysis. Lancet Haematol 3:e526–e536

Bauer RJ (2011) NONMEM 7.2 user manual. Available at https://iconplc.com

Bieri S, Roosnek E, Ozsahin H et al (2011) Outcome and risk factors for late-onset complications 24 months beyond allogeneic hematopoietic stem cell transplantation. Eur J Haematol 87:138–147

Boelens JJ, Aldenhoven M, Purtill D et al (2013) Outcomes of transplantation using a various cell source in children with hurlers syndrome after myelo-ablative conditioning. an eurocord-EBMT-CIBMTR collaborative study. Blood 121:3981–3987

Bosch M, Dhadda M, Hoegh-Petersen M et al (2012) Immune reconstitution after anti-thymocyte globulin-conditioned hematopoietic cell transplantation. Cytotherapy 14:1258–1275

Brentjens RJ, Davila ML, Riviere I et al (2013) CD19-targeted T cells rapidly induce molecular remissions in adults with chemotherapy-refractory acute lymphoblastic leukemia. Sci Transl Med 5:177ra38

Brink MH, Ackaert O, Zwaveling J et al (2014) Pharmacokinetics of treosulfan in pediatric patients undergoing hematopoietic stem cell transplantation. Ther Drug Monit 36:465–472

Bruno B, Gooley T, Hackman RC, Davis C, Corey L, Boeckh M (2003) Adenovirus infection in hematopoietic stem cell transplantation: effect of ganciclovir and impact on survival. Biol Blood Marrow Transplant 9:341–352

Call SK, Kasow KA, Barfield R et al (2009) Total and active rabbit antithymocyte globulin (rATG; Thymoglobulin) pharmacokinetics in pediatric patients undergoing unrelated donor bone marrow transplantation. Biol Blood Marrow Transplant 15:274–278

Chiesa R, Gilmour K, Qasim W et al (2012) Omission of in vivo T-cell depletion promotes rapid expansion of naïve CD4+ cord blood lymphocytes and restores adaptive immunity within 2 months after unrelated cord blood transplant. Br J Haematol 156:656–666

Claas FHS et al (2016) Europdonor annual report 2015. Available at https://www.matchis.nl

Corbacioglu S, Cesaro S, Faraci M et al (2012) Defibrotide for prophylaxis of hepatic veno-occlusive disease in paediatric haemopoietic stem-cell transplantation: an open-label, phase 3, randomised controlled trial. Lancet 379:1301–1309

Davies SM, Ramsay NKC, Klein JP et al (2000) Comparison of preparative regimens in transplants for children with acute lymphoblastic leukemia. J Clin Oncol 18:340–347

de Haar C, Plantinga M, Blokland NJ et al (2015) Generation of a cord blood-derived Wilms Tumor 1 dendritic cell vaccine for AML patients treated with allogeneic cord blood transplantation. Oncoimmunology 4:e1023973

de Koning C, Admiraal R, Nierkens S, Boelens JJ (2017) Immune reconstitution and outcomes after conditioning with anti-thymocyte-globulin in unrelated cord blood transplantation; the good, the bad, and the ugly. Stem Cell Investig 4:38

Deol A, Lum LG (2010) Role of donor lymphocyte infusions in relapsed hematological malignancies after stem cell transplantation revisited. Cancer Treat Rev 36:528–538

Eapen M, Rocha V, Sanz G et al (2010) Effect of graft source on unrelated donor haemopoietic stem-cell transplantation in adults with acute leukaemia: a retrospective analysis. Lancet Oncol 11:653–660

El-Jawahri A, Li S, Ballen KK et al (2016) Phase II trial of reduced-intensity busulfan/clofarabine conditioning with allogeneic hematopoietic stem cell transplantation for patients with acute myeloid leukemia, myelodysplastic syndromes, and acute lymphoid leukemia. Biol Blood Marrow Transplant 22:80–85

EMEA (2007) Guideline on reporting the results of population pharmacokinetic analyses. Available at https://www.ema.europa.eu

Falkenburg JHF, Warren EH (2011) Graft versus leukemia reactivity after allogeneic stem cell transplantation. Biol Blood Marrow Transplant 17:S33–S38

FDA (1999) Guidance for industry, population pharmacokinetics. Available at https://www.fda.gov/

Ferrara JL, Levine JE, Reddy P, Holler E (2009) Graft-versus-host disease. Lancet 373:1550–1561
Filipovich AH, Weisdorf D, Pavletic S et al (2005) National Institutes of health consensus development project on criteria for clinical trials in chronic graft-versus-host disease: I. Diagnosis and staging working group report. Biol Blood Marrow Transplant 11:945–956
Friberg LE, Henningsson A, Maas H, Nguyen L, Karlsson MO (2002) Model of chemotherapy-induced myelosuppression with parameter consistency across drugs. J Clin Oncol 20:4713–4721
Glucksberg H, Storb R, Fefer A et al (1974) Clinical manifestations of graft-versus-host disease in human recipients of marrow from HL-A-matched sibling donors. Transplantation 18:295–304
Gotoh M, Yoshizawa S, Katagiri S et al (2014) Human herpesvirus 6 reactivation on the 30th day after allogeneic hematopoietic stem cell transplantation can predict grade 2-4 acute graft-versus-host disease. Transpl Infect Dis 16:440–449
Gratwohl A, Passweg J, Baldomero H, Hermans J, Urbano-Ispizua A (2000) Hematopoietic stem cell transplantation in Europe 1998. Hematol J 1:333–350
Green DM, Kawashima T, Stovall M et al (2009) Fertility of female survivors of childhood cancer: a report from the childhood cancer survivor study. J Clin Oncol 27:2677–2685
Grimwade D, Freeman SD (2014) Review article defining minimal residual disease in acute myeloid leukemia: which platforms are ready for "prime time"? Blood 124:3345–3355
Grupp SA, Kalos M, Barrett D et al (2013) Chimeric antigen receptor–modified T cells for acute lymphoid leukemia. N Engl J Med 368:1509–1518
Gyurkocza B, Sandmaier BM (2014) Conditioning regimens for hematopoietic cell transplantation: one size does not fit all. Blood 124:344–353
Heemskerk MBA, van Walraven SM, Cornelissen JJ et al (2005) How to improve the search for an unrelated haematopoietic stem cell donor. Faster is better than more! Bone Marrow Transplant 35:645–652
Hiwarkar P, Gaspar HB, Gilmour K et al (2013) Impact of viral reactivations in the era of pre-emptive antiviral drug therapy following allogeneic haematopoietic SCT in paediatric recipients. Bone Marrow Transplant 48:803–808
Hiwarkar P, Qasim W, Ricciardelli I et al (2015) Cord blood T cells mediate enhanced anti-tumor effects compared with adult peripheral blood T cells. Blood 126:2882–2891
Holtick U, Albrecht M, Chemnitz JM et al (1996) Bone marrow versus peripheral blood allogeneic haematopoietic stem cell transplantation for haematological malignancies in adults. Cochrane Database Syst Rev 4:CD010189
Hough R, Danby R, Russell N et al (2015) Recommendations for a standard UK approach to incorporating umbilical cord blood into clinical transplantation practice: an update on cord blood unit selection, donor selection algorithms and conditioning protocols. Br J Haematol:360–370
Ince I, de Wildt SN, Tibboel D, Danhof M, Knibbe CAJ (2009) Tailor-made drug treatment for children: creation of an infrastructure for data-sharing and population PK – PD modeling. Drug Discov Today 14:316–320
Jol-van der Zijde C, Jansen-Hoogendijk A, Raaijmakers S et al (2009) Kinetics of active and total thymoglobulin in paediatric stem cell transplantation. Bone Marrow Transplant 43:S126–S127
Kakhniashvili I, Filicko J, Kraft WK, Flomenberg N (2005) Heterogeneous clearance of antithymocyte globulin after CD34+-selected allogeneic hematopoietic progenitor cell transplantation. Biol Blood Marrow Transplant 11:609–618
Kanda J (2013) Effect of HLA mismatch on acute graft-versus-host disease. Int J Hematol 98:300–308
Kanda J, Chiou LW, Szabolcs P et al (2012) Immune recovery in adult patients after myeloablative dual umbilical cord blood, matched sibling, and matched unrelated donor hematopoietic cell transplantation. Biol Blood Marrow Transplant 18:1664–1676.e1
Kearns GL, Abdel-Rahman SM, Alander SW, Blowey DW, Leeder JS, Kauffman RE (2003) Developmental pharmacology—drug disposition, action and therapy in infants and children. New Engl J Med drug Ther 349:1157–1167

Kimland E, Odlind V (2012) Off-label drug use in pediatric patients. Clin Pharmacol Ther 91:796–801

Knechtli CJC, Goulden NJ, Hancock JP et al (2014) Minimal residual disease status before allogeneic bone marrow transplantation is an important determinant of successful outcome for children and adolescents with acute lymphoblastic leukemia. Blood 92:4072–4079

Knibbe CAJ, Danhof M (2011) Individualized dosing regimens in children based on population PKPD modelling: are we ready for it? Int J Pharm 415:9–14

Knibbe CAJ, Krekels EHJ, Danhof M (2011) Advances in paediatric pharmacokinetics. Expert Opin Drug Metab Toxicol 7:1–8

Krejci O, van der Velden VHJ, Bader P et al (2003) Level of minimal residual disease prior to haematopoietic stem cell transplantation predicts prognosis in paediatric patients with acute lymphoblastic leukaemia: a report of the Pre-BMT MRD Study Group. Bone Marrow Transplant 32:849–851

Krenger W, Blazar BR, Holländer GA (2011) Thymic T-cell development in allogeneic stem cell transplantation. Blood 117:6768–6776

Laínez JM, Orcun S, Pekny JF et al (2014) Comparison of an assumption-free bayesian approach with optimal sampling schedule to a maximum a posteriori approach for personalizing cyclophosphamide dosing. Pharmacotherapy 34:330–335

Lalmohamed A, Bartelink I, van Reij L et al (2015) Studying the optimal intravenous busulfan exposure in pediatric allogeneic hematopoietic cell transplantation (alloHCT) to improve clinical outcomes: a multicenter study. Biol Blood Marrow Transplant 21:S102–S103

Langenhorst JB, Dorlo TPC, van Maarseveen EM et al (2019a) Population pharmacokinetics of fludarabine in children and adults during conditioning prior to allogeneic hematopoietic cell transplantation. Clin Pharmacokinet 58:627–637

Langenhorst JB, van Kesteren C, van Maarseveen EM et al (2019b) Fludarabine exposure in the conditioning prior to allogeneic hematopoietic cell transplantation predicts outcomes. Blood Adv 3(14):2179–2187

Lankester A, Bierings M, van Wering E et al (2010) Preemptive alloimmune intervention in high-risk pediatric acute lymphoblastic leukemia patients guided by minimal residual disease level before stem cell transplantation. Leukemia 24:1462–1469

Leader A, Lishner M, Michaeli J, Revel A (2011) Fertility considerations and preservation in haemato-oncology patients undergoing treatment. Br J Haematol 153:291–308

Lee DW, Kochenderfer JN, Stetler-Stevenson M et al (2015) T cells expressing CD19 chimeric antigen receptors for acute lymphoblastic leukaemia in children and young adults: a phase 1 dose-escalation trial. Lancet 385:517–528

Lindemans CA, Chiesa R, Amrolia PJ et al (2014) Impact of thymoglobulin prior to pediatric unrelated umbilical cord blood transplantation on immune reconstitution and clinical outcome. Blood 123:126–132

Lindemans CA, Calafiore M, Mertelsmann AM et al (2015) Interleukin-22 promotes intestinal-stem-cell-mediated epithelial regeneration. Nature 528:560–564

Locatelli F, Lucarelli B, Merli P (2014) Current and future approaches to treat graft failure after allogeneic hematopoietic stem cell transplantation. Expert Opin Pharmacother 15:23–36

Long-Boyle JR, Green KG, Brunstein CG et al (2011) High fludarabine exposure and relationship with treatment-related mortality after nonmyeloablative hematopoietic cell transplantation. Bone Marrow Transplant 46:20–26

Louis CU, Savoldo B, Dotti G et al (2011) Antitumor activity and long-term fate of chimeric antigen receptor – positive T cells in patients with neuroblastoma. Blood 118:6050–6056

Lucchini G, Perales M-A, Veys P (2015) Immune reconstitution after cord blood transplantation: peculiarities, clinical implications and management strategies. Cytotherapy 17:711–722

Lund TC, Liegel J, Bejanyan N et al (2015) Second allogeneic hematopoietic cell transplantation for graft failure: poor outcomes for neutropenic graft failure. Am J Hematol 90:892–896

Mank AP, Davies M (2008) Examining low bacterial dietary practice: a survey on low bacterial food. Eur J Oncol Nurs 12:342–348

Marsh JC, Pearce RM, Koh MBC et al (2014) Retrospective study of alemtuzumab vs ATG-based conditioning without irradiation for unrelated and matched sibling donor transplants in acquired severe aplastic anemia: a study from the British Society for Blood and Marrow Transplantation. Bone Marrow Transplant 49:42–48

Maude SL, Frey N, Shaw PA et al (2014) Chimeric antigen receptor T cells for sustained remissions in leukemia. N Engl J Med 371:1507–1517

McCune JS, Vicini P, Salinger DH et al (2014a) Population pharmacokinetic/dynamic model of lymphosuppression after fludarabine administration. Cancer Chemother Pharmacol 75:67–75. https://doi.org/10.1007/s00280-014-2618-2

McCune JS, Jacobson P, Wiseman A, Militano O (2014b) Optimizing drug therapy in pediatric SCT: focus on pharmacokinetics. Bone Marrow Transplant 50:1–8

Mohty M (2007) Mechanisms of action of antithymocyte globulin: T-cell depletion and beyond. Leukemia 21:1387–1394

Mohty M, Malard F, Savani BN (2014) High-dose total body irradiation and myeloablative conditioning before allogeneic stem cell transplantation: time to rethink? Biol Blood Marrow Transplant 21:1–5

Molineux G, Pojda Z, Hampson IN, Lord BI, Dexter TM (1990) Transplantation potential of peripheral blood stem cells induced by granulocyte colony-stimulating factor. Blood 76:2153–2158

Nagler A, Savani BN, Labopin M et al (2015) Outcomes after use of two standard ablative regimens in patients with refractory acute myeloid leukaemia: A retrospective, multicentre, registry analysis. Lancet Haematol:384–392

Nash RA, Antin JH, Karanes C et al (2000) Phase 3 study comparing methotrexate and tacrolimus with methotrexate and cyclosporine for prophylaxis of acute graft-versus-host disease after marrow transplantation from unrelated donors. Blood 96:2062–2068

O'Grady NP, Alexander M, Dellinger EP et al (2002) Guidelines for the prevention of intravascular catheter-related infections. Am J Infect Control 30:476–489

Oshrine BR, Li Y, Teachey DT, Heimall J, Barrett DM, Bunin N (2013) Immunologic recovery in children after alternative donor allogeneic transplantation for hematologic malignancies: comparison of recipients of partially T cell-depleted peripheral blood stem cells and umbilical cord blood. Biol Blood Marrow Transplant 19:1581–1589

Pai S-Y, Logan BR, Griffith LM et al (2014) Transplantation outcomes for severe combined immunodeficiency, 2000–2009. N Engl J Med 371:434–446

Palucka K, Banchereau J (2013) Dendritic-cell-based therapeutic cancer vaccines. Immunity 39:38–48

Park M, Lee YH, Lee SH et al (2014) Cytomegalovirus infection in seropositive unrelated cord blood recipients: a study of 349 Korean patients. Ann Hematol 94:481–489

Parkman R, Cohen G, Carter SL et al (2006) Successful immune reconstitution decreases leukemic relapse and improves survival in recipients of unrelated cord blood transplantation. Biol Blood Marrow Transplant 12:919–927

Pasquini M, Zhu X (2018) Current uses and outcomes of hematopoietic cell transplantation (HCT): CIBMTR summary slides. Available at https://www.cibmtr.org

Passweg JR, Baldomero H, Peters C et al (2014) Hematopoietic SCT in Europe: data and trends in 2012 with special consideration of pediatric transplantation. Bone Marrow Transplant 49:744–750

Passweg JR, Labopin M, Cornelissen J et al (2015) Conditioning intensity in middle-aged patients with AML in first CR: No advantage for myeloablative regimens irrespective of the risk group-an observational analysis by the Acute Leukemia Working Party of the EBMT. Bone Marrow Transplant 50:1063–1068

Petersen SL, Ryder LP, Björk P et al (2003) A comparison of T-, B- and NK-cell reconstitution following conventional or nonmyeloablative conditioning and transplantation with bone marrow or peripheral blood stem cells from human leucocyte antigen identical sibling donors. Bone Marrow Transplant 32:65–72

Ponce DM, Eapen M, Sparapani R et al (2015) In vivo T-cell depletion with myeloablative regimens on outcomes after cord blood transplantation for acute lymphoblastic leukemia in children. Biol Blood Marrow Transplant 21:2173–2179

Porter DL, Levine BL, Kalos M, Bagg A, June CH (2011) Chimeric antigen receptor-modified T cells in chronic lymphoid leukemia. N Engl J Med 365:725–733

Rambaldi A, Grassi A, Masciulli A et al (2015) Busulfan plus cyclophosphamide versus busulfan plus fludarabine as a preparative regimen for allogeneic haemopoietic stem-cell transplantation in patients with acute myeloid leukaemia: An open-label, multicentre, randomised, phase 3 trial. Lancet Oncol 16:1525–1536

Ratanatharathorn V, Nash RA, Przepiorka D et al (1998) Phase III study comparing methotrexate and tacrolimus (prograf, FK506) with methotrexate and cyclosporine for graft-versus-host disease prophylaxis after HLA-identical sibling bone marrow transplantation. Blood 92:2303–2314

Riechmann L, Clark M, Waldmann H, Winter G (1988) Reshaping human antibodies for therapy. Nature 332:323–327

Robinson PD, Lehrnbecher T, Phillips R, Dupuis LL, Sung L (2016) Strategies for empiric management of pediatric fever and neutropenia in patients with cancer and hematopoietic stem-cell transplantation recipients: a systematic review of randomized trials. J Clin Oncol. https://doi.org/10.1200/JCO.2015.65.8591

Sayan M, Cassidy RJ, Butker EE et al (2016) Gonadal shielding technique to preserve fertility in male pediatric patients treated with total body irradiation for stem cell transplantation. Bone Marrow Transplant:1–2

Sengsayadeth S, Savani BN, Blaise D, Malard F, Nagler A, Mohty M (2015) Reduced intensity conditioning allogeneic hematopoietic cell transplantation for adult acute myeloid leukemia in complete remission – a review from the acute leukemia working party of the EBMT. Haematologica 100:859–869

Servais S, Lengline E, Porcher R et al (2014) Long-term immune reconstitution and infection burden after mismatched hematopoietic stem cell transplantation. Biol Blood Marrow Transplant 20:507–517

Sheiner L, Beal S (1980) Evaluation of methods for estimating population pharmacokinetics parameters. I. Michaelis-Menten model: routine clinical pharmacokinetic data. J Pharmacokinet Biopharm 8:553–571

Sheinerm L (1984) The population approach to pharmacokinetic data analysis: rationale and standard data analysis methods. Drug Metab Rev 15(1–2):153–171

Shulman HM, Sullivan KM, Weiden PL et al (1980) Chronic graft-versus-host syndrome in man. A long-term clinicopathologic study of 20 Seattle patients. Am J Med 69:204–217

Soiffer RJ, Lerademacher J, Ho V et al (2011) Impact of immune modulation with anti – T-cell antibodies on the outcome of reduced-intensity allogeneic hematopoietic stem cell transplantation for hematologic malignancies Impact of immune modulation with anti – T-cell antibodies on the outcome of reduc. Blood 117:6963–6970

Storek J, Mohty M, Boelens JJ (2015) Rabbit anti–T cell globulin in allogeneic hematopoietic cell transplantation. Biol Blood Marrow Transplant 21:959–970

Szabolcs P, Niedzwiecki D (2007) Immune reconstitution after unrelated cord blood transplantation. Cytotherapy 9:111–122

Theurich S, Fischmann H, Chakupurakal G et al (2013) Anti-thymocyte globulins for post-transplant graft-versus-host disease prophylaxis-A systematic review and meta-analysis. Crit Rev Oncol Hematol 88:178–186

Tolar J, Mehta PA, Walters MC (2012) Hematopoietic cell transplantation for nonmalignant disorders. Biol Blood Marrow Transplant 18:S166–S171

Uberti JP, Agovi M, Tarima S et al (2011) Comparative analysis of BU and CY versus CY and TBI in full intensity unrelated marrow donor transplantation for AML, CML and myelodysplasia. Bone Marrow Transplant 46:34–43

Van Kesteren C, Zandvliet AS, Karlsson MO et al (2005) Semi-physiological model describing the hematological toxicity of the anti-cancer agent indisulam. Invest New Drugs 23:225–234

Veys P, Wynn RF, Ahn KW et al (2012) Impact of immune modulation with in vivo T cell depletion and myleoablative total body irradiation conditioning regimen on outcomes after unrelated donor transplantation for acute lymphoblastic leukemia in children. Blood 119:6155–6162

Wagner JE, Eapen M, Carter S et al (2014) One-unit versus two-unit cord-blood transplantation for hematologic cancers. N Engl J Med 371:1685–1694

Waller EK, A a L, Lonial S et al (2003) Pharmacokinetics and pharmacodynamics of anti-thymocyte globulin in recipients of partially HLA-matched blood hematopoietic progenitor cell transplantation. Biol Blood Marrow Transplant 9:460–471

Wang L, Gu Z, Zhai R et al (2015) The efficacy and safety of sirolimus-based graft-versus-host disease prophylaxis in patients undergoing allogeneic hematopoietic stem cell transplantation: a meta-analysis of randomized controlled trials. Transfusion 55:2134–2141

Willemsen L, Jol-van der Zijde CM, Admiraal R et al (2015) Impact of serotherapy on immune reconstitution and survival outcomes after stem cell transplantations in children: thymoglobulin versus alemtuzumab. Biol Blood Marrow Transplant 21:473–482

Williams K, Hakim FT, Gress RE (2008) T-cell immune reconstitution following lymphodepletion. Semin Immunol 19:318–330

Zhou X, Di Stasi A, Tey S-K et al (2014) Long-term outcome and immune reconstitution after haploidentical stem cell transplant in recipients of allodepleted-T-cells expressing the inducible caspase-9 safety transgene. Blood 123(25):3895–3905. https://doi.org/10.1182/blood-2014-01-551671

Narcotic-Sparing Approaches and the Shift Toward Paracetamol in Neonatal Intensive Care

Karel Allegaert, Dick Tibboel, and John van den Anker

Contents

K. Allegaert (✉)
Department of Pediatrics, Division of Neonatology, Erasmus MC Sophia Children's Hospital, Rotterdam, The Netherlands

Department of Development and Regeneration, KU Leuven, Leuven, Belgium

Neonatal Intensive Care Unit, University Hospital, Leuven, Belgium
e-mail: karel.allegaert@uzleuven.be

D. Tibboel
Intensive Care, Erasmus MC-Sophia Children's Hospital, Rotterdam, The Netherlands

Department of Pediatric Surgery, Erasmus MC-Sophia Children's Hospital, Rotterdam, The Netherlands
e-mail: d.tibboel@erasmusmc.nl

J. van den Anker
Intensive Care, Erasmus MC-Sophia Children's Hospital, Rotterdam, The Netherlands

Division of Pediatric Pharmacology and Pharmacometrics, University Children's Hospital, Basel, Switzerland

Division of Clinical Pharmacology, Children's National Health System, Washington, DC, USA
e-mail: Jvandena@childrensnational.org

W. Kiess et al. (eds.), *Pediatric Pharmacotherapy*,
Handbook of Experimental Pharmacology 261, https://doi.org/10.1007/164_2019_207

Abstract

Effective analgesia in neonates is relevant not only because of ethical aspects or empathy, but it is a crucial and integral part of medical and nursing care. However, there is also emerging evidence – although mainly in animal models – on the relation between the exposure to narcotics and impaired neurodevelopmental outcome, resulting in a CATCH-22 scenario. Consequently, a balanced approach is needed with the overarching intention to attain adequate pain management with minimal side effects. Despite the available evidence-based guidance on narcotics in ventilated neonates, observations on drug utilization still suggest an overall increase in exposure with extensive variability between units. This increased exposure over time and the extensive variability is concerning given the limited evidence of benefits and potential harm.

Implementation strategies are effective to reduce exposure to narcotics but result in increased paracetamol exposure. We therefore summarized the evidence on paracetamol use in procedural pain management, in minor to moderate as well as major pain syndromes in neonates. While there are sufficient data on short-term safety, there are still concerns on long-term side effects. These concerns relate to neurobehavioral outcome, atopy or fertility, and are at present mainly driven by epidemiological perinatal observations, together with postulated mechanisms.

We conclude that future clinical research objectives should still focus on the need to develop better assessment tools to quantify pain and on the need for high-quality data on long-term outcome of therapeutic interventions – also for paracetamol – and exploration of the mechanisms involved.

Keywords

Narcotics · Newborn · Outcome · Pain management · Paracetamol

1 Introduction: The CATCH-22 of Neonatal Pain and Stress Management

The paradigm that immaturity of pain processing systems in (pre)term infants protected them from pain- and stress-related adverse events was rejected when Anand et al. demonstrated that untreated perioperative pain resulted in increased short-term mortality and morbidity (Anand et al. 1987). As a consequence of these pivotal observations and the subsequent accumulating evidence, it became obvious that effective analgesia in neonates is a crucial part of any treatment during neonatal admission: *effective analgesia is relevant not only because of ethical reflections or empathy, but it is a crucial and integral part of medical and nursing care*.

However, there is also emerging evidence on the relation between the exposure to narcotics and impaired neurodevelopmental outcome, resulting in a CATCH-22 scenario (Schiller et al. 2018; van den Bosch et al. 2017). These findings are further supported by a variety of animal experimental observations related to exposure to narcotics such as altered apoptosis, axonal growth, or synaptogenesis (van den Bosch et al. 2017; Andropoulos 2018). In the human neonate, it has been suggested that the limbic system is a specific vulnerable target structure for overexposure to pain, stress, or narcotics. This can be explained based on the observation that the limbic system undergoes rapid development in the third trimester of pregnancy and early infancy, while related to this structure, the hippocampus and its connections are crucial for encoding, consolidation, and retrieval of memory. These deficits are commonly reported in NICU graduates (Schiller et al. 2018).

The long-term outcome results further add to the available short-term side effects of narcotics – mainly morphine – that were observed and quantified as safety outcome data of randomized controlled trials in ventilated neonates and relate to respiratory depression, hypotension, intestinal hypoperistalsis, and urinary retention. The respiratory depression has been quantified and results in prolonged (+1 day, 7 (4–20) instead of 6 (3–19) days) duration of ventilation (Bhandari et al. 2005). The available data on hypotension reported in different studies likely reflect differences in morphine doses. Simons et al. were unable to document differences in arterial blood pressure, the use of inotropics, or blood pressure variability related to the morphine maintenance infusion (10 μg/kg/h), irrespective of the postmenstrual age (Simons et al. 2006). In contrast, the morphine maintenance infusion (10–30 μg/kg/h), additional morphine administration, and lower age have been associated with hypotension in the NEOPAIN study (Anand et al. 2004). Similarly, morphine delayed the attainment of full enteral feeds (+3 days, 20 (13–29) instead of 17 (12–26) days) in the NEOPAIN trial (Menon et al. 2008). Finally, data on the incidence and extent of urinary retention were not retrieved but have been observed in the clinical setting.

This CATCH-22 scenario results in the need of a balanced approach, considering wanted as well as side effects with the overarching intention to attain adequate pain management with minimal side effects caused by either pain itself or the kind or amount of narcotics administered. Besides neurodevelopment, other compound-specific side effects (e.g., bleeding tendency, hepatic impairment, atopy, renal impairment, blood pressure) should also be considered. Moreover, assessment of pain in neonates as pharmacodynamic outcome variable is at best based on pain scales that do not go beyond intersubjectivity at present. Finally, new pharmacological options such as intravenous paracetamol, locoregional techniques, clonidine, or dexmedetomidine to treat pain became available and have been introduced in the neonatal intensive care, commonly off-label and with limited data on efficacy and safety (Thewissen and Allegaert 2011). This is also true for intravenous paracetamol. Likely because of the uncertainties related to the assessment of the analgesic effects (PD validity of assessment tools) during registration studies, the product failed registration in the United States, while registration in Europe is still limited to term neonates. However, there is extensive off-label use of this product in neonates (Pacifici and Allegaert 2014; van den Anker and Allegaert 2018).

In this review, we aim to provide the reader with an overview on drug utilization on narcotics in neonatal intensive care to show how scientific evidence is implemented or not in clinical practice. This will be followed by a focused overview on the currently available data on pharmacokinetics, safety, and efficacy of paracetamol in neonates to treat pain, to subsequently highlight some knowledge gaps, and to suggest a research agenda. We will not discuss the more recent trend to use paracetamol for treatment of a patent ductus arteriosus and refer the interested reader to other recent reviews on this topic (Jasani et al. 2018; Aranda et al. 2017).

2 Drug Utilization Research on Narcotics in Neonatal Intensive Care

Drug utilization research is a tool to assess whether pharmacotherapy is rational. In neonates, this goal is obviously hampered because of the extensive off-label and unlicensed prescription practices. For research on drug utilization of narcotics, the anatomic therapeutic chemical (ATC, N02) classification can be applied, be it that newborn-specific indications exist for ibuprofen or paracetamol for noncentral nervous system-related indications, like patent ductus arteriosus closure (Jasani et al. 2018; Aranda et al. 2017). Still, *quality* (compare practices to guidelines, local drug formularies), *patterns* (extent or profiles of drug use, trends), *outcomes* (health outcomes, both benefits and adverse effects) of drug utilization, or *determinants* (prescriber characteristics, impact of interventions) can be explored to describe patterns on narcotics used and provide early signals of potential irrational drug utilization, benchmarking, or to guide research priorities (Rosli et al. 2017).

In the latest meta-analysis on the appropriateness to use opioids in ventilated preterm neonates ('Neopain studies'), Bellu et al. concluded almost a decade ago that there is good evidence *not* to administer routinely opioids to these neonates (Bellu et al. 2010). Instead, the authors suggested that opioids should only be administered selectively, when indicated by clinical evaluation of pain indicators. Based on this meta-analytic evidence, one may anticipate that this has resulted in reduced exposure to narcotics and more homogeneity in prescription practices. However, evidence in itself does not result in better practices and lower exposure but necessitate implementation strategies. To further illustrate this, we report on recent publications on drug utilization of narcotics in neonates to provide data on *trends over time*, on variability *between units*, and on the *impact of implementation of guidelines* on practices.

2.1 Trends in Prescription Practices over Time for Narcotics

The Pediatrix consortium reported on medication use in two consecutive time intervals (1997–2004 and 2005–2010), exploring a prospectively collected administrative database. When we compare both databases, it is worth to notice that fentanyl and morphine were in the top 30 list (19 and 25/30) with an estimated exposure of 56 and 35/1000 admitted neonates in the 1997–2004 cohort, to increase to positions 7 and 14 with an estimated exposure of 70 and 51/1000 admitted neonates, with appearance of paracetamol on position 16 with 43/1000 in the more recent (2005–2010) analysis (Clark et al. 2006; Hsieh et al. 2014). Using the same Pediatrix database with focus on the use of sedatives, analgesics, and paralytics in preterm neonates (<1,500 g, <32 weeks' gestational age, 1997–2012, $n = 85{,}911$ ventilated preterm neonates), Zimmerman et al. documented that – despite the meta-analytical evidence – the exposure to opioids and sedatives increased, respectively, from 5% to 32% and 5% to 24% of ventilated infant days (Zimmerman et al. 2017). Similarly, a recent Canadian network analysis on 20,744 preterm neonates (2010–2014, <33 weeks' gestational age) documented that, respectively, 17%, 23%, and 29% of neonates were exposed to either a sedative, a narcotic, or one of these compounds as continuous infusion (Borenstein-Levin et al. 2017).

2.2 Variability Between Units in Prescription Practices for Narcotics

In the Canadian network analysis, extensive variability in practices between units was observed (2–48% for sedatives, 3–41% for narcotics), not explained by clinical characteristics (Borenstein-Levin et al. 2017). A similar pattern with extensive variability between units and common exposure to opioids (26%), sedatives/hypnotics (12%), or paracetamol (14%) has been described in the EUROPAIN prospective cohort (243 units, 6,680 neonates) study (Carbajal et al. 2015). Exposure was much more common in cases with tracheal ventilation, when compared to noninvasive ventilation or spontaneous ventilation (Carbajal et al. 2015). Finally, large differences in neonatal drug use were observed between Dutch neonatal units, and these differences were most pronounced for nervous system (ATC)-related drugs with a range of 919–2,278 (2.5-fold) prescriptions per 1,000 neonates (Flint et al. 2017).

Increased exposure to narcotics over time and the extensive variability is concerning given the limited evidence of benefit and the potential for harm (Clark et al. 2006; Hsieh et al. 2014; Zimmerman et al. 2017; Borenstein-Levin et al. 2017; Carbajal et al. 2015; Flint et al. 2017). This is line with the opioid epidemic across the globe, as reflected in the significant increase in the incidence of newborns diagnosed with neonatal withdrawal syndrome up to 2–6/1,000 newborns (Allegaert and van den Anker 2016).

2.3 Implementation Strategies Are Effective Tools to Reduce Exposure to Narcotics

Implementation of guidelines on the use of opioids and sedatives is effective to reduce the utilization of these drugs and its variability (Rana et al. 2017). This reduction in exposure was reflected in the number of patients (63–33%) and the cumulative dose (morphine −68%; midazolam −37%). Interestingly, this intervention also resulted in a significant reduction in the number of cases (−75%) requiring methadone treatment for iatrogenic opioid withdrawal (Rana et al. 2017). Unfortunately, the authors have not provided information on paracetamol consumption, but the appendices of their paper suggest that this protocol resulted in an increased paracetamol exposure, both in number of cases and in duration (Rana et al. 2017). Along the same line, Baarslag et al. documented that adherence to clinical implementation of intravenous paracetamol as primary analgesia after major surgery resulted in a similar low additional morphine exposure when compared to the observations collected during the original placebo-controlled randomized trial on the effect of intravenous paracetamol on postoperative morphine requirements in non-cardiac surgery newborns and infants (Baarslag et al. 2018; Ceelie et al. 2013).

In essence, both examples resulted in a reduction of exposure to narcotics and a parallel increase in exposure to paracetamol, reflecting some rational for the earlier-mentioned increase in paracetamol exposure in neonates (Hsieh et al. 2014). This makes it valuable to summarize the currently available evidence on the efficacy and safety of paracetamol in neonates, taking into account that intravenous paracetamol is still off-label in the United States for all neonates and on label in Europe from term neonates onward, but not in preterm neonates (Pacifici and Allegaert 2014).

3 Paracetamol for Pain Management in Neonates: In Search for the Available Evidence

3.1 Pharmacokinetics and Metabolism of Paracetamol in Neonates

Data on the pharmacokinetics and metabolism of paracetamol disposition have been described for the full range of gestational age and weight, except for perhaps very specific clinical settings like cardiac bypass and extracorporeal membrane oxygenation. Pooled pharmacokinetic analyses have been reported for both intravenous and enteral (oral, rectal) administration, including external validation efforts (Anderson et al. 2002; Allegaert et al. 2011; Cook et al. 2016a). Obviously, intravenous administration hereby avoids the additional absorption-related variability following oral or rectal administration (Anderson et al. 2002, Allegaert et al. 2011, Cook et al. 2016a). Besides overall clearance, detailed information on the various routes of elimination (glucuronidation, sulfation, oxidation, renal) and their maturational trends have been reported (Cook et al. 2016b). More recently, Flint et al. described the gestational age-driven increase in glucuronidation without evidence for saturation of a specific pathway as there was a proportional increase in exposure of paracetamol and its metabolites in extreme preterm neonates between 24 and 32 weeks' gestational age (Flint et al. 2017).

3.2 Paracetamol for Procedural Pain Management in Neonates: A Misguided Rocket

The data on paracetamol-related pain management for procedural pain in neonates are relatively limited but overall suggest that there is no analgesic effect when used for procedural pain relief. To further illustrate this, Table 1 provides an overview of reported randomized studies on the use of paracetamol for procedural pain for heel lancing (4 studies, 352 cases) or eye examination during screening for retinopathy of prematurity (3 studies, 252 cases) in (pre)term neonates. Compared to placebo, there was no benefit in the cases exposed to paracetamol, while the effect of paracetamol was inferior when compared to non-pharmacological interventions (like sucrose or dextrose).

These findings are in line with the Cochrane review on interventions to reduce needle- and vaccine injection-related pain in infants, since this analysis confirmed the positive impact of breastfeeding, topical anesthetics, and sweet-tasting solutions on acute distress in infants, while there was no benefit for paracetamol or ibuprofen (Shah et al. 2015). Similarly, Roofthooft et al. also concluded that intravenous paracetamol is not suitable as analgesic for PICC placement in preterm neonates, despite the fact that paracetamol target concentration was reached (Roofthooft et al. 2017). So in conclusion, paracetamol is not effective for procedural pain management.

3.3 Minor to Moderate Pain Syndromes

The effects of paracetamol to treat minor to moderate pain syndromes in (pre)term neonates has been described after minor surgery (1 study, circumcision) or following birth-related trauma (vacuum extraction, bruising, 3 studies) (Table 2). Paracetamol (oral, 15 mg/kg, q6h for 24 h) was not effective to reduce immediate postoperative pain during and following circumcision but provided some benefit (postoperative comfort score lower) after this immediate postoperative period (>6–24 h) (Howard et al. 1994). In a randomized, placebo-controlled study design in 122 neonates delivered by vacuum extraction, a single dose of paracetamol (20 mg/kg, rectal) significantly improved the initial clinical condition (e.g., drinking behavior), but without difference in pain scores. Subsequent doses of paracetamol did not show any additional effect (van Lingen et al. 2001). Using a similar design in 123 (near)term neonates (20–25 mg/kg, rectal at 2 and 8 h after delivery) following assisted vaginal delivery, early neonatal pain score were low, irrespective of paracetamol exposure. Intriguingly, neonates exposed to paracetamol after birth displayed an aggravated subsequent stress response during heel lancing on days 2–3 of postnatal life (Tinner et al. 2013). Both these studies used a preemptive approach.

In contrast, an open-label intravenous paracetamol study in neonates with elevated pain scores following birth-related trauma in 19 cases resulted in lower pain scores within 30 min after administration, with a slight increase in pain scores

Table 1 Overview of studies investigating the use of paracetamol for procedural pain (heel prick, eye examination) in (pre)term neonates

Reference	Study design and pain model	Paracetamol dosing	Results
Shah et al. (1998)	Double-blind placebo-controlled trial 75 term neonates, *heel prick* Facial action pain scores and cry score	Single oral paracetamol 20 mg/kg or placebo, 60–90 min before prick	No differences in facial action pain scores or in cry score
Bonetto et al. (2008)	Prospective randomized trial 76 term neonates, *heel prick* Pain scores (NIPS neonatal infant pain score > 4)	Placebo, dextrose (25%), lidocaine-prilocaine (EMLA) cream, or oral paracetamol (20 mg/kg, 60 min before prick)	NIPS < 4 similar between placebo, paracetamol, and EMLA (47%, 42%, and 63%) Oral dextrose was most effective (84% NIPS < 4, NNT 2.7)
Badiee and Torcan (2009)	Randomized placebo-controlled trial in 72 preterm (mean 32 weeks) neonates, *heel prick* PIPP (premature infant pain profile) score	Single (high dose) oral paracetamol (40 mg/kg) 90 min before prick	PIPP scores placebo (9, 7, SD 4.2) were similar to paracetamol (11.1, SD 3.8)
Foronda et al. (2014)	Randomized, single-blind study in 129 neonates, *heel prick*, NIPS and PIPP score, paracetamol ($n = 42$) to dextrose ($n = 47$) or placebo ($n = 40$)	No information on paracetamol dose used	PIPP and NIPS score lower in dextrose group Duration of crying shorter in dextrose group (30 instead of 79 s)
Kabatas et al. (2016)	Blinded, placebo-controlled trial, 114 preterm neonates, *eye examination retinopathy of prematurity*. PIPP score	Topical anesthetics + paracetamol (15 mg/kg, oral, 60 min before prick) or placebo	Significant lower PIPP in paracetamol exposed cases [12(9–13) vs 14(13–15)] but very modest effect (cutoff PIPP score < 7)
Seifi et al. (2013)	Prospective randomized trial, 120 preterm neonates, *eye examination retinopathy of prematurity*. PIPP score	Sucrose 25% vs oral paracetamol (15 mg/kg) vs placebo	Sucrose was effective, paracetamol not when compared to placebo at eye examination
Manjunatha et al. (2009)	Double blind, randomized, placebo controlled. *Eye examination retinopathy of prematurity*, 18 preterms recruited (63 intended), PIPP	Oral morphine (200 μg/kg), or paracetamol (20 mg/kg) or placebo	Morphine cases tended to have lower pain scores (PIPP), but no significant differences (underpowered study)

Table 2 Overview of studies investigating the use of paracetamol for different minor to moderate pain syndromes in (pre)term neonates

Reference	Study design and pain model	Paracetamol dosing	Results
Van Lingen et al. (2001)	Randomized placebo-controlled trial 122 term neonates *after vacuum extraction* Facies scale + objective clinical symptoms	Rectal (20 mg/kg. q6h) 24 h, paracetamol or placebo after delivery	No differences in pain scores, objective Clinical symptoms (nurse assessment) only better in para-group 1 h after first dose
Tinner et al. (2013)	Randomized double-blind placebo-controlled trial. EDIN (Echelle de douleur et d'inconfort du nouveau né) score in the 24 h *after vacuum extraction* in 123 (near)term neonates	Rectal paracetamol (20–25 mg/kg) 2 and 8 h after delivery	No differences in mean EDIN score No differences in EDIN score ≥ 5
	In the same group, BPSN (Bernese pain score) *after heel prick* on days 2–3	0.2 mL sucrose in all cases No other interventions	BPSN after heel prick higher in the "former" paracetamol group [5 (3–9) vs 3 (0–6)]
Howard et al. (1994)	Randomized double-blind placebo-controlled trial in 44 healthy term neonates, undergoing *neonatal circumcision* (Gomco), postoperative comfort score	Oral paracetamol 15 mg/kg.q6h for 24 h start 2 h before surgery	No effects during circumcision Postoperative score similar until 6 h when paracetamol group scored better
Allegaert et al. (2013)	Open-label intravenous paracetamol in the PARANEO study (19/60 monotherapy) *Vacuum extraction or medical condition* with LNPS (Leuven neonatal pain score) above threshold	Loading dose of intravenous paracetamol (20 mg/kg)	Decrease in LNPS from 30 min onward, with a slight increase in pain scores from 5 h onward

from 5 h onward after administration (Allegaert et al. 2013). So in conclusion, these data suggest that paracetamol is likely an effective therapeutic intervention when minor to moderate pain is present, but not when used as part of a preventive strategy.

3.4 Paracetamol Has Opioid-Sparing Effects to Treat Major Pain, Also in Neonates

Systematic reviews support the opioid-sparing effect of perioperative nonsteroidal anti-inflammatory drugs (NSAIDs) and paracetamol for perioperative pain management in children (Wong et al. 2013). However, the evidence for a relevant reduction in opioid-related adverse effects is much less robust, and data in neonates were only more recently reported after major non-cardiac surgery (Ceelie et al. 2013). Using a placebo-controlled randomized study design, Ceelie et al. indeed documented a clinical significant (−66%) morphine-sparing effect in neonates and infants co-treated with intravenous paracetamol after major, non-cardiac surgery (Ceelie et al. 2013). This reduction was most pronounced in neonates. The morphine-sparing effect (−54% for the cumulative morphine dose, −59% for the number of morphine boluses administered) has also been observed in a retrospective analysis on morphine consumption in preterm neonates (<32 weeks) before and after introduction of intravenous paracetamol in one single Finnish unit (Härmä et al. 2016).

3.5 Short- and Long-Term Safety of Paracetamol in Neonates

3.5.1 Short-Term Safety

Short-term side effects of paracetamol described in other populations mainly relate to *hepatotoxicity* or *hemodynamic* effects. Prospective data suggest good hepatic tolerance, but individual cases with hepatic toxicity potential related to paracetamol in newborns have been observed, and more advanced tools for pharmacovigilance have been suggested. Similarly, hemodynamic effects of paracetamol in neonates are modest with the suggestion to be more careful in the specific setting of impaired hemodynamics in neonates (Allegaert and van den Anker 2017; Pacifici and Allegaert 2014).

3.5.2 Long-Term Safety

While short-term safety has been well documented, there is active research going on exploring potential associations and causal links between perinatal (mainly prenatal) paracetamol exposure and neurobehavioral issues, increased incidence of atopy, or reduced fertility. For readers who want to have a more complete overview on the data as published, we refer to a recently published overview on the available epidemiological data, while here we focus on mechanisms that may support causality (Allegaert and van den Anker 2017; Bauer et al. 2018).

Neurodevelopmental Outcome The available studies suggested an association between prenatal paracetamol exposure and indicators (attention deficit hyperactivity disorder, autism spectrum disorders, less intelligence) of neurodevelopmental outcome. Signals were strongest for hyperactivity and attention deficits. Moreover, a relationship between the extent of exposure and outcome was documented, irrespective of the maternal indication (Allegaert and van den Anker 2017, Bauer et al. 2018). Suggested mechanisms relate to cerebral inflammation or to metabolites like cannabinoids. Intriguingly, in an animal experimental model, paracetamol and Δ(9)-tetrahydrocannabinol, but not ibuprofen, resulted in developmental neurotoxicity (Philippot et al. 2016, 2018). Animal experimental observations documented differences in serotonin and non-adrenaline degradation products in different regions of the central nervous system, including the cerebellum, spinal cord, and medulla oblongata (Blecharz-Klin et al. 2016; Mian and Allegaert 2017). However, it is not yet clear to what extent these prenatal observations also can be extrapolated to early neonatal exposure (Allegaert and van den Anker 2017). Moreover, the Food and Drug Administration (FDA) and European Medicine Agency (EMA) examined the available observations in 2016 and 2014, respectively, and concluded that the clinical relevance of these potential associations is still unknown, leading to the decision not to change their advices (Mian and Allegaert 2017).

Atopy Epidemiological studies suggest a link between fetal/maternal exposure and atopy (eczema, nutrition driven allergy, wheezing) during infancy. Interestingly, maternal antioxidant gene polymorphisms (e.g., nuclear erythroid 2 p45-related factor 2 (Nrf2) polymorphism, glutathione S-transferase (GST)) in mothers and their offspring may modify this relation between prenatal paracetamol exposure and childhood asthma, strengthening evidence for causality (Shaheen et al. 2010). Furthermore, it has been suggested that these atopy-driven effects are based on the nonselective inhibitory action on peripheral cyclooxygenase activity of paracetamol. This action is besides its central action and only occurs in the absence of inflammation and in a low prostaglandin environment. In this setting, and related to maturational immunity (T_H1 vs T_H2 lymphocytes), this may affect the normal development of tolerance and may induce autoimmune deviations (Langhendries et al. 2016).

Fertility Epidemiological cohort studies also have generated evidence for an association between prenatal paracetamol exposure and subsequent risk for cryptorchidism (NNH = 32), or hypospadias in second trimester of pregnancy, or shorter anogenital distance in male infants as marker for impaired masculinization after first trimester paracetamol exposure (Kilcoyne and Mitchell 2017; Allegaert and van den Anker 2017). The suggested mechanism explaining impaired masculinization relates to reduced fetal testicular testosterone production following fetal paracetamol exposure (Fisher et al. 2016). Genitals of male mammals are actively masculinized during fetal and early postnatal life by androgens and prostaglandins, and both androgens and prostaglandins are known to be inhibited by paracetamol exposure (Hay-Schmidt et al. 2017). Again, it is not clear to what extent these fetal observations are causal and if so, to what extent these findings also apply to (extreme) preterm neonates.

4 Paracetamol in Neonates: Toward a Better Benefit-Risk Balance

Effective analgesia is a crucial and valid part of the care provided to neonates. However, there is emerging evidence on the amount of exposure to narcotics in neonates and impaired neurodevelopmental outcome, in addition to some short-term outcome side effects. Consequently, a balanced approach is needed with the overarching intention to attain adequate pain management with minimal side effects caused by pain or narcotics.

Despite the available guidance on narcotics in ventilated neonates, observations on drug utilization still suggest an overall increase in exposure with extensive variability in practices. Implementation strategies are effective to reduce exposure to narcotics but result in increased paracetamol exposure.

As illustrated by the papers on implementation strategies, a structured approach is needed to translate knowledge into good practice (Rana et al. 2017; Baarslag et al. 2018). Such a structural pain management plan should be based on *prevention*, *assessment*, and *treatment* followed by a *reassessment*. Effective pain control is based on preventive strategies including the decrease of the number of painful procedures and environmental stress, driven by systematic assessment of pain based on a validated assessment tool, and followed by titrated administration of the best fitted analgesic and subsequent reassessment. The most appropriate approach should start with the routine use of a validated pain assessment score for the given age group, followed by a condition-specific pain management protocol with a limited number of compounds ("tool box") of which caregivers are aware of (side) effects. Moreover, such a pain management protocol should also focus on the titration of analgesics, including a decision tree on when and how to increase and decrease exposure to analgesics. For each of these levels, a research agenda is needed.

We summarized the evidence on paracetamol use in procedural pain management, in minor to moderate as well as major pain syndromes in neonates. We hereby concluded that the absence of benefit of paracetamol for procedural analgesia has consistently been shown, irrespective of dose or route of administration. For minor to moderate pain syndromes, there are data that support the use of a symptomatic, but not a preemptive approach. For major pain syndromes, relevant opioid-sparing effects have been documented after major non-cardiac surgery in term neonates and infants and have been suggested for preterm neonates.

While there are sufficient data on short-term safety, there are still concerns on long-term side effects. These concerns relate to neurobehavioral outcome, atopy or fertility, and are at present mainly driven by epidemiological perinatal observations, supported by postulated mechanisms and animal experimental observations. So even more than three decades after the pivotal findings of Anand et al. (1987), we are still in search for a better benefit-risk balance, also for an old compound like paracetamol.

At present, assessment of pain in neonates as pharmacodynamic outcome variable is at best based on pain scales that do not go beyond intersubjectivity, while real reflection of the nociceptive stimulus on the nervous system is far from clear. A relationship between nociceptive brain activity, spinal reflex withdrawal, and behavior in newborn infants has been described in an effort to shift form clinical behavioral to electrophysiological signal analysis as more objective tool to assess pain or nociception (Hartley et al. 2015). Interestingly, the same group recently reported on the maturational changes in both clinical behavioral and electrophysiological signal analysis following procedural pain in neonates, resulting in discrepancies in pain behavior and electrophysiological pain signals, most pronounced in extreme preterm neonates. Although these observations reflect objective changes, the question still remains whether conscious input also occurs especially in the youngest neonates.

Another line of research should focus on long-term outcome data following exposure to narcotics and paracetamol, with additional focus on the mechanisms related to the variability observed. This exploration on mechanisms should cross talk with animal experimental studies. This research should be conducted using the best available research models (prospective, multivariable, valid measurements) and should be supported by data on human perinatal physiology and pharmacology (e.g., placental transfer and metabolism) and animal experimental studies (dose, models) relevant to the human setting. Such animal experimental studies should be tailored to the clinical needs and practices and therefore should include, e.g., the effects of repetitive painful procedures, assess the outcome (mechanical sensitivity, post-injury hypersensitivity, microstructures) at adult equivalent age, or assess the effect of paracetamol (van den Hoogen et al. 2017). To illustrate the potential relevance of such a cross talk between clinical and experimental studies, it was documented that paracetamol administration in the neonatal rat had no effect upon short-term mechanical hypersensitivity during the first postnatal week or upon long-term baseline sensitivity from 3 to 8 weeks in a procedural pain prick model. However, neonatal paracetamol administration significantly reduced the postoperative mechanical hypersensitivity in young adults, caused by repetitive needle pricking (van den Hoogen et al. 2016). Within this context the choice of the most suited animal model is fundamental as many suggestions are based on carrageen induced chronic inflammation as a model (Ruda et al. 2000). In the clinical setting, however, a chronic osteomyelitis model is not commonly applicable to the neonatal pain events since this hardly even occurs in clinical practice (van den Hoogen et al. 2016).

In conclusion, effective analgesia in neonates is relevant not only because of ethics or empathy, but it is a crucial and integral part of medical and nursing care. However, there is emerging evidence on the relation between the exposure to narcotics and impaired neurodevelopmental outcome, resulting in a CATCH-22 scenario. Consequently, a balanced approach is needed. Future clinical research objectives should focus on the need to develop better assessment tools to quantify pain and on the need for high-quality data on long-term outcome of therapeutic interventions – also for paracetamol – and exploration of the mechanisms involved.

References

Allegaert K, van den Anker JN (2016) Neonatal withdrawal syndrome: reaching epidemic proportions across the globe. Arch Dis Child Fetal Neonatal Ed 101:F2–F3

Allegaert K, van den Anker JN (2017) Perinatal and neonatal use of paracetamol for pain relief. Semin Fetal Neonatal Med 22:308–313

Allegaert K, Palmer GM, Anderson BJ (2011) The pharmacokinetics of intravenous paracetamol in neonates: size matters most. Arch Dis Child 96:575–580

Allegaert K, Naulaers G, Vanhaesebrouck S et al (2013) The paracetamol concentration-effect relation in neonates. Paediatr Anaesth 23:45–50

Anand KJ, Sippell WG, Aynsley-Green A (1987) Pain, anaesthesia, and babies. Lancet 2(8569):1210

Anand KJ, Hall RW, Desai N et al (2004) Effects of morphine analgesia in ventilated preterm neonates: primary outcomes from the NEOPAIN randomised trial. Lancet 363:1673–1682

Anderson BJ, van Lingen RA, Hansen TG et al (2002) Acetaminophen developmental pharmacokinetics in premature neonates and infants: a pooled population analysis. Anesthesiology 96:1336–1345

Andropoulos DB (2018) Effect of anesthesia on the developing brain: infant and fetus. Fetal Diagn Ther 43:1–11

Aranda JV, Salomone F, Valencia GB et al (2017) Non-steroidal anti-inflammatory drugs in newborns and infants. Pediatr Clin N Am 64:1327–1340

Baarslag MA, Ista E, de Leeuw T et al (2018) Clinically effective implementation of intravenous paracetamol as primary analgesia after major surgery in neonates and young infants. Arch Dis Child 103:1168–1169. https://doi.org/10.1136/archdischild-2018-315379

Badiee Z, Torcan N (2009) Effects of high dose orally administered paracetamol for heel prick pain in premature infants. Saudi Med J 30:1450–1453

Bauer AZ, Kriebel D, Herbert MR et al (2018) Prenatal paracetamol exposure and child neurodevelopment: a review. Horm Behav 101:125–147

Bellu R, de Waal K, Zanini R (2010) Opioids for neonates receiving mechanical ventilation: a systematic review and meta-analysis. Arch Dis Child Fetal Neonatal Ed 95:F241–F251

Bhandari V, Bergqvist LL, Kronsberg SS et al (2005) Morphine administration and short-term pulmonary outcomes among ventilated preterm infants. Pediatrics 116:352–359

Blecharz-Klin K, Joniec-Maciejak I, Jawna-Zboinska K et al (2016) Cerebellar level of neurotransmitters in rats exposed to paracetamol during development. Pharmacol Rep 68:1159–1164

Bonetto G, Salvatico E, Varela N et al (2008) Pain prevention in term neonates: randomized trial for three methods. Arch Argent Pediatr 106:392–396

Borenstein-Levin L, Synnes A, Grunau RE et al (2017) Narcotics and sedative use in preterm neonates. J Pediatr 180:92–98.e1

Carbajal R, Eriksson M, Courtois E et al (2015) Sedation and analgesia practices in neonatal intensive care units (EUROPAIN): results from a prospective cohort study. Lancet Respir Med 3:796–812

Ceelie I, de Wildt SN, van Dijk M et al (2013) Effect of intravenous paracetamol on postoperative morphine requirements in neonates and infants undergoing major noncardiac surgery: a randomized controlled trial. JAMA 309:149–154

Clark RH, Bloom BT, Spitzer AR et al (2006) Reported medication use in the neonatal intensive care unit: data from a large national data set. Pediatrics 117:1979–1987

Cook SF, Roberts JK, Samiee-Zafarghandy S et al (2016a) Population pharmacokinetics of intravenous paracetamol (acetaminophen) in preterm and term neonates: model development and external evaluation. Clin Pharmacokinet 55:107–119

Cook SF, Stockmann C, Samiee-Zafarghandy S et al (2016b) Neonatal maturation of paracetamol (acetaminophen) glucuronidation, sulfation, and oxidation based on a parent-metabolite population pharmacokinetic model. Clin Pharmacokinet 55:1395–1411

Fisher BG, Thankamony A, Hughes IA et al (2016) Prenatal paracetamol exposure is associated with shorter anogenital distance in male infants. Hum Reprod 31:2642–2650

Flint RB, Roofthooft DW, van Rongen A et al (2017) Exposure to acetaminophen and all its metabolites upon 10, 15 and 20 mg/kg intravenous acetaminophen in very-preterm infants. Pediatr Res 82:678–684

Foronda O, Rocha S, Grandy G (2014) Efficacies of paracetamol and glucose in pain reduction in newborns: a randomized, controlled and single blind study. Pediatr Res 75:A473

Härmä A, Aikio O, Hallman M, Saarela T (2016) Intravenous paracetamol decreases requirements of morphine in very preterm infants. J Pediatr 168:36–40

Hartley C, Goksan S, Poorun R et al (2015) The relationship between nociceptive brain activity, spinal reflex withdrawal and behaviour in newborn infants. Sci Rep 5:12519

Hay-Schmidt A, Finkielman OTE, Jensen BAH et al (2017) Prenatal exposure to paracetamol/acetaminophen and precursor aniline impairs masculinisation of male brain and behaviour. Reproduction 154:145–152

Howard CR, Howard FM, Weitzman ML (1994) Acetaminophen analgesia in neonatal circumcision: the effect on pain. Pediatrics 93:641–646

Hsieh EM, Hornik CP, Clark RH et al (2014) Medication use in the neonatal intensive care unit. Am J Perinatol 31:811–821

Jasani B, Weisz DE, McNamara PJ (2018) Evidence-based use of acetaminophen for hemodynamically significant ductus arteriosus in preterm infants. Semin Perinatol 42:243–252

Kabatas EU, Dursun A, Beken S et al (2016) Efficacy of single dose oral paracetamol in reducing pain during examination for retinopathy of prematurity: a blinded randomized controlled trial. Indian J Pediatr 83:22–26

Kilcoyne KR, Mitchell RT (2017) Assessing the impact of in-utero exposures: potential effects of paracetamol on male reproductive development. Arch Dis Child 102:1169–1175

Langhendries JP, Allegaert K, van den Anker JN et al (2016) Possible effects of repeated exposure to ibuprofen and acetaminophen on the intestinal immune response in young infants. Med Hypotheses 87:90–96

Manjunatha CM, Ibhanesebhor SE, Rennix C et al (2009) Pain control during retinopathy of prematurity screening: double-blind, randomised, placebo-controlled study. Infant 5:155–158

Menon G, Boyle EM, Bergqvist LL et al (2008) Morphine analgesia and gastrointestinal morbidity in preterm infants: secondary results from the NEOPAIN trial. Arch Dis Child Fetal Neonatal Ed 93:F362–F367

Mian P, Allegaert K (2017) Fetal and neonatal rats paracetamol dosage and the perinatal human setting: lost in translation ? Pharmacol Rep 69:371–372

Pacifici GM, Allegaert K (2014) Clinical pharmacology of paracetamol in neonates: a review. Curr Ther Res Clin Exp 77:24–30

Philippot G, Nyberg F, Gordh T et al (2016) Short-term exposure and long-term consequences of neonatal exposure to Δ(9)-tetrahydrocannabinol (THC) and ibuprofen in mice. Behav Brain Res 307:137–144

Philippot G, Hallgren S, Gordh T et al (2018) A cannabinoid receptor type 1 (CB1R) agonist enchance the developmental neurotoxicity of acetaminophen (paracetamol). Toxicol Sci 166:203–212. https://doi.org/10.1093/toxsci/kfy199

Rana D, Bellflower B, Sahni J et al (2017) Reduced narcotic and sedative utilization in a NICU after implementation of pain management guidelines. J Perinatol 37:1038–1042

Roofthooft DWE, Simons SHP, van Lingen RA et al (2017) Randomized controlled trial comparing different doses of intravenous paracetamol for placement of peripherally inserted central catheters in preterm infants. Neonatology 112:150–158

Rosli R, Dali AF, Abd Aziz N et al (2017) Drug utilization on neonatal wards: a systematic review of observational studies. Front Pharmacol 8:27

Ruda MA, Ling QD, Hohmann AG et al (2000) Altered nociceptive neuronal circuits after peripheral inflammation. Science 289:628–631

Schiller J, Allegaert K, van den Bosch GE et al (2018) Analgesics and sedatives in critically ill newborns and infants: the impact on long-term neurodevelopment. J Clin Pharmacol 58:S140–S150

Seifi F, Peirovifar A, Gharehbaghi MM (2013) Comparing the efficacy of oral sucrose and acetaminophen in pain relief for ophthalmologic screening of retinopathy of prematurity. Am J Med Sci Med 1:24–27

Shah V, Taddio A, Ohlsson A (1998) Randomised controlled trial of paracetamol for heel prick pain in neonates. Arch Dis Child Fetal Neonatal Ed 79:F209–F211

Shah V, Taddio A, McMurtry CM et al (2015) Pharmacological and combined interventions to reduce vaccine injection pain in children and adults: systematic review and meta-analysis. Clin J Pain 31(10 Suppl):S38–S63

Shaheen SO, Newson RB, Ring SM et al (2010) Prenatal and infant acetaminophen exposure, antioxidant gene polymorphisms, and childhood asthma. J Allergy Clin Immunol 126:1141–1148.e7

Simons SH, Roofthooft DW, van Dijk M et al (2006) Morphine in ventilated neonates: its effects on arterial blood pressure. Arch Dis Child Fetal Neonatal Ed 91:F46–F51

Thewissen L, Allegaert K (2011) Analgosedation in neonates: do we still need additional tools after 30 years of clinical research? Arch Dis Child Educ Pract Ed 96:112–118

Tinner EM, Hoesli I, Jost K et al (2013) Rectal paracetamol in newborn infants after assisted vaginal delivery may increase pain response. J Pediatr 162:62–66

van den Anker JN, Allegaert K (2018) Acetaminophen in the neonatal intensive care unit: shotgun approach or silver bullet. J Pediatr 198:10–11

van den Bosch GE, Dijk MV, Tibboel D et al (2017) Long-term effects of early exposure to stress, pain, opioids and anaesthetics on pain sensitivity and neurocognition. Curr Pharm Des 23:5879–5886

Van den Hoogen NJ, Tibboel D, Honig WM et al (2016) Neonatal paracetamol treatment reduces long-term nociceptive behaviour after neonatal procedural pain in rats. Eur J Pain 20:1309–1318

Van den Hoogen NJ, Patijn J, Tibboel D et al (2017) Neonatal plasticity of the nociceptive system: mechanisms, effects, and treatment of repetitive painful procedures during NICU admittance. Curr Pharm Des 23:5902–5910

Van Lingen RA, Quak CM, Deinum HT et al (2001) Effects of rectally administered paracetamol on infants delivered by vacuum extraction. Eur J Obstet Gynecol Reprod Biol 94:73–78

Wong I, St John-Green C, Walker SM (2013) Opioid-sparing effects of perioperative paracetamol and nonsteroidal anti-inflammatory drugs (NSAIDs) in children. Paediatr Anaesth 23:475–495

Zimmerman KO, Smith PB, Benjamin DK et al (2017) Sedation, analgesia, and paralysis during mechanical ventilation of premature infants. J Pediatr 180:99–104.e1

Disorders of Puberty: Pharmacotherapeutic Strategies for Management

Margaret Zacharin

Contents

M. Zacharin (✉)
Department of Endocrinology, Royal Children's Hospital, Parkville, VIC, Australia
e-mail: margaret.zacharin@rch.org.au

W. Kiess et al. (eds.), *Pediatric Pharmacotherapy*,
Handbook of Experimental Pharmacology 261, https://doi.org/10.1007/164_2019_208

Abstract

During puberty, with activation of the hypothalamic pituitary axis that has been quiescent since the neonatal period, linear growth accelerates, secondary sexual characteristics develop, and adult fertility potential and bone mass are achieved, together with psychosocial and emotional maturation.

Disordered pubertal onset and progress, either early or late, presents frequently for endocrine care. Where a disorder is found, due either to a central hypothalamic pituitary cause or to primary gonadal failure, pharmacotherapeutic interventions are required to alter the trajectory of disturbed pubertal onset or progress and for maintenance of adolescent and adult sex hormone status. This paper describes pharmacologic interventions used for pubertal disorders but is not intended to address the diagnostic cascade in detail.

Keywords

Aromatase inhibitor · Estrogen · Gonadotropin · Hormone replacement · Progestin · Puberty induction · SERM · Testosterone

Introduction

Puberty is a time of major changes in linear growth, development of secondary sexual characteristics and bone mass accrual, together with attainment of adult fertility potential, psychosocial and emotional maturation.

The average onset of puberty occurs around age 10–12 in girls, characterized by breast development rather than pubic hair, and by age 11–13 in boys, with testicular enlargement of 4 mL or more. Disordered pubertal onset occurs when puberty starts below age 8 in girls and 10 in boys or after age 13 in girls and 14 in boys. Puberty occurs upon reactivation of the hypothalamic pituitary gonadal axis, normally inactive after the first 4–6 months of infancy.

Disorders of the hypothalamic pituitary gonadal axis may occur in relation to early onset of puberty, due either to structural or functional changes within the HPG axis or to peripheral sex hormone secretion, adrenal or gonadal in origin.

Conversely, puberty will be delayed, arrested or absent if any part of the HPG axis fails to function, due either to central hypothalamic pituitary disorders or to primary gonadal failure. Hypogonadism may also result from a chronic illness or its treatment.

Pharmacotherapies used to alter the trajectory of disturbed pubertal onset or progress and for maintenance of adolescent and adult sex hormone status will be reviewed in this paper, intended as a guide to management strategies but not as a pathway to diagnosis.

Precocious Puberty

When a child has apparent pubertal onset at an age earlier than expected, endocrine referral is common. Thorough clinical assessment is essential, to establish whether there may be a familial, central or peripheral cause. A careful history to include features of age of onset, change in linear growth parameters, rapidity of pubertal progress and examination for concordance or discordance between the breast and pubic hair in girls or testicular size and virilization in boys will provide a useful pathway for preliminary investigation.

1 Pharmacotherapies Used for Precocious Puberty

1.1 GnRH Agonist

1.1.1 Structure

GnRH agonists are structural analogues of natural GnRH, all commonly sharing a hydrophobic D-amino acid substituting for glycine 6, with higher receptor binding than natural GnRH. Further structural modifications differ between agonists but are not required for effect (Perrin et al. 1980). Bioactivity is dependent on resistance to enzymatic degradation.

1.1.2 Pharmacokinetics

Microcapsules or micro-granules of a biodegradable polymer, coupled to the agonist, release peptide progressively for several weeks in two phases: immediate release of peptide molecules on the surface of the microcapsules and a slower, long-lasting release of the internal peptide molecules. After initial rapid release, a stable serum level of agonist is achieved (Lahlou et al. 2000; Roger et al. 1986) until the end of 4 weeks. Of injected triptorelin, 38% is released during the first 13 days, and 0.9% is released daily thereafter, with a similar profile seen for leuprolide (Happ et al. 1987).

1.1.3 Mechanism of Action

In contrast to pulsatile GnRH that stimulates pituitary gonadotropin secretion, continuous GnRH has been thought to reduce secretion. Frequency and amplitude of GnRH pulses are not altered by agonist use, and desensitization of the hypothalamus does not occur. Increase in alpha subunit and decrease in beta subunit secretion of endogenous LH occur, with inhibition of gonadotropin secretion (Lahlou et al. 2000).

1.1.4 Clinical Trials

A number of non-randomized trials of GnRH agonists to try to increase final adult height outcome in short stature have not demonstrated effectiveness. Attempts to increase the height achieved by treatment of girls with normal but early puberty have also not been effective (Bertelloni et al. 2017; Lazar et al. 2002). Recent clinical trial meta-analysis of GnRH agonist plus growth hormone studies [6 RCTs (162 patients) and 6 controlled studies (247 patients)] indicated a very small mean increase (2.81 cm) in overall height achieved, with combination treatment (Liu et al. 2016; Paul et al. 1995).

1.1.5 Early Use

Studies comparing actual height outcome to predicted height are limited by the complexities of prediction capacity, possible other hormone deficiencies, secular changes in height with time and severity at time of first presentation. Results have been conflicting, ranging from little to no change in height achieved compared to height prediction, to several cm increase in treated versus non-randomized untreated cohorts (Carel et al. 2009). The key features of outcome relate to early age of commencement of puberty, early intervention and underlying condition if any, in terms of achieving a better height outcome (Cisternino et al. 2000; Kauli et al. 1997; Kletter and Kelch 1994; Palmert et al. 1999; Paul et al. 1995).

1.1.6 Long-Term Use

By contrast with attempts to increase height in girls with early puberty, GnRH agonists have been used for treatment of progressive CPP for 40 years and have consistently been shown to have been of benefit in terms of reduced gonadotropin and growth velocity, slowing skeletal maturation, with a mean increase in predicted final height of around 4 cm, although in many studies compared to target, final height was 0.4–5.2 cm shorter than target height. A comprehensive critical review of outcomes is referenced (Bereket 2017).

1.1.7 Dosing Recommendations

Representative preparations are given although others are available: (Teutonico et al. 2012).

Triptorelin (leuprolide) 4 weekly IMI 3.75 mg, 12 weekly IMI 7.5 mg, 11.25 mg, and 15 mg 11.25 mg and 30 mg for 3-month administration. It is recommended that dosing and follow-up should be performed in an informed healthcare facility, due to delivery difficulties with current preparations.

Goserelin s/c delivery, 4 weekly, 3.6 mg and 10.8 mg 12 weekly.

1.1.8 Adverse Effects

Leuprolide and histrelin have been associated with sterile abscess formation (Miller and Shukla 2010). Careful mixing of solid with liquid phase of preparation may diminish risk.

1.1.9 Availability

GnRH agonists are available in most countries to treat CPP but are frequently extremely costly, with patient access curtailed by cost constraint. Government subsidy in some countries improves accessibility. Monthly, three monthly long-acting and occasionally six monthly preparations are used.

1.2 Progestins (Progestogens): Oral and Parenteral

Medroxyprogesterone acetate and cyproterone acetate are the only two progestins likely to be considered for menstrual suppression in children with precocious puberty. Further information can be found in Sect. 2.2.

1.2.1 Structure

Progestins, as synthetic forms of progesterone, are steroid hormones, activities varying from agonist (medroxyprogesterone acetate [MPA]) to antagonist (cyproterone acetate[CPA]) depending on side chain form. CPA functions both as progestin and anti-androgen. MPA is a synthetic pregnane steroid, a derivative of progesterone and 17α-hydroxyprogesterone (6α-methyl-17α-acetoxyprogesterone).

1.2.2 Mechanism of Action

Progestins bind to the progesterone receptor, resulting in receptor phosphorylation and transcription activation via interaction with transcription factors, lowering estrogen levels via reduction of the number of estrogen receptors, together with increasing estrogen metabolism. Endometrium is attenuated. However, MPA acts as an agonist for progesterone, androgen and glucocorticoid receptors with little effect on the estrogen receptor (Schindler et al. 2008). It has therefore been used as an inhibitor of both central and peripheral precocious puberty.

1.2.3 Pharmacokinetics

Oral MPA is almost all bioavailable, with a T1/2 around 30 h. Depo-Provera has a T1/2 of 40 days. Doses of Depo-Provera of 25, 50, 100 and 150 mg administered to women demonstrated a longer mean time for return of follicular and luteal activity with increasing doses (Fotherby et al. 1980). No woman receiving 50 or 100 mg Depo-Provera had return of luteal function within 100 days of injection.

Cyproterone acetate (CPA) is also almost all bioavailable, with steady-state levels reached after about 8 days, most studies having been performed using low doses of 2 mg in reverse sequential OCP (Miller and Jacobs 1986).

1.2.4 Early Use

Progestins have been used for menstrual suppression for over 30 years in children, largely supplanted by the more efficient GnRH agonists (Brito et al. 2008; Laron and Kauli 2000; Neumann 1994).

1.2.5 Long-Term Use

MPA has a central effect on inhibition of the hypothalamic-pituitary-adrenal (HPA) and hypothalamic-pituitary-gonadal (HPG) axes, with suppression of gonadotropin, androgen, estrogen, adrenocorticotropic hormone (ACTH) and cortisol levels.

Both MPA and CPA can be used in combination with GnRH agonist if persistent bleeding occurs (Brito et al. 2008). In countries where GnRH agonist is not available or is not a viable proposition, due to cost factors, progestins are a useful alternative and may not only cause endometrial atrophy but have a central effect as well, with relative switch off of the hypothalamic-pituitary-gonadal axis.

CPA has been used for suppression of gonadotropin stimulation over the first month of GnRH use but has not been reported to usefully prevent withdrawal bleeding (Seminara et al. 2010). It has been used for male-limited familial precocious puberty with moderate effect on pubertal control (Almeida et al. 2008).

1.2.6 Dosing Recommendations

MPA 2.5, 5 and 10 mg tabs. 10–20 mg/day provides menstrual suppression in most children with CPP.

CPA 50 mg, 100 mg tabs. For menstrual suppression 50 mg/day is adequate for most children.

1.2.7 Adverse Effects

These are usually limited to a degree of fluid retention with occasional headache or altered mood, but CPA has rarely been reported to have risk for B12 deficiency and at high dose for adrenal suppression (Ramsay and Rushton 1990).

1.2.8 Availability

Both MPA and CPA are widely available, at accessible cost in most countries. CPA may not be available or approved for use in the USA. Whilst not as efficient as GnRH agonist, progestins are a useful alternative option for menstrual control in CPP.

1.3 Aromatase Inhibitors

Aromatase, cytochrome P-450 CYP19A1, catalyzes conversion of C-19 androgens to C-18 estrogens, as the rate-limiting step in conversion of testosterone to estradiol and androstenedione to estrone. It is primarily expressed in ovary and is also found in fat, muscle, liver and breast. Aromatase inhibitors can be steroidal, with irreversible action, or non-steroidal with reversible action.

1.3.1 Structure of Non-steroidal Aromatase Inhibitors

Anastrozole 2,2′[5-(1H-1,2,4-triazol-1-ylmethyl)1,3-phenylene] bis-(2-methyl propiononitrile).

Letrozole (4,4′-[(1H-1,2,4- -1-yl) methylene] bis-benzonitrile.

1.3.2 Mechanism of Action

The third-generation non-steroidal aromatase inhibitors are highly selective competitive inhibitors of the aromatase enzyme, with 98% aromatase inhibition in humans (Geisler 2011; Geisler et al. 1996), resulting in more than 90% suppression of plasma estrogen. Letrozole 2.5 mg daily resulted in more estrogen suppression compared with 1.0 mg anastrozole (Bhatnagar et al. 2001).

1.3.3 Pharmacokinetics

After oral administration, letrozole is rapidly and completely absorbed and extensively distributed to tissues where approximately 60% is bound to plasma proteins, mainly to albumin (55%). Studies have been performed in healthy postmenopausal female volunteers or women with breast cancer. The half-life (T1/2) of letrozole is 42 h, with a steady state of plasma levels reached in 2–6 weeks (Sioufi et al. 1997). Hepatic metabolism is responsible for roughly 85% elimination of anastrozole, with around 11% contribution from renal excretion.

1.3.4 Clinical Trials

Clinical trials in children with peripheral precocious puberty have been limited, due to rarity of these conditions, mainly reported for children with McCune-Albright syndrome, most use being directed towards attempts to improve final height in conditions of short stature (Feuillan et al. 2007). A Cochrane database review of four randomized controlled trials (RCTs) of boys with these conditions, for only 84 children, suggested height to be greater in boys with constitutional delay in growth and puberty (CGDP) and did not report in relation to pubertal changes (McGrath and O'Grady 2015).

A prospective study of anastrozole for treatment of PP in 27 girls with MAS reported that it was not effective to stop menstruation or to attenuate growth or bone age advance (Mieszczak and Eugster 2007; Mieszczak et al. 2008; Neyman and Eugster 2017).

A more recent long-term study of 28 letrozole-treated girls demonstrated slowed skeletal maturation with sustained improvement in predicted adult height, without change in ovarian volume or uterine size. No adverse events were reported over years of study (Estrada et al. 2016).

Treatment of boys with MAS is rarely reported and has utilized multiple treatment modalities together (Messina et al. 2015; Schoelwer and Eugster 2016).

Use for male-limited familial precocious puberty in children reported reduced growth and rate of bone age advance.

1.3.5 Dosing Recommendations

Oral doses of letrozole 1.5–2 mg/m^2/day or 1 mg/day anastrazole.

1.3.6 Adverse Effects

Early concerns were raised, regarding abnormalities of vertebral endplate in rats treated with anastrazole (Bajpai et al. 2010). Vertebral body morphology changes were seen in 5/11 (45%) adolescents with idiopathic short stature who were prepubertal prior to treatment with aromatase inhibitor, compared to none in the placebo group (Hero et al. 2010). These changes were not seen in boys after treatment who had constitutional delay in puberty, perhaps due to older age and shorter duration of treatment (Eugster et al. 2003; Wickman et al. 2003).

A small retrospective study of 21 boys treated for short stature has raised concerns regarding an adverse effect of increased testosterone levels on haematocrit, acne and BMI, without reduction in estradiol level (Ferris and Geffner 2017).

Nausea, vomiting, abdominal pain, diarrhoea, headache, erythrocytosis, bone pain, arthralgia and skin rashes have been reported in adults, but no reports of similar conditions other than a single case of cyclical vomiting have been seen in a child. Due to mode of excretion, avoidance of use in renal or hepatic disorders has been recommended.

Rare reports of men with aromatase deficiency suggest a possibility of adverse effects on bone mass accrual and hyperlipidaemia, but these have not been seen in children, where use is limited to a few years.

1.3.7 Availability

Aromatase inhibitors are available in many countries, but use may be restricted to special access or government-authorized prescription. They may be purchased easily between countries where local access is limited.

1.4 Anti-androgens and Selective Estrogen Receptor Modulators (SERMS)

These are discussed together as most use has been in multiple drug combinations for gonadotropin-independent precocious puberty.

1.4.1 Mechanism of Action

Anti-androges

1. *Bicalutamide*, as a potent non-steroidal anti-androgen, binds to the androgen receptor, inhibits its action and increases its degradation.
2. *Spironolactone* is a steroidal mineralocorticoid antagonist, with a short T1/2 after oral administration of 1.4 h, mainly metabolized in the liver to metabolites with a longer T1/2 that allows effective drug response, with renal excretion.
3. *Ketoconazole* inhibits both adrenal and testicular androgen biosynthesis.

SERMs

1. *Tamoxifen* is a selective estrogen receptor modulator acting by competitive binding.
2. *Fulvestrant*, a synthetic estrane steroid, as an anti-estrogen, acting by antagonizing and degrading the estrogen receptor.

1.4.2 Clinical Trials

Girls with McCune-Albright syndrome were treated with 20 mg tamoxifen/day, with reported improvement in growth velocity and reduced rate of bone age advance, together with marked reduction in menstruation. Increase in uterine size raised possible concerns regarding stromal tumours. Surveillance is recommended with long-term use (Eugster et al. 2003).

Bicalutamide has been used for boys with testotoxicosis in combination with aromatase inhibitors (Lenz et al. 2010; Reiter et al. 2010).

Fulvestrant has also been reported to slow puberty and growth in girls with McCune-Albright syndrome (Sims et al. 2012).

1.4.3 Early Use

The majority of reports have been confined to treatment of girls:

A retrospective review of girls aged 3–8 years with McCune-Albright syndrome reported reduced rate of bone age advance, menstrual suppression and possible improvement in final height but, in some, less than predicted (de Passone et al. 2015).

1.4.4 Long-Term Use

Reports are mainly for girls (Neyman and Eugster 2017), but a report of combined tamoxifen with spironolactone in boys with familial male-limited precocious puberty suggested good response with pubertal arrest and without adverse effects over several years (Leschek et al. 1999). A single case report of combined treatment with an aromatase inhibitor suggested a good response in a boy with McCune-Albright syndrome (Tessaris et al. 2012).

Ketoconazole has been used successfully to treat small numbers of boys with gonadotropin-independent precocious puberty since its first description in 1985 (Almeida et al. 2008; Holland et al. 1985; Soriano-Guillen et al. 2005).

1.4.5 Dosing Recommendations

Bicalutamide 2 mg/kg, once daily.
Spironolactone 100–150 mg/day (5 mg/kg).
Ketoconazole reported at 16.2 mg/kg/day.
Tamoxifen, 10–20 mg/day in two doses.

1.4.6 Availability

Spironolactone is universally available.

Bicalutamide has limited availability and approval in some countries. Whilst ketoconazole is available in some countries, it has been withdrawn from the market in others, due to safety concerns.

SERMs are generally available in most countries at modest cost, although use for management of precocious puberty is off label.

1.4.7 Adverse Effects

Gynecomastia and breast pain are reported. Hepatotoxicity that may be severe is reported with ketoconazole.

Delayed Puberty

Delayed puberty in males is probably the most common reason for referral to an endocrinologist. Although equally prevalent in girls, fewer attend for similar complaints, probably related to the discrepancy in timing of pubertal onset and linear growth spurt between sexes. Although constitutional delay in puberty numerically far outweighs all other diagnoses, establishing a possible underlying cause remains of paramount importance. The need for hormonal support to induce puberty or to sustain pubertal progress must be determined by diagnosis and by individual requirement, such as failure to enter puberty, versus pubertal arrest or late pubertal failure.

HRT, where needed, should aim to provide normal linear growth, together with an appropriate rate of feminization or virilization in keeping with that of peers, thus maximizing bone mass accrual and ensuring emotional and social maturation. Management should encompass adolescent sexual health and consideration for optimizing capacity for future fertility. Long-term maintenance of adult hormonal status is required for many conditions of hypogonadism. Attention must be given to preferred hormone formulation and delivery modality, in order to meet needs for compliance, and for harm minimization in terms of adverse and side effects, plus contraception if needed.

2 Pharmacotherapies Used for Delayed Puberty in Girls

2.1 Estrogens

2.1.1 Oral

Structure

Estrogen as a steroid hormone is usually presented as 17 beta estradiol (estradiol 17β-estra-1,3,5(10)-triene-3,17β-diol 17β-pentanoate), an esterified form of natural estradiol, improving absorption and bioavailability after oral administration.

Pharmacokinetics

Estradiol is rapidly absorbed after oral administration, dose dependent, with 95% of estradiol metabolized via the first pass in the liver with less than 5% systemic availability (Longcope et al. 1985; Stanczyk et al. 2013). Most is excreted in urine, as glucuronide. Similar rapid absorption is seen for estradiol valerate. Conjugated equine estrogens contain more than 100 estrogen moieties, and no pharmacokinetic studies are available.

Clinical Trials

Controversy continues to exist regarding optimal methods for inducing puberty and maintaining HRT in girls with hypogonadism, the most studied group being those with Turner syndrome. In general, transdermal estrogen is considered the most physiological choice with best absorption and least adverse effect on lipid or coagulation profiles, but local skin allergy, patient choice and adherence to treatment can limit use. Comparison of pharmacokinetics and pharmacodynamics of oral and transdermal 17β-estradiol in girls with Turner syndrome confirmed the transdermal route as most approximating natural estrogen, but effects on IGF1 and lipid profile were inconclusive in terms of absolute levels (Mauras et al. 2012; Taboada et al. 2011; Torres-Santiago et al. 2013).

Linear growth has been demonstrated to be better if estrogen replacement is not delayed (Ross et al. 2011).

Long-Term Use

Once an adult dose of 2 mg/day has been reached, this can be continued long term, with cyclical addition of progestogen for regular withdrawal bleeds. For either primary or secondary hypogonadism, continuous estrogen is necessary to prevent bone loss during a "pill-free" week, as occurs with oral contraceptive pill (OCP) use.

Dosing Recommendations

Estradiol valerate:

For pubertal induction: 0.5 mg second daily for 3 months, increasing to 0.5 mg/day for 6–12 months, depending upon rate of clinical response, then to 1 mg/day for 12–18 months until linear growth is near complete and the majority of adult feminization has been achieved. Dose should then be increased to 2 mg/day, with addition of progestin at that time.

For adult maintenance: 2 mg/day continuous.

Availability

Estradiol valerate is inexpensive and available in most countries.

Transdermal preparations are infrequently available in developing countries, have problems of adherence in tropical or hot climates and must be imported outside of regulatory authorities if needed for specific patients. Conjugated equine estrogens (Premarin) remain the most commonly prescribed estrogen for pubertal induction and later HRT despite the availability of 17 beta estradiol, the latter not being widely recognized as available and a cheaper option.

2.1.2 Transdermal (TD) Patch

Structure

Three layers: translucent polyethylene film, estradiol as estra-1,3,5(10)-triene-3 and 17ß-diol with a cover of siliconized or fluoropolymer-coated polyester film to be removed prior to application.

Mechanism of Action, Pharmacokinetics

The skin is permeable to estradiol, with diffusion of drug, directly absorbed into capillaries. A depot effect in the skin and subcutaneous fat allows continuous delivery into the circulation and a constant level of plasma estradiol for the duration on patch life, usually 7 days with most modern patches (T1/2 36 h). The skin lacks enzymes to metabolize estradiol. Adhesive plastic matrix patches release approximately 25 μg 17β-estradiol/24 h. Active ingredient per patch: Climara 25 contains 2 mg of estradiol, Climara 50: 3.8 mg of estradiol, Climara 75: 5.7 mg of estradiol and Climara 100: 7.6 mg of estradiol.

Clinical Trials

Although TD patches have been used for years for pubertal induction, particularly in girls with Turner syndrome (Klein et al. 2018), few RCTs of their use have been performed (Shah et al. 2014). Most studies (Norjavaara et al. 2016) have been performed in girls with Turner syndrome, who have particular potential risks for hepatic steatosis and metabolic syndrome. Those reports may not be representative of other hypogonadal populations (Nabhan and Eugster 2013).

Increasing evidence suggests possible overall benefit over oral estrogen for long-term HRT, to be negotiated with patients regarding preferred delivery modality. See Sect. 4.1.2.

Dosing Recommendations

These are described for a commonly available preparation. Others are available also.

For pubertal induction:

Commencing dose is usually 0.5 mg/week = 1/4 of a Climara 25 patch, increasing slowly over 2–2.5 years to an adult dose of 3.8–5.7 mg estradiol/week, to mimic a normal pattern of linear growth and feminization.

Availability Varies Between Countries

Generally obtainable at competitive pricing compared with oral preparations. Limited access in many countries.

Adverse Effects

Skin allergy is common and may prevent ongoing use. Even if available in tropical climates or hot weather, poor adhesion and allergy may preclude ongoing use.

2.1.3 Transdermal Gel

Gels are not commonly used for pubertal induction. Although absorption is satisfactory, dosing can be erratic and is user dependent for successful application. Gels are rejected by some girls as messy and time-consuming to use.

Early Use

TD gel was first described as successful for pubertal induction nearly 30 years ago (Piippo et al. 2004), mimicking normal pubertal growth and rate of development.

2.2 Progestins (Progestogens)

Also see Sect. 1.2.

2.2.1 Structure

Two classes of progestins are used most commonly, either as progestin alone or in combination with estrogen as an OCP: 17α-acetoxyprogesterone derivatives (pregnanes) include medroxyprogesterone acetate(MPA). Estranes are norethindrone derivatives (lynestrenol, norgestrel, norgestimate, desogestrel, norethindrone, norethynodrel, norethindrone acetate, ethynodiol diacetate and desogen).

2.2.2 Oral

During pubertal induction and early months of HRT for hypogonadism, progestins are not required. Once an adult dose of estrogen has been reached, addition of progestin is required to ensure adequacy of endometrial shedding. MPA or norethisterone acetate are the commonest choices for initial management.

Menorrhagia is common during adolescence. A recent addition to the choices available for these girls includes a combined contraceptive pill containing estradiol valerate plus dienogest, with trials demonstrating significant reduction in menstrual losses, both for menorrhagia and for girls with normal periods (Fraser et al. 2011).

2.2.3 Dosing Recommendations

MPA (Provera) 10 mg/day for 14 days every second or third calendar month is usually sufficient to ensure regular endometrial shedding without breakthrough bleeding. Monthly use is possible if patients wish.

NEA (norethisterone acetate) 5 mg/day in the same regime as MPA.

2.2.4 Availability

Progestins are inexpensive and generally available in all countries.

2.2.5 Adverse Effects

Headache, weight gain and fluid retention are common, but side effects differ widely between individuals. Choice of progestin relates solely to any side effects experienced. Changing to an alternative preparation usually is effective.

3 Pharmacotherapies Used for Delayed Puberty in Boys

Constitutional delay in growth and puberty (CDGP) in boys is the commonest reason for referral to a paediatric endocrinologist. Often, assessment and reassurance suffice, and no intervention is required. However, extreme pubertal delay, usually accompanied by short stature, may need a short course of testosterone, aimed to prime the HPG axis. Differentiation from primary hypogonadism should not be difficult to differentiate from CDGP by adolescence, as gonadotropins are likely to be raised by then, but central hypogonadism can be difficult to diagnose with certainty prior to puberty because even a GnRH test may not accurately predict permanent hypogonadism at that time. It may be necessary to complete pubertal induction to the end of linear growth and full adult virilization in some cases and then cease treatment to reassess. This option may also be needed for chronic disease with pubertal delay or arrest.

3.1 Testosterone Preparations

3.1.1 Testosterone Undecanoate (Oral)

Structure

C17β undecylate (undecanoate) ester of testosterone.

Mechanism of Action

Pharmacokinetics

Peak plasma total testosterone occurred 2–7 h after a 40 mg dose of testosterone undecanoate in prepubertal boys (Geere et al. 1980; Nieschlag et al. 1975).

Dosing Recommendations

For pubertal induction, 40 mg of oral testosterone undecanoate should be administered second daily for 3 months, then 40 mg/day for 6–12 months depending on clinical effect, increases to be judged on linear growth and virilization rate of bone age advance, increasing progressively to 80, 120 mg/day by 18–24 months from commencement. A change to parenteral testosterone is usually made above this dose.

Availability

Variable. Widely available in many countries, limited in some developing countries.

3.1.2 Testosterone Esters

Structure

Androstane esterified steroids.

Mechanism of Action

Testosterone binds to and activates the androgen receptor. Hepatic metabolism to inactive metabolites.

Pharmacokinetics

Rapid increase to supraphysiological levels of testosterone is achieved after a single injection of 250 mg, decreasing to a hypogonadal range by 14 days (Behre et al. 2004). Measured plasma testosterone and LH after 25 mg testosterone remained in an adult range for 1 day, for 2 days after 50 and 14 days after 250 mg testosterone enanthate (Nieschlag et al. 1976).

Uses

1. Priming prior to growth hormone testing are usually around 100–125 mg.
2. For short-term treatment of boys with constitutional delay in growth and puberty (CDGP) (Howard and Dunkel 2016).
3. For pubertal induction when oral androgens are unavailable.

Dosing Recommendations

1. For priming*:* Doses of testosterone esters used for priming prior to growth hormone testing are usually around 100–125 mg.
2. For CDGP: Several different regimes are used. A common choice is 100 mg/month for 6 months, with clinical review to assess for spontaneous entry to puberty. An alternate option is 125 mg as a first dose then two further doses of 250 mg, 3–4 weeks apart, with review after 6 months.
3. For puberty induction: 50–100 mg monthly, increasing to 250 mg every month, rate of dose change predicated by linear growth and virilization rate and rate of bone age advance, 250 mg every 2 weeks if needed for long-term treatment.

Recent data has suggested that subcutaneous administration of testosterone esters may be equally effective to induce virilization, compared with intramuscular injection (Spratt et al. 2017).

Adverse Events

Priapism has been reported rarely even after a single dose of 100–125 mg (Albrecht et al. 2018).

Availability

Worldwide.

3.1.3 Testosterone Undecanoate (Parenteral)

See Long-Term Use

Due to prolonged duration of action of parenteral T undecanoate, it is not recommended for pubertal induction as is likely to advance bone age too rapidly with a potential for truncating final height. Its use should be limited to boys with hypogonadism who have completed the majority of their linear growth potential.

3.1.4 Testosterone Gel

Structure

Hydroalcoholic gel (Sitruk-Ware 1989; Wang et al. 2000).

Direct rapid skin absorption to a reservoir state in the stratum corneum, with steady-state levels reached over several hours.

Pharmacokinetics

Testosterone gel 1.62% was evaluated in a randomized controlled study of men aged 18–80. Normal adult range testosterone levels were seen in 81.6% after 16 weeks administration. Similar pharmacokinetics were seen using a pump actuation of 2% gel (Efros et al. 2016; Kaufman et al. 2012).

Clinical Trials

A recent comparison between IM testosterone and testosterone gel for pubertal induction over 6 months suggested gel to be comparable, at least in the short term (Chioma et al. 2018).

Dosing Recommendations

Unknown to date.

Availability

Widely available in many countries.

Adverse Events

See long-term use adverse events.

If a female parent/carer is administering testosterone gel to an adolescent boy, she must be advised to wear protective gloves.

3.2 Gonadotropins (Human Chorionic Gonadotropin (hCG) and Follicle-Stimulating Hormone (FSH))

3.2.1 Structure

hCG

hCG is a 237 heterodimeric amino acid glycoprotein, sharing an alpha subunit identical to LH, FSH and TSH but a unique beta subunit.

FSH

FSH is also a glycoprotein heterodimer, sharing an alpha subunit as above, with a unique 111 amino acid beta subunit.

3.2.2 Mechanism of Action

Both hCG and FSH act via interaction with their specific hormone receptor, for downstream signaling and hormonal response.

3.2.3 Pharmacokinetics

(1) hCG

The T1/2 of hCG has been estimated as approximately 30 h, with doses equal to or greater than 125 mcg, with a shorter T1/2 for a low dose of 25 mcg of 2 h, with a uni-phasic response in testosterone in hypogonadal men and a biphasic response in normal men who had a pool of active Leydig cells. Response occurred 12 h after administration with testosterone levels not returning to baseline by 8 days (Trinchard-Lugan et al. 2002).

(2) FSH

After IM compared with subcutaneous administration of 75 or 150 IU, peak plasma levels of FSH achieved were reported as later, due to slower absorption, but levels achieved were the same by 21 h, within a eugonadal range (Handelsman et al. 1995).

3.2.4 Early Use

hCG and FSH use has been reported in mixed cohorts of childhood and adult onset hypogonadism for 20 years, limiting conclusions as to benefits for those solely with childhood onset hypogonadism.

Childhood onset male hypothalamic hypogonadism is reported to be associated with poorer adult fertility outcomes. FSH has a key role in spermatogonial development and Sertoli cell proliferation and function. FSH and endogenous testosterone are required for normal spermatogenesis. Prolonged use of androgen administration alone for puberty induction and HRT prevents spermatogenesis and may reduce efficiency of future fertility induction.

3.2.5 Clinical Trials

In the past 10 years, small cohorts with childhood onset hypogonadism, prepubertal prior to hCG exposure, had puberty induction with hCG, FSH being added to induce fertility. Linear growth and virilization mimicked natural puberty; spermatogenesis was achieved after 6–9 months of combination treatment. Testicular imprinting at puberty may reduce duration of later fertility induction treatment (Rohayem et al. 2017; Zacharin et al. 2012).

A survey of men on long-term treatment for these disorders reported a lasting impact on psychosexual functioning despite adequate physical management, adding to need for reviewing methods of pubertal induction (Dwyer et al. 2015; Zacharin 2015).

3.2.6 Dosing Recommendations

hCG for pubertal induction in hypothalamic hypogonadism: 500 mg × 2/week for 6 months, increasing to 1,000 u × 2/week for 12–8 months, dose increases to be made judged by linear growth, rapidity of virilization and bone age advance. Further increase to 1,500 u × 2/week should only be made if virilization is incomplete and plasma testosterone is below adult levels. NB hCG is more efficient than exogenous testosterone, so intermittent measurement of testosterone levels will help guide need for dosage change.

Once testosterone is in the adult range, FSH can be added at 150 IU × 3/week. Observation of increasing testicular size is of more value than frequent measurement of Inhibin B, but a rising Inhibin B guides timing of semen analysis or possible need to increase FSH to 300 IU × 3/week for adequate spermatogenesis. Once this has occurred, preferably with semen storage, HRT can be maintained using testosterone preparations.

3.2.7 Availability

hCG is more generally available, but FSH use is severely curtailed by expense and thus lack of access in many places. Subsidized treatment can be obtained for fertility induction in some countries.

Long-Term Hormone Replacement Pharmacotherapies

Many of the following preparations have been described in detail for pubertal induction. Those preparations will be discussed, regarding evidence for long-term use and beneficial and possible adverse effects. Detailed analysis of oral and parenteral contraceptive agents is beyond the scope of this article. Many thousands of publications exist. Recent reviews are referenced.

4 Pharmacotherapies Used for Long-Term Hormone Replacement in Girls

4.1 Estrogen

4.1.1 Oral

Dosing Recommendations

Estradiol valerate 2 mg/day on a continuous basis. See Sect. 2.1.

For Turner syndrome or other conditions where there may be a significant risk for hypertension, a natural estrogen is preferred long term, and OCP containing ethinyl estradiol should not be used as the ethinyl radical induces renin substrate at 40 times the rate of natural estrogens (Crane and Harris 1969; Crane et al. 1966).

4.1.2 Transdermal Patch

Clinical Trials

Recent Information

New data compared stored plasma samples from girls who had been treated with oral or TD estrogen with normal controls on no medication. LCMSMS measurement of 12 estrogen metabolites demonstrated several estrogen metabolites at higher, unphysiologic levels in those who had oral estrogen, increasing concerns regarding first pass effect in the liver (Mauras et al. 2018).

A meta-analysis of available trials has confirmed an overall benefit of transdermal estrogen patches as the optimal method of estrogen delivery in girls with Turner syndrome, in terms of improved lipid profile, but no statistically significant differences were seen between oral and TD preparations IGF1, BMI, fat mass, fasting insulin, estradiol or estrone levels. However, compliance and patient preference remain significant factors in choice of HRT agent. An apparent increase in BMD z score should be interpreted with caution as adult BMD values are not currently available between groups (Zaiem et al. 2017).

Availability

Transdermal Gel and Estrogen Spray

These are not used in adolescent practice in most countries and will not be addressed.

4.1.3 Oral Contraceptive Pills (OCP) Summary

Structure and Pharmacokinetics

Estrogen, as ethinyl estradiol, is rapidly absorbed after oral ingestion, with levels 90–130 pg/mL found within 1–2 h after intake, levels being proportionate to dose. After the first pass effect in the liver, metabolism being less than that of natural estrogen, there remains around 45% bioavailability, variable between women (Fotherby 1982).

Progestins used in most OCPs are commonly 19-nortestosterone derivatives estranes (NEA) or acetoxyprogesterone derivatives pregnanes (medroxyprogesterone acetate (MPA) and megestrol acetate). Drospirenone is derived from spironolactone, with anti-androgenic and antimineralocorticoid activity, and reported to be less androgenic than estranes (Dragoman et al. 2018; Stanczyk et al. 2013).

Mechanism of Action

Inhibition of ovulation.

Dosing Recommendations

Combined OCPs have been used for over 50 years. Reduction in estrogen content has clearly contributed to reduced thromboembolic risk in users. First-generation progestogens remain as likely the safest in this regard (Dragoman et al. 2018), although recent formulations may change recommendations (Bastianelli et al. 2017; Farris et al. 2017).

The lowest dose that achieves menstrual control without breakthrough bleeding or side effects should be the primary aim of treatment.

Attention to specific individual needs is of particular importance in the adolescent age range, such as anticonvulsant use increasing rate of estrogen metabolism (lamotrigine) or via enzyme induction (phenobarbitone, phenytoin, carbamazepine and oxcarbazepine), in women with epilepsy, where increased seizure activity, with adverse brain effects, is reported (Reddy 2017). Unintended pregnancy was also more commonly seen in younger women with epilepsy using OCP, compared with other contraceptive modalities (Herzog et al. 2017). Alternatively, if OCP is the preferred method of contraception, high estrogen dose preparation (50 mcg ethinyl estradiol) should be given.

Antibiotics do not interfere with estrogen metabolism, except for rifampicin and griseofulvin which increase hepatic metabolism via the CYP450 enzyme. OCP use should be avoided in women taking these drugs.

Migraine may be a contraindication to use of the OCP, but level of evidence from all studies is low. A recent consensus is inconclusive, recommending that desogestrel OCP may be a preferred option if OCP use is undertaken for this group. Confirmation is needed regarding a recent report which described a sixfold increase in stroke risk in OCP users who have migraine with aura but not those without (Champaloux et al. 2017).

Menstrual migraine during the pill-free week may be ameliorated by addition of an estrogen patch, but published evidence is lacking (Sacco et al. 2018).

When choosing a contraceptive option for the adolescent, adherence capacity, risk-taking behaviours and potentially interfering medications must be carefully weighed. OCP is often prescribed for control of dysfunctional uterine bleeding in adolescents, as well as for contraception. Mood disturbance may be induced or exacerbated by any OCP. Careful evaluation as to possible contribution from OCP may require a change to a preparation containing a different progestin.

Availability

OCP are available worldwide, but in many developing countries, access is limited to a very few preparations – usually containing 30 mcg ethinyl estradiol plus L norgestel or NEA.

Depot Preparations of Estrogen Are Not Commonly Used or Available in Adolescence and Will Not Be Discussed

4.2 Progestins

4.2.1 Oral

See Sect. 2.1.1.

4.2.2 Parenteral

Comprehensive reviews of long-acting reversible contraceptive agents (IUD and implants) used in women less than age 25 indicated that high 12-month continuation of these options exists and that this type of contraception should be offered to all adolescents as a first-line option (Curtis and Peipert 2017; Diedrich et al. 2017).

4.2.3 Subcutaneous Progestin-Bearing Rod

Structure

Implantable plastic rod impregnated with etonogestrel, an estrane derivative of norethisterone.

Pharmacokinetics

Steady-state levels are reached within a week of implant, with 100% bioavailability. Implants need replacement every 3 years.

Early Use

The Implanon rod was first used 20 years ago, effective as a long-acting reversible contraceptive, but with problems of continued irregular bleeding, including polymenorrhoea in around 10% of users. Weight gain, depression and acne are usually cited as reasons for early removal although a recent study did not support differences in weight after 12 months use between Implanon and other long-acting contraceptive agents (Silva Dos Santos et al. 2017).

Availability

Widely available in many countries.

Adverse Events

Rod migration has been reported, into areas distant from insertion site. Including vasculature and the lung (Kang et al. 2017).

4.2.4 Intramuscular: Depot

Depot medroxyprogesterone acetate (DMPA).

Long-Term Use

DMPA has a significant central progestin action and often switches off the hypothalamic pituitary ovarian axis. The FDA instituted a black box warning on DMPA packaging in 2004. This is of particular importance in an adolescent who has a major disability, where this secondary effect will further reduce bone mass accrual and predispose to osteoporotic fracture, in a high-risk population where DMPA may be used long term. A study reported improvement to normal bone density after discontinuation, over 2–3 years in adolescent girls who had used DMPA, and adult studies were reported to provide similar reassurance (Harel et al. 2010; Isley and Kaunitz 2011). A recent study of college students reported lower BMD in DMPA users (Nieves et al. 2016). Caution should be exercised in considering DMPA in girls who have not achieved peak bone mass or who intend DMPA as a long-term contraceptive option. A recent report suggested possible shift in management choices for this group, with none of 80 adolescents with disability using DMPA (Chuah et al. 2017).

Dosing Recommendations

MPA 150 mg IMI every 12 weeks will usually result in complete amenorrhoea.

Availability

Depo-Provera is widely available at low cost in almost all countries.

4.2.5 Transdermal Patch

See Sect. 4.1.2.

4.2.6 Intra-uterine system

The major use of IUDs in this age group is for menstrual control in adolescent girls who have a major physical or intellectual disability and where amenorrhoea is desired, along with contraception. IUD may be first choice, particularly in presence of anticonvulsant use or considered after OCP failure for any reason.

Structure

Plastic T shaped device coated with a membrane containing L-norgestrel (Luukkainen 1991).

Mechanism of Action

The L-norgestrel IUD acts via causing change in cervical mucus, thus impairing sperm penetration. It may have some additional effect on ovulation in some women (Xiao et al. 1990). More recently marketed devices are smaller, allowing easier insertion in a nulliparous cervix.

Pharmacokinetics

Slow continuous release of L-norgestrel over 3–5 years, most over 5 years. The gold standard Mirena IUD contains 52 mg L-norgestrel, continuously released. A newer device, Kyleena (Bayer Healthcare, Whippany, NJ, USA), contains 19.5 mg of LNG released at 17.5 μg/day after 24 days, decreasing progressively to 9.8 μg/day after 1 year and 7.4 μg/day after 5 years, with an average of 9 μg/day over 5 years (Grandi et al. 2018).

Recent Information

Analysis of nine studies of IUD adherence and acceptance for women under age 25 versus other long-acting methods of contraception, from an extensive database search, suggests better acceptance of this method (Usinger et al. 2016). Evidence from a systematic review of safety suggests that the risk of adverse outcomes related to infection, heavy bleeding, pregnancy, perforation or removals among young IUD users is low but that expulsion rate is higher than for older women raising need for awareness regarding alternative contraceptive (Jatlaoui et al. 2017).

Availability

IUDs are available worldwide, limited only by cost and importation restrictions in certain countries.

4.2.7 Vaginal Ring

The vaginal rings used for contraception are uncommonly prescribed in adolescence and will not be discussed in detail. They contain norgestrel progestins (desogestrel, levonorgestrel, etonogestrel, gestodene, norgestimate), acting via transmucosal absorption. Due to need for regular replacement, compliance is required for efficacy.

5 Pharmacotherapies Used for Long-Term Hormone Replacement in Boys

5.1 Testosterone Esters

5.1.1 Long-Term Use

Largely supplanted by long-acting testosterone undecanoate, wherever available.

Dosing Recommendations

Testosterone esters: 250 mg IMI every 14–21 days.

Availability

Worldwide.

Adverse Effects

High endogenous T concentrations are not associated with increased risk of VTE, DVT or PE (Holmegard et al. 2014; Roetker et al. 2018). However all parenterally administered testosterone has a risk for progressively increasing haemoglobin, particularly seen with the long-acting preparations, presumably related to more steady-state maintenance of androgen levels compared with the peaks and troughs of shorter-acting testosterone esters. Regular full blood count assessment should be undertaken, with consideration for possible interventions of dose reduction, longer intervals between doses and occasional need for regular venesection (Ponce et al. 2018).

5.2 Testosterone Undecanoate Oral

5.2.1 Long-Term Use

As oral administration of this form of testosterone requires at least twice daily dosing, with multiple capsules/day, long-term use in adolescent boys with hypogonadism is likely to be limited by acceptability and compliance issues.

5.2.2 Dosing Recommendations

Doses around 160–240 mg/day are usually required to maintain testosterone levels in an adult range. Occasional dose reductions may be considered if there is problem of excessive, disinhibited, sexualized behaviour in boys who have intellectual disability. Provided the testosterone level can be maintained above 5–6 nmol/L, bone health should not deteriorate, but BMD evaluation would be desirable in this small group. Alternative medications to reduce behavioural disorder should be considered if needed rather than rendering the boy hypogonadal.

5.2.3 Adverse Events

Inadvertent transfer of gel to female children or partners or other male children due to skin contact of administered areas has been reported several times, with potential for virilization (Hewitt and Zacharin 2012).

5.3 Testosterone Undecanoate Parenteral

5.3.1 Recent Information

Many studies have demonstrated safety and tolerability (Minnemann et al. 2007).

5.3.2 Adverse Events

Long-acting preparations have been linked with microembolization of the oil vehicle, most frequently resulting in acute cough (Middleton et al. 2015). Drug delivery should be administered in a facility with available facilities for management of an emergency situation.

5.3.3 Dosing Recommendations

Parenteral testosterone undecanoate 1,000 mg by deep intramuscular injection, preferably in the far lateral buttock, delivered slowly over at least 90 s, using a 21 gauge needle will help prevent haematoma and embolization.

5.3.4 Availability

Widely available but availability is currently limited in many developing countries.

5.4 Testosterone Gel

This is only likely to be a treatment choice during adolescent years for boys who have a complex disability, where parents and carers may have preference for a non-invasive method of androgen delivery for a boy who has permanent hypogonadism of any cause or where chronic illness and low body weight preclude regular HPG axis function. Inability to maintain adult sex hormone levels after puberty has been reported in patients attending young adult cerebral palsy clinics (Trinh et al. 2016).

5.5 Testosterone Spray

This preparation is not used in adolescent practice.

5.6 Testosterone Pellets

These pellets are only available in a few countries and are not commonly used in the adolescent population due to surgical requirement for insertion.

5.7 Gonadotropins FSH/hCG

See Sect. 3.2 for further information.

5.7.1 Dosing Recommendations

FSH and hCG are used for fertility induction at any post-pubertal age, dosing at same levels as the final adult dose used during pubertal induction:

Parenteral testosterone should be ceased prior to administration of hCG.

hCG 1,500 IU × 2/week s/c until a level of testosterone in the normal adult range has been achieved. Addition of FSH 150 IU × 3/week, increasing to 300–450 IU × 3/week as required after at least 4 months of observation of testicular size increase, with measurement of inhibin B to predict onset of spermatogenesis.

Combined treatment should be continued until confirmed pregnancy, at 12 weeks gestation. IM testosterone can then be substituted until future fertility is desired.

Disclosure Prof Zacharin has from time to time received unrestricted educational grants from Novartis, Pfizer, Ipsen and Bessins. She participated in a symposium on precocious puberty, sponsored by Sandoz, at the 2014 53rd Annual Meeting of the European Society of Paediatric Endocrinology. She has no conflicts of interest to disclose in relation to this paper.

References

Albrecht A, Penger T, Marx M, Hirsch K, Dorr HG (2018) Short-term adverse effects of testosterone used for priming in prepubertal boys before growth hormone stimulation test. J Pediatr Endocrinol Metab 31(1):21–24. https://doi.org/10.1515/jpem-2017-0280

Almeida MQ, Brito VN, Lins TS, Guerra-Junior G, de Castro M, Antonini SR et al (2008) Long-term treatment of familial male-limited precocious puberty (testotoxicosis) with cyproterone acetate or ketoconazole. Clin Endocrinol 69(1):93–98. https://doi.org/10.1111/j.1365-2265.2007.03160.x

Bajpai A, Simm PJ, McPherson SJ, Russo VC, Azar WJ, Wark JD et al (2010) Peripubertal aromatase inhibition in male rats has adverse long-term effects on bone strength and growth and induces prostatic hyperplasia. J Endocrinol 207(1):27–34. https://doi.org/10.1677/JOE-10-0006

Bastianelli C, Farris M, Rosato E, Brosens I, Benagiano G (2017) Pharmacodynamics of combined estrogen-progestin oral contraceptives: 1. Effects on metabolism. Expert Rev Clin Pharmacol 10 (3):315–326. https://doi.org/10.1080/17512433.2017.1271708

Behre HM, C W, Handelsman DJ, Nieschlag E (2004) Pharmacology of testosterone preparations. In: Testosterone, action, deficiency, substitution. Cambridge University Press, Cambridge, pp 405–444

Bereket A (2017) A critical appraisal of the effect of gonadotropin-releasing hormone analog treatment on adult height of girls with central precocious puberty. J Clin Res Pediatr Endocrinol 9(Suppl 2):33–48. https://doi.org/10.4274/jcrpe.2017.S004

Bertelloni S, Massart F, Miccoli M, Baroncelli GI (2017) Adult height after spontaneous pubertal growth or GnRH analog treatment in girls with early puberty: a meta-analysis. Eur J Pediatr 176 (6):697–704. https://doi.org/10.1007/s00431-017-2898-8

Bhatnagar AS, Brodie AM, Long BJ, Evans DB, Miller WR (2001) Intracellular aromatase and its relevance to the pharmacological efficacy of aromatase inhibitors. J Steroid Biochem Mol Biol 76(1–5):199–202

Brito VN, Latronico AC, Arnhold IJ, Mendonca BB (2008) Update on the etiology, diagnosis and therapeutic management of sexual precocity. Arq Bras Endocrinol Metabol 52(1):18–31

Carel JC, Eugster EA, Rogol A, Ghizzoni L, Palmert MR, ESPE-LWPES GnRH Analogs Consensus Conference Group et al (2009) Consensus statement on the use of gonadotropin-releasing hormone analogs in children. Pediatrics 123(4):e752–e762. https://doi.org/10.1542/peds.2008-1783

Champaloux SW, Tepper NK, Monsour M, Curtis KM, Whiteman MK, Marchbanks PA, Jamieson DJ (2017) Use of combined hormonal contraceptives among women with migraines and risk of ischemic stroke. Am J Obstet Gynecol 216(5):489.e1–489.e7. https://doi.org/10.1016/j.ajog.2016.12.019

Chioma L, Papucci G, Fintini D, Cappa M (2018) Use of testosterone gel compared to intramuscular formulation for puberty induction in males with constitutional delay of growth and puberty: a preliminary study. J Endocrinol Investig 41(2):259–263. https://doi.org/10.1007/s40618-017-0726-7

Chuah I, McRae A, Matthews K, Maguire AM, Steinbeck K (2017) Menstrual management in developmentally delayed adolescent females. Aust N Z J Obstet Gynaecol 57(3):346–350. https://doi.org/10.1111/ajo.12595

Cisternino M, Arrigo T, Pasquino AM, Tinelli C, Antoniazzi F, Beduschi L et al (2000) Etiology and age incidence of precocious puberty in girls: a multicentric study. J Pediatr Endocrinol Metab 13(Suppl 1):695–701

Crane MG, Harris JJ (1969) Plasma renin activity and aldosterone excretion rate in normal subjects. II. Effect of oral contraceptive agents. J Clin Endocrinol Metab 29(4):558–562. https://doi.org/10.1210/jcem-29-4-558

Crane MG, Heitsch J, Harris JJ, Johns VJ Jr (1966) Effect of ethinyl estradiol (estinyl) on plasma renin activity. J Clin Endocrinol Metab 26(12):403–406

Curtis KM, Peipert JF (2017) Long-acting reversible contraception. N Engl J Med 376(5):461–468. https://doi.org/10.1056/NEJMcp1608736

de Passone GBC, Kuperman H, Cabral de Menezes-Filho H, Spassapan Oliveira Esteves L, Lana Obata Giroto R, Damiani D (2015) Tamoxifen improves final height prediction in girls with McCune-Albright syndrome: a long follow-up. Horm Res Paediatr 84(3):184–189. https://doi.org/10.1159/000435881

Diedrich JT, Klein DA, Peipert JF (2017) Long-acting reversible contraception in adolescents: a systematic review and meta-analysis. Am J Obstet Gynecol 216(4):364.e1–364.e2. https://doi.org/10.1016/j.ajog.2016.12.024

Dragoman MV, Tepper NK, Fu R, Curtis KM, Chou R, Gaffield ME (2018) A systematic review and meta-analysis of venous thrombosis risk among users of combined oral contraception. Int J Gynaecol Obstet 141(3):287–294. https://doi.org/10.1002/ijgo.12455

Dwyer AA, Quinton R, Pitteloud N, Morin D (2015) Psychosexual development in men with congenital hypogonadotropic hypogonadism on long-term treatment: a mixed methods study. Sex Med 3(1):32–41. https://doi.org/10.1002/sm2.50

Efros M, Carrara D, Neijber A (2016) The efficacy, bioavailability and safety of a novel hydroalcoholic testosterone gel 2% in hypogonadal men: results from phase II open-label studies. Andrologia 48(6):637–645. https://doi.org/10.1111/and.12493

Estrada A, Boyce AM, Brillante BA, Guthrie LC, Gafni RI, Collins MT (2016) Long-term outcomes of letrozole treatment for precocious puberty in girls with McCune-Albright syndrome. Eur J Endocrinol 175(5):477–483. https://doi.org/10.1530/EJE-16-0526

Eugster EA, Rubin SD, Reiter EO, Plourde P, Jou HC, Pescovitz OH, McCune-Albright Study G (2003) Tamoxifen treatment for precocious puberty in McCune-Albright syndrome: a multicenter trial. J Pediatr 143(1):60–66. https://doi.org/10.1016/S0022-3476(03)00128-8

Farris M, Bastianelli C, Rosato E, Brosens I, Benagiano G (2017) Pharmacodynamics of combined estrogen-progestin oral contraceptives: 2. Effects on hemostasis. Expert Rev Clin Pharmacol 10 (10):1129–1144. https://doi.org/10.1080/17512433.2017.1356718

Ferris JA, Geffner ME (2017) Are aromatase inhibitors in boys with predicted short stature and/or rapidly advancing bone age effective and safe? J Pediatr Endocrinol Metab 30(3):311–317. https://doi.org/10.1515/jpem-2016-0219

Feuillan P, Calis K, Hill S, Shawker T, Robey PG, Collins MT (2007) Letrozole treatment of precocious puberty in girls with the McCune-Albright syndrome: a pilot study. J Clin Endocrinol Metab 92(6):2100–2106. https://doi.org/10.1210/jc.2006-2350

Fotherby K (1982) Pharmacokinetics of ethynyloestradiol in humans. Methods Find Exp Clin Pharmacol 4(2):133–141

Fotherby K, Koetsawang S, Mathrubutham M (1980) Pharmacokinetic study of different doses of Depo Provera. Contraception 22(5):527–536

Fraser IS, Romer T, Parke S, Zeun S, Mellinger U, Machlitt A, Jensen JT (2011) Effective treatment of heavy and/or prolonged menstrual bleeding with an oral contraceptive containing estradiol valerate and dienogest: a randomized, double-blind phase III trial. Hum Reprod 26 (10):2698–2708. https://doi.org/10.1093/humrep/der224

Geere G, Jones J, Atherden SM, Grant DB (1980) Plasma androgens after a single oral dose of testosterone undecanoate. Arch Dis Child 55(3):218–220

Geisler J (2011) Differences between the non-steroidal aromatase inhibitors anastrozole and letrozole – of clinical importance? Br J Cancer 104(7):1059–1066. https://doi.org/10.1038/bjc.2011.58

Geisler J, King N, Dowsett M, Ottestad L, Lundgren S, Walton P et al (1996) Influence of anastrozole (Arimidex), a selective, non-steroidal aromatase inhibitor, on in vivo aromatisation and plasma oestrogen levels in postmenopausal women with breast cancer. Br J Cancer 74 (8):1286–1291

Grandi G, Farulla A, Sileo FG, Facchinetti F (2018) Levonorgestrel-releasing intra-uterine systems as female contraceptives. Expert Opin Pharmacother 19(7):677–686. https://doi.org/10.1080/14656566.2018.1462337

Handelsman DJ, Turner L, Boylan LM, Conway AJ (1995) Pharmacokinetics of human follicle-stimulating hormone in gonadotropin-deficient men. J Clin Endocrinol Metab 80(5):1657–1663. https://doi.org/10.1210/jcem.80.5.7745014

Happ J, Schultheiss H, Jacobi GH, Wenderoth UK, Buttenschön K, Miesel K, Spahn H, Hör G (1987) Pharmacodynamics, pharmacokinetics and bioavailability of the prolonged LH-RH agonist decapeptyl-SR. In: Paridaens R, Klijn JMG, Foekens JA (eds) Hormonal manipulation of cancer: peptide, growth factors and new (anti) steroidal agents. Raven Press, New York, pp 249–253

Harel Z, Johnson CC, Gold MA, Cromer B, Peterson E, Burkman R et al (2010) Recovery of bone mineral density in adolescents following the use of depot medroxyprogesterone acetate contraceptive injections. Contraception 81(4):281–291. https://doi.org/10.1016/j.contraception.2009.11.003

Hero M, Toiviainen-Salo S, Wickman S, Makitie O, Dunkel L (2010) Vertebral morphology in aromatase inhibitor-treated males with idiopathic short stature or constitutional delay of puberty. J Bone Miner Res 25(7):1536–1543. https://doi.org/10.1002/jbmr.56

Herzog AG, Mandle HB, Cahill KE, Fowler KM, Hauser WA (2017) Predictors of unintended pregnancy in women with epilepsy. Neurology 88(8):728–733. https://doi.org/10.1212/WNL.0000000000003637

Hewitt JK, Zacharin MR (2012) Adverse effects of adult topical androgen use on children. Med J Aust 197(9):490

Holland FJ, Fishman L, Bailey JD, Fazekas AT (1985) Ketoconazole in the management of precocious puberty not responsive to LHRH-analogue therapy. N Engl J Med 312(16):1023–1028. https://doi.org/10.1056/NEJM198504183121604

Holmegard HN, Nordestgaard BG, Schnohr P, Tybjaerg-Hansen A, Benn M (2014) Endogenous sex hormones and risk of venous thromboembolism in women and men. J Thromb Haemost 12 (3):297–305. https://doi.org/10.1111/jth.12484

Howard S, Dunkel L (2016) Sex steroid and gonadotropin treatment in male delayed puberty. Endocr Dev 29:185–197. https://doi.org/10.1159/000438891

Isley MM, Kaunitz AM (2011) Update on hormonal contraception and bone density. Rev Endocr Metab Disord 12(2):93–106. https://doi.org/10.1007/s11154-011-9180-6

Jatlaoui TC, Riley HE, Curtis KM (2017) The safety of intrauterine devices among young women: a systematic review. Contraception 95(1):17–39. https://doi.org/10.1016/j.contraception.2016.10.006

Kang S, Niak A, Gada N, Brinker A, Jones SC (2017) Etonogestrel implant migration to the vasculature, chest wall, and distant body sites: cases from a pharmacovigilance database. Contraception 96(6):439–445. https://doi.org/10.1016/j.contraception.2017.08.009

Kaufman JM, Miller MG, Fitzpatrick S, McWhirter C, Brennan JJ (2012) One-year efficacy and safety study of a 1.62% testosterone gel in hypogonadal men: results of a 182-day open-label extension of a 6-month double-blind study. J Sex Med 9(4):1149–1161. https://doi.org/10.1111/j.1743-6109.2011.02630.x

Kauli R, Galatzer A, Kornreich L, Lazar L, Pertzelan A, Laron Z (1997) Final height of girls with central precocious puberty, untreated versus treated with cyproterone acetate or GnRH analogue. A comparative study with re-evaluation of predictions by the Bayley-Pinneau method. Horm Res 47(2):54–61. https://doi.org/10.1159/000185432

Klein KO, Rosenfield RL, Santen RJ, Gawlik AM, Backeljauw PF, Gravholt CH et al (2018) Estrogen replacement in turner syndrome: literature review and practical considerations. J Clin Endocrinol Metab 103(5):1790–1803. https://doi.org/10.1210/jc.2017-02183

Kletter GB, Kelch RP (1994) Clinical review 60: effects of gonadotropin-releasing hormone analog therapy on adult stature in precocious puberty. J Clin Endocrinol Metab 79(2):331–334. https://doi.org/10.1210/jcem.79.2.8045943

Lahlou N, Carel JC, Chaussain JL, Roger M (2000) Pharmacokinetics and pharmacodynamics of GnRH agonists: clinical implications in pediatrics. J Pediatr Endocrinol Metab 13(Suppl 1):723–737

Laron Z, Kauli R (2000) Experience with cyproterone acetate in the treatment of precocious puberty. J Pediatr Endocrinol Metab 13(Suppl 1):805–810

Lazar L, Kauli R, Pertzelan A, Phillip M (2002) Gonadotropin-suppressive therapy in girls with early and fast puberty affects the pace of puberty but not total pubertal growth or final height. J Clin Endocrinol Metab 87(5):2090–2094. https://doi.org/10.1210/jcem.87.5.8481

Lenz AM, Shulman D, Eugster EA, Rahhal S, Fuqua JS, Pescovitz OH, Lewis KA (2010) Bicalutamide and third-generation aromatase inhibitors in testotoxicosis. Pediatrics 126(3): e728–e733. https://doi.org/10.1542/peds.2010-0596

Leschek EW, Jones J, Barnes KM, Hill SC, Cutler GB Jr (1999) Six-year results of spironolactone and testolactone treatment of familial male-limited precocious puberty with addition of deslorelin after central puberty onset. J Clin Endocrinol Metab 84(1):175–178. https://doi.org/10.1210/jcem.84.1.5413

Liu S, Liu Q, Cheng X, Luo Y, Wen Y (2016) Effects and safety of combination therapy with gonadotropin-releasing hormone analogue and growth hormone in girls with idiopathic central precocious puberty: a meta-analysis. J Endocrinol Investig 39(10):1167–1178. https://doi.org/10.1007/s40618-016-0486-9

Longcope C, Gorbach S, Goldin B, Woods M, Dwyer J, Warram J (1985) The metabolism of estradiol; oral compared to intravenous administration. J Steroid Biochem 23(6A):1065–1070

Luukkainen T (1991) Levonorgestrel-releasing intrauterine device. Ann N Y Acad Sci 626:43–49

Mauras N, Torres-Santiago L, Taboada M, Santen R (2012) Estrogen therapy in Turner syndrome: does the type, dose and mode of delivery matter? Pediatr Endocrinol Rev 9(Suppl 2):718–722
Mauras N, Torres-Santiago L, Santen R, Mericq V, Ross J, Colon-Otero G et al (2018) Impact of route of administration on genotoxic oestrogens concentrations using oral vs transdermal oestradiol in girls with Turner syndrome. Clin Endocrinol 90:155–161. https://doi.org/10.1111/cen.13869
McGrath N, O'Grady MJ (2015) Aromatase inhibitors for short stature in male children and adolescents. Cochrane Database Syst Rev 10:CD010888. https://doi.org/10.1002/14651858.CD010888.pub2
Messina MF, Aversa T, de Sanctis L, Wasniewska M, Valenzise M, Pajno GB et al (2015) Adult height following a combined treatment of ketoconazole – cyproterone acetate – leuprolide depot in a boy with atypical McCune-Albright syndrome. Hormones (Athens) 14(2):286–292. https://doi.org/10.14310/horm.2002.1515
Middleton T, Turner L, Fennell C, Savkovic S, Jayadev V, Conway AJ, Handelsman DJ (2015) Complications of injectable testosterone undecanoate in routine clinical practice. Eur J Endocrinol 172(5):511–517. https://doi.org/10.1530/EJE-14-0891
Mieszczak J, Eugster EA (2007) Treatment of precocious puberty in McCune-Albright syndrome. Pediatr Endocrinol Rev 4(Suppl 4):419–422
Mieszczak J, Lowe ES, Plourde P, Eugster EA (2008) The aromatase inhibitor anastrozole is ineffective in the treatment of precocious puberty in girls with McCune-Albright syndrome. J Clin Endocrinol Metab 93(7):2751–2754. https://doi.org/10.1210/jc.2007-2090
Miller JA, Jacobs HS (1986) Treatment of hirsutism and acne with cyproterone acetate. Clin Endocrinol Metab 15(2):373–389
Miller BS, Shukla AR (2010) Sterile abscess formation in response to two separate branded long-acting gonadotropin-releasing hormone agonists. Clin Ther 32(10):1749–1751. https://doi.org/10.1016/j.clinthera.2010.09.009
Minnemann T, Schubert M, Hubler D, Gouni-Berthold I, Freude S, Schumann C et al (2007) A four-year efficacy and safety study of the long-acting parenteral testosterone undecanoate. Aging Male 10(3):155–158. https://doi.org/10.1080/13685530701437510
Nabhan Z, Eugster EA (2013) Hormone replacement therapy in children with hypogonadotropic hypogonadism: where do we stand? Endocr Pract 19(6):968–971. https://doi.org/10.4158/EP13101.OR
Neumann F (1994) The antiandrogen cyproterone acetate: discovery, chemistry, basic pharmacology, clinical use and tool in basic research. Exp Clin Endocrinol 102(1):1–32. https://doi.org/10.1055/s-0029-1211261
Neyman A, Eugster EA (2017) Treatment of girls and boys with McCune-Albright syndrome with precocious puberty – update 2017. Pediatr Endocrinol Rev 15(2):136–141. https://doi.org/10.17458/per.vol15.2017.nau.treatmentgirlsboys
Nieschlag E, Mauss J, Coert A, Kicovic P (1975) Plasma androgen levels in men after oral administration of testosterone or testosterone undecanoate. Acta Endocrinol 79(2):366–374
Nieschlag E, Cuppers HJ, Wiegelmann W, Wickings EJ (1976) Bioavailability and LH-suppressing effect of different testosterone preparations in normal and hypogonadal men. Horm Res 7(3):138–145. https://doi.org/10.1159/000178721
Nieves JW, Ruffing JA, Zion M, Tendy S, Yavorek T, Lindsay R, Cosman F (2016) Eating disorders, menstrual dysfunction, weight change and DMPA use predict bone density change in college-aged women. Bone 84:113–119. https://doi.org/10.1016/j.bone.2015.12.054
Norjavaara E, Ankarberg-Lindgren C, Kristrom B (2016) Sex steroid replacement therapy in female hypogonadism from childhood to young adulthood. Endocr Dev 29:198–213. https://doi.org/10.1159/000438892
Palmert MR, Malin HV, Boepple PA (1999) Unsustained or slowly progressive puberty in young girls: initial presentation and long-term follow-up of 20 untreated patients. J Clin Endocrinol Metab 84(2):415–423. https://doi.org/10.1210/jcem.84.2.5430

Paul D, Conte FA, Grumbach MM, Kaplan SL (1995) Long-term effect of gonadotropin-releasing hormone agonist therapy on final and near-final height in 26 children with true precocious puberty treated at a median age of less than 5 years. J Clin Endocrinol Metab 80(2):546–551. https://doi.org/10.1210/jcem.80.2.7852518

Perrin MH, Rivier JE, Vale WW (1980) Radioligand assay for gonadotropin-releasing hormone: relative potencies of agonists and antagonists. Endocrinology 106(4):1289–1296

Piippo S, Lenko H, Kainulainen P, Sipila I (2004) Use of percutaneous estrogen gel for induction of puberty in girls with Turner syndrome. J Clin Endocrinol Metab 89(7):3241–3247. https://doi.org/10.1210/jc.2003-032069

Ponce OJ, Spencer-Bonilla G, Alvarez-Villalobos N, Serrano V, Singh-Ospina N, Rodriguez-Gutierrez R et al (2018) The efficacy and adverse events of testosterone replacement therapy in hypogonadal men: a systematic review and meta-analysis of randomized, placebo-controlled trials. J Clin Endocrinol Metab. https://doi.org/10.1210/jc.2018-00404

Ramsay ID, Rushton DH (1990) Reduced serum vitamin B12 levels during oral cyproterone-acetate and ethinyl-oestradiol therapy in women with diffuse androgen-dependent alopecia. Clin Exp Dermatol 15(4):277–281

Reddy DS (2017) Do oral contraceptives increase epileptic seizures? Expert Rev Neurother 17 (2):129–134. https://doi.org/10.1080/14737175.2016.1243472

Reiter EO, Mauras N, McCormick K, Kulshreshtha B, Amrhein J, De Luca F et al (2010) Bicalutamide plus anastrozole for the treatment of gonadotropin-independent precocious puberty in boys with testotoxicosis: a phase II, open-label pilot study (BATT). J Pediatr Endocrinol Metab 23(10):999–1009

Roetker NS, MacLehose RF, Hoogeveen RC, Ballantyne CM, Basu S, Cushman M, Folsom AR (2018) Prospective study of endogenous hormones and incidence of venous thromboembolism: the atherosclerosis risk in communities study. Thromb Haemost 118(11):1940–1950. https://doi.org/10.1055/s-0038-1673613

Roger M, Chaussain JL, Berlier P, Bost M, Canlorbe P, Colle M et al (1986) Long term treatment of male and female precocious puberty by periodic administration of a long-acting preparation of D-Trp6-luteinizing hormone-releasing hormone microcapsules. J Clin Endocrinol Metab 62 (4):670–677. https://doi.org/10.1210/jcem-62-4-670

Rohayem J, Hauffa BP, Zacharin M, Kliesch S, Zitzmann M, German Adolescent Hypogonadotropic Hypogonadism Study Group (2017) Testicular growth and spermatogenesis: new goals for pubertal hormone replacement in boys with hypogonadotropic hypogonadism? – a multicentre prospective study of hCG/rFSH treatment outcomes during adolescence. Clin Endocrinol 86 (1):75–87. https://doi.org/10.1111/cen.13164

Ross JL, Quigley CA, Cao D, Feuillan P, Kowal K, Chipman JJ, Cutler GB Jr (2011) Growth hormone plus childhood low-dose estrogen in Turner's syndrome. N Engl J Med 364 (13):1230–1242. https://doi.org/10.1056/NEJMoa1005669

Sacco S, Merki-Feld GS, Ægidius KL, Bitzer J, Canonico M, Gantenbein AR et al (2018) Effect of exogenous estrogens and progestogens on the course of migraine during reproductive age: a consensus statement by the European Headache Federation (EHF) and the European Society of Contraception and Reproductive Health (ESCRH). J Headache Pain 19(1):76. https://doi.org/10.1186/s10194-018-0896-5

Schindler AE, Campagnoli C, Druckmann R, Huber J, Pasqualini JR, Schweppe KW, Thijssen JH (2008) Classification and pharmacology of progestins. Maturitas 61(1–2):171–180

Schoelwer M, Eugster EA (2016) Treatment of peripheral precocious puberty. Endocr Dev 29:230–239. https://doi.org/10.1159/000438895

Seminara S, Nanni L, Generoso M, Mirri S, Leonardi V, Slabadzianiuk T et al (2010) Effect of treatment with cyproterone acetate on uterine bleeding at the beginning of GnRH analogue therapy in girls with idiopathic central precocious puberty. Horm Res Paediatr 73(5):386–389. https://doi.org/10.1159/000308172

Shah S, Forghani N, Durham E, Neely EK (2014) A randomized trial of transdermal and oral estrogen therapy in adolescent girls with hypogonadism. Int J Pediatr Endocrinol 2014(1):12. https://doi.org/10.1186/1687-9856-2014-12

Silva Dos Santos PN, Madden T, Omvig K, Peipert JF (2017) Changes in body composition in women using long-acting reversible contraception. Contraception 95(4):382–389. https://doi.org/10.1016/j.contraception.2016.12.006

Sims EK, Garnett S, Guzman F, Paris F, Sultan C, Eugster EA, Fulvestrant McCune-Albright Study Group (2012) Fulvestrant treatment of precocious puberty in girls with McCune-Albright syndrome. Int J Pediatr Endocrinol 2012(1):26. https://doi.org/10.1186/1687-9856-2012-26

Sioufi A, Gauducheau N, Pineau V, Marfil F, Jaouen A, Cardot JM et al (1997) Absolute bioavailability of letrozole in healthy postmenopausal women. Biopharm Drug Dispos 18 (9):779–789

Sitruk-Ware R (1989) Transdermal delivery of steroids. Contraception 39(1):1–20

Soriano-Guillen L, Lahlou N, Chauvet G, Roger M, Chaussain JL, Carel JC (2005) Adult height after ketoconazole treatment in patients with familial male-limited precocious puberty. J Clin Endocrinol Metab 90(1):147–151. https://doi.org/10.1210/jc.2004-1438

Spratt DI, Stewart II, Savage C, Craig W, Spack NP, Chandler DW et al (2017) Subcutaneous injection of testosterone is an effective and preferred alternative to intramuscular injection: demonstration in female-to-male transgender patients. J Clin Endocrinol Metab 102(7):2349–2355. https://doi.org/10.1210/jc.2017-00359

Stanczyk FZ, Archer DF, Bhavnani BR (2013) Ethinyl estradiol and 17beta-estradiol in combined oral contraceptives: pharmacokinetics, pharmacodynamics and risk assessment. Contraception 87(6):706–727. https://doi.org/10.1016/j.contraception.2012.12.011

Taboada M, Santen R, Lima J, Hossain J, Singh R, Klein KO, Mauras N (2011) Pharmacokinetics and pharmacodynamics of oral and transdermal 17beta estradiol in girls with Turner syndrome. J Clin Endocrinol Metab 96(11):3502–3510. https://doi.org/10.1210/jc.2011-1449

Tessaris D, Matarazzo P, Mussa A, Tuli G, Verna F, Fiore L, Lala R (2012) Combined treatment with bicalutamide and anastrozole in a young boy with peripheral precocious puberty due to McCune-Albright syndrome. Endocr J 59(2):111–117

Teutonico D, Montanari S, Ponchel G (2012) Leuprolide acetate: pharmaceutical use and delivery potentials. Expert Opin Drug Deliv 9(3):343–354. https://doi.org/10.1517/17425247.2012.662484

Torres-Santiago L, Mericq V, Taboada M, Unanue N, Klein KO, Singh R et al (2013) Metabolic effects of oral versus transdermal 17beta-estradiol (E(2)): a randomized clinical trial in girls with Turner syndrome. J Clin Endocrinol Metab 98(7):2716–2724. https://doi.org/10.1210/jc.2012-4243

Trinchard-Lugan I, Khan A, Porchet HC, Munafo A (2002) Pharmacokinetics and pharmacodynamics of recombinant human chorionic gonadotrophin in healthy male and female volunteers. Reprod Biomed Online 4(2):106–115

Trinh A, Wong P, Fahey MC, Brown J, Churchyard A, Strauss BJ et al (2016) Musculoskeletal and endocrine health in adults with cerebral palsy: new opportunities for intervention. J Clin Endocrinol Metab 101(3):1190–1197. https://doi.org/10.1210/jc.2015-3888

Usinger KM, Gola SB, Weis M, Smaldone A (2016) Intrauterine contraception continuation in adolescents and young women: a systematic review. J Pediatr Adolesc Gynecol 29(6):659–667. https://doi.org/10.1016/j.jpag.2016.06.007

Wang C, Berman N, Longstreth JA, Chuapoco B, Hull L, Steiner B et al (2000) Pharmacokinetics of transdermal testosterone gel in hypogonadal men: application of gel at one site versus four sites: a General Clinical Research Center study. J Clin Endocrinol Metab 85(3):964–969. https://doi.org/10.1210/jcem.85.3.6437

Wickman S, Kajantie E, Dunkel L (2003) Effects of suppression of estrogen action by the p450 aromatase inhibitor letrozole on bone mineral density and bone turnover in pubertal boys. J Clin Endocrinol Metab 88(8):3785–3793. https://doi.org/10.1210/jc.2002-021643

Xiao BL, Zhou LY, Zhang XL, Jia MC, Luukkainen T, Allonen H (1990) Pharmacokinetic and pharmacodynamic studies of levonorgestrel-releasing intrauterine device. Contraception 41 (4):353–362

Zacharin M (2015) Pubertal induction in hypogonadism: current approaches including use of gonadotrophins. Best Pract Res Clin Endocrinol Metab 29(3):367–383. https://doi.org/10.1016/j.beem.2015.01.002

Zacharin M, Sabin MA, Nair VV, Dabadghao P (2012) Addition of recombinant follicle-stimulating hormone to human chorionic gonadotropin treatment in adolescents and young adults with hypogonadotropic hypogonadism promotes normal testicular growth and may promote early spermatogenesis. Fertil Steril 98(4):836–842. https://doi.org/10.1016/j.fertnstert.2012.06.022

Zaiem F, Alahdab F, Al Nofal A, Murad MH, Javed A (2017) Oral versus transdermal estrogen in turner syndrome: a systematic review and meta-analysis. Endocr Pract 23(4):408–421. https://doi.org/10.4158/EP161622.OR

The manufacturer's authorised representative in the EU is Springer Nature Customer Service Centre GmbH, Europaplatz 3, 69115 Heidelberg, Germany. If you have any concerns regarding our products, please contact ProductSafety@springernature.com

Printed and bound by CPI Group (UK) Ltd, Croydon, CR0 4YY
05/10/2026
02228123-0015